Translational and Clinical Research in Urology

Translational and Clinical Research in Urology

Editor: Timothy Lawson

AMERICAN
MEDICAL PUBLISHERS
www.americanmedicalpublishers.com

AMERICAN
MEDICAL PUBLISHERS
www.americanmedicalpublishers.com

Cataloging-in-Publication Data

Translational and clinical research in urology / edited by Timothy Lawson.
p. cm.
Includes bibliographical references and index.
ISBN 979-8-88740-525-4
1. Urology. 2. Urology--Research. 3. Genitourinary organs--Diseases. 4. Urinary organs--Diseases. I. Lawson, Timothy.
RC871 .T73 2023
616.6--dc23

American Medical Publishers,
41 Flatbush Avenue,
1st Floor, New York,
NY 11217, USA

ISBN 979-8-88740-525-4 (Hardback)

Contents

Preface

Urology is a medical specialty that focuses on the diseases affecting the male and female urinary tract systems. The main organs of urinary tract include bladder, kidneys and ureters. Urological diseases are typically associated with problems of prostate, kidneys, urethra, testes, bladder and ureters. Some urologic conditions are temporary while others are chronic, and treatment of these conditions entails determining and treating the underlying symptoms or causes. Painkillers and self-care techniques are some of the potential remedies for these disorders. Other treatment options include chemotherapy, surgery, radiation therapy, as well as the usage of antibiotics and medications for relaxing the bladder. Current clinical trials in the field of urology involve researching novel therapeutic drugs and treatments for a variety of conditions, such as overactive bladder, incontinence, urinary tract cancer, kidney stones, etc. This book aims to shed light on the translational and clinical researches in urology. It presents researches and studies performed by experts across the globe. Those in search of information to further their knowledge will be greatly assisted by this book.

All of the data presented henceforth, was collaborated in the wake of recent advancements in the field. The aim of this book is to present the diversified developments from across the globe in a comprehensible manner. The opinions expressed in each chapter belong solely to the contributing authors. Their interpretations of the topics are the integral part of this book, which I have carefully compiled for a better understanding of the readers.

At the end, I would like to thank all those who dedicated their time and efforts for the successful completion of this book. I also wish to convey my gratitude towards my friends and family who supported me at every step.

Editor

1

Relationship between alterations of urinary microbiota and cultured negative lower urinary tract symptoms in female type 2 diabetes patients

Jiawei Chen[1†], Jie Zhao[2†], Ying Cao[3], Guihao Zhang[1], Yang Chen[1], Jialei Zhong[1], Weina Huang[1], Jiarong Zeng[1] and Peng Wu[1*]

Abstract

Background: Lower urinary tract symptoms (LUTS) is the most common complication of diabetes. However, the underlying pathogenesis of cultured negative LUTS (cn-LUTS) in diabetic patients has not been well understood. Numerous evidence indicates that urinary dysbiosis is related to urologic disorders. We aim to study alterations of the urinary microbiota of cn-LUTS in type 2 diabetes (T2D) patients.

Methods: Female T2D patients and controls were recruited and requested to finish the American Urological Association Symptom Index. Mid-stream urine was collected for culturing and extracting DNA. Microbial diversity and composition were analyzed by targeting to 16S rDNA. Linear discriminant analysis effect size (LEfSe) was carried out to identify significantly different bacteria.

Results: 32 female T2D patients and 26 controls were enrolled. No significant differences in alpha diversity were observed between patients and controls. However, statistically decreased richness (ACE index and Chao 1 index, 85.52(13.75, 204.84) vs. 129.82(63.89, 280.30) and 83.86(11.00, 210.77) vs. 125.19(62.00, 251.77), $P = 0.005$; Observed Species, 76(10, 175) vs. 98(54, 234), $P = 0.011$) and decreased species diversity (Shannon index, 1.37(0.04, 3.48) vs. 2.09(0.98, 3.43), $P = 0.033$; Simpson index, 0.46 (0.06, 0.99) vs. 0.23(0.07, 0.64), $P = 0.029$) were shown in moderate-to-severe LUTS group and high Hemoglobin A1c group, respectively. A significant difference of beta diversity was found between T2D patients and controls and T2D patients with different severity of cn-LUTS as well as the different level of Hemoglobin A1c. LEfSe revealed that 10 genera (e.g., *Escherichia-Shigella* and *Klebsiella*) were increased and 7 genera were decreasing in T2D patients, 3 genera (e.g., *Escherichia-Shigella* and *Campylobacter*) were increased and 16 genera (e.g., *Prevotella*) were reduced in moderate-to-severe LUTS group, 2 genera (*Escherichia-Shigella* and *Lactobacillus*) were over-represented and 10 genera (e.g., *Prevotella*) were under-represented in high Hemoglobin A1c group. Finally, Hemoglobin A1c was found positively correlated with the total score of the American Urological Association Symptom Index ($r = 0.509$, $P = 0.003$).

Conclusions: Urinary dysbiosis may be related to cn-LUTS in female T2D patients. A better understanding of urinary microbiota in the development and progression of cn-LUTS in female T2D patients was necessary. The severity of cn-LUTS was correlated to hyperglycemia and chronic hyperglycemia might induce or promote cn-LUTS by influencing urinary microbiota.

Keywords: Diabetes mellitus, Lower urinary tract symptoms, Urinary microbiota, Hemoglobin A1c

* Correspondence: doctorwupeng@gmail.com
[†]Jiawei Chen and Jie Zhao contributed equally to this work.
[1]Department of Urology, Nanfang Hospital, Southern Medical University, Guangzhou 510515, China
Full list of author information is available at the end of the article

Background

Diabetes is burgeoning worldwide due to an increase in aging population and changes in eating habits [1]. Chronic hyperglycemia is associated with damage, dysfunction, and failure of multiple organ systems, including the genitourinary system. 80% of individuals with diabetes are accompanied by lower urinary tract symptoms (LUTS) [1, 2]. Although diabetes-induced LUTS is not life-threatening, it seriously affects patients' life quality. Most diabetic patients are likely suffering from LUTS without evidence of urinary tract infections (UTI), which are refractory and hardly benefit from the conventional treatment. For these patients, it is supposed that the potential pathogenesis of LUTS may be linked to polyuria, oxidative stress and autonomic neuropathy induced by chronic hyperglycemia [3]. However, the underlying pathogenesis of cultured negative LUTS (cn-LUTS) induced by diabetes has not been fully appreciated.

Microbiota has been increasingly considered as an essential factor in human health and disease [4–8]. Traditionally, specimens from mid-stream urine were usually considered being sterile for not enough uropathogens were yielded under standard clinical cultivation procedures. However, the dogma of 'sterile urine' has been broken. Recent studies have revealed that urine samples from healthy individuals inhabit numerous microorganisms [9]. Moreover, alterations of urinary microbiota were found in various urologic disorders [10–13]. Decreasing diversity and richness of urinary microbiota were found in female overactive bladder patients in our previous study [10]. Pearce et al. found that, compared to healthy controls, the proportion of *Gardnerella* in urge urinary incontinence patients was increased while the proportion of *Lactobacillus* was decreasing [11]. Siddiqui et al. reported that the diversity of urinary microbiota in interstitial cystitis patients was lower than that in healthy individuals and the proportion of *Lactobacillus* was increased [12].

An increased level of urine glucose induced by chronic hyperglycemia changes the microenvironment of the urinary tract which might further change the urinary microbiota. Liu et al. reported that urine specimens collected from female Type 2 diabetes (T2D) patients had a decreasing diversity and richness urinary microbiota [14]. They also found that increased *Actinobacteria* phylum and decreasing *Akkermansia muciniphila* was associated with the level of fasting blood glucose levels [14]. Accordingly, we suggested that alterations of urinary microbiota might also take part in the occurrence of cn-LUTS in diabetic patients. The goal of our study was to characterize urinary microbiota in Chinese T2D females by comparing the alpha and beta diversity as well as the specific genus and to explore the potential pathogenesis of diabetes-induced cn-LUTS from the characteristics of urinary microbiota.

Methods

Patient enrollment and urinary samples collection

This study was subject to approval by the Ethical Committee of Southern Medical University. From June 2017 to December 2017, females who diagnosed with T2D and healthy female volunteers, age between 40 and 70, were approached for participation. Participants with medical conditions that could interfere with voiding function such as presence of UTI, known abnormal anatomical abnormalities of urinary tract, hereditary and congenital diseases (spina bifida, spinal meninges, etc.), neurological diseases (Guillain-Barré syndrome, multiple sclerosis, etc.), LUTS caused by drug abuse, history of spinal injury, history of hysterectomy, previous major pelvis surgery and evidence of vaginal prolapse were excluded. Patients during the menstrual period or with medical conditions which may interfere with urinary microbiota such as recent antibiotics usage or indwelling catheter (within one month) were also excluded. All participants were requested to offer demographic information and complete the AUA-SI to evaluate the severity of LUTS. Before evaluation, all participants were briefed on the procedure and asked to write informed consent. Mid-stream urine (50 ml) was collected with the labial separation which was supervised by the author (Weina Huang) and 20 ml was left for standard cultivation to exclude UTI. Within 1 h, the rest specimens were immediately shifted to the laboratory and centrifuged at 16,000 g for 10 min. Pellets were kept at – 80 °C until further processing.

DNA extraction, PCR, and MiSeq sequencing

DNA extraction was carried out using the cultured cells protocol supplied with the DNeasy Blood and Tissue Kit (Qiagen, Germany) in a laminar flow hood to avert contamination. The concentration of extracted DNA was tested by the Nanodrop ND-1000 spectrophotometer (Thermo Electron Corporation, USA). Specific primer sets for V3-V4 regions were chosen to perform PCR amplification of 16S rDNA. To assess the contribution of extraneous DNA from reagents, extraction negative controls (no urine) and PCR negative controls (no template) were included as the blank controls. Qiaquick PCR purification kit (Qiagen, Valencia, CA) was selected for purifying the final PCR products from unincorporated nucleotides and primers. Purified samples were normalized to equal DNA concentration and sequenced by Illumina Miseq sequencer (Illumina, Inc., USA).

Statistical analysis

Differences in the demographic and clinical characteristics between groups were tested by Student's *t*-test or

Mann-Whitney U test (for continuous variables) as well as Pearson's chi-square test or Fisher's exact test (for count data). Pearson's correlation was implemented to detect the relations between clinical data and indices of bacterial bioinformatics. All data were analyzed using SPSS (version 22). All tests were two-sided and P-values < 0.05 was considered statistically significant. PASS programme (PASS 11, NCSS, Kaysville UT, USA) provides estimates of power by simulation.

Bioinformatics analysis

Quantitative Insights Into Microbial Ecology (QIIME, version 1.80) was applied to create an operational taxonomic units (OTUs) table at a default similarity level of 97% based on the 16S rDNA sequence data [15, 16]. Subsequently, chimera detection was performed through the UCHIME method [17]. The representative sequence of each OTU was aligned to Silva and Greengenes database using Ribosomal Database Project Classifier [18].

Five alpha diversity was calculated by mothur software (version 1.31.2) indexes in QIIME including the Observed Species, Chao 1 index, ACE index, Shannon index, and Simpson index. The difference of alpha diversity was evaluated by Mann-Whitney U test in R (version 3.03). Observed Species, Chao1 index, and ACE index represented bacterial richness, while Shannon index and Simpson index were quantitative measures of bacterial diversity that reflecting both species richness and evenness.

To compare microbial composition between groups, principal coordinate analysis (PCoA) was applied on Bray Curtis, weighted UniFrac and unweighted UniFrac distance metrics to generate three-dimensional plots in QIIME. Multiple Response Permutation Procedure (MRPP, a nonparametric test which applied to test beta diversity values between groups) was performed to test the differences of Bray Curtis, weighted UniFrac, unweighted UniFrac distance metrics between groups in QIIME.

Significant bacteria on the relative abundance was tested by Metastats Test. Initial p-value was corrected with the method of Benjamini-Chochberg in R [19]. False discovery rate (FDR) represented the corrected p-value and FDR < 0.05 was considered significant. To identify significantly different bacteria as biomarkers between groups, taxa summaries were reformatted and inputted into Linear discriminant analysis effect size (LEfSe) via the Huttenhower Lab Galaxy Server [20]. Firstly, the Kruskal-Wallis rank sum test and Mann-Whitney U test were applied to identify the significantly different bacteria. Subsequently, linear discriminant analysis (LDA) was used to score the effect size of the different bacteria. Only taxa with logarithmic LDA score greater than 2 were considered significantly enriched.

Results

Demographic and clinical characteristics of participants

Sixty five female volunteers were enrolled, including 35 T2D patients and 30 healthy controls. All the urine samples from these participants were verified cultured negative during the standard culture procedure. However, 3 samples from patients and 4 from controls were excluded due to the sequencing reads could not be achieved. With 32 patients in diabetes group and 26 subjects in the control group ($\alpha = 0.05$; $\beta = 0.2$), we would have 95% power to detect differences at the 0.05 significance level (alpha) using a two-sided Mann-Whitney U test and have 96% power to detect differences at the 0.05 significance level (alpha) using a two-sided Student's t-test. Detailed comparisons between T2D patients and healthy controls were shown in Table 1. Except for fasting blood glucose, no significant differences were observed in the demographic and clinical characteristics between diabetes group and control group (for example, age, 56.969 ± 8.014 vs. 57.615 ± 9.239; body mass index, 23.739 ± 4.379 vs. 24.298 ± 3.120; hypertension rate, 14(43.8%) vs. 8(30.8%); etc.). Besides, higher scores of American Urological Association Symptom Index (AUA-SI) (total score, 9.219 ± 6.904 vs. 2.846 ± 3.319; storage score, 5.375 ± 4.612 vs. 1.846 ± 1.617; emptying score, 3.844 ± 4.573 vs. 1.000 ± 2.482) were found in T2D patients ($P < 0.05$).

Comparisons of bioinformatics between T2D patients and controls

All reads were classified into 6212 operational taxonomic units (OTUs). 3070 OTUs were identified in T2D patients and 3142 OTUs were identified in controls. Comparisons of alpha diversity between T2D patients and controls were shown in Table 1. There were no significant differences in Observed Species (88(11, 245) vs. 135(15, 258)), Chao 1 index (103.60(14.00, 272.00) vs. 149.50(29.00, 339.00)), ACE index 104.30(16.50, 416.70) vs. 146.10(40.70, 428.60), Shannon index (1.70(0.04, 3.48) vs. 1.78(0.01, 3.54)) and Simpson index (0.31(0.06, 0.99) vs. 0.38(0.07,1.00)) between diabetes group and control group (Table 1, Fig. 1a, e), which indicated that neither bacterial richness nor species diversity was not significantly changed in the T2D cohort.

As shown in Fig. 1f – h, we found urinary microbiota in diabetes group and control group mainly clustered together in the different area of the PCoA plots, respectively. Statistical differences were noted in weighted UniFrac ($P = 0.045$) as well as unweighted

Table 1 Comparisons of demographic and clinical characteristics as well as bacterial alpha diversity between diabetes group and control group

	Diabetes ($n = 32$)	Control ($n = 26$)	*P* value
Demographic Characteristics			
Age (y)	56.969 ± 8.014	57.615 ± 9.239	0.776
Body mass index (kg/m2)	23.739 ± 4.379	24.298 ± 3.120	0.587
Menstrual status [no.(%)]			0.600
Premenopausal	8 (25.0%)	5 (19.2%)	
Postmenopausal	24 (75.0%)	21 (80.8%)	
Reproductive status [no.(%)]			0.448
Fertile	32 (100%)	25 (96.2%)	
Sterile	0 (0%)	1 (3.8%)	
Clinical Characteristics			
Duration of diabetes (y)	6.906 ± 4.748	N/A	
Fasting blood glucose (mmol/L)	7.913 ± 3.264	5.182 ± 0.592	< 0.001
Hemoglobin A1c (%)	8.088 ± 2.168	N/A	
Retinopathy [no.(%)]	10 (31.3%)	N/A	
Peripheral neuropathy [no.(%)]	27 (84.4%)	N/A	
Hypertension [no.(%)]	14 (43.8%)	8 (30.8%)	0.311
Creatinine (μmol/L)	65.156 ± 52.802	58.423 ± 8.420	0.178
Estimated glomerular filtration rate (ml/min/1.73m^2)	104.513 ± 38.578	94.576 ± 16.170	0.193
American Urological Association Index			
Total score	9.219 ± 6.904	2.846 ± 3.319	< 0.001
Storage score	5.375 ± 4.612	1.846 ± 1.617	0.001
Emptying score	3.844 ± 4.573	1.000 ± 2.482	0.001
Parameter of Bacterial Alpha Diversity			
Observed species	88 (11, 245)	135 (15, 258)	0.166
Chao1	103.60 (14.00, 272.00)	149.50 (29.00, 339.00)	0.107
ACE index	104.30 (16.50, 416.70)	146.10 (40.70, 428.60)	0.077
Shannon index	1.70 (0.04, 3.48)	1.78 (0.01, 3.54)	0.552
Simpson index	0.31 (0.06, 0.99)	0.38 (0.07, 1.00)	0.381

Data were presented as mean ± SD for continuous variables and n (%) for counts in demographic and clinical characteristics. Parameters of bacterial alpha diversity were reported as median (range). N/A, not applicable. ※No data were missing

UniFrac ($P = 0.010$) distance metrics. However, the difference in Bray Curtis distance metrics could not reach statistical significance (Fig. 1h, $P = 0.053$).

We found that 10 genera were over-represented in the T2D cohort including *Escherichia-Shigella, Klebsiella, Aerococcus, Delftia, Enterococcus, Alistipes, Stenotrophomonas, Micrococcus, Deinococcus* and *Rubellimicrobium,* while 7 genera were under-represented including *Gallicola, Arcobacter, Arcanobacterium, Kocuria, Murdochiella, Solitalea* and *Peptoniphilus* (Fig. 1i). Among the genera mentioned above, Metastats algorithm shown the significantly altered in *Delftia, Enterococcus, Stenotrophomonas, Micrococcus, Deinococcus, Solitalea* and *Peptoniphilus* (Additional file 1: Table S1).

Comparisons of bioinformatics between T2D patients with no to mild LUTS and those with moderate to severe LUTS

In order to detect the specific bacteria associated with the severity of LUTS, we next studied whether the urinary microbial profile was different between T2D patients with no to mild LUTS (LS group, total AUA-SI score ≤ 7) and T2D patients with moderate to severe LUTS (HS group, total AUA-SI score > 7). Higher Observed Species (Fig. 2a, 76(10, 175) vs. 98(54, 234), $P = 0.011$), Chao1 index (Fig. 2b, 83.86(11.00, 210.77) vs. 125.19(62.00, 251.77), $P = 0.005$), ACE index (Fig. 2c, 85.52(13.75, 204.84) vs. 129.82(63.89, 280.30), $P = 0.005$) were presented in the LS group, while no significant differences

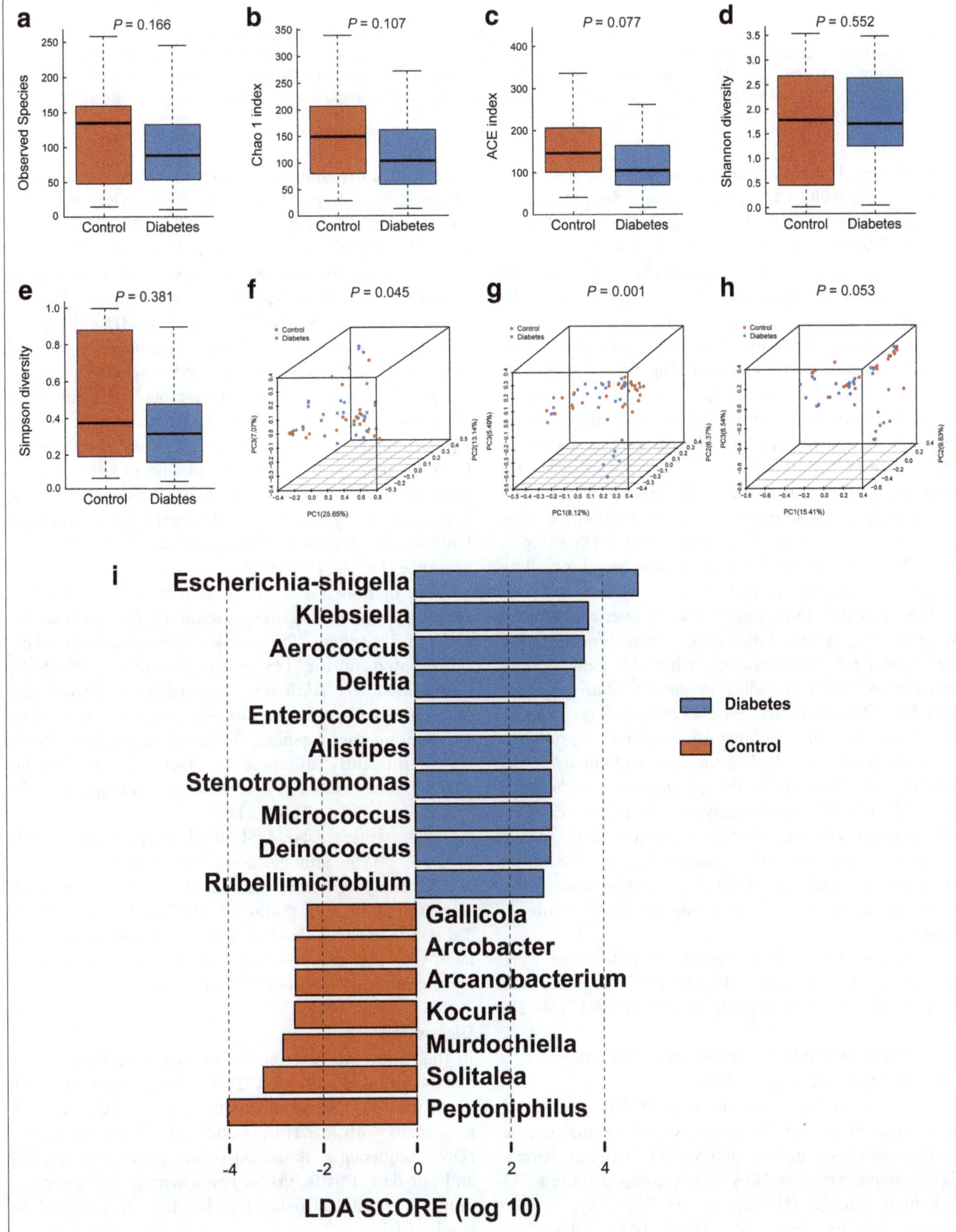

Fig. 1 (See legend on next page.)

(See figure on previous page.)
Fig. 1 Alpha diversity and principal coordinate analysis for the control group and diabetes group urinary microbiota. Observed Species **(a)**; Chao1 index**(b)**; ACE index **(c)**; Shannon index **(d)**; Simpson index **(e)**. Principal coordinate analysis plots of the urinary microbiota based on the weighted UniFrac **(f)**, unweighted UniFrac **(g)** and Bray-Curtis **(h)** distance metrics. Association of specific microbiota taxa with the diabetes group and control group was analyzed by LEfSe **(i)**. Genera enriched for controls in red and enriched for patients in blue. Only genera meeting a linear discriminant analysis score threshold > 2 are shown

were observed in Shannon index (Fig. 2d, 1.40(0.04, 3.48) vs. 2.01(0.98, 3.43), $P = 0.132$) and Simpson index (Fig. 2e, 0.44(0.06, 0.99) vs. 0.28(0.07, 0.64), $P = 0.202$). This indicated that significantly decreasing bacterial richness was found in the HS group (Table 2). However, no correlation was observed between AUA-SI and alpha diversity.

PCoA plots demonstrated that samples from different groups were clustered together respectively and suggested that the urinary microbiota composition of LS group was distinct from that of HS group (Fig. 2f, h). Statistically differences were observed in MRPP test ($P = 0.002$, $P = 0.024$, $P = 0.001$ for weighted UniFrac, unweighted UniFrac and Bray Curtis distance metrics, respectively). In addition, a clear hierarchical clustering of LS samples and HS samples was observed on dendrogram which based on Bray Curtis distance metrics (Fig. 3).

LEfSe revealed that 3 genera were over-represented in the HS group including *Escherichia-Shigella, Campylobacter, Megasphaera*, while 16 genera were under-represented including *Prevotella, Dialister, Leptotrichia, Anaerococcus, Fusobacterium, Prevotella_6, Fastidiosipila, Varibaculum, Mycoplasma, Peptoniphilus, Porphyromonas, Fodinicola, Brevundimonas, Candidatus-Nomurabacteria, Paracoccus* and *Rhodococcus* (Fig. 2i). The Metastats analysis shown that *Escherichia-Shigella* was significantly more abundant in the HS group, while *Prevotella, Leptotrichia, Varibaculum, Mycoplasma,* and *Candidatus-Nomurabacteria* were more abundant in the LS group (Additional file 1: Table S1).

Of interest was that no significant differences were noted in clinical characteristics except Hemoglobin A1c (HbA1c) between the LS group and HS group (Table 2).

Comparisons of bioinformatics between T2D patients with low HbA1c and high HBA1c

Due to the significant difference of HbA1c was found between LS group and HS group, we further analysis the characteristics of urinary microbiota between female T2D patients with low HbA1c (LH group, HbA1c ≤ 7%) and high HbA1c (HH group, HbA1c > 7%). Higher Shannon index (Fig. 4d, 1.369(0.044, 3.478) vs. 2.089(0.979, 3.429), $P = 0.033$) and lower Simpson index (Fig. 4e, 0.461(0.055, 0.987) vs. 0.229(0.069, 0.640), $P = 0.029$) were presented in LH group, while no significantly difference in Observed Species, Chao1 index and ACE index (Fig. 4a, 77(10,204) vs. 86(54, 234), $P = 0.157$; Fig. 4b, 97.00(11.00, 213.55) vs. 115.67(63.89,245.84), $P = 0.105$; Fig. 4c, 94.87(0.26, 3.32) vs. 121.30(63.89, 280.30), $P = 0.089$). Comparison of alpha diversity indicated that significantly decreasing species diversity was discovered in HH cohort.

PCoA plots demonstrated that LH group samples and HH group samples were clustered respectively, which suggested that the urinary microbiota composition of LH group differed from that of HH group (Fig. 4f and Fig. 4h). MRPP test shown that the observed differences in PCoA plots were statistically significant ($P = 0.001$ for weighted UniFrac and Bray Curtis distance metrics, respectively). However, the difference in unweighted UniFrac distance metrics could not reach statistical significance (Fig. 4g, P = 0.078).

LEfSe demonstrated that 2 genera were over represented in the HH group, including *Escherichia-Shigella* and *Lactobacillus*, while 10 genera were over-represented in the LH group, including *Prevotella, Campylobacter, Dialister, Anaerococcus, Peptoniphilus, Porphyromonas, Fodinicola, Negativicoccus* (Fig. 4i). Among these genera, Metastats algorithm shown the significantly different in *Anaerococcus, Fodinicola, Lactobacillus, Peptoniphilus, Senegalimassilia* (Additional file 1: Table S1).

Higher scores of AUA-SI (total score, 13.059 ± 6.805 vs. 4.867 ± 3.796; storage score, 7.824 ± 4.825 vs. 2.600 ± 2.230; emptying score, 5.235 ± 5.118 vs. 2.267 ± 3.369) were found in HH group ($P < 0.05$, Additional file 2: Table S2). Besides, HbA1c was found positively correlated with the total score of AUA-SI based on Pearson's correlation (Fig. 5, $r = 0.509$, $P = 0.003$).

Discussion

In this study, we describe the urinary microbiota in the female with and without T2D, female T2D patients with no to mild LUTS and moderate to severe LUTS as well as patients with low HbA1c and high HBA1c using 16S rDNA sequencing. Based on other reports [10, 11, 21] and our data, this is further confirmation that the commonly held clinical belief that healthy urine should be sterile is false.

Consented with Liu's study, our results indicated that the composition of urinary microbiota may be impacted by diabetes [14]. (1) Samples from T2D patients and

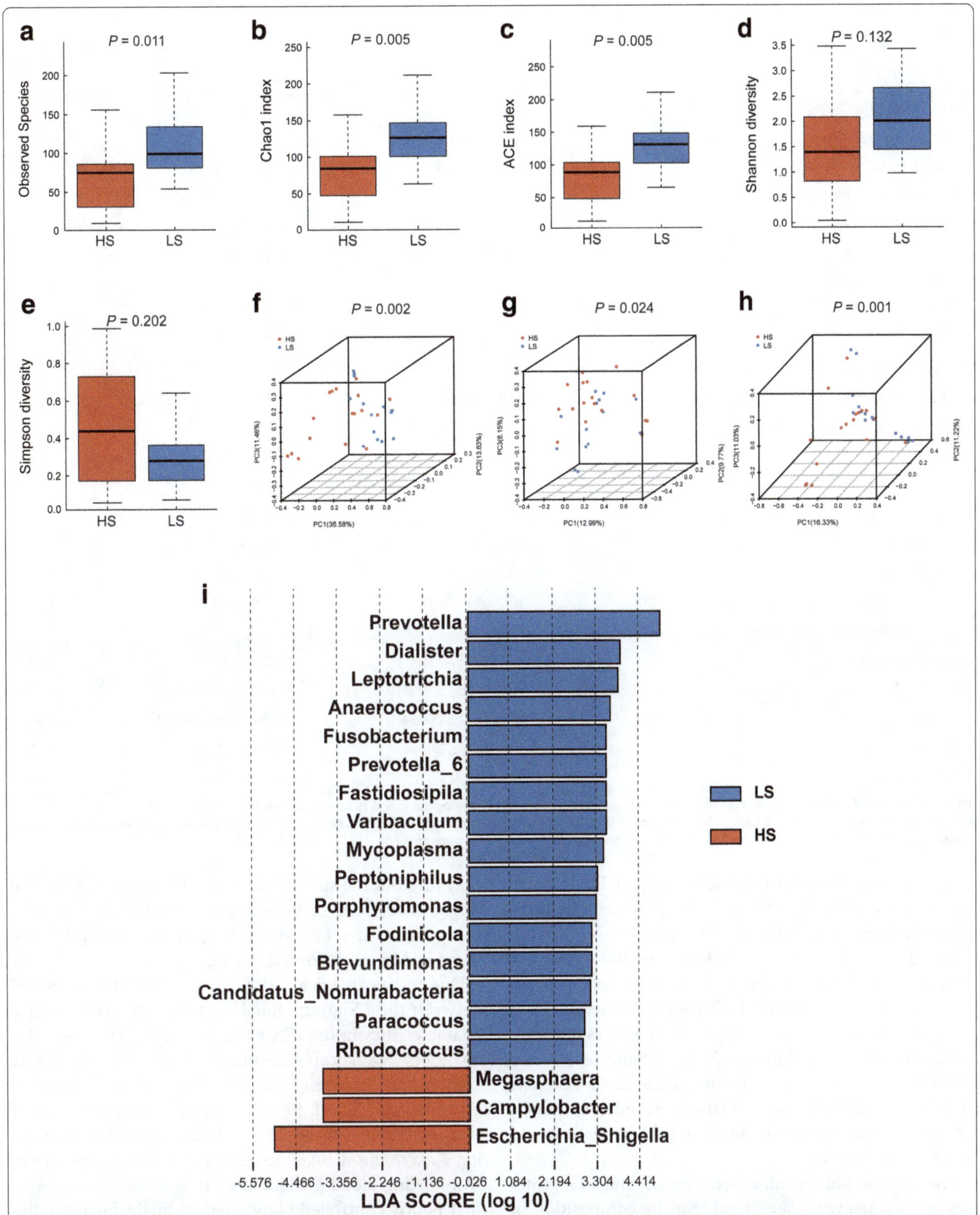

Fig. 2 Alpha diversity and principal coordinate analysis for the HS group and LS group urinary microbiota. Observed Species **(a)**; Chao1 index **(b)**; ACE index **(c)**; Shannon index **(d)**; Simpson index **(e)**. Principal coordinate analysis plots of the urinary microbiota based on the weighted UniFrac **(f)**, unweighted UniFrac **(g)** and Bray-Curtis **(h)** distance metrics. Association of specific microbiota taxa with the HS group and LS group was analyzed by LEfSe **(i)**. Genera enriched for HS in red and enriched for LS in blue. Only genera meeting a linear discriminant analysis score threshold > 2 are shown

Table 2 Comparisons of demographic and clinical characteristics as well as bacterial alpha diversity between HS group and LS group

	HS ($n = 17$)	LS ($n = 15$)	P value
Demographic Characteristics			
Age (y)	57.882 ± 8.230	55.933 ± 7.914	0.501
Body mass index (kg/m2)	23.715 ± 4.320	23.766 ± 4.596	0.975
Menstrual status [no.(%)]			1.000
Premenopausal	4 (23.5%)	4 (26.7%)	
Postmenopausal	13 (76.5%)	11 (73.3%)	
Reproductive status [no.(%)]			N/A
Fertile	17 (100%)	15 (100%)	
Sterile	0 (0%)	0 (0%)	
Clinical Characteristics			
Duration of diabetes (y)	6.882 ± 5.278	6.933 ± 4.250	0.976
Fasting blood glucose (mmol/L)	8.148 ± 3.798	7.647 ± 2.640	0.672
Hemoglobin A1c (%)	9.294 ± 2.044	6.720 ± 1.364	< 0.001
Retinopathy [no.(%)]	5 (29.4%)	5 (33.3%)	1.000
Peripheral neuropathy [no.(%)]	15 (88.2%)	12 (80.0%)	0.645
Hypertension [no.(%)]	7 (41.2%)	7 (46.7%)	0.755
Creatinine (μmol/L)	70.177 ± 68.789	59.467 ± 26.465	0.852
Estimated glomerular filtration rate (ml/min/1.73m^2)	101.304 ± 34.613	108.150 ± 43.583	0.624
Parameter of Bacterial Alpha Diversity			
Observed species	76 (10, 175)	98 (54, 234)	0.011
Chao1	83.86 (11.00, 210.77)	125.19 (62.00, 251.77)	0.005
ACE index	85.52 (13.75, 204.84)	129.82 (63.89, 280.30)	0.005
Shannon index	1.40 (0.04, 3.48)	2.01 (0.98, 3.43)	0.132
Simpson index	0.44 (0.06, 0.99)	0.28 (0.07, 0.64)	0.202

Data were presented as mean ± SD for continuous variables and n (%) for counts in demographic and clinical characteristics. Parameters of bacterial alpha diversity were reported as median (range). HS, female type 2 diabetes patients with moderate to severe lower urinary tract symptoms. LS, female type 2 diabetes patients with no to mild lower urinary tract symptoms. N/A, not applicable. ※No data were missing

those from controls clustered separately in PCoA plots (Fig. 1f, h), which suggested a common urinary dysbiosis was associated to diabetes; (2) 10 genera were over-represented in T2D patients, including common pathogens such as *Escherichia-Shigella, Klebsiella* and *Enterococcus;* (3) it is found that female T2D patients suffering from much serious LUTS. Taken together, these results indicated that urinary dysbiosis (e.g. significantly increasing pathogens) may contribute to the initiation or development of cn-LUTS in type 2 diabetic patients. Common pathogens that over-represented in T2D patients would be discussed below.

Urinary microbial profile between LS and HS group was further analyzed. We found that the composition of urinary microbiota in the LS group was also significantly different from that in the HS group (Fig. 2f, 2i, Fig. 3). Hence, this raises the possibility that specific microbial patterns may be associated with more serious LUTS or the progression of LUTS in the female T2D patients. We may find out the specific urinary microbiota (Fig. 2i) that might exacerbate diabetes-induced cn-LUTS. The relatively increasing and decreasing genus would be also discussed in the following passage.

Due to the significant difference of HbA1c was found between the LS group and HS group, urinary microbial characteristics in the HH group and LH group were also analyzed. Statistical differences of urinary microbiota composition between HH and LH cohort were found in our analysis (Fig. 4f, i). In Liu et al.'s study, they found that increased *Actinobacteria* phylum as well as decreasing *Akkermansia muciniphila* were positively correlated with fasting blood glucose [14]. It is therefore suggested that poorly controlled blood glucose might further influence the composition of urinary microbiota. Furthermore, we found that most patients in the HH group suffered from more serious LUTS and HbA1c was positively correlated with AUA-SI. These raise the possibility that poorly controlled blood glucose might exacerbate

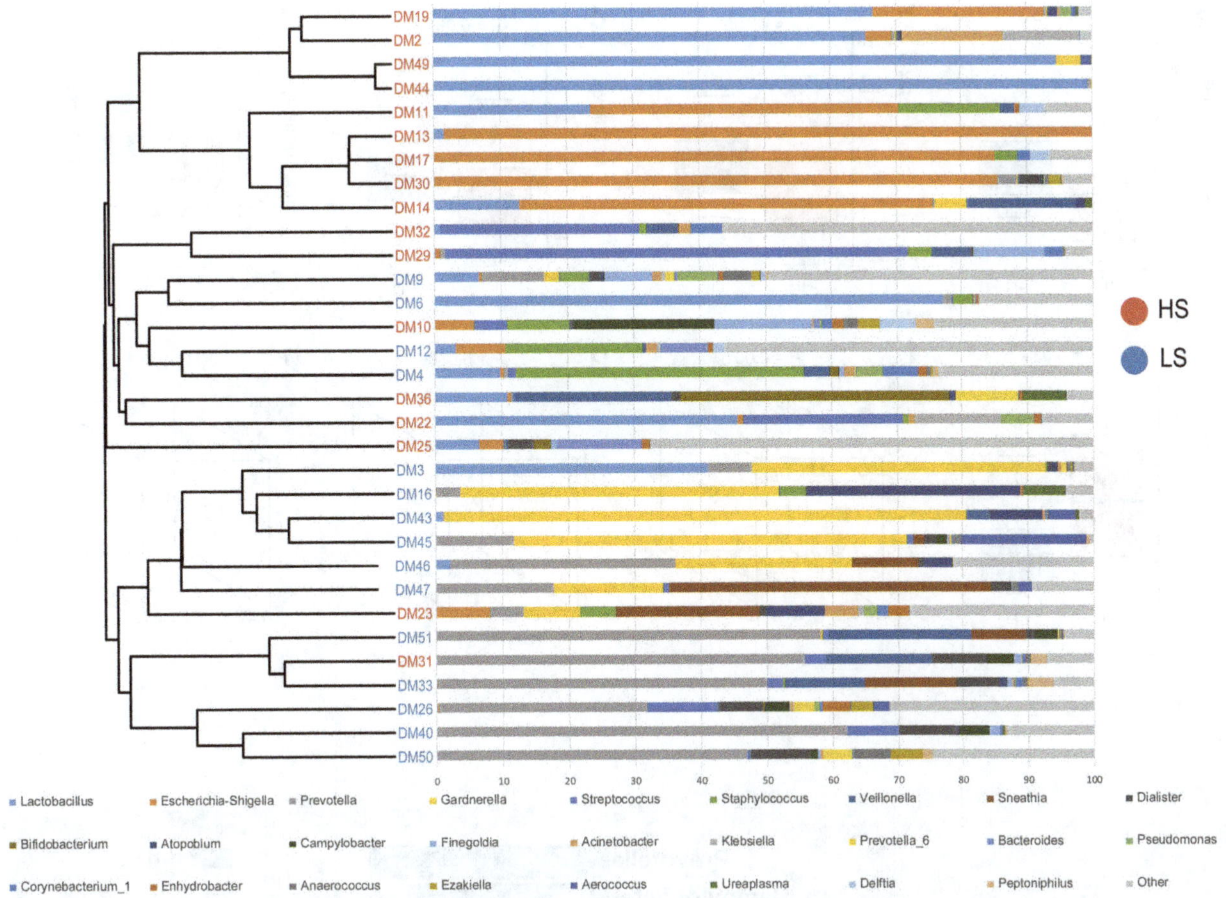

Fig. 3 A clear hierarchical clustering of HS samples was observed in the dendrogram at the genus level (left; based on Bray Curtis distance metrics). In the histogram (right), each colored box represents a bacterial taxon and each bar, a subject. The height of a colored box represents the relative abundance of each organism in the sample. Bacterial genera with a relative abundance < 0.5% and unclassified genera are grouped as "Other"

cn-LUTS. As a result, we suggested the intriguing hypothesis that chronic hyperglycemia might induce or deteriorate cn-LUTS in T2D patients through influencing the urinary microbiota composition. Although the cause-effect relationship among hyperglycemia, urinary microbiota and cn-LUTS cannot be determined under our study, it is worth further researching.

In both cohorts, one or two genera dominated most of the sequence profiles. *Escherichia-Shigella* was relatively increased in diabetes group and HS group. *Klebsiella* and *Enterococcus* were relatively increased in the diabetes group. *Klebsiella* is a common conditional pathogenic bacterium that causing respiratory and urinary tract infections when host immunity is impaired [22]. *Enterococcus* is a nosocomial pathogen which can cause UTI and endocarditis [23]. Increased TNF-α, a proinflammatory cytokine, was discovered in the bladder tissue of T2D mice [24]. Toll-like receptors 4 pathway was also activated in type 1 diabetes rats induced by Streptozotocin [25]. It was a strong indication that inflammation existed in the bladder tissue of diabetic animals. In the present study, diabetic patients that included were suffered from cn-LUTS. As for these patients, standard clinical cultivation procedures have a too low sensitivity to detect the uropathogens. 16S rDNA sequencing of mid-stream urine samples might represent a novel method for diagnosing "UTI" (urinary dysbiosis).

The trends of *Prevotella* abundance changes were variable in different researches. In our study, *Prevotella* was decreasing in HS cohort and our previous study shown that decreasing *Prevotella* was found in overactive bladder patients [10]. However, Pearce et al. revealed that enrichment of *Prevotella* was observed in urgency urinary incontinence patients [11]. 16S rDNA sequencing-based approach can't identify bacteria well at the species level and over 20 species have been already classified into *Prevotella*. It is hypothesized that various species play distinct roles in different disorders, leading to the contradiction mentioned before. Thus, it may be necessary to explore

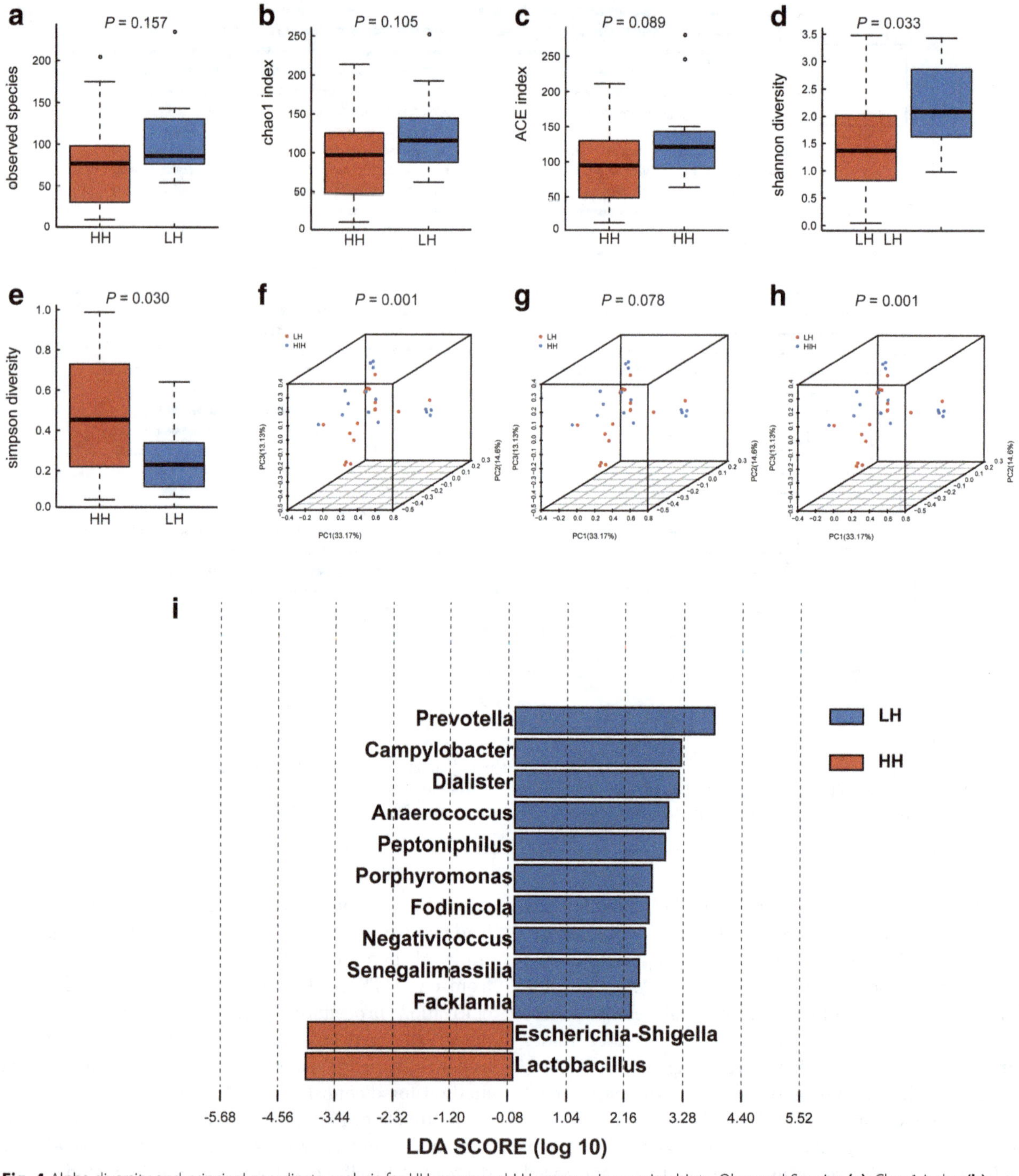

Fig. 4 Alpha diversity and principal coordinate analysis for HH group and LH group urinary microbiota. Observed Species **(a)**; Chao1 index **(b)**; ACE index **(c)**; Shannon index **(d)**; Simpson index **(e)**. Principal coordinate analysis plots of the urinary microbiota based on the weighted UniFrac **(f)**, unweighted UniFrac **(g)** and Bray-Curtis **(h)** distance metrics. Association of specific microbiota taxa with HH group and LH group was analyzed by LEfSe **(i)**. Genera enriched for HH in red and enriched for LH in blue. Only genera meeting a linear discriminant analysis score threshold > 2 are shown

the role of *Prevotella* in urologic disorders via whole genome shotgun sequencing or expanded urine culture.

Enrichment of *Lactobacillus* was presented in the HH group. *Lactobacillus* is considered being low virulence, hardly causing infections in human beings [12]. It is best known for its dominance in vaginal microbiota and it can prevent vaginitis by maintaining a physiological acidic environment in the vagina. Because of these

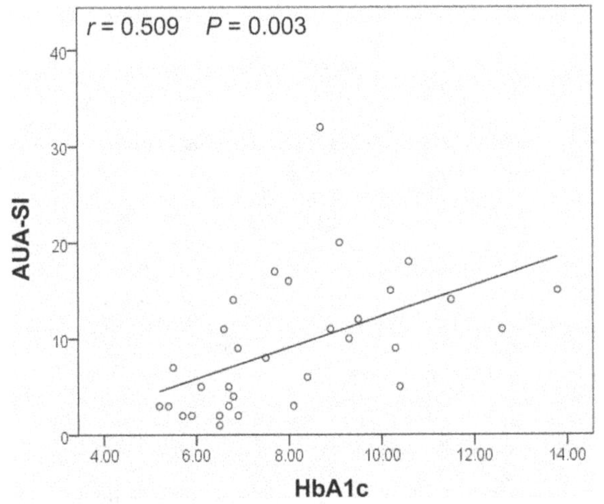

Fig. 5 Correlations between AUA-SI and Hemoglobin A1c in female type 2 diabetes patients. Higher Hemoglobin A1c positively correlated with the AUA-SI score

properties, *Lactobacillus* has been applied to prevent or even treat UTI [26]. However, there is increasing evidence that specific *Lactobacillus spp* may be pathogenic and linked to UTI [27, 28]. It has been suggested that *Lactobacillus* is resistant to the widely used antibiotics, which can reproduce during the treatment of UTI and invade the bladder to induce inflammation [29]. In addition, several studies found that *Lactobacillus* was closely associated with cn-LUTS [27, 28]. For example, Maskell et al. found that *Lactobacillus* gradually disappeared (detected by special culture techniques) as symptoms subsided after the use of antibiotics for treating LUTS in the female patients who had a negative urine culture before [30]. The result suggested that a shift in the microbial community towards *Lactobacillus* in the HH group may be an important etiological factor for the more serious LUTS reported by the patients.

In this study, no significant differences in alpha diversity were found between T2D patients and controls but decreased richness as well as species diversity were shown in HS and HH group, respectively. Although a reduction in alpha diversity has been thought as a feature of gastrointestinal diseases, such as ulcerative colitis, Crohn's disease and colorectal cancer [31–33] as well as an increased vaginal microbiota diversity was associated with bacterial vaginitis [34]. No consistent changes in alpha diversity were found in urologic disorders. Increased alpha diversity was observed in urgency urinary incontinence [11], decreasing alpha diversity was demonstrated in overactive bladder [10], while no significant difference was noted in prostate cancer [35]. In Liu et al.'s study, they reported that urinary microbiota diversity and richness were lower in female T2D patients [14]. Demographic features, exclusive criteria and less microbial species in the urinary tract may be the reasons leading to this contradiction between Liu's study and ours [14].

Owing to the urine samples may be contaminated with microbiota surrounding the urethral orifice, mid-stream urine was collected by the clean catch method with labial separation supervised by the author (Weina Huang). Catheter-derived urine samples were suggested as an alternative method, but the method was considered being invasive and was not ethically workable in patients who do not have a clinical indication for it. Comparison of results from Siddiqui et al.'s urinary microbiota study on female mid-stream urine with the consequences of suprapubic aspirate by Wolfe et al. shown that the major findings were the same [12]. It was a strong indication that results from mid-stream urinary microbiota were reliable.

Participants who used antibiotics recently have been excluded, however, numerous drugs may influence gut microbiota composition, and their effect may be present even in the urinary microbiota. Anti-diabetic drugs, particularly metformin, also have a well-known effect on the gut microbiota composition [36]. Although all the T2D patients included in our study were hospitalized and most of them were treated with insulin (data not shown), we could not fully avoid the interference of anti-diabetic drugs. The correlation between urinary microbiota and anti-diabetic drugs should be studied.

Our study is not devoid of limitations. Firstly, it is impossible to determine the cause-effect relationship between symptoms and bioinformatics indicators in this cross-sectional study. Thus, prospective studies with a larger sample and animal experimentation will be needed to clarify the role of urinary microbiota in the development and progression of cn-LUTS in female T2D patients. Secondly, we cannot confirm that the urinary microbes characterized by 16S rDNA sequencing were actually viable. We should add expanded urine culture as a complementary method and make a comprehensive analysis of information that provided by expanded urine culture and 16S sequencing in the future. Finally, the heterogeneity of our cohort should not be ignored because of wide the range of age and duration of diabetes in our cohort. Thus, patients might be stratified by age and time of symptoms in a larger cohort.

Conclusions

We have comprehensively profiled the urinary microbiota associated with cn-LUTS in female T2D patients. The link between urinary microbiota and cn-LUTS in female T2D patients without evidence of UTI has been established but the cause-effect relationship is still unclear. A better understanding of urinary microbiota in the development and progression of cn-LUTS in female T2D patients was necessary, which might provide novel diagnostic biomarkers as well as microbiota-targeted therapeutic options. The severity of cn-LUTS might be related to hyperglycemia and chronic hyperglycemia might induce or promote cn-LUTS by influencing the composition of urinary microbiota.

Additional files

Additional file 1: Table S1. Differences of urinary microbiota between groups at genus level based on Metastats algorithm (XLSX 12 kb)

Additional file 2: Table S2. Comparisons of demographic and clinical characteristics between HH group and LH group (DOCX 16 kb)

Abbreviations

AUA-SI: American Urological Association Symptom Index questionnaire; cn-LUTS: Cultured negative lower urinary tract symptoms; HbA1c: Hemoglobin A1c; LEfSe: Linear discriminant analysis effect size; LUTS: Lower urinary tract symptoms; MRPP: Multiple Response Permutation Procedure; OTUs: Operational taxonomic units; PCoA: Principal coordinate analysis; QIIME: Quantitative Insights Into Microbial Ecology; T2D: Type 2 diabetes; UTI: Urinary tract infections

Acknowledgments

Not applicable.

Authors' contributions

PW (Peng Wu), JC (Jiawei Chen) and JZ1 (Jie Zhao) were involved in study design; JC, YC1 (Ying Cao) and GZ (Guihao Zhang) processed the samples and carried out the molecular techniques; JC, JZ2 (Jialei Zhong) and YC2 (Yang Chen) performed the bioinformatics and taxonomic analysis; PW, JC and JZ1 drafted the manuscript; PW, GZ and WH (Weina Huang) performed the critical revision of the manuscript; JZ3 (Jiarong Zeng) performed the statistical analysis. All authors read and approved the final manuscript.

Author details

[1]Department of Urology, Nanfang Hospital, Southern Medical University, Guangzhou 510515, China. [2]School of Pharmaceutical Sciences, Southern Medical University, Guangzhou, China. [3]Department of Endocrinology and Metabolism, Nanfang Hospital, Southern Medical University, Guangzhou 510515, China.

References

1. Kirschner-Hermanns R, Daneshgari F, Vahabi B, Birder L, Oelke M, Chacko S. Does diabetes mellitus-induced bladder remodeling affect lower urinary tract function? ICI-RS 2011. Neurourol Urodyn. 2012;31:359–64.
2. Golbidi S, Laher I. Bladder dysfunction in diabetes mellitus. Front Pharmacol. 2010;1:136.
3. Daneshgari F, Liu G, Birder L, Hanna-Mitchell AT, Chacko S. Diabetic bladder dysfunction: current translational knowledge. J Urol. 2009;182(Suppl):18–26.
4. Young VB. The role of the microbiome in human health and disease: an introduction for clinicians. BMJ. 2017;15:j831.
5. Darveau RP. Periodontitis: a polymicrobial disruption of host homeostasis. Nat Rev Microbiol. 2010;8:481–90.
6. Irrazábal T, Belcheva A, Girardin SE, Martin A, Philpott DJ. The multifaceted role of the intestinal microbiota in colon cancer. Mol Cell. 2014;54:309–20.
7. Chu H, Khosravi A, Kusumawardhani IP, Kwon AH, Vasconcelos AC, Cunha LD, et al. Gene-microbiota interactions contribute to the pathogenesis of inflammatory bowel disease. Science. 2016;352:1116–20.
8. Urbaniak C, Gloor GB, Brackstone M, Scott L, Tangney M, Reid G. The microbiota of breast tissue and its association with breast Cancer. Appl Environ Microbiol. 2016;82:5039–48.
9. Wolfe AJ, Toh E, Shibata N, Rong R, Kenton K, Fitzgerald M, et al. Evidence of uncultivated bacteria in the adult female bladder. J Clin Microbiol. 2012; 50:1376–83.
10. Wu P, Chen Y, Zhao J, Zhang G, Chen J, Wang J, et al. Urinary microbiome and psychological factors in women with overactive bladder. Front Cell Infect Microbiol. 2017;7:488.
11. Pearce MM, Hilt EE, Rosenfeld AB, Zilliox MJ, Thomas-White K, Fok C, et al. The female urinary microbiome: a comparison of women with and without urgency urinary incontinence. MBio. 2014;5:e01283–14.
12. Siddiqui H, Lagesen K, Nederbragt AJ, Jeansson SL, Jakobsen KS. Alterations of microbiota in urine from women with interstitial cystitis. BMC Microbiol. 2012;12:205.
13. Fouts DE, Pieper R, Szpakowski S, Pohl H, Knoblach S, Suh MJ, et al. Integrated next-generation sequencing of 16S rDNA and metaproteomics differentiate the healthy urine microbiome from asymptomatic bacteriuria in neuropathic bladder associated with spinal cord injury. J Transl Med. 2012;10:174.
14. Liu F, Ling Z, Xiao Y, Lv L, Yang Q, Wang B, et al. Dysbiosis of urinary microbiota is positively correlated with type 2 diabetes mellitus. Oncotarget. 2017;8:3798–810.
15. Caporaso JG, Kuczynski J, Stombaugh J, Bittinger K, Bushman FD, Costello EK, et al. QIIME allows analysis of high-throughput community sequencing data. Nat Methods. 2010;7:335–6.
16. Edgar RC. UPARSE: highly accurate OTU sequences from microbial amplicon reads. Nat Methods. 2013;10:996–8.
17. Edgar RC, Haas BJ, Clemente JC, Quince C, Knight R. UCHIME improves sensitivity and speed of chimera detection. Bioinformatics. 2011;27: 2194–200.
18. Wang Q, Garrity GM, Tiedje JM, Cole JR. Naive Bayesian classifier for rapid assignment of rRNA sequences into the new bacterial taxonomy. Appl Environ Microbiol. 2007;73:5261–7.
19. White JR, Nagarajan N, Pop M. Statistical methods for detecting differentially abundant features in clinical metagenomic samples. PLoS Comput Biol. 2009;5:e1000352.
20. Segata N, Izard J, Waldron L, Gevers D, Miropolsky L, Garrett WS, et al. Metagenomic biomarker discovery and explanation. Genome Biol. 2011; 12:R60.
21. Wu P, Zhang G, Zhao J, Chen J, Chen Y, Huang W, et al. Profiling the urinary microbiota in male patients with bladder Cancer in China. Front Cell Infect Microbiol. 2018;8:167.
22. Dehshiri M, Khoramrooz SS, Zoladl M, Khosravani SA, Parhizgari N, Motazedian MH, et al. The frequency of Klebsiella pneumonia encoding genes for CTX-M, TEM-1 and SHV-1 extended-spectrum beta lactamases enzymes isolated from urinary tract infection. Ann Clin Microbiol Antimicrob. 2018;17(1):4.
23. Fisher K, Phillips C. The ecology, epidemiology and virulence of Enterococcus. Microbiology. 2009;155:1749–57.
24. Wang Z, Cheng Z, Cristofaro V, Li J, Xiao X, Gomez P, et al. Inhibition of TNF-α improves the bladder dysfunction that is associated with type 2 diabetes. Diabetes. 2012;61:2134–45.
25. Szasz T, Wenceslau CF, Burgess B, Nunes KP, Webb RC. Toll-like receptor 4 activation contributes to diabetic bladder dysfunction in a murine model of type 1 diabetes. Diabetes. 2016;65:3754–64.
26. Falagas ME, Betsi GI, Tokas T, Athanasiou S. Probiotics for prevention of recurrent urinary tract infections in women: a review of the evidence from microbiological and clinical studies. Drugs. 2006;66:1253–61.
27. Darbro BW, Petroelje BK, Doern GV. Lactobacillus delbrueckii as the cause of urinary tract infection. J Clin Microbiol. 2009;47:275–7.
28. Imirzalioglu C, Hain T, Chakraborty T, Domann E. Hidden pathogens uncovered: metagenomic analysis of urinary tract infections. Andrologia. 2008;40:66–71.
29. Maskell RM. The natural history of urinary tract infection in women. Med Hypotheses. 2010;74:802–6.
30. Maskell R, Pead L, Sanderson RA. Fastidious bacteria and the urethral syndrome: a 2-year clinical and bacteriological study of 51 women. Lancet. 1983;2:1277–80.
31. Ahn J, Sinha R, Pei Z, Dominianni C, Wu J, Shi J, et al. Human gut microbiome and risk for colorectal cancer. J Natl Cancer Inst. 2013;105: 1907–11.
32. Lepage P, Häsler R, Spehlmann ME, Rehman A, Zvirbliene A, Begun A, et al. Twin study indicates loss of interaction between microbiota and mucosa of patients with ulcerative colitis. Gastroenterology. 2011;141:227–36.

33. Gevers D, Kugathasan S, Denson LA, Vázquez-Baeza Y, Van Treuren W, Ren B, et al. The treatment-naive microbiome in new-onset Crohn's disease. Cell Host Microbe. 2014;15:382–92.
34. Liu MB, Xu SR, He Y, Deng GH, Sheng HF, Huang XM, et al. Diverse vaginal microbiomes in reproductive-age women with vulvovaginal candidiasis. PLoS One. 2013;8:e79812.
35. Shrestha E, White JR, Yu SH, Kulac I, Ertunc O, De Marzo AM, et al. Profiling the urinary microbiome in men with positive versus negative biopsies for prostate Cancer. J Urol. 2018;199:161–71.
36. Tong X, Xu J, Lian F, Yu X, Zhao Y, Xu L, et al. Structural alteration of gut microbiota during the amelioration of human type 2 diabetes with hyperlipidemia by metformin and a traditional Chinese herbal formula: a multicenter, randomized. Open Label Clinical Trial MBio. 2018;9:e02392–17.

2

Long-term outcomes of two types of metal stent for chronic benign ureteral strictures

Joongwon Choi[1], Kyung Jin Chung[2], Seol Ho Choo[3] and Deok Hyun Han[1*]

Abstract

Background: We aimed to compare the results of long-term use of two types of metal stent for chronic benign ureteral strictures.

Methods: Our study included 46 ureter units (UUs) that underwent metal stent placement from 2010 to 2017. We included benign ureteral strictures causes by variety reasons that could not be solved by other treatment and malignant obstructions were excluded. Covered mesh stent (Uventa™) and a thermo-expandable stent (Memokath 051™) were used. Primary success was defined as maintaining patency without procedures and overall success was defined as maintaining patency with additional procedures.

Results: We placed covered mesh stents in 25 UUs and thermo-expandable stents in 21 UUs. The mean follow-up duration of each stent was 41.4 ± 23.1 and 34.4 ± 16.5 months ($p = 0.250$). In the first year of stent insertion, primary success was achieved in 54.9 and 70.4% ($p = 0.204$). Overall success was achieved in 78.7 and 75.4% in same duration, respectively ($p = 0.586$). Longer stent placement had positive predictive value on both success rates (HR = 0.185, $p = 0.047$ and HR = 0.111, $p = 0.018$). Prior radiation therapy and non-pelvic ureter stricture both adversely affected the overall success rate (HR = 5.412, $p = 0.048$ and HR = 4.203, $p = 0.030$). Previous PCN status had negative predictive value for both success rates (HR = 4.014, $p = 0.003$ and HR = 3.064, $p = 0.035$).

Conclusions: The treatment outcomes of two types of metal stent were comparable, especially in the first year of stent insertion.

Keywords: Benign ureteral stricture, Mesh, Metal stent, Success rate, Thermo-expandable

Background

Ureteral strictures can occur in a wide variety of benign and malignant diseases. Benign strictures have various etiologies, including radiation therapy, retroperitoneal fibrosis, and ureter stones. When urinary diversion is not effective, ureteral strictures can turn chronic, causing serious problems. Conventional polymer stents can also introduce several problems, such as encrustation, stone formation, pain, infection, reflux and migration [1]. Open urinary diversions were gradually abandoned because of their technical difficulty with associated risk [2]. After metal stents were successfully used in vascular and biliary systems, they began to be used in urinary diseases. Milroy et al. [3] inserted the first metal stents in urethral stricture patients in 1988. Since then, many metal stents have been developed, but identifying the best stent for specific conditions is difficult because each stent has a different mechanism.

Malignant ureteral strictures are caused by extrinsic compression or direct invasion by a primary or metastatic tumor and lymphadenopathy [4]. The nature of strictures caused by direct tumor invasion can be very different from strictures caused by benign diseases.

Comparing the effects of metal stents in a benign environment allows us to eliminate complexity and make relatively objective comparisons. Thus, we compared two metal stent types—the covered mesh stent and the thermo-expandable stent. The Uventa™ model (Taewoong Medical, Seoul, Korea) was chosen as the mesh stent, and the Memokath 051™ model (PNN Medical, Glostrup, Denmark) was chosen as the thermo-expandable stent.

* Correspondence: dhhan@skku.edu
[1]Department of Urology, Samsung Medical Center, Sungkyunkwan University School of Medicine, 81 Irwon-ro, Gangnam-gu, Seoul 06351, South Korea
Full list of author information is available at the end of the article

Early metal stent models had a problem with tissue ingrowth, which led to ureteral lumen occlusion and increased the difficulty of endoscopic removal [5]. To solve this problem, an externally coated single-layered segmental stent (Passager; Boston Scientific, Miami, FL, USA) was developed for ureteral strictures. However, the polytetrafluoroethylene (PTFE) membrane covering the stent reduced the stent's ability to obtain firm adhesion, which caused high rates of stent migration—as much as 81.0% [6].

Uventa was developed in response to these problems. It has a triple-layered mesh construction, and the PTFE is stacked with nitinol above and below. The outer stent has a high friction coefficient to prevent migration, while the PTFE membrane prevents tissue ingrowth [7]. Its diameter is 7 mm, and the length ranges from 6 to 16 cm.

Memokath 051™ has a closed spiral structure which can prevent urothelial ingrowth. Its tight spiral and metal alloy hold the stricture site without urothelial overgrowth [5]. Its titanium component has the ability to resist corrosion in the urinary system [1]. Stoller et al. [8] reported that the spiral stent yielded higher flow rates than the conventional polymer stent. The products are available in lengths of 3, 6, 10, 15, 20, and 25 cm.

A previous study compared the two stents [9], but did not distinguish between benign and malignant causes, and complications were not systematically classified. The study also did not compare the primary success rate with the overall success rate. The aim of this study is to improve those limitations and compare two type of stent, and identified the risk factors for keep patency.

Methods

The Institutional Review Board of Samsung Medical Center approved this study (IRB No.: 2018–05–106-001). We retrospectively obtained data from the medical records of patients who presented with chronic benign ureteral strictures and received metal stent placement. From May 2010 to December 2017, 36 patients (14 men and 22 women), with a total of 46 ureter units, underwent metal stent placement. We included benign ureteral strictures that were caused by radiation therapy, retroperitoneal fibrosis, ureter stone, pelvic surgery, ureteropelvic junction (UPJ) obstruction, renal tuberculosis, fibromatosis, and pelvic abscess. We excluded obstructions caused by direct malignant invasion.

To compare the efficacy and safety of mesh and thermo-expandable stents, we examined all medical records, including age, gender, previous pelvic radiation therapy (RT), side (right or left ureter), stricture length, lesion crossing the ureterovesical (UVJ) junction, previous balloon dilatation, previous double J (D-J) stenting, and previous percutaneous nephrostomy (PCN) catheter insertion.

We tended to insert a mesh stent if the sticture length was long (> 10 cm) or expected to be difficult to insert, which is easier to insert because it allows us to insert separate smaller stents.

We defined primary success as maintaining patency after the first stenting without an additional procedure. And overall success was defined as maintaining patency after further salvage procedures during the observed period. For example, if patency was maintained after the stent change or removed small debris from the ureteroscopy, it was considered as an overall success. Chung et al. first proposed this methodology [10].

Baumgarten et al. [11] defined stent failure as a need for PCN insertion, increasing hydronephrosis with a metal ureteral stent, or deteriorating renal function that is suspected to be post-renal in nature. We define this as failure. If patient have to keep a PCN with a metal stent, it is considered a failure.

We divided the ureteral stricture location into a pelvic ureter and non-pelvic ureter, according to the international anatomical system.

Statistical analysis

All results are presented as number with percent, mean with standard deviation, or median with interquartile range. We used the Kolmogorov-Smirnov statistic to analyze continuous variables for normality. We used the Mann-Whitney U-test to analyze descriptive variables, except age, stricture length, and follow-up months, which were calculated using the independent t-test. We estimated time to primary and overall failure using Kaplan-Meier curves and the log-rank test. We analyzed risk factors for primary and overall success with Cox regression analysis. Data were analyzed using SPSS version 21.0 (IBM, Chicago, IL, USA) and MedCalc version 14 (MedCalc Software, Ostend, Belgium).

Results

Table 1 shows the basic clinical characteristics. There were no differences between the groups except prior radiation therapy (RT, $p = 0.008$) and stricture length ($p = 0.010$). The most common motivation for replacement of the existing stent with a metal stent was inconvenience of frequent replacement (56.0 and 76.2%) followed by D-J malfunction (36.0 and 19.0%). Few people wanted to change to a metal stent to manage irritation symptoms from their existing D-J stent.

The underlying causes of metal stent placements are presented in Table 2. Radiation therapy was the most common cause (40.0%) for mesh stenting, followed by idiopathic (20.0%) and retroperitoneal fibrosis (20.0%). For thermo-expandable stenting, pelvic surgery was the most common cause (28.6%).

Table 1 Basic clinical characteristics of the mesh and thermo-expandable stent groups

Characteristics	*Mesh (n = 25)*	*Thermo-expandable (n = 21)*	*p-value*
Age, yr	62.7 ± 15.3	59.1 ± 12.6	0.394
Gender, n (%)			0.430
Male	9 (36.0)	10 (47.6)	
Female	16 (64.0)	11 (52.4)	
Previous pelvic radiation therapy	13 (52.0)	3 (14.3)	0.008
Side, n (%)			0.980
Right	13 (52.0)	11 (52.4)	
Left	12 (48.0)	10 (47.6)	
Stricture length (cm)	12.7 ± 6.3	7.8 ± 6.0	0.010
Reason for placement			0.159
D-J malfunction	9 (36.0)	4 (19.0)	
Irritation symptoms of D-J	2 (8.0)	1 (4.8)	
Inconvenience of frequent replacement	14 (56.0)	16 (76.2)	
Prior diversion, n (%)			
D-J	24 (96.0)	19 (90.5)	0.455
PCN	12 (48.0)	13 (61.9)	0.351

D-J double-J stent, *PCN* percutaneous nephrostomy

Intraoperative factors are compared in Table 3. The two stent groups were statistically different with regard to stent length ($p = 0.008$). Mesh stents are technically capable of being inserted as a set of overlapping multiple stents, while thermo-expandable stents are designed to be inserted as a single.

Time to primary failure is presented in Fig. 1. The median time to primary failure was 15.6 (9.3–21.5) months for mesh stents and 30.9 (15.2–39.9) months for thermo-expandable stents ($p = 0.204$). Figure 2 shows time to overall failure. The median time to overall failure was 29.0 (21.5–65.8) and 54.3 (20.6–54.3) months, respectively ($p = 0.586$).

The treatment outcomes for the mesh and thermo-expandable stent groups were comparable (Table 4). There was no statistical difference in follow-up months between the two groups ($p = 0.250$). Primary success was achieved for 12.0% of mesh stents and 28.6% of thermo-expandable stents throughout the entire observation period ($p = 0.204$). The overall success rates were 40.0 and 57.1%, respectively ($p = 0.586$). Thermo-expandable stents had better durability for primary success, especially in the second and third years.

Table 5 shows the risk factors affecting primary and overall success. Although stent type did not have a statistically significant effect on success rate, thermo-expandable stents generally yielded more favorable results for primary success (HR = 0.393, $p = 0.052$). Previous PCN status negatively impacted both primary (HR = 4.014, $p = 0.003$) and overall success (HR = 3.064, $p = 0.035$). However, longer stents had a positive effect on primary (HR = 0.185, $p = 0.047$) and overall success (HR = 0.111, $p = 0.018$). Prior radiation therapy and non-pelvic ureteral stricture adversely affected the overall success rate (HR = 5.412, $p = 0.048$). Additionally, risk factors of mesh and thermo-expandable stent were analyzed separately. The female gender was identified as the protective factor of primary success (HR = 0.136, $p = 0.024$) in mesh stent (Additional file 1: Table S1). In thermo-expandable stent, non-pelvic ureter (HR = 6.134, p = 0.048), previous PCN (HR = 10.192, $p = 0.013$) was risk factors (Additional file 2: Table S2) and stent length more than 15 cm reduce risk of primary failure (HR = 0.010, $p = 0.037$). Factors that showed multicollinearity were excluded.

Table 6 shows the types and numbers of failure events for both stents. If migration occurred but patency was

Table 2 Underlying Causes of Chronic Benign Strictures

	Mesh (n = 25)	*Thermo-expandable (n = 21)*
Idiopathic	5 (20.0)	1 (4.8)
Radiation therapy	10 (40.0)	3 (14.3)
Retroperitoneal fibrosis	5 (20.0)	4 (19.0)
Ureter stone	0 (0.0)	4 (19.0)
Pelvic surgery	2 (8.0)	6 (28.6)
UPJ obstruction	0 (0.0)	2 (9.5)
Renal tuberculosis	0 (0.0)	1 (4.8)
Fibromatosis	1 (4.0)	0 (0.0)
Pelvic abscess	2 (8.0)	0 (0.0)

UPJ ureteropelvic junction

Table 3 Intraoperative Factors of the Mesh and Thermo-Expandable Stent Groups

Characteristics	*Mesh (n = 25)*	*Thermo-expandable (n = 21)*	*p-value*
Stent length			0.008
< 10 cm	2 (8.0)	9 (42.9)	
10–15 cm	12 (48.0)	8 (38.1)	
> 15 cm or multiple[a]	11 (44.0)	4 (19.0)	
Location			0.060
Upper	2 (8.0)	4 (19.0)	
Mid	1 (4.0)	4 (19.0)	
Lower	4 (16.0)	5 (23.8)	
Upper-mid	5 (20.0)	1 (4.8)	
Mid-lower	4 (16.0)	2 (9.5)	
Upper-lower	9 (36.0)	5 (23.8)	
Across UVJ	10 (40.0)	4 (19.0)	0.128
Ballooning			0.521
Before stent placement	4 (16.0)	7 (33.3)	
After stent placement	5 (20.0)	0 (0.0)	

[a]more than two stents
UVJ Ureterovesical junction

maintained, we did not define it as a failure; this was relevant for one case in our study. The number of complication events was 31 for mesh stents and 15 for thermo-expandable stents; this difference was borderline significant ($p = 0.08$). The numbers of severe complications (above grade 3) were 12 and 10, respectively, which were not significantly different ($p = 0.96$).

Discussion

There have been a number of conflicting evaluations of metal stents. While early studies were generally promising [12–14], the reports shifted from mixed to unfavorable for both mesh [7, 9, 10] and thermo-expandable stents [2].

We used metal stents for benign strictures because we experienced acceptable results with malignant obstructions. In Korea, benign ureteral stricture is included in the indication of metal stent placement and It has also been reported that the metal stent is effective in the benign ureteral stricture [15]. Patients included in this study had sufficient discussion on the choice of treatment policies, and include cases who do not want to have repeated reconstructive surgery or it was not adaptive. Two UPJ stricture included in this study were

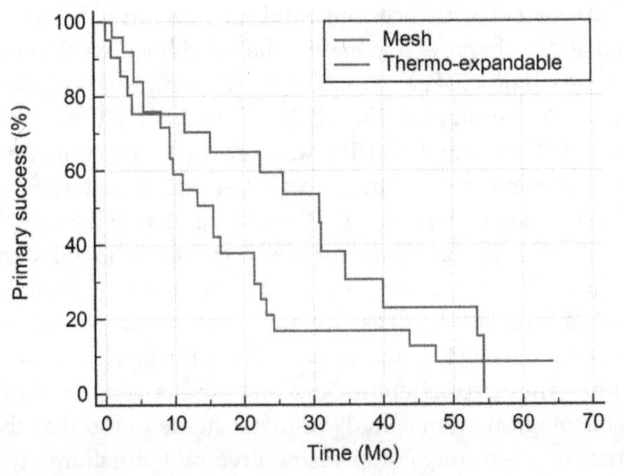

Fig. 1 Kaplan-Meier curves for primary success rates of the mesh and thermo-expandable metal stents: The medians (95% CI) for the two groups were 15.6 (9.3–21.5) and 30.9 (15.2–39.9), respectively ($p = 0.204$)

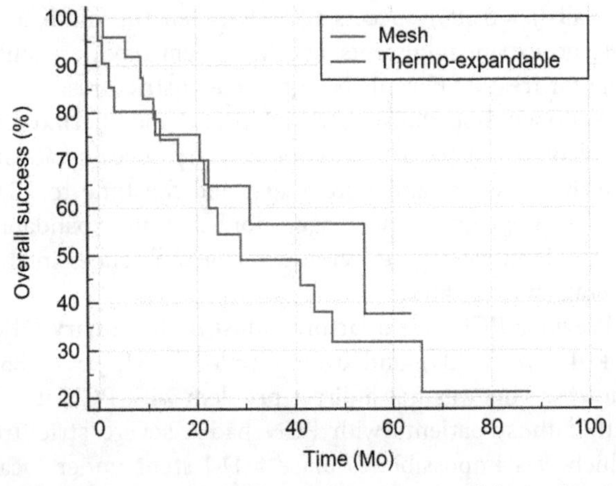

Fig. 2 Kaplan-Meier curves for overall success rates of the mesh and thermo-expandable metal stents: The medians (95% CI) for the two groups were 29.0 (21.5–65.8) and 54.3 (20.6–54.3), respectively ($p = 0.586$)

Table 4 Treatment Outcomes of the Mesh and Thermo-Expandable Stent Groups

	Mesh (n = 25)		*Thermo-expandable (n = 21)*	
	Primary	*Overall*	*Primary*	*Overall*
Follow-up months[a]	41.4 ± 23.1		34.4 ± 16.5	
Success rate[b], n (%)				
First year (%)	13 (54.9)	18 (78.7)	14 (70.4)	15 (75.4)
Second year (%)	4 (16.9)	10 (54.5)	11 (59.5)	12 (64.6)
Third year (%)	4 (16.9)	9 (49.1)	4 (30.6)	7 (56.5)
Time to 50% failure (month)	15.6	29.0	30.9	54.3
Cause of failure, n (%)				
Patency-related failure				
Migration	4 (16.0)	4 (16.0)	2 (9.5)	1 (4.8)
Hyperplasia	14 (56.0)	5 (20.0)	3 (14.3)	5 (23.8)
Encrustation	1 (4.0)	2 (8.0)	9 (42.9)	3 (14.3)
Patency-unrelated failure				
Concomitant change[c]	0 (0.0)	0 (0.0)	1 (4.8)	0 (0.0)
Fistula	2 (8.0)	3 (12.0)	0 (0.0)	0 (0.0)
Pseudoaneurysm	1 (4.0)	1 (4.0)	0 (0.0)	0 (0.0)

[a]Follow-up months for the two groups were comparable ($p = 0.250$)
[b]Success rate is an estimate, and the standard error is omitted. Neither the primary nor the overall rates were statistically significant ($p = 0.204$, 0.586)
[c]Concomitant change refers to the exchange of one obstructed stent as well as the other unobstructed stent due to concerns over future obstruction

recurred after pyeloplasty cases. One case was recurred after an additional endoureterotomy, and the other was who had history of multiple balloon dilatation after recur. The treatment policy was determined after sufficient consultation.

Since urinary tract reconstruction is not possible for every patient, metal stenting became a useful option in our practice. We wanted to identify effective metal stent for chronic benign ureteral strictures, especially between two commonly used stent in our hospital. There were no significant differences in primary ($p = 0.204$) and overall ($p = 0.586$) success rates between the mesh and thermo-expandable stents, and both stent types are suitable for treating chronic benign ureteral strictures.

Although not statistically significant, the thermo-expandable stent yielded a better primary success rate in the first, second, and third years, and the time to 50% failure was generally longer for thermo-expandable stents. However, there were no major differences in the overall success rates.

Previous PCN was a factor against both primary (HR = 4.014, $p = 0.003$) and overall (HR = 3.064, $p = 0.035$) success. This was not a direct problem with PCN itself; rather most patients with PCN had a severe stricture which was impossible to place a D-J stent under local anesthesia.

It is interesting that stent length longer than 15 cm and multiple stent insertions were positive factors for primary and overall success (HR = 0.185, $p = 0.047$ and HR = 0.111, $p = 0.018$). We suspect that sufficient lengthy stent insertion warrants favorable results rather than inserting a short stent that fits in a stricture segment.

Our study shows that the success rate is high when including the pelvic ureter. According to our search, the risk difference in stricture location is not clear. Pelvic ureter receives blood supplies from a much wider variety of vessels than abdominal ureter such as internal iliac artery, superior vesical artery, middle rectal artery, and inferior vesical artery. Which may have an effect, but further research is needed.

Consistent with previous studies, we found that prior radiation therapy decreased the likelihood of overall success [HR = 5.412, $p = 0.048$] [4, 7]. However, Liatsikos et al. [16] evaluated the effect of external RT in a pig model. They found that RT was safe for tissue containing a metal stent, but placing a metal stent in an ureter which was weakened by previous RT may cause tissue damage.

In our study, age was not a risk factor for metal stent failure. However, another study discussed age-related biomechanical changes in the ureter. According to Petsepe et al. [17], the muscle layer thickens with age, unlike the ureteral epithelium and lamina propria. Also, a histological animal study of metal stents found that the stent wire severely compressing ureteral epithelium [18]. It is possible that resistance of the ureter to a metal stent could decrease with age.

The overall trend was similar when risk factors were verified according to the stent type, but there were some

Table 5 Risk Factors Affecting Primary and Overall Success Rates

	Primary		*Overall*	
	HR	*p-value*	*HR*	*p-value*
Stent type				
Mesh	1.000	—	1.000	—
Thermo-expandable	0.393	0.052	0.680	0.468
Age (yr)	0.983	0.298	0.966	0.095
Gender				
Male	1.000	—	1.000	—
Female	0.469	0.131	0.640	0.462
Stricture location				
Pelvic ureter	1.000	—	1.000	—
Non-pelvic ureter[a]	2.631	0.062	4.203	0.030*
Stricture length (cm)				
≤10 cm	1.000	—	1.000	—
> 10 cm	2.925	0.077	1.789	0.430
Stent length		0.138		0.058
< 10 cm	1.000	—	1.000	—
10–15 cm	0.425	0.144	0.388	0.140
> 15 cm or multiple[b]	0.185	0.047*	0.111	0.018*
Prior radiation therapy				
No	1.000	—	1.000	—
Yes	2.155	0.198	5.412	0.048*
Previous PCN				
No	1.000	—	1.000	—
Yes	4.014	0.003*	3.064	0.035*
Balloon dilatation				
No	1.000	—	1.000	—
Yes	0.980	0.963	0.978	0.970

*Statistically significant ($p < 0.05$)
[a]upper ureteral stricture only
[b]more than two stents
HR hazard ratio, *PCN* percutaneous nephrostomy

Table 6 Numbers of All Types of Complication Events

Complications	*Modified Clavien classification*						
	Total	I	II	IIIa	IIIb	IV	V
Mesh ($n = 25$)		8	11	1	9	1	1
Persistent pain	3 (12.0%)	3					
Lower urinary tract symptoms	5 (20.0%)	5					
Urinary tract infection	9 (36.0%)		8				1
Persistent hematuria	3 (12.0%)		3				
Ureteroenteric fistula	3 (12.0%)				2	1	
Stent migration	5 (20.0%)				5		
Encrustation	2 (8.0%)				2		
Iliac artery pseudoaneurysm	1 (4.0%)			1			
Thermo-expandable ($n = 21$)		2	3	0	10	0	0
Persistent pain	1 (4.8%)	1					
Lower urinary tract symptoms	1 (4.8%)	1					
Urinary tract infection	2 (9.5%)		2				
Persistent hematuria	1 (4.8%)		1				
Ureteroenteric fistula	0 (0.0%)						
Stent migration	3 (14.3%)				3		
Encrustation	7 (33.3%)				7		
Iliac artery pseudoaneurysm	0 (0.0%)						

differences in two groups. Mesh stent showed favorable results when used in female gender (HR = 0.136), and was not affected by other risk factors. On the other hand, the primary failure was increased in the non-pelvic ureter with thermo-expandable stent (HR = 6.134). And it showed a favorable result when stent longer than 15 cm was inserted (HR = 0.010). In subgroup analysis, there were no factors affecting overall success.

Hsu et al. [19] reported antegrade insertion and response to cancer treatment as factors predicting immediate stent failure. Kim et al. [7] reported that female, cervical cancer, stricture length over 6 cm, and post-procedure follow-up over two years were risk factors for severe complications.

The mesh stent tended to caused more severe complications in our study. Overall, three fistulas and one pseudoaneurysm occurred in the mesh stent group. One patient had a stent placement because of radiation fibrosis, and the stent was exposed to the rectum for 21.5 months after the procedure, which was removed by open surgery. Another patient also had radiation fibrosis, and a left ureterosigmoid fistula was discovered only 9.3 months after the procedure; emergency exploration was performed and stent was removed. Another patient visited the emergency room with gross hematuria 13.3 months after metal stent insertion. In this case, CT findings revealed a pseudoaneurysm along the left distal ureter to the proximal sigmoid colon; the patient underwent immediate open nephrectomy, stent was removed and colon was repaired. Song et al. [20] reported three types of fistula after metal stent placements, including ureteroarterial fistula, ureteroenteral fistula, and ureterovaginal fistula. When a patient with a metal stent visits the emergency room with a gross hematuria, fistula should be highly suspected.

Generally, metal stents are contraindicated in renal stone formers. We used metal stent in four ureter stone cases, but the all patients were recurred cases after ureteroplasty or endopyelotomy. According to Wang et al. [21], it is not recommended to use metal stents in patients with stones because it is more likely to form encrustation and stones. Sountoulides et al. [2] also pointed out that most encrustation was occurred in former stone disease patients.

The impact of our findings is limited by retrospective nature and relatively small sample size. However, this is not a small number in the paper about metal stent, especially when limited to benign strictures. And baseline characteristics are not comparable in radiation treatment history and stricture length between two groups. But we analyzed the risk factors with multivariate analysis and able to offset some of the limitations. Multivariate analysis provides comprehensive information between the two groups and it was verified that there was no difference in success rates between two metal stents.

The treatment outcomes from mesh and thermo-expandable stents for chronic benign ureteral strictures were comparable. Although the primary and overall success rates were not significantly different between the stent groups, the thermo-expandable stent yielded more favorable results for primary success. Non-pelvic ureteral stricture, prior radiation therapy, and previous PCN had a negative effect on success. Longer stents had a positive effect on stent success. Both stents are suitable for treating chronic benign ureteral strictures, but more systematic and detailed research is needed to estimate success rates. There is no established optimal indication or strategy for selecting metal stents, but we expect our findings to contribute to that effort.

Conclusions

Both mesh and thermo-expandable stents are useful as a treatment for chronic benign ureteral strictures. There was no significant difference between the primary and overall success rates of the both stents, especially in the first year of stent insertion.

Additional files

Additional files 1: Table S1. Risk factors affecting success rates for covered mesh stent (DOCX 19 kb)

Additional files 2: Table S2. Risk factors affecting success rates for thermo-expandable stent (DOCX 19 kb)

Abbreviations

DJ: Double J stenting; PCN: Percutaneous nephrostomy; RT: Radiation therapy; UU: Ureter units; UVJ: Ureterovesical junction

Acknowledgements

Not applicable.

Authors' contributions

JC analyzed and interpreted the patient data, and was a major contributor in writing the manuscript. KC performed data acquisition. SC was in charge of conception and design. DH revised the manuscript critically. All authors read and approved the final manuscript.

Author details

[1]Department of Urology, Samsung Medical Center, Sungkyunkwan University School of Medicine, 81 Irwon-ro, Gangnam-gu, Seoul 06351, South Korea. [2]Department of Urology, Gachon University Gil Medical Center, Gachon University School of Medicine, 21, Namdong-daero 774beon-gil, Namdong-gu, Incheon 21565, South Korea. [3]Department of Urology, Ajou University Medical Center, Ajou University School of Medicine, 164, World cup-ro, Yeongtong-gu, Suwon 16499, South Korea.

References

1. Arya M, Mostafid H, Patel HRH, et al. The self-expanding metallic ureteric stent in the long-term management of benign ureteric strictures. BJU Int. 2001;88:339–42.
2. Sountoulides P, Kaplan A, Kaufmann OG, et al. Current status of metal stents for managing malignant ureteric obstruction. BJU Int. 2010;105:1066–72.
3. Milroy EJ, Chapple CR, Cooper JE, et al. A new treatment for urethral strictures. Lancet. 1988;1:1424–7.
4. Khoo CCK, Abboudi H, Cartwright R, et al. Metallic Ureteric Stents in Malignant Ureteric Obstruction: a Systematic Review. Urology. 2018;118:12–20.
5. Kellett MJ. Interventional uroradiology: an update. BJU Int. 2000;86:164–73.
6. Barbalias GA, Liatsikos EN, Kalogeropoulou C, et al. Externally coated ureteral metallic stents: an unfavorable clinical experience. Eur Urol. 2002;42:276–80.
7. Kim M, Hong B, Park HK. Long-term outcomes of double-layered polytetrafluoroethylene membrane-covered self-expandable segmental metallic stents (Uventa) in patients with chronic ureteral obstructions: is it really safe? J Endourol. 2016;30:1339–46.
8. Stoller ML, Schwartz BF, Frigstad JR, et al. An in vitro assessment of the flow characteristics of spiral-ridged and smooth-walled JJ ureteric stents. BJU Int. 2000;85:628–31.
9. Kim KS, Choi S, Choi YS, et al. Comparison of efficacy and safety between a segmental thermo-expandable metal alloy spiral stent (Memokath 051) and a self-expandable covered metallic stent (UVENTA) in the management of ureteral obstructions. J Laparoendosc Adv Surg Tech A. 2014;24:550–5.
10. Chung KJ, Park BH, Park B, et al. Efficacy and safety of a novel, double-layered, coated, self-expandable metallic mesh stent (Uventa) in malignant ureteral obstructions. J Endourol. 2013;27:930–5.
11. Baumgarten AS, Hakky TS, Carrion RE, et al. A single-institution experience with metallic ureteral stents: a cost-effective method of managing deficiencies in ureteral drainage. Int Braz J Urol. 2014;40:225–31.
12. Kulkarni B. A new thermo-expandable shape-memory nickel-titanium alloy stent for the management of ureteric strictures. BJU Int. 1999;83:755–9.
13. Wakui M, Takeuchi S, Isioka J, et al. Metallic stents for malignant and benign ureteric obstruction. BJU Int. 2000;85:227–32.
14. Pandian SS, Hussey JK, McClinton S. Metallic ureteric stents: early experience. Br J Urol. 1998;82:791–7.
15. Lopez-Huertas HL, Polcari AJ, Acosta-Miranda A, et al. Metallic ureteral stents: a cost-effective method of managing benign upper tract obstruction. J Endourol. 2010;24:483–5.
16. Liatsikos E, Kyriazis I, Kallidonis P, et al. Ureteric response to abdominal radiotherapy and metallic double-pigtail ureteric stents: a pig model. BJU Int. 2009;104:862–6.
17. Petsepe DC, Kourkoulis SK, Papadodima SA, et al. Regional and age-dependent residual strains, curvature, and dimensions of the human ureter. Proc Inst Mech Eng H. 2018;232:149–62.
18. Nishino S, Goya N, Ishikawa N, et al. An experimental study of self-expanding ureteric metallic stents: macroscopic and microscopic changes in the canine ureter. BJU Int. 2002;90:730–5.
19. Hsu JS, Huang CY, Liu KL, et al. Risk factors for primary failure of metallic ureteral stents: experience from a tertiary center. J Endourol. 2018. https://doi.org/10.1089/end.2017.0611.
20. Song G, Lim B, Han KS, et al. Complications after polymeric and metallic ureteral stent placements including three types of fistula. J Endourol. 2015;29:485–9.
21. Wang HJ, Lee TY, Luo HL, et al. Application of resonance metallic stents for ureteral obstruction. BJU Int. 2011;108:428–32.

3

The resonance® metallic ureteral stent in the treatment of malignant ureteral obstruction

Jun Miyazaki[1*], Mizuki Onozawa[1], Satoshi Takahashi[2], Yuka Maekawa[3], Mitsuru Yasuda[3], Koichiro Wada[4], Yuji Maeda[5], Takuro Masaki[6], Akito Yamaguchi[6], Masahiko Suzuki[7], Yasuyuki Sakai[8], Tomokazu Kimura[9], Manabu Takai[10], Kensaku Seike[11], Takahiko Hashimoto[12] and Shingo Yamamoto[12]

Abstract

Background: To study the outcomes and experiences of using metallic stents in treating patients with malignant ureteral obstruction (MUO), we examined the effects of metallic ureteral stenting using the Cook Resonance® stent in the treatment of MUO.

Methods: All patients who had a Resonance metallic stent inserted between April 2015 and March 2018 at one of multiple facilities were prospectively observed with a 1-year follow-up. The primary outcome was the patency rate of the metallic ureteral stent. The secondary outcomes included the complications (e.g., infection and fever).

Results: Although stent insertion was attempted in 50 patients, the stent could not be inserted as a ureteral stent in three patients due to severe ureteral stricture, and one ureteral cancer patient was excluded from the analysis. The remaining 46 patients' median age was 67 years (range 28–85 years) (16 males, 30 females). Twenty-four patients died during the study; their median survival time was 226 days. The median follow-up period for the censored patients was 355 days (range 16–372 days), and just seven patients were still alive without Resonance failure > 1 year later. The women's IPSS scores tended to be lower than those of the men. Regarding the OABSS score, although the women's total score tended to be low, the difference between the men's and women's scores was nonsignificant. The bacteria detected from urine culture after stent insertion were more gram-positive than gram-negative.

Conclusion: Metallic ureteric stenting using the Resonance stent is safe and effective for treating MUO. Subjective symptoms were relatively less in the female patients.

Keywords: Metal stent, Malignant ureteral obstruction, Ureteral stent, Metallic ureteric stenting, Resonance stent

Background

A malignant ureteral obstruction (MUO) can be caused by a malignancy that compresses the ureter externally. MUO has been reported to be an indicator of poor prognosis, and the median life expectancy of patients with metastatic cancer that causes a ureteral obstruction is generally < 1 year [1–3]. Immediate urinary diversion using a ureteral stent and the preservation of renal function are required for an MUO, especially when further chemotherapy is considered [4, 5].

The Resonance® Metallic Ureteral Stent (hereafter, 'the Resonance;' Cook Medical, Bloomington, IN, USA) is the first metal ureteral stent (MRI-compatible) available for use in Japan. Made of a Ni-Co-Cr-M alloy (corrosion-resistant and resistant to calculus adhesion), the Resonance has a tightly wound wire coil structure, with no side hole openings at either end. The Resonance enables continuous drainage as urine passes through the

* Correspondence: jmiyazaki@iuhw.ac.jp
[1]Department of Urology, International University of Health and Welfare, 6-1-14 Kounodai, Ichikawa City, Chiba 272-0827, Japan
Full list of author information is available at the end of the article

stent from gaps in the tightly wound coil and exits the stent; this stent is extremely resistant to collapsing and kinking from extrinsic pressure [6]. Since Borin et al. reported the initial experiences with the Resonance metallic stent [7], it was approved in 2007 in many countries. It is resistant to migration and dislodgement because it is placed along the entire length of the ureter. In addition, like the existing products, the Resonance is easy to deploy and remove, and problems with long-term placement (e.g., stent occlusion, calculus formation on the surface, migration, and dislodgement) have been rectified, enabling the urinary tract to be secured for a maximum of 12 months without changing the stent, even in patients with an MUO.

The Resonance has an occluded end design, which results in urine draining through small gaps between the spirally wound coils [5]. This provides reduced stent encrustation that requires only an annual exchange. The Resonance was also confirmed to be more cost-effective than standard polymer stenting [8]. However, the published experience with the Resonance is limited and includes case series with small numbers of patients [9–17]. We conducted the present study to evaluate the efficacy and safety of the Resonance in the treatment of MUO, in a multicenter prospective study. We report the treatment outcomes based on our multicenter prospective study cohort of 50 patients with indwelling metallic stents against MUO, and we identify an indicator of stent patency in these patients.

Patients and methods

This study protocol was approved by the Tsukuba University Protocol Review Committee (H26–168), the Tsukuba Clinical Research & Development Organization (T-CReDO), and the institutional review board of each participating hospital before the initiation of the study. This study was performed in accordance with the international ethical recommendations stated in the Declaration of Helsinki [18] and the Japanese Ethical Guidelines for Epidemiological Research. The T-CReDO conducted central monitoring to ensure the integrity of the data submission and patient eligibility and on-schedule study progress.

Study design

This prospective observational study was conducted at 10 centers by volunteer members of or related to the Stent Committee of the Japanese Society of Endourology. The clinical data accumulation was performed by T-CReDO. Cook Medical Co. paid T-CReDO for the data collection costs.

The inclusion criterion for the patients with a first ureteral obstruction due to extrinsic underlying disease was a ureteral obstruction due to a gastrointestinal, gynecological, or urological tumor (excluding cases in which the primary disease was ureteral cancer or renal pelvic cancer). Between December 2014 and March 2018, we enrolled 50 patients with MUOs who were referred to a participating hospital for retrograde stenting. The study endpoint was the patency rate of the metallic ureteral stent. The secondary endpoints were the complications, e.g., infection and fever. When a patient's renal function was shown to be impaired by a blood test or imaging test, the patient's case was classified as stent obstruction. Stent failure was also defined as unanticipated stent exchange or nephrostomy placement for signs of ureteral obstruction based on imaging (ultrasound of CT scans) conducted every 3 months or on a blood test (creatinine).

All Resonance stents were placed in standard retrograde fashion with the use of X-ray guidance, a guidewire, and a coaxial inner sheath and outer catheter under spinal anesthesia or local anesthesia. The stent was inserted through the sheath after the guidewire and inner catheter were removed. The length of the Resonance was determined depending on each institution's guideline or by the treating physician. After the placement of the Resonance stent, the patients were followed for up to 1 year or until obstruction of the ipsilateral ureter, death, or an adverse event requiring management occurred.

On the day before the stent placement and at 3, 6, 9, and 12 months post-placement, follow-up imaging, creatinine measurement, urine cultures, and testing for the patient's International Prostate Symptom Score (IPSS) and Overactive Bladder Symptom Score (OABSS) were carried out in stable patients. For the actual follow-up visit date, deviations of approx. 4 weeks from the scheduled date were allowed. The IPSS, developed by Barry et al. [19], was initially used to assess the symptom severity of benign prostatic hyperplasia [20]. It was subsequently noted that the IPSS is neither sex-specific nor disease-specific for benign prostatic hyperplasia [21, 22]. Many clinician have already used the IPSS in daily practice and/or epidemiologic surveys of lower urinary tract symptoms (LUTS) in female patients [23, 24].

The IPSS can be subdivided into the IPSS voiding subscore (IPSS-V) and the IPSS storage subscore (IPSS-S) [25, 26]. The IPSS-V is the sum of the answers to question 1 (incomplete emptying), question 3 (intermittency), question 5 (weak stream), and question 6 (straining to void). The IPSS-S is the sum of the answers to question 2 (frequency), question 4 (urgency), and question 7 (nocturia) (the sum of the voiding and post-void symptom subscores is obtained). When patients were alive > 1 year after stent placement, the follow-up was completed.

Statistical analyses

The Wilcoxon rank sum test was used to compare the quantitative or ordinal data between groups. Since this study dealt with competing risks (i.e., death, obstruction, and other events), cumulative incidences in each risk were estimated by the Aalen-Johansen approach using the package 'survival' and 'prodlim' in R according to the reference manual (versions 2.44–1.1. and 2018.04.18, respectively). Open-source software, i.e., R ver. 3.5.2 [27], was used for all statistical analyses. All tests were two-sided, and a p-value < 0.05 was considered significant.

Results

A total of 50 patients were enrolled in the study; a Resonance stent was placed in 47 of these patients. Figure 1 is a flow chart with the patient survival/outcomes. In the remaining three patients, a Resonance could not be implanted due to severe ureteral obstruction. With the exception of the three patients with stent insertion failure, there was no problem with the stent insertions. Of the 47 patients, one patient with ureteral cancer was excluded from the analysis because of a protocol violation.

The clinical characteristics of the 46 patients (30 females, 16 males) are summarized in Table 1. The median patient age was 67 years (range 28–85 years). The most common primary malignancy causing the MUO was gastrointestinal cancer (27 patients, 58.7%) followed by gynecological cancer (13 patients, 28.3%). Twenty-six patients had lymph node metastases, ten had peritoneal involvement, and five had bone metastasis. Of the 46 patients, two patients had at least one complication associated with the Resonance (migration, $n = 1$; febrile urinary tract infection, n = 1) and their stents were removed. Twenty-four patients died during the study period. The median overall survival time was 226 days. The median follow-up period for the censored patients was 355 days (range 16–372 days), and just seven patients (six females, one male) were still alive without Resonance failure > 1 year after their stent implantation (Fig. 2).

Stent obstruction occurred in eight patients: six females and two males (Fig. 1). Although four of these eight patients underwent percutaneous nephrostomy construction and the other two patients were treated by ureteral stent exchange, two patients needed no further intervention because of their short life expectancy. The

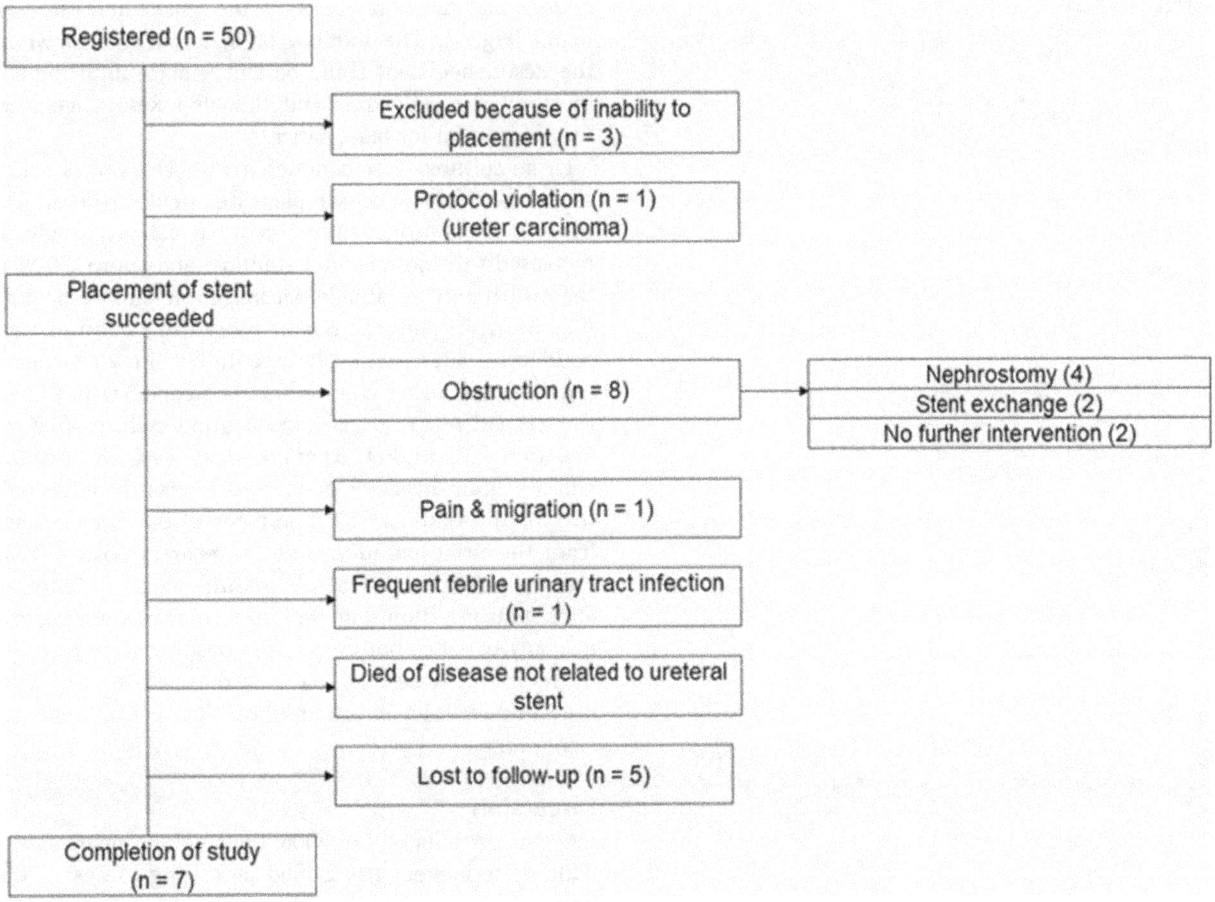

Fig. 1 Flow chart with the patient survival/outcomes

Table 1 Characteristics of the 46 patients with a Resonance stent for MUO

	Total (*n* = 46)	Female (*n* = 30)	Male (*n* = 16)
Age			
Min.	28	28	43
Median	67	66	68.5
Max.	85	81	85
ECOG performance status			
0	26	16	10
1	14	9	5
2	4	3	1
3	2	2	0
Origin			
Gastrointestinal	27	12	15
Bile/pancreas	6	3	3
Colon	12	7	5
Esophagus	1	0	1
Stomach	8	2	6
Gynecological	13	13	(–)
Ovary	4	4	(–)
Uterine cervix	9	9	(–)
Other	6	5	1
Breast	2	2	0
Malignant Lymphoma	1	1	0
Peritoneum	1	1	0
Prostate	1	(–)	1
Unknown	1	1	0
Metastasis			
No	4	2	2
Yes	42	28	14
Lymph node	26	17	9
Peritoneum	10	7	3
Pelvic organ	3	3	0
Liver	2	1	1
Bone	5	3	2
Lung	7	4	3
Ascites			
No	30	23	7
Yes	16	7	9
Pleural effusion			
No	36	25	11
Yes	10	5	5

cumulative stent obstruction incidence at 3, 6, 9, and 12 months after the procedure was 8.9% (95%CI: 0.2–16.8), 16.3% (95%CI: 4.5–26.7), 16.3% (95%CI: 4.5–26.7), and 18.8% (95%CI: 6.1–29.7), respectively (Fig. 2).

The median serum creatinine level before stenting was 1.15 mg/dL (range 0.44–9.90 mg/dL), which decreased to 0.81 mg/dL (range 0.50–1.54 mg/dL) at 3 months post-stenting ($p = 0.0003$) (Fig. 3). In two patients, the creatinine level had risen sharply at 9 months post-stenting, and these two patients died of cancer. The other nine patients had stable creatinine levels up to 12 months (Fig. 3).

The IPSS scores tended to be lower for the female patients than the males. In particular, the IPSS voiding subscores of the female patients were lower than those of the males, suggesting that the Resonance stent resulted in little discomfort regarding female urination (Fig. 4). Although the female patients' storage subscores tended to be lower than those of the males, the difference was not significant (Fig. 4). The quality of life (QOL) score was approx. 3 for both the female and male patients (a nonsignificant difference) (Fig. 4). With regard to the OABSS score, although the female patients' total scores tended to be low, there was not a large difference in total scores between the female and male patients (Fig. 4). The number of male patients in whom the Resonance stent could be left in place until the end of study was only one, and thus the Resonance stent may be painful for male patients.

Urine cultures were conducted with 41 samples before stent insertion and 45 samples after stent insertion. The proportion of urine culture-positive patients gradually increased to 9 months after stenting, and approx. 60% of the 46 patients eventually became urine culture-positive (Fig. 5). In 21 patients, one or more urine cultures were conducted after stent placement, but in 25 patients, post-stenting urine culture was not conducted. Among the 21 patients who provided a urine culture after the insertion, 17 (81.0%) experienced at least one positive culture: gram-negative only ($n = 4$), gram-positive only ($n = 8$), and both ($n = 5$). The types of bacteria detected from the urine cultures were more gram-positive than gram-negative strains at all months except 12 months after stent insertion (Fig. 5). Urine cultures were positive in many patients, but despite the positive urine cultures, no fever was observed except in one patient with a febrile urinary tract infection whose Resonance stent was removed.

Discussion

Since its introduction in 2006, the Cook Resonance® metallic ureteric stent has gained increasing use as an option for relieving ureteric obstruction from a malignant tumor. The management of an MUO is difficult, as

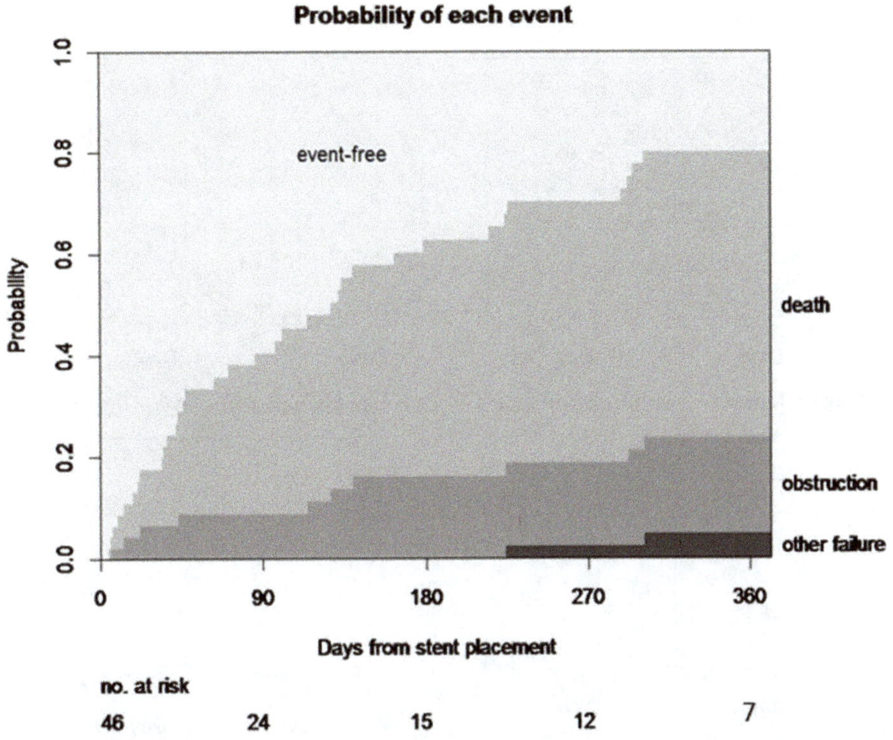

Fig. 2 Cumulative incidence curve for each event. The cumulative incidence curves are stacked, and the distance between the two curves at a particular point in time represents the probability of the indicated event

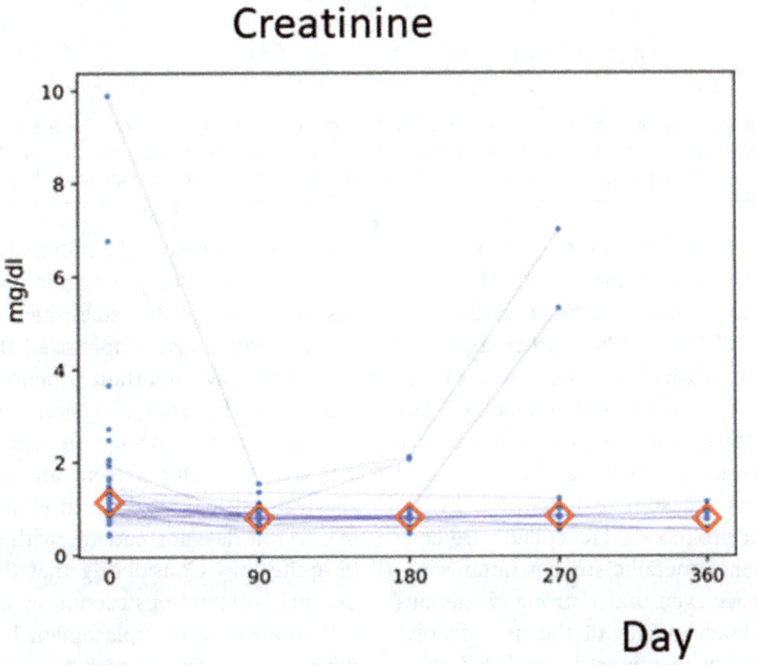

Fig. 3 Renal function before (00 M) and after the insertion of a Resonance stent. After insertion, blood samples were collected every 3 months for 12 months. Values from individual patients are shown by lines. The *red diamonds* represent the median at each point in time

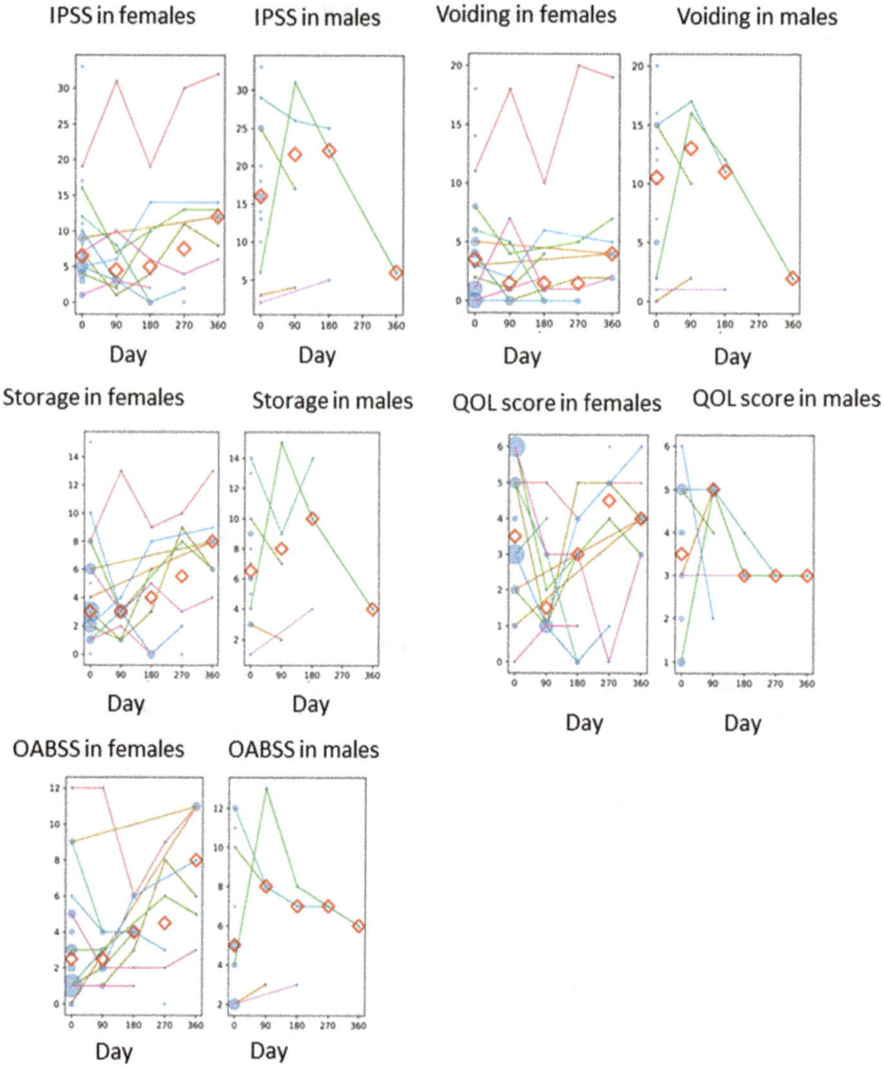

Fig. 4 IPSS, storage, and voiding symptom subdomains and the OABSS before and after the insertion of a Resonance stent. After the insertion, symptoms were reported every 3 months for 12 months. Values from individual patients are shown by lines. The *red diamonds* represent the median at each time point (days from intervention). The size of each circle represents the number of patients. Males, $n = 16$; females, $n = 30$

urologists must balance renal preservation, patient QOL, and the risk of complications in the setting of a poor prognosis. No consensus has been reached regarding the proper management of MUOs [28, 29]. Earlier studies of the Resonance examined relatively small cohorts, and almost all of the studies were retrospective analyses. We thus examined the treatment outcomes of the Resonance stents for MUO in a prospective study, and we evaluated the relationship between the stent patency rate in the MUO patients and their prognoses. The coiled wire construction of the Resonance metallic stent maintains patency and urinary drainage even under strong exogenous pressure. One of the disadvantages of the use of polymeric stents in Japan is that they must be replaced every 3–6 months, whereas metallic stents can be maintained in place for 12 months before they must be replaced.

Wong et al. reported a minimal benefit regarding overall survival after decompression in patients who had metastases or a previously established diagnosis of MUO [2]. Another study also emphasized that no other factors appeared to play important prognostic roles which patients would benefit from diversion [29]. Asakawa et al. [30] showed that the median survival time of MUO patients was 210 days. Our present analysis revealed the median survival time of 226 days. In clinical settings, the number of survival days for patients with an MUO is expected to be quite low. Considering that the median survival with extrinsic ureteral obstruction as a result of malignancy is < 12 months, stent replacement is probably not necessary during the survival of such patients [3].

Our present findings demonstrated that the treatment success rate for MUO was 77.3% at 6 months and 70.3%

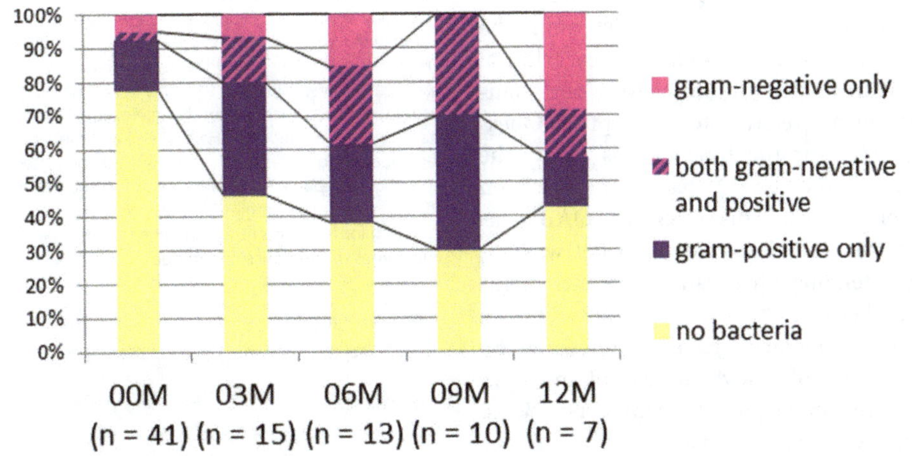

Fig. 5 Pathogens isolated from the 46 patients with a Resonance stent

at 1 year; these results are similar to those of previous reports [10, 30, 31]. It has also been observed that stent replacement is not necessary in most MUO cases, as we also observed herein. In light of the above-described findings, it is apparent that the frequent replacement of a stent can be avoided, thereby improving patients' quality of life and reducing medical costs [8, 32].

Medical costs are important to consider when deciding whether to use the Resonance or a conventional polymeric stent. In Japan, stent insertion is permitted by the national health insurance system. The costs of stents are currently as follows: metal ureteral stent, 139,000 yen; polymeric stent, 23,800 yen; and the stent insertion, 34, 000 yen. The cost of inserting a polymeric stent twice is 115,600 yen, which is cheaper than a metal ureteral stent, but if a polymeric stent must be used three times, it will be 173,400 yen, which is higher than the cost of inserting the Resonance stent (173,000 yen).

In our study, stent failure occurred in eight (17%) patients. A previous retrospective study [30] reported that 15.4% of their patients experienced stent failure. Moreover, the failure rate of conventional polymeric stents is higher (25–40%) [33]. The Resonance is stiffer than a normal polymeric stent, and it has thus been considered difficult to remove the Resonance. However, in our experience, it was possible to remove the Resonance without adhesion of calculi, and it was also possible to replace the Resonance with a polymeric ureteral stent.

Although the effect of the Resonance stent on patients' quality of life might vary among individuals, there are no studies using validated questionnaires to assess the stent's subjective tolerability. In our present cohort, the IPSS voiding subscore was lower in the female patients than the male patients. Indwelling of the stent was considered to have no significant discomfort for urination in the female patients. Although there was not much difference between our female and male patients in the storage subscore or the QOL score, the storage subscore worsened with time in the females. Similarly, the OABSS score did not differ significantly between the female and male patients, but the OABSS scores of the female patients tended to deteriorate over time.

Regarding the patients' renal function, there was no relationship between the preoperative serum creatinine levels and stent occlusion. Serum creatinine is affected mostly by the patient's general condition and/or contralateral renal function, and it might not reflect the stent patency rate.

Although bacterial colonization of indwelling ureteral stents is an important issue and colonization rates of 42–90% have been reported [34, 35], in the present study the only significant correlation noted was between urine culture and stenting duration [36]. There is a great discrepancy between urine and catheter cultures [36]. Of the 250 patients in a prior study [37], the risk of bacteriuria and colonization of the ureteral stent tip was significantly associated with the duration of stent retention, patient sex, and the systemic disease (including diabetic nephropathy and chronic kidney disease without dialysis). As mentioned above, in the present study, approx. 81.0% of the patients were positive for urine culture: gram-negative only ($n = 4$), gram-positive only ($n = 8$), and both ($n = 5$). A wide variety of bacteria such as gram-positive bacteria including MRSA and also gram-negative bacteria were detected. However, although the culture results were positive, the patients did not necessarily show signs of infection, and symptoms such as fever related to infection were not observed.

There are several limitations in our study. We could not compare treatment outcomes of the metallic stent and polymeric stents by a randomized control study, as a standard cohort study requires one group of patients with metallic stents and another group with polymeric stents as their initial management. We tried to eliminate potential confounders by conducting a prospective study. This study design also made it possible to determine the patency rate of the Resonance stent in real clinical settings. Second, stent-related symptoms were not evaluated with the use of a Ureteric Stent Symptom Questionnaire (USSQ) [38]. At the time of this study, the Japanese version of the USSQ had not yet been validated. We therefore used the IPSS and OABSS as substitutes. Third, since the length of the stent was determined by the attending physician, symptoms might have been present because the stent was long. Fourth, since there was only one male patient who could be followed up to the end of study, our use of the IPSS score and QOL score cannot provide many conclusions. Fifth, although this was a prospective study, the number of cases was small.

However, compared to other investigations, our study has several advantages. First, the results of this prospective study confirmed that there are many MUO patients with poor prognoses in clinical practice. Second, by using the IPSS, QOL, and OABSS values of MUO patients, we were able to determine the changes in the patients' quality of life, and we observed that the female patients had less deterioration in the voiding subscore in a real-life setting. Third, although urine cultures from MUO patients are often positive, urine culture positivity did not necessarily represent a serious infection.

In summary, our findings provide a valid argument that a metallic stent is appropriate for MUO patients. It also seems reasonable that a metallic stent should be preferred for female patients. Further research is required to further test metallic stents' superiority in randomized controlled studies.

Conclusion

The Resonance stent is effective and safe for relieving MUOs, and 70–80% of our patients with a Resonance stent did not need to have their stent changed at 1 year. In our female patients, the IPSS and OABSS scores were also within self-control during the study period.

Abbreviations

IPSS: International Prostate Symptom Score; IPSS-S: IPSS storage subscore; IPSS-V: IPSS voiding subscore; MUO: Malignant ureteral obstruction; OABSS: Overactive Bladder Symptom Score; QOL: Quality of life; T-CReDO: Tsukuba Clinical Research & Development Organization; USSQ: Ureteric Stent Symptom Questionnaire

Acknowledgments

None.

Authors' contributions

JM, ST, MO and SY performed the development of study design, and the original literature search, and participated in drafting the manuscript. JM and MO participated in the design of the study and performed the statistical analysis. JM, ST, YM1, MY, KW, YM2, TM, AY, MS, YS, TK, MT, KS, TH and SY participated in Data acquisition and analysis. All authors read and approved the final manuscript.

Ethics approval and consent to participate

This study protocol was approved by the Tsukuba University Protocol Review Committee (H26–168), the Tsukuba Clinical Research & Development Organization (T-CReDO), and the institutional review board of each participating hospital before the initiation of the study. This study was performed in accordance with the international ethical recommendations stated in the Declaration of Helsinki [19] and the Japanese Ethical Guidelines for Epidemiological Research. The T-CReDO conducted central monitoring to ensure the integrity of the data submission and patient eligibility and the study's on-schedule progress.
Written informed consent was obtained from all participants.

Full names of the ethics committees

Ethics committees
International University of Health and Welfare
Sapporo Medical University School of Medicine
Gifu University Graduate School of Medicine
Okayama University Graduate School of Medicine
Public Central Hospital of Matto Ishikawa
Harasanshin Hospital
Kasumigaura Medical Center
National Cancer Center East
Faculty of Medicine, University of Tsukuba
Hyogo College of Medicine

Author details

[1]Department of Urology, International University of Health and Welfare, 6-1-14 Kounodai, Ichikawa City, Chiba 272-0827, Japan. [2]Department of Infection Control and Laboratory Medicine, Sapporo Medical University School of Medicine, S1 W16, Chuo-ku, Sapporo 060-8543, Japan. [3]Department of Urology, Gifu University Graduate School of Medicine, 1-1 Yanagido, Gifu City 501-1194, Japan. [4]Department of Urology, Okayama University Graduate School of Medicine, Dentistry and Pharmaceutical Sciences, 2-5-1 Shikata-cho, Kita-ku, Okayama 700-8558, Japan. [5]Department of Urology, Public Central Hospital of Matto Ishikawa, 3-8 Kuramitsu, Hakusan-shi, Ishikawa 924-0865, Japan. [6]Department of Urology, Harasanshin Hospital, 1-8 Taihaku-machi, Hakata-ku, Fukuoka City, Fukuoka 812-0033, Japan. [7]Department of Urology, Kasumigaura Medical Center, 2-7-14 Shimotakatsu, Tsuchiura City, Ibaraki 300-0812, Japan. [8]Department of Urology, National Cancer Center East, 6-5-1 Kashiwanoha, Kashiwa-shi, Chiba 277-8577, Japan. [9]Department of Urology, Faculty of Medicine, University of Tsukuba, Tennodai 1-1-1, Tsukuba City, Ibaraki 305-8575, Japan. [10]Department of Urology, Kizawa Memorial Hospital, 590 Shimokobi, Kobicho, Minokamo, Gifu 505-8503, Japan. [11]Department of Urology, Chuno Kosei Hospital, 5-1 Wakakusadori, Seki-city, Gifu 501-3802, Japan. [12]Department of Urology, Hyogo College of Medicine, 1-1 Mukogawa-cho, Nishinomiya City, Hyogo 663-8501, Japan.

References

1. Kouba E, Wallen EM, Pruthi RS. Management of ureteral obstruction due to advanced malignancy: optimizing therapeutic and palliative outcomes. J Urol. 2008;180(2):444–50.
2. Wong LM, Cleeve LK, Milner AD, Pitman AG. Malignant ureteral obstruction: outcomes after intervention. Have things changed? J Urol. 2007;178(1):178–83 discussion 183.
3. Jeong IG, Han KS, Joung JY, Seo HK, Chung J. The outcome with ureteric stents for managing non-urological malignant ureteric obstruction. BJU Int. 2007;100(6):1288–91.
4. Feng MI, Bellman GC, Shapiro CE. Management of ureteral obstruction secondary to pelvic malignancies. J Endourol. 1999;13(7):521–4.
5. Blaschko SD, Deane LA, Krebs A, Abdelshehid CS, Khan F, Borin J, Nguyen A, McDougall EM, Clayman RV. In-vivo evaluation of flow characteristics of novel metal ureteral stent. J Endourol. 2007;21(7):780–3.

6. Wah TM, Irving HC, Cartledge J. Initial experience with the resonance metallic stent for antegrade ureteric stenting. Cardiovasc Intervent Radiol. 2007;30(4):705–10.
7. Borin JF, Melamud O, Clayman RV. Initial experience with full-length metal stent to relieve malignant ureteral obstruction. J Endourol. 2006;20(5):300–4.
8. Lopez-Huertas HL, Polcari AJ, Acosta-Miranda A, Turk TM. Metallic ureteral stents: a cost-effective method of managing benign upper tract obstruction. J Endourol. 2010;24(3):483–5.
9. Liatsikos E, Kallidonis P, Kyriazis I, Constantinidis C, Hendlin K, Stolzenburg JU, Karnabatidis D, Siablis D. Ureteral obstruction: is the full metallic double-pigtail stent the way to go? Eur Urol. 2010;57(3):480–6.
10. Kadlec AO, Ellimoottil CS, Greco KA, Turk TM. Five-year experience with metallic stents for chronic ureteral obstruction. J Urol. 2013;190(3):937–41.
11. Nagele U, Kuczyk MA, Horstmann M, Hennenlotter J, Sievert KD, Schilling D, Walcher U, Stenzl A, Anastasiadis AG. Initial clinical experience with full-length metal ureteral stents for obstructive ureteral stenosis. World J Urol. 2008;26(3):257–62.
12. Wang HJ, Lee TY, Luo HL, Chen CH, Shen YC, Chuang YC, Chiang PH. Application of resonance metallic stents for ureteral obstruction. BJU Int. 2011;108(3):428–32.
13. Modi AP, Ritch CR, Arend D, Walsh RM, Ordonez M, Landman J, Gupta M, Knudsen BE. Multicenter experience with metallic ureteral stents for malignant and chronic benign ureteral obstruction. J Endourol. 2010;24(7):1189–93.
14. Garg T, Guralnick ML, Langenstroer P, See WA, Hieb RA, Rilling WS, Sudakoff GS, O'Connor RC. Resonance metallic ureteral stents do not successfully treat ureteroenteric strictures. J Endourol. 2009;23(7):1199–201 discussion 1202.
15. Benson AD, Taylor ER, Schwartz BF. Metal ureteral stent for benign and malignant ureteral obstruction. J Urol. 2011;185(6):2217–22.
16. Goldsmith ZG, Wang AJ, Banez LL, Lipkin ME, Ferrandino MN, Preminger GM, Inman BA. Outcomes of metallic stents for malignant ureteral obstruction. J Urol. 2012;188(3):851–5.
17. Gayed BA, Mally AD, Riley J, Ost MC. Resonance metallic stents do not effectively relieve extrinsic ureteral compression in pediatric patients. J Endourol. 2013;27(2):154–7.
18. Williams JR. The ethics activities of the world medical association. Sci Eng Ethics. 2005;11(1):7–12.
19. Barry MJ, Fowler FJ Jr, O'Leary MP, Bruskewitz RC, Holtgrewe HL, Mebust WK, Cockett AT. The American urological association symptom index for benign prostatic hyperplasia. The measurement Committee of the American Urological Association. J Urol. 1992;148(5):1549–57 discussion 1564.
20. Okamura K, Nojiri Y, Osuga Y, Tange C. Psychometric analysis of international prostate symptom score for female lower urinary tract symptoms. Urology. 2009;73(6):1199–202.
21. Chai TC, Belville WD, McGuire EJ, Nyquist L. Specificity of the American urological association voiding symptom index: comparison of unselected and selected samples of both sexes. J Urol. 1993;150(5 Pt 2):1710–3.
22. Chancellor MB, Rivas DA. American urological association symptom index for women with voiding symptoms: lack of index specificity for benign prostate hyperplasia. J Urol. 1993;150(5 Pt 2):1706–8 discussion 1708-1709.
23. Boyle P, Robertson C, Mazzetta C, Keech M, Hobbs FD, Fourcade R, Kiemeney L, Lee C, UrEpik Study G. The prevalence of lower urinary tract symptoms in men and women in four centres. The UrEpik study. BJU Int. 2003;92(4):409–14.
24. Terai A, Matsui Y, Ichioka K, Ohara H, Terada N, Yoshimura K. Comparative analysis of lower urinary tract symptoms and bother in both sexes. Urology. 2004;63(3):487–91.
25. Lim JS, Sul CK, Song KH, Na YG, Shin JH, Oh TH, Kim YH. Changes in urinary symptoms and tolerance due to long-term ureteral double-J stenting. Int Neurourol J. 2010;14(2):93–9.
26. Zhang HL, Huang ZG, Qiu Y, Cheng X, Zou XQ, Liu TT. Tamsulosin for treatment of lower urinary tract symptoms in women: a systematic review and meta-analysis. Int J Impot Res. 2017;29(4):148–56.
27. TeamR RC: R. A Language and Environment for Statistical Computing. Vienna, Austria: R Foundation for Statistical Computing; 2017.
28. Ganatra AM, Loughlin KR. The management of malignant ureteral obstruction treated with ureteral stents. J Urol. 2005;174(6):2125–8.
29. Shekarriz B, Shekarriz H, Upadhyay J, Banerjee M, Becker H, Pontes JE, Wood DP Jr. Outcome of palliative urinary diversion in the treatment of advanced malignancies. Cancer. 1999;85(4):998–1003.
30. Asakawa J, Iguchi T, Tamada S, Ninomiya N, Kato M, Yamasaki T, Nakatani T. Outcomes of indwelling metallic stents for malignant extrinsic ureteral obstruction. Int J Urol. 2018;25(3):258–62.
31. Asakawa J, Iguchi T, Tamada S, Ninomiya N, Kato M, Yamasaki T, Nakatani T. Treatment outcomes of ureteral stenting for malignant extrinsic ureteral obstruction: a comparison between polymeric and metallic stents. Cancer Manag Res. 2018;10:2977–82.
32. Polcari AJ, Hugen CM, Lopez-Huertas HL, Turk TM. Cost analysis and clinical applicability of the resonance metallic ureteral stent. Exp Rev Pharmacoecon Outcomes Res. 2010;10(1):11–5.
33. Sountoulides P, Kaplan A, Kaufmann OG, Sofikitis N. Current status of metal stents for managing malignant ureteric obstruction. BJU Int. 2010; 105(8):1066–72.
34. Kehinde EO, Rotimi VO, Al-Hunayan A, Abdul-Halim H, Boland F, Al-Awadi KA. Bacteriology of urinary tract infection associated with indwelling J ureteral stents. J Endourol. 2004;18(9):891–6.
35. Reid G, Denstedt JD, Kang YS, Lam D, Nause C. Microbial adhesion and biofilm formation on ureteral stents in vitro and in vivo. J Urol. 1992; 148(5):1592–4.
36. Klis R, Korczak-Kozakiewicz E, Denys A, Sosnowski M, Rozanski W. Relationship between urinary tract infection and self-retaining double-J catheter colonization. J Endourol. 2009;23(6):1015–9.
37. Kehinde EO, Rotimi VO, Al-Awadi KA, Abdul-Halim H, Boland F, Al-Hunayan A, Pazhoor A. Factors predisposing to urinary tract infection after J ureteral stent insertion. J Urol. 2002;167(3):1334–7.
38. Joshi HB, Newns N, Stainthorpe A, MacDonagh RP, Keeley FX Jr, Timoney AG. Ureteral stent symptom questionnaire: development and validation of a multidimensional quality of life measure. J Urol. 2003;169(3):1060–4.

4

Conservative treatment for urinary fistula following ileal conduit urinary diversion: A simple method

Yun-lin Ye[1†], Hai-tao Liang[1†], Lei Tan[1,2†], Xia Zheng[1], Dan Xiong[1,3], Kang-hua Xiao[1] and Zi-ke Qin[1*]

Abstract

Background: The presence of urinary fistula after ileal conduit urinary diversion is a challenging complication, and this study investigated the role of the intra-conduit negative pressure system (NPS) in the presence of urinary fistula following ileal conduit (IC) urinary diversion as a conservative treatment.

Methods: Using the intra-conduit NPS, a minor drainage tube was placed within a silicon tube to suck urine from the conduit with consistent negative pressure. Patients with urinary fistula following IC from August 2012 to July 2017 were recorded, and the clinical characteristics and outcome were retrospectively analyzed.

Results: The intra-conduit NPS was used as a primarily conservative treatment for 13 patients who suffered from urinary fistula and presented with a large amount of abdominal/pelvic drainage without other significant morbidities. The median age was 60 years old (42–74 years), and 7patients were male. The median duration between the IC operation and the presence of urinary fistula was 15 days (2–28 days), and elevated creatinine levels were detected in the abdominal/pelvic drainage with a median level of 2114 μmol/L (636–388 μmol/L). A significant decrease in abdominal/pelvic drainage was identified in 12 patients. The median time that the NPS was used was 9 days (7–11 days). The other patient did not show any improvements after 2 days of observation and then underwent open surgery. With ureteral stenting, 2 abdominal drainage tubes and the intra-conduit NPS were placed during operation, no urine leakage was observed in the abdominal/pelvic field, and the patient was cured in 9 days. With a median follow-up of 22 months, no fistula recurrence or hydronephrosis was detected.

Conclusion: The intra-conduit negative pressure system is a feasible and promising way to cure urinary fistula following ileal conduit urinary diversion. Because this procedure is a mini-invasive and simple approach, it might represent an alternative in selected patients.

Keywords: Urinary fistula, Ileal conduit, Negative pressure system, Intra-conduit, Conservative treatment

Background

Cystectomy and urinary diversion are some of the most complicated procedures in urological operations, with a nearly 40% perioperative morbidity rate. The presence of urinary fistula after ileal conduit urinary diversion is rare, but the management of this complication is challenging [1–4]. Although ureteroenteric anastomosis and conduit closure both carry the risk of urine leakage, management is simple as follows: evaluate and ensure urinary fistula, drain the urine, and then repair the fistula actively or conservatively [4–8]. Compared to surgical approaches, retrograde stent placement and nephrostomy are more common mini-invasive approaches than surgical approaches for addressing the presence of urinary fistula following ileal conduit urinary diversion [8–11]. A contrastographic study before nephrostomy can be used to comprehensively evaluate abdominal/pelvic ureter and ureterointestinal anastomoses. However, sometimes urine cannot be completely drained, and a balloon is used to obstruct the ureter during nephrostomy. Although completeness has been

* Correspondence: qinzk@sysucc.org.cn
[†]Yun-lin Ye, Hai-tao Liang and Lei Tan contributed equally to this work.
[1]Department of Urology, Sun Yat-sen University Cancer Center, State Key Laboratory of Oncology in South China, Collaborative Innovation Center for Cancer Medicine, Guangzhou 510060, Guangdong, China
Full list of author information is available at the end of the article

favorable in recent studies, it is a complicated mini-invasion procedure in clinical practice.

Negative pressure system (NPS) drainage has generally been used to cure complicated wounds [12–14]. In a sparse number of reports, NPS drainage has also been revealed as a promising outcome in the management of urinary fistula [15–17]. Therefore, we tried to use an intra-conduit NPS as a conservative way to cure patients who had suffered from urine leakage after ileal conduit urinary diversion since 2012. Initially, the NPS was only recommended for patients with good performance as an alternative for retrograde stenting or nephrostomy. We now report our preliminary experiences using the intra-conduit NPS to address the presence of urinary fistula after ileal conduit urinary diversion.

Methods

Patients who underwent ileal conduit urinary diversion in our center were retrospectively reviewed from August 2012 to July 2017. Urine leakage was diagnosed by imaging and/or the amount of abdominal/pelvic drainage reported in drainage creatinine studies. For patients who did not present with significant abdominal infection or other severe morbidities, the intra-conduit negative pressure system was set as the conservative treatment. If this treatment did not work within 2 days, subsequent treatments such as the retrograde placement of ureter stents, nephrostomy or open surgery would be performed. Informed contest was confirmed after a comprehensive consultation.

A sterile silicon tube (F18 abdominal drainage tube) with lateral holes was reset into the conduit in patients who had this tube removed after the operation. Then, a mini-plastic tube (F12 stomach tube) with lateral holes was also placed into the silicon tube and was tied to a negative pressure system (Figure 1). During this process, if the ureteral stents had not been previously removed, they were now kept, and the silicon tube was gently placed into the ileal conduit (Additional file 1: Figure S1). When the negative pressure system had a pressure of 20–25 cmH_2O, urine was drained out continuously, and the abdominal/pelvic drainage decreased significantly. Most of the time, the NPS was supplied by the central negative pressure system; when the patients were released from the hospital bed, a negative pressure machine with a battery was administered. This process could be accomplished at the bedside and would work for approximately one week, where no urine leakage was detected by clinical evaluation as characterized by the dose of urine, the amount of abdominal drainage, the creatinine drainage level, patient complaints, etc.

The perioperative clinical features were retrospectively analyzed, and the final follow-up was completed in October 2018. Survival status was recorded, and imaging of

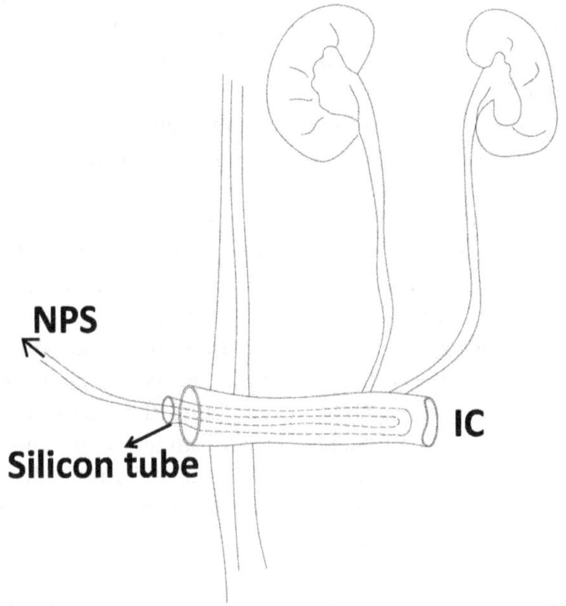

Fig. 1 Sketch of the intra-conduit negative pressure system NPS: negative pressure system; IC: ileal conduit.

the upper urinary tract was retrieved during follow-up of patients with primary cancer.

Results

During these 5 years, 446 cases of ileal conduit urinary diversion were completed following radical cystectomy or pelvic exenteration in our center. All ureterointestinal anastomoses were performed using Bricker ureteral implantation, and 18 patients suffered from urine leakage 30 days after this difficult procedure. Of these patients, 13 presented with a high amount of abdominal/pelvic drainage and decreased urine output from the ileal conduit without significantly severe morbidities. An intra-conduit negative pressure system was first chosen as the conservative treatment for these patients.

The median age was 60 years old (42–74 years), and 7patients were male. The primary diagnosis was bladder cancer in 11 patients. The median interval between IC and the diagnosis of urinary fistula was 15 days (2–28 days), and elevated creatinine levels were detected in the abdominal/pelvic drainage with a median level of 2114 μmol/L (636-3852 μmol/L). Abdominal X-ray was performed in 4 patients to identify the locations of the ureteric stents, and abdominal/pelvic contrast-enhanced CT was performed in 2 patients without positive findings. An intravenous pyelogram confirmed 1 ureterointestinal anastomotic fistula, but this method was not used in the first 2 weeks after the operation. Additionally, an ileal conduit contrastographic study confirmed 2 conduit fistulas. When the intra-conduit NPS was used as the primary treatment, a significant decrease in abdominal/pelvic drainage was identified in 12 patients. For these patients, the median time that the NPS was used was9 days (7–11 days), and then the fistula was cured (Table 1).

The other patient showed no improvement after 2 days of observation and then underwent open surgery for the combination of consistent ileus and suspicious abdominal infection. Preoperative contrast imaging showed a significant leak at the location of the distal conduit. During the reoperation, stickiness made it difficult to repair a 1-cm hole linked to the left ureterointestinal anastomosis. During this operation, we found that a sticky belt pressed over the distal third of the ileal conduit, and the silicon tube of the NPS did not cross this stricture to suck urine out completely. Double ureter stents and 2 abdominal drainage tubes were placed, and a new silicon tube was placed to the end of the ileal conduit. No urine leaked into the abdominal/pelvic field, and the patient was cured 9 days after the operation.

With a median follow-up of 22 months (16–46 months), 1 patient died of cervical cancer 41 months after NPS treatment. No hydronephrosis was detected, and no recurrence of fistula occurred.

Discussion

Urinary fistula following ileal conduit urinary diversion is rather rare, but it is associated with severe comorbidities such as abdominal infection, ileus, and metabolism impairment. Treatment is challenging, especially when it is administered following complicated pelvic organ resection and urinary diversion [6, 8, 9]. For these fragile patients, the management of urinary fistula should be as minimally invasive as possible. A surgical approach is usually avoided due to postoperative complications and stickiness. In recent years, several approaches including a retrograde ureteral approach and percutaneous nephrostomy have been developed in the field of endourology to address this complicated consequence, but neither of these two options is easy to accomplish [18–21].

In this cohort, most (12/13) patients with urinary fistulas following ileal conduit urinary diversion were cured with the intra-conduit NPS, which was a time-consuming (7–11 days) but an extremely simple, safe and mini-invasive method. For these selected patients, the use of the intra-conduit NPS as a conservative treatment was compatible and tolerated, as this bedside process was nearly noninvasive. It was easy to evaluate the effect of the NPS via the decreases in abdominal/pelvic drainage and the normalized creatinine level. For the patient who experienced failure of NPS, we found that the ileal conduit was pressed by a sticky belt during the operation so that the silicon tube could not reach the end of the conduit. This may have resulted in the inability of urine to be successfully and completely suctioned. When the silicon tube was successfully placed during the second operation, the NPS worked efficiently after the operation. In fact, most urine leakage following ileal conduit urinary diversion was due to ureteroenteric anastomosis and conduit closure, so the drainage of urine out of the conduit was critical to cure urine leakage, and the intra-conduit NPS might be a good procedure to accomplish this purpose.

In recent years, an increasing number of studies have demonstrated that endourology approaches are feasible for dealing with upper urinary tract lesions. Olson Land

Table 1 Clinical characteristics of patients underwent intra-conduit negative pressure system

No.	Age (year)	Primary cancer	Major operation	Interval (day)[a]	Status of Ureter stent	Time of NPS (day)	Outcome
1	< 60	Epithelioid trophoblastic tumor of the uterine	Pelvic exenteration	21	Kept	9	Cured
2	< 60	Cervical cancer	Pelvic exenteration	28	Moved	10	Cured
3	< 60	Bladder Cancer	Radical cystectomy	2	Kept	7	Cured
4	< 60	Bladder Cancer	Radical cystectomy	3	Kept	7	Cured
5	< 60	Bladder Cancer	Radical cystectomy	15	Kept	9	Cured
6	> 60	Bladder Cancer	Radical cystectomy	24	Moved	10	Cured
7	> 60	Bladder Cancer	Radical cystectomy	8	Kept	9	Cured
8	> 60	Bladder Cancer	Radical cystectomy	3	Kept	7	Cured
9	< 60	Bladder Cancer	Radical cystectomy	14	Kept	9	Cured
10	> 60	Bladder Cancer	Radical cystectomy	18	Moved	10	Cured
11	> 60	Bladder Cancer	Radical cystectomy	17	Moved	10	Cured
12	> 60	Bladder Cancer	Radical cystectomy	15	Moved	2	Failed[bb]
13	> 60	Bladder Cancer	Radical cystectomy	4	Kept	11	Cured

NPS Negative pressure system
[a]Time between fistula and surgery
[bb]Transformed to surgical approach

colleagues reported that the success rate was approximately 74%(40/54) during retrograde endourological management of upper urinary tract abnormalities [10]. An antegrade percutaneous flexible endoscopic approach also demonstrated favorable outcomes [11].

In clinical practice, percutaneous nephrostomy is feasible and relatively safe for ureteroenteric anastomosis stricture. However, for patients with urine leakage following ileal conduit urinary diversion, there is often no obstruction of the ureter. Without hydronephrosis, nephrostomy is deemed to be a difficult procedure, and it is not very safe for patients following radical cystectomy/pelvic exenteration and ileal conduit urinary diversion. Therefore, this procedure should be performed only in high-volume centers by experienced surgeons. Retrograde stenting is much safer than nephrostomy, but exploration of the ureteral anastomosis is time-consuming, and mucosal edema of the ileal conduit and ureter makes the procedure difficult. Additionally, this process has a potential risk of invasive abdominal infection.

Compared to endourology approaches and transperitoneal surgery, the intra-conduit NPS is a more mini-invasive and convenient approach [9, 18]. It is a bedside procedure, but we can't see the details of the conduit during this process, and the placement of the silicon tube might not be deep enough for certain reasons. Additionally, this procedure should be performed by a surgeon who is familiar with the operation details for each patient. If this procedure is not successful, further management, such as ureteral stenting and/or nephrostomy and even surgery might be needed. Moreover, for 8 patients, the ureteral stent was not removed when urinary fistula was diagnosed. Therefore, retrograde ureteral stenting might not be very reliable for some patients.

Although there is no recommendation of the NPS in the treatment of urinary fistula following ileal conduit urinary diversion, the NPS has often been used in complicated wounds, and its uniform negative pressure can enhance wound healing. In some complicated cases of urine leakage, the NPS was associated with a favorable outcome [15, 16]. In this study, the use of the intra-conduit NPS also resulted in a favorable outcome as a conservative procedure. Therefore, the NPS might be a good alternative for curing urinary fistula following ileal conduit urinary diversion. Compared to other approaches, the intra-conduit NPS is a mini-invasive and compatible approach, and caregivers should attempt its use in clinical practice in selected patients.

This retrospective study did not strictly define the indications of the NPS, and selection bias was inevitable because all patients were in good conditions when they chose the intra-conduit NPS as a conservative treatment for urine leakage. In terms of the rarity of urine leakage, the population was limited, and no control group was recorded. As the NPS is a new approach for treating urine leakage following ileal conduit urinary diversion, advanced studies and long-term follow-up periods are needed. All of these patients were reviewed in our single center, a university-affiliated hospital. Furthermore, these patients received good supportive treatment and consistent observation and evaluation. To our knowledge, this is the largest report of the use of the NPS for urinary fistula. As a conservative treatment, the intra-conduit negative pressure system is a mini-invasive and compatible approach for selected patients with urine leakage following ileal conduit urinary diversion.

Conclusion

The intra-conduit negative pressure system is a feasible and promising way to cure urinary fistula following ileal conduit urinary diversion. As this system is a mini-invasive and simple approach, it might represent an alternative for nephrostomy in selected patients. Further advanced studies are needed.

Supplementary information

Additional file 1. The installation of negative pressure system

Abbreviations
IC: Ileal conduit; NPS: Negative pressure system

Acknowledgments
Not applicable.

Author's contribution
ZKQ, YLY, XZ: Protocol/project development; HTL, LT, XZ, KHX: Data collection or management; YLY, HTL, LT, XZ, DX: Data analysis; YLY, ZKQ, HTL, DX, LT: Manuscript writing. All authors have read and approved the manuscript.

Author details
[1]Department of Urology, Sun Yat-sen University Cancer Center, State Key Laboratory of Oncology in South China, Collaborative Innovation Center for Cancer Medicine, Guangzhou 510060, Guangdong, China. [2]Department of Urology, the First Affiliated Hospital of Sun Yat-sen University, Guangzhou 510080, Guangdong, China. [3]Medical Laboratory of The Third affiliated Hospital of Shenzhen University, Shenzhen 518000, Guangdong, China.

References

1. Novara G, Catto JW, Wilson T, et al. Systematic review and cumulative analysis of perioperative outcomes and complications after robot-assisted radical cystectomy. Eur Urol. 2015;67:376–401.
2. Bochner BH, Dalbagni G, Sjoberg DD, et al. Comparing open radical cystectomy and robot-assisted laparoscopic radical cystectomy: a randomized clinical trial. Eur Urol. 2015;67:1042–50.
3. Sathianathen NJ, Kalapara A, Frydenberg M, et al. Robotic assisted radical cystectomy vs open radical cystectomy: systematic review and meta-analysis. J Urol. 2019;201:715–20.
4. Lee RK, Abol-Enein H, Artibani W, et al. Urinary diversion after radical cystectomy for bladder cancer: options, patient selection, and outcomes. BJU Int. 2014;113:11–23.

5. Gill HS. Diagnosis and surgical management of uroenteric fistula. Surg Clin North Am. 2016;96:583–92.
6. Kuetting D, Pieper CC. Percutaneous treatment options of lower urinary tract fistulas and leakages. Rofo. 2018;190:692–700.
7. Brown KG, Koh CE, Vasilaras A, Eisinger D, Solomon MJ. Clinical algorithms for the diagnosis and management of urological leaks following pelvic exenteration. Eur J Surg Oncol. 2014;40:775–81.
8. Smith ZL, Johnson SC, Golan S, McGinnis JR, Steinberg GD, Smith ND. Fistulous complications following radical cystectomy for bladder cancer: analysis of a large modern cohort. J Urol. 2018;199:663–8.
9. Msezane L, Reynolds WS, Mhapsekar R, Gerber G, Steinberg G. Open surgical repair of ureteral strictures and fistulas following radical cystectomy and urinary diversion. J Urol. 2008;179:1428–31.
10. Olson L, Satherley H, Cleaveland P, et al. Retrograde endourological management of upper urinary tract abnormalities in patients with Ileal conduit urinary diversion: a dual-center experience. J Endourol. 2017;31:841–6.
11. Stuurman RE, Al-Qahtani SM, Cornu JN, Traxer O. Antegrade percutaneous flexible endoscopic approach for the management of urinary diversion-associated complications. J Endourol. 2013;27:1330–4.
12. Montori G, Allievi N, Coccolini F, et al. Negative pressure wound therapy versus modified barker vacuum pack as temporary abdominal closure technique for open abdomen management: a four-year experience. BMC Surg. 2017;17(1):86.
13. Driver VR, Eckert KA, Carter MJ, French MA. Cost-effectiveness of negative pressure wound therapy in patients with many comorbidities and severe wounds of various etiology. Wound Repair Regen. 2016:241041–58.
14. Glass GE, Murphy GF, Esmaeili A, Lai LM, Nanchahal J. Systematic review of molecular mechanism of action of negative-pressure wound therapy. Br J Surg. 2014;101:1627–36.
15. Yetisir F, Salman AE, Aygar M, Yaylak F, Aksoy M, Yalcin A. Management of fistula of ileal conduit in open abdomen by intra-condoit negative pressure system. Int J Surg Case Rep. 2014;5:385–8.
16. Freeman JJ, Storto DL, Berry-Caban CS. Repair of a vesicocutaneous fistula using negative-pressure wound therapy and urinary diversion via a nephrostomy tube. J Wound Ostomy Continence Nurs. 2013;40:536–8.
17. Heap S, Mehra S, Tavakoli A, Augustine T, Riad H, Pararajasingam R. Negative pressure wound therapy used to heal complex urinary fistula wounds following renal transplantation into an ileal conduit. Am J Transplant. 2010;10:2370–3.
18. Asvadi NH, Arellano RS. Transrenal antegrade ureteral occlusion: clinical assessment of indications, technique and outcomes. J Urol. 2015;194:1428–32.
19. Natarajan V, Boucher NR, Meiring P, Spencer P, Parys BT, Oakley NE, Stent (Society for Endourology in North Trent) Group. Ureteric embolization: an alternative treatment strategy for urinary fistulae complicating advanced pelvic malignancy. BJU Int. 2007;99:147–9.
20. Horenblas S, Kroger R, van Boven E, Meinhardt W, Newling DW. Use of balloon catheters for ureteral occlusion in urinary leakage. Eur Urol. 2000;38:613–7.
21. Forde JC, O'Connor KM, Fanning DM, Guiney MJ, Lynch TH. Management of a persistent ileo-ureteric anastomotic leak with bilateral ureteric occlusion using angioplasty balloon catheters. Can J Urol. 2010;17:5397–400.

5

Testicular Cancer mortality in Brazil: Trends and predictions until 2030

Samara Carollyne Mafra Soares[1†], Katarina Márcia Rodrigues dos Santos[2†], Fabia Cheyenne Gomes de Morais Fernandes[1], Isabelle Ribeiro Barbosa[3] and Dyego Leandro Bezerra de Souza[3*]

Abstract

Background: Despite the fact that testicular cancer presents good prognosis, wide variations in mortality rates have been reported internationally. In Brazil, mortality trends and estimates have not been fully assessed. The objective of the study presented herein is to analyze the mortality trends for testicular cancer in Brazil in the period 2001–2015 and calculate mortality predictions for the period 2016–2030.

Methods: This is a population-based ecological study that utilized information of the Mortality Information System, on testicular cancer-related deaths in Brazil. Mortality trends were analyzed by Joinpoint regression, and Nordpred was utilized for the calculation of predictions.

Results: The mortality rate for men, standardized to the world population, varied between 0.36/100,000 for the year 2001, to 0.41/100,000 for the year 2015. There was an increasing trend for Brazil (APC = 1.3% CI95% 0.6; 2.0) and the Southeast region (APC = 1.5% CI95%0.2; 2.7). When analyzing Brazilian data for the period 2016–2030, predictions indicate 2888 deaths due to testicular cancer, which corresponds to a 26.6% change when compared to the 2011–2015 period. This change is mostly explained by an increase in the risk of death (14.2%) when compared with modifications in the demographic structure (12.4%).

Conclusions: Testicular cancer mortality in Brazil presents increasing trends, and until 2030 these rates continue to increase.

Keywords: Mortality, Predictions, Public health, Testicular neoplasm, Time series studies

Background

In recent years, testicular cancer incidence has increased, especially in developed countries, where Europe and North America correspond to approximately 50% of the new cases registered in the world, in 2018 (6.2/100,000 men and 5.1/100,000 men, respectively). The age standardized world incidence rate for testicular cancer by world standard population was 1.7/100,000 men, in 2018 [1].

Testicular cancer is considered rare, and usually affects young men (aged between 15 and 39 years) [1]' representing approximately 0.7% of all cancers [2]. Although this type of tumor affects a relatively small share of the population, it affects a productive and sexually active age group, with negative impacts on social and economic aspects. It must be highlighted that this type of cancer is usually aggressive, but presents high chances of cure when detected early [3], justifying the importance of its study to public health.

The age standardized world mortality rate for testicular cancer by world standard population was 0.23/100,000 men. In 2018, world estimates reported the incidence of 71,105 new cases and approximately 9507 deaths, of which only 2131 occurred in the most developed regions of the world [1]. Although the highest incidence rates occurred in more developed regions, approximately 80% of the deaths attributed to testicular cancer occurred in developing countries, with Latin

* Correspondence: dysouz@yahoo.com.br
†Samara Carollyne Mafra Soares and Katarina Márcia Rodrigues dos Santos contributed equally to this work.
[3]Graduate Program in Collective Health, Universidade Federal do Rio Grande do Norte/Federal University of Rio Grande do Norte. Programa de Pós-Graduação em Saúde Coletiva, Avenida Senador Salgado Filho 1787, CEP: 59010-000 Lagoa Nova, Natal, RN, Brazil
Full list of author information is available at the end of the article

America and the Caribbean presenting very high rates (0.55 deaths/100,000 men) [4].

Testicular cancer presents a strong genetic component in its development, and is 4 to 5 times more prevalent in Causasians than in Afrodescendant populations. It usually affects young men, with the following risk factors: cryptorchidism, infertility, family history (heritability varies between 37 and 49%) and also associated with the Klinefelter syndrome [2].

Testicular tumors are histologically classified in seminoma and non-seminoma. Approximately 70% of diagnosis are made in initial stages, with excellent cure rates due to its high sensitivity to chemotherapy and radiotherapy, especially if detected early [5]. Five-year survival rates also vary by histological type, from 48 to 92%. [6].

Because testicular cancer presents significant mortality in developing countries, comprehension of its geographic distribution and behavior of rates throughout time is very relevant. Analysis of the epidemiological situation is necessary as an instrument to support the planning of public health policies for the most vulnerable groups. There is a lack in the scientific literature on the epidemiology of testicular cancer in South America, especially in Brazil.

The objective of this study was to analyze the temporal trends of testicular cancer mortality in Brazil and its geographic regions between 2001 and 2015 and estimate mortality predictions for the period 2016–2030.

Methods

An ecological study of temporal series is presented herein, based on secondary data collected prior to this research and available online, from the Mortality Information System (SIM) of the Informatics Department of the Unified Health System (Brazil's publicly funded health system). Deaths due to malignant testicular neoplasm (C62) were analyzed, categorized from the International Classification of Diseases, 10th Revision (ICD-10) and performed equivalence for the ICD- 9, occurred in Brazil in the period 2001–2015 and analyzed according to age groups and geographic regions (five geographic regions).

According to SIM [7], secondary data at regional level for "Ill-defined causes in cause-of-death registration (%)" and "Civil registration coverage of cause-of-death" are, respectively: North (12.56%/81.21%), Northeast (10.96%/ 84.1%), Southeast (11.76%/88.05%), South (9.73%/ 91.86%), Midwest (8.43%/ 90.33%). The mortality information system of Brazil and its geographical regions can be classified as presenting intermediate quality [8]. In recent years, although the quality of registries within SIM has improved considerably, the utilization of secondary data on mortality is still subject to under-registry. Information was utilized from the redistribution of deaths by chapter, corrected by active search [9], to account for the under-registry of deaths due to malignant testicular neoplasms. This is an initiative of the Brazilian Ministry of Health, with data made available at the website of the Informatics Department of the Unified Health System (http://datasus.saude.gov.br/informacoes-de-saude/tabnet) [9].

The percentage difference between the amount of notified deaths to SIM and the amount of redistributed deaths, based on chapter II (neoplasms) of ICD-10, was obtained from a correction factor calculated for each age group, time period, and geographic region [10].This difference was expressed in decimal values, with 1 corresponding to a 100% change, for example. Higher values are possible, as the redistributed amount of deaths could present higher values than what was reported to SIM. When the redistributed value was lower than what was reported to SIM, a negative difference was obtained.

$$D = \frac{\mathbf{NR{-}NS}}{\mathbf{NS}}$$

D = difference between the redistributed deaths and those reported to SIM due to neoplasms, in relation to the number of deaths reported to SIM due to neoplasms; NR = number of deaths redistributed due to neoplasms; and NS = number of deaths reported to SIM due to neoplasms.

The difference obtained was added to the value 1 to calculate the correction factor, as the number 1 is a neutral factor in multiplications:

$$F = 1 + D$$

F = correction factor for chapter II (neoplasms); and D = difference between the redistributed deaths and those reported to SIM due to neoplasms, in relation to the number of deaths reported to SIM due to neoplasms.

This factor was multiplied by the number of cancer-related deaths. Therefore, it was considered that the correction factor for chapter II could be applicable to testicular cancer:

$$DC = F \times NDS$$

DC = corrected number of deaths due to testicular malignant neoplasms), NDS = number of deaths reported to SIM due to testicular malignant neoplasms), and F.

With information on the readjusted number of deaths, standardized mortality rates were calculated, adjusted in accordance with the world population, per 100,000 men [11]. Population data by region and age group were obtained from demographic census information and intercensus predictions, from the website of the Brazilian Institute of Geography and Statistics [12].

Temporal mortality trends for testicular cancer were calculated for Brazil and its geographic regions, and mortality predictions were estimated until 2030, in five-year periods (2016–2020, 2021–2025 and 2026–2030).

Analysis of mortality trends employed Joinpoint regression, utilizing the software *Joinpoint Regression Program*, Version 4.4.0, 2017. The objective is to identify the occurrence of possible joinpoints, where significant changes in trends have occurred.

The method employed identified joinpoints based on the model with a maximum of three change points. The final selected model was the most adjusted model, with *Annual Percentage Change* (APC) based on the trend of each segment, estimating whether these values were statistically significant to a 0.05 level, to describe the terms "significant increase" or "significant decrease". The significance levels utilized herein are based on the Monte Carlo permutation method and on the calculation of the annual percentage change of the ratio, utilizing the logarithm of the ratio [13].

Nordpred (Cancer Registry of Norway, Oslo, Norway), inscribed within statistical program R, was employed to calculate the predictions for each period, utilizing the age-period-cohort. Data were compiled in 5-year blocks and the limit age group considered for analysis was the first with more than 10 cases for the combined period.

Future rates were predicted, until 2030, using the average trend of all observed data (15-year cohorts). Observed and predicted rates for each five-year period were compiled for the population of men in the age groups of 0–14, 15–39 and over 40 years old. The projection of the recent linear trend for the last ten years was attenuated in the drift parameter of 25% in the second and 50% in third 5-year period prediction periods.

The results of the predictions are presented for the total of observed and expected deaths for each period, for Brazil and its five geographic regions. For each period, adjusted mortality rates based on the world standard population were calculated for global comparisons, expressed per 100,000 inhabitants/year (ASW/100, 000 inhab) [11].

Annual changes in the number of deaths in the last predicted period (2026–2030) were calculated in comparison with the last observed period (2011–2015), where the proportion of this change was verified in terms of changes in risks or demographics (size or structure of the population). These components can be different from zero and present a positive or negative direction. Calculation is expressed as [14].

$$\Delta_{tot} = \Delta_{risk} + \Delta_{pop} = (N_{fff} - N_{off}) + (N_{off} - N_{ooo})$$

Δtot = total change, Δrisk = change in function of risk, Δpop = change in function of the population, *Nooo* = number of observed cases, *Nfff* = number of predicted cases, Noff = number of expected cases when mortality cases increase during the observed period.

Results

For the period 2001–2015, there were 4075 deaths due to malignant testicular neoplasm in Brazil. The mortality rate standardized to the world population varied between 0.36 deaths/100,000 men in 2001, to 0.41 deaths/100,000 men in 2015. Mortality rates higher than the overall Brazilian average were registered for the Southern and Northern regions of the country (Fig. 1). When analyzing the historical series of mortality rates, increasing trends were detected for Brazil (APC of 1.3%) and the Southeastern region (APC of 1.5%) ($p < 0.05$) with stability for the remaining geographic regions, with no joinpoints (Table 1).

Table 2 presents the number of deaths and standardized mortality rates for the observed and predicted periods. Data analysis for the 5-year period 2026–2030 in Brazil predicted the occurrence of 2888 deaths due to testicular cancer. Predictions indicate that mortality is increasing in Brazil and the South, North and Northeast regions, while there is stability for the Southeast region and slight reduction in rates until 2030 for the Midwest.

Figure 2 presents the mortality rates for testicular cancer, in the observed and estimated periods, according to the influence of risks and population structure of Brazil and its geographic regions. For Brazil, there will be a 26.6% increase in the number of deaths due to testicular cancer in the period 2026–2030 when compared with 2011–2015, and this change is explained mostly by an increase in the risk of death (14.2%), followed by modifications in the demographic structure of the country (12.4%). For the South region, predictions indicate an increase of 71.3% in the number of deaths, explained mostly by an increase in the risk of dying from the disease (58.2%). For the North region, the increase will be of 45.1%, explained by changes in demographic structure (24.3%) as well as by risk of death (20.8%).

Discussion

This study revealed increasing trends for testicular cancer mortality in Brazil, and that until 2030, the mortality burden will continue to increase; for this period, a change of approximately 30% will be recorded in the number of deaths due to this disease. For this type of cancer, it is observed that in areas where high incidences were historically registered, there are actually decreasing trends. However, in most countries of Latin America and some parts of Asia, South Africa and southern Europe, testicular cancer starts to emerge as an important cause of morbidity and mortality in young men [15, 16].

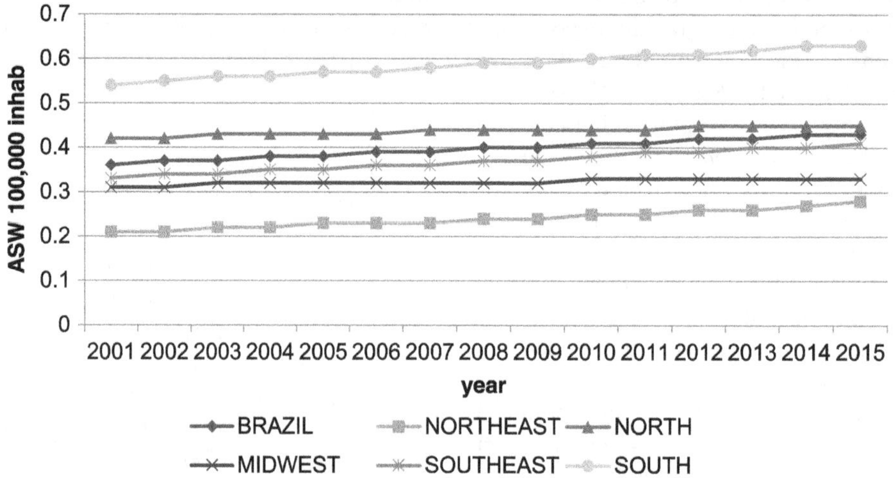

Fig. 1 Standardized testicular mortality rates for Brazil and its geograpphic regions, for the period 2001–2015. Brazil, 2018

In 2012, incidence rates for testicular cancer varied more than 44 times around the world. The highest rates were detected in Western Europe (8.7 cases/100,000 men), Northern Europe (7.2 cases/100,000 men) and Australia/New Zealand (6.8 cases/100,000 men), while the lowest rates were observed in Middle Africa (0.2 cases/100,000 men) [17]. The estimates for year 2018 show that the highest incidence rates remained in the same regions: Western Europe (9.7 cases/100,000 men), Northern Europe (7.2 cases/100,000 men) and Australia/ New Zealand (7.4 cases/100,000 men), while the lowest rates were found in Middle Africa (7.2 cases/100,000 men) [18]. Incidence trends, within the last 10 years before 2012, showed persistent increases in the majority of countries of the world, except for China (APC = – 0.3%). The most pronounced increasing trends were registered in Southern Europe, with APC = 6.8% in Croatia and 6.1% in Spain [17]. This increasing trend for Southern Europe has already been present in the 10 years before 2008 [14].

In 2012, the highest mortality estimates of the world were found in Latin America/the Caribbean (0.55 deaths/ 100,000 men), followed by Europe (0.4 deaths/ 100,000 men) [17]. Estimated data for 2018 remained in the same perspective [1]. The highest value of the ASR-World mortality was reached in the estimates for 2018 in Chile and Georgia (1.1/100,000, both), followed by Niger (0.91/100,000), and Argentina (0.85/100,000). The lowest mortality rates were Dominican Republic and Singapore (0.02/100,000, both), and in many African and Asian countries [18]. The most recent trend, analyzing the 10 years before 2012, verified that most countries presented a reduction in mortality, especially China, which presented a significant decrease in mortality (APC = – 6.1%). Croatia, Brazil, USA and Colombia were exceptions, with increasing testicular cancer mortality (APC = 1.7, 1.8, 0.9 and 0.9%, respectively). Although Europe presents a secondary position regarding global mortality rates, these are still relatively low when compared with high incidence, differently from what is observed in regions of Africa and Asia, where mortality rates are close to the incidence rates [17].

As observed herein and when comparing global rates, Brazilian mortality rates that are lower than those of

Table 1 Temporal trends for testicular cancer mortality in Brazil and its geographic regions: number of deaths, *Annual Percentage Change* (APC), confidence interval and year of joinpoint occurrence, with the total number of deaths over the 15 years, for the period 2001–2015. Brazil, 2018

	Number of deaths	APC (CI 95%)	Joinpoint	Annual population size
Brazil	5996	1.3*(0.6; 2.0)	–	94.558.522
Northeast	957	2.0 (−0.1; 4.3)	–	
North	530	0.5 (−3.7; 4.8)	–	
Midwest	339	0.5 (−3.5; 4.6)	–	
Southeast	2441	1.5* (0.2; 2.7)	–	
South	1303	1.1 (−0.3; 2.4)	–	

*Statistical significance $p < 0.05$
APC Annual percentage change; 95% CI, 95% confidence interval

Table 2 Testicular cancer mortality in Brazil: number of observed and projected deaths per age group and mortality rates adjusted to the world population (ASW/100,000 inhab)

	Observed			Projected		
	2001–2005	2006–2010	2011–2015	2016–2020	2021–2025	2026–2030
BRAZIL						
Age (years)						
0–14	22	18	22	18	17	16
15–39	1189	1520	1645	1817	1876	1896
≥ 40	472	494	614	697	831	976
ASW	0.36	0.39	0.41	0.44	0.45	0.47
Northeast						
Age (years)						
0–14	5	6	12	8	8	7
15–39	189	207	240	256	269	275
≥ 40	65	118	115	145	167	186
ASW	0.2	0.25	0.25	0.27	0.28	0.29
North						
Age (years)						
0–14	0	2	3	2	2	2
15–39	81	155	163	192	207	222
≥ 40	47	30	49	51	66	88
ASW	0.41	0.45	0.47	0.48	0.5	0.53
Midwest						
Age (anos)						
0–14	3	0	2	1	1	1
15–39	53	88	95	91	84	80
≥ 40	33	33	32	43	41	51
ASW	0.29	0.32	0.31	0.28	0.26	0.26
Southeast						
Age (years)						
0–14	9	6	3	4	4	4
15–39	478	649	668	706	699	671
≥ 40	190	196	242	257	297	350
ASW	0.33	0.38	0.38	0.39	0.39	0.39
South						
Age (years)						
0–14	3	3	1	2	2	2
15–39	249	279	349	429	472	496
≥ 40	129	120	170	231	313	394
ASW	0.55	0.53	0.63	0.77	0.87	0.96

some developed countries and some Latin American countries, but with increasing predictions until 2030.

When evaluating the trends and predictions for testicular cancer mortality in Brazil, different patterns were identified across the geographic regions, demonstrating the epidemiological diversity of the country. The highest rates were registered in the South region, while the lowest rates were identified in the Northeast region. Trend analysis demonstrated that, in the last 15 years, there were significant increases in the overall Brazilian rates and for the Southeast region, with stable trends for the remaining regions. It must be highlighted that, although

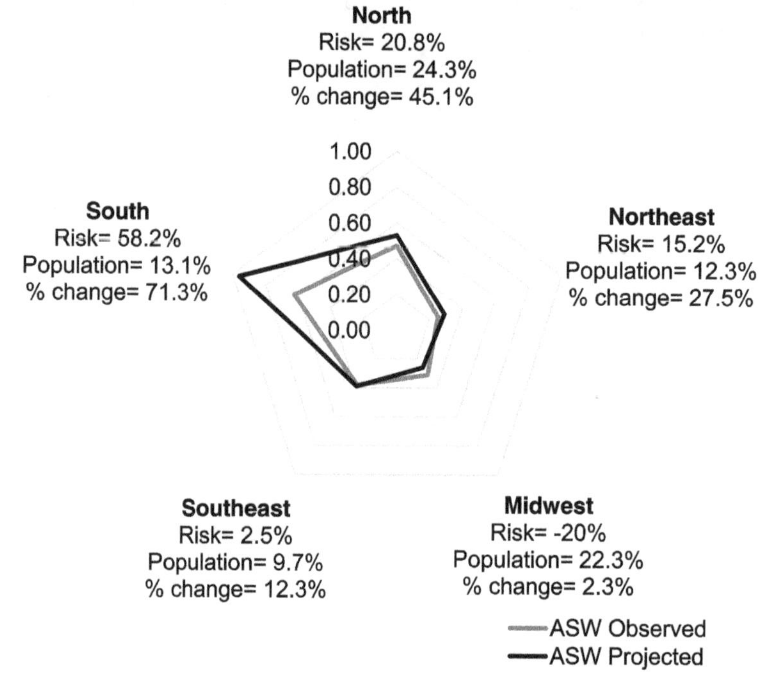

Fig. 2 Testicular cancer mortality rates (ASW) (world standard) in Brazilian regions for 2001–2015 (observed period) and 2026–2030 (projected period), total change (change), change due to change in risk (risk), and change due to demographic alterations (population)

there were different patterns for mortality trends, the predictions indicated increases in the crude number of deaths for all regions. This fact is justified mainly by changes in the size and structure of the population. Predictions for 2030 indicate increasing mortality rates for Brazil and for the South, North and Northeast regions. Decreasing rates should occur for the Midwest region, with stability for the Southeast.

The worst social and economic conditions are concentrated in the North and Northeast regions of Brazil. The most developed regions of the country, South and Southeast, present better per capita income, lower illiteracy rate and overall better infrastructure of health services. The Midwest region presents an intermediate condition [19].

It is difficult to explain the geographic and temporal variations observed in population levels and translate these to the testicular cancer mortality rates in the absence of well-defined risk determinants. However, there is a direct relationship between mortality reduction and the organization of urological care services and the introduction and availability of cisplatin-based therapies in the 1970s. The reduction in mortality rates experienced by the majority of European countries in the most recent decades and in the United States was associated with improvements in diagnosis and efficacy of chemotherapy, with the inclusion of cisplatin in treatment regimes [20].

The epidemiological transition of Brazil has defined a picture of epidemiological polarization, where infectocontagious diseases share space with an increase in noncommunicable chronic diseases, such as cancer [21]. Besides, there is also significant inequity regarding access to cancer diagnosis and treatment services in large urban centers and in more interior locations, as occurs in other South American countries [22, 23]. In Brazil, there is a concentration of oncological services in large urban centers that present better socioeconomic levels (Southeast and South regions). This inequality in the distribution of services contributes to delays in diagnosis and treatment of patients in the least wealthy regions, which in the end present worse prognosis when compared with patients that live in urban centers. This also increases the pressure on medical reference centers due to the migration of patients to larger cities [21].

One of the causes related to cancer mortality in a defined population is the prevalence and distribution of related risk factors [24]. For testicular cancer, ethnicity appears as a risk factor for the increase of incidence and, consequently, affects mortality rates. In the USA, incidence is almost five times higher in Caucasians (9.1 cases per 100,000 men/year) than in Afrodescendants (2.0 cases per 100,000 men/year). In this aspect, the high mortality rates predicted for testicular cancer in the South region of Brazil could be partly explained by the phenotypic characteristics of that population. The South presents a predominance of European descendants, with a high proportion of Caucasians (more than 70% of the population), while the North and Northeast regions present Caucasian percentages under 40% [25, 26]. Another possible explanation for the mortality trends detected for the South region of Brazil could be the better structure of epidemiological cancer vigilance services, characteristic of well-developed regions, which results in better quality of death registries [23].

Nevertheless, the increasing rates observed for the poorest regions of Brazil could be a result of acquiescence and challenging access to the health service network in these areas [27], as prophylactic actions and availability and access to diagnosis and treatment methods affect cancer survival and mortality rates of a population [28].

Considering that 5-year localized testicular cancer survival is 99.2%, minimization of the impact that this type of cancer could cause in the future should count with special attention to the detection of early stage lesions [29]. The high level of survival of testicular cancer patients in the Slovak Republic in comparison with several other countries of eastern Europe with worse survival rates were probably influenced by the massive education of physicians of first examining the testis within the framework of preventive physical examinations [30]. Priority should be given to primary assistance within public health strategies through the implementation of primary prevention measures, and especially, of educational and active vigilance measures that favor self-examination. The advances and improvements in treatment techniques and protocols are very relevant, along with better access and availability to treatment in due time, and training of health professionals so that these can effectively promote health awareness and early detection of suspected cases [29].

A limitation of this study is the utilization of secondary data on mortality, which is subject to under-registry. However, considerable improvements have been attained recently regarding the quality of SIM in Brazil. This study applied data correction, which reduces this potential bias. Cancer predictions should be interpreted with caution, as diagnosis and therapeutic conditions can change in the future and, consequently, mortality trends could be slightly modified. However, the currently employed methods have certified validity, and some authors have pointed differences between 10 and 20% between estimates and registries of events [31].

Conclusions

The findings of this study reveal increasing trends for testicular cancer mortality in Brazil for the 15 years analyzed, and these rates will continue to increase until 2030, also indicating that there are inequalities in the distribution of testicular cancer mortality across Brazilian regions. In this aspect, the phenotypic profile of the Brazilian population is considered along with inequalities in the offer and access to prevention, vigilance, diagnosis and treatment of cancer in Brazil. With the aim of reducing the possible disparities in testicular cancer mortality across Brazil, it is paramount to implement public health policies directed to the most affected populations, associated with a decrease in social inequalities and improvement of access to primary prevention, early diagnosis and effective treatments.

Abbreviations

APC: Annual Percentage Change; BIGS: Brazilian Institute of Geography and Statistics; HDI: Human Development Indices; ICD-10: International Classification of Diseases, 10th Revision; SIM: Mortality Information System

Acknowledgements

Not applicable.

Authors' contributions

KMRS, SCMS, DLBS and IRB developed and planned the study. KMRS, SCMS and FCGMF contributed to data acquisition. SCMS and KMRC drafted the first and successive versions of the manuscript. DLBS and FCGMF analyzed and interpreted data. IRB contributed to the analyses and interpretation of results. SCMS contributed to the interpretation of the results. All authors read and approved the final manuscript.

Author details

[1]Student in the Graduate Program in Collective Health, Health Science Faculty of Trairi, Federal University of Rio Grande do Norte (UFRN), Natal, Brazil. [2]Undergraduate student in Nursing, Health Science Faculty of Trairi, Federal University of Rio Grande do Norte (UFRN), Natal, Brazil. [3]Graduate Program in Collective Health, Universidade Federal do Rio Grande do Norte/ Federal University of Rio Grande do Norte. Programa de Pós-Graduação em Saúde Coletiva, Avenida Senador Salgado Filho 1787, CEP: 59010-000 Lagoa Nova, Natal, RN, Brazil.

References

1. Ferlay J, Colombet M, Soerjomataram I, Mathers C, Parkin DM, Piñeros M, et al. Estimating the global cancer incidence and mortality in 2018: GLOBOCAN sources and methods. Int J Cancer. 2018.
2. Wang Z, McGlynn KA, Rajpert-De Meyts E, Bishop DT, Chung CC, Dalgaard MD, et al. Meta-analysis of five genome-wide association studies identifies multiple new loci associated with testicular germ cell tumor. Nat Genet. 2017;49:1141–7. https://doi.org/10.1038/ng.3879.
3. Smith ZL, Werntz RP, Eggener SE. Testicular Cancer: Epidemiology, Diagnosis, and Management Med Clin North Am. 2018;102:251–64.
4. Stewart BW, Wild CP. World cancer report 2014. France: Lyon; 2014.
5. Albers P, Albrecht W, Algaba F, Bokemeyer C, Cohn-Cedermark G, Fizazi K, et al. EAU guidelines on testicular cancer: 2011 update. Eur Urol. 2011;60:304–19.
6. Albers P, Albrecht W, Algaba F, Bokemeyer C, Cohn-Cedermark G, Fizazi K, et al. Guidelines on testicular Cancer: 2015 update. Eur Urol. 2015;68:1054–68.
7. Ministério da Saúde Brasil. http://datasus.saude.gov.br/informacoes-de-saude/tabnet. Accessed 22 Mar 2019.
8. Mathers CD, Fat DM, Inoue M, Rao C, Lopez AD. Counting the dead and what they died from: an assessment of the global status of cause of death data. Bull World Health Organ. 2005;83:171–7.
9. Brasil M da S. Mortalidade: Redistribuição por Capítulos dos Óbitos corrigidos pela Pesquisa de Busca Ativa. 2015. http://datasus.saude.gov.br/sistemas-e-aplicativos/eventos-v/sim-sistema-de-informacoes-de-mortalidade. Accessed 1 May 2018.
10. Santos, CA, Souza, DLB. Melanoma mortality in brazil: Trends and projections (1998-2032). Cien Saude Colet [periódico na internet] (2017/Jul). [Citado em 26/06/2019]. http://www.cienciaesaudecoletiva.com.br/artigos/melanoma-mortality-in-brazil-trends-and-projections-19982032/16311?id=16311.
11. Doll R, Payne P, Waterhouse J. Cancer incidence in five continents. v. 1. Geneva, Berlim: UICC: Springer; 1966.
12. IBGE IB de G e E. https://www.ibge.gov.br/. Accessed 20 Mar 2019.
13. Kim HJ, Fay MP, Feuer EJ, Midthune DN. Permutation tests for joinpoint regression with applications to cancer rates. Stat Med. 2000;19:335–51.

14. Møller B, Fekjær H, Hakulinen T, Sigvaldason H, Storm HH, Talbäck M, et al. Prediction of cancer incidence in the Nordic countries: empirical comparison of different approaches. Stat Med. 2003;22:2751–66.
15. Verhoeven RHA, Gondos A, Janssen-heijnen MLG, Saum KU, Brewster DH, Holleczek B, et al. Testicular cancer in Europe and the USA: survival still rising among older patients. Ann Oncol. 2013;24:508–13.
16. Le Cornet C, Lortet-Tieulent J, Forman D, Béranger R, Flechon A, Fervers B, et al. Testicular cancer incidence to rise by 25% by 2025 in Europe? Model-based predictions in 40 countries using population-based registry data. Eur J Cancer. 2014;50:831–9.
17. Park JS, Kim J, Elghiaty A, Ham WS. Recent global trends in testicular cancer incidence and mortality. Medicine (Baltimore). 2018;97:e12390.
18. Ferlay J, Ervik M, Lam F, Colombet M, Mery L, Piñeros M, et al. The Globocan Cancer observatory. Global Cancer observatory: Cancer today. Lyon, France: International Agency for Research on. Cancer. 2018; https://gco.iarc.fr/today. Accessed 20 Mar 2019.
19. Barbosa IR, Costa I do CC, Pérez MB, Souza DLB de. SOCIOECONOMIC INEQUALITY AND CANCER MORTALITY : AN ECOLOGICAL STUDY IN BRAZIL Desigualdades socioeconômicas e mortalidade por câncer : um estudo ecológico no Brasil Desigualdades socioeconómicas y mortalidad por cáncer : un estudio ecológico en Brasil. 2016;29:350–356.
20. Bosetti C, Bertuccio P, Chatenoud L, Negri E, La Vecchia C, Levi F. Trends in mortality from urologic cancers in Europe, 1970-2008. Eur Urol. 2011;60:1–15.
21. Souza DLB, Jerez-Roig J, Cabral FJ, De Lima JRF, Rutalira MK, Costa JAG. Colorectal cancer mortality in Brazil: predictions until the year 2025 and cancer control implications. Dis Colon Rectum. 2014;57:1082–9.
22. Goss PE, Lee BL, Badovinac-Crnjevic T, Strasser-Weippl K, Chavarri-Guerra Y, Louis JS, et al. Planning cancer control in Latin America and the Caribbean. Lancet Oncol. 2013;14:391–436.
23. Barbosa IR, Costa I do CC, Bernal MM, de SDLB. PRINCIPAIS CAUSAS DE ÓBITOS POR CÂNCER NO BRASIL , trends in mortality rates of the ten leading causes death cancer in Brazil , 1996-2012. Rev Ciência Plur. 2016;2:3–16.
24. Antunes JLF, Toporcov TN, Biazevic MGH, Boing AF, Bastos JL. Gender and racial inequalities in trends of oral cancer mortality in Sao Paulo, Brazil. Rev Saude Publica. 2013;47:470–8.
25. Xavier R. Brasil. Instituto Brasileiro de Geografia e Estatística. Paz YLA: Claros M. Censo; 2010. p. 2013. https://censo2010.ibge.gov.br/
26. American Cancer Society. Cancer Facts and Figures 2017. 2017. doi:https://doi.org/10.1101/gad.1593107.
27. Barros MB de A, Francisco PMSB, Zanchetta LM, César CLG. Tendências das desigualdades sociais e demográficas na prevalência de doenças crônicas no Brasil, PNAD: 2003- 2008. Cien Saude Colet. 2011;16:3755–68. https://doi.org/10.1590/S1413-81232011001000012.
28. Sharpe KH, McMahon AD, Raab GM, Brewster DH, Conway DI. Association between socioeconomic factors and cancer risk: a population cohort study in Scotland (1991-2006). PLoS One. 2014;9.
29. Stevenson SM, Lowrance WT. Epidemiology and diagnosis of testis Cancer. Urol Clin North Am. 2015;42:269–75.
30. Ondrus D, Ondrusova M, Dusek L. Recent patterns in testicular cancer incidence, mortality and survival in the Slovak Republic with reference to international comparisons. Cancer Investig. 2012;30:545–51.
31. Bernal M, Romero FJ, Souza DLB, Gómez-Bernal FJ, Gómez-Bernal GJ. Estimation of the projections of incidence rates, prevalence and mortality due to prostate cancer in Aragon (Spain). Actas Urol españolas. 2011;35: 470–4.

6

Quantitative proteomic characterization of human sperm cryopreservation: Using data-independent acquisition mass spectrometry

Longlong Fu[1,2], Qi An[1,2,3], Kaishu Zhang[4], Ying Liu[5], Yue Tong[1,2,3], Jianfeng Xu[1,2], Fang Zhou[1,2], Xiaowei Wang[1,2], Ying Guo[1,2], Wenhong Lu[1,3*], Xiaowei Liang[2] and Yiqun Gu[1,2,3*]

Abstract

Background: Human sperm cryopreservation is a simple and effective approach for male fertility preservation.

Methods: To identify potential proteomic changes in this process, data-independent acquisition (DIA), a technology with high quantitative accuracy and highly reproducible proteomics, was used to quantitatively characterize the proteomics of human sperm cryopreservation.

Results: A total of 174 significantly differential proteins were identified between fresh and cryoperservated sperm: 98 proteins decreased and 76 proteins increased in the cryopreservation group. Bioinformatic analysis revealed that metabolic pathways play an important role in cryopreservation, including: propanoate metabolism, glyoxylate and dicarboxylate metabolism, glycolysis/gluconeogenesis, and pyruvate metabolism. Four different proteins involved in glycolysis were identified by Western blotting: GPI, LDHB, ADH5, and PGAM1.

Conclusions: Our work will provide valuable information for future investigations and pathological studies involving sperm cryopreservation.

Keywords: Cryopreservation, Fertility preservation, Reproductive techniques, assisted, Metabolic networks and pathways

Background

Human sperm cryopreservation plays an important role in the treatment of male infertility when the male partner has severe abnormalities in semen parameters [1]. Furthermore, this technique is a simple and effective approach to male fertility preservation [2, 3], and is the only approach used in the clinic in many countries [4]. However, the cryopreservation protocols will induce a notable decrease in sperm motility, as well as affecting other parameters, including: membrane and acrosome integrity, DNA fragment, and reactive oxygen species [5, 6]. Certain intracellular and extracellular factors have been shown to lead to cryo-damage [7, 8]. However, the related pathogenesis of sperm cryo-damage during the process of cryopreservation shaould be clarified by further study.

Proteomics, especially sperm proteomics, is a new field in human reproduction studies. Ptoteomics can elucidate complex biological systems, including sperm motility and fertilization, and it can discover the potential pathogenic mechanisms and the biomarkers associated with male infertility [9, 10]. Data-independent acquisition (DIA) is, a novel proteomics technology, based on acquiring fragment ion information for all precursor ions within a certain range of m/z values [11]. Different from data-dependent acquisition (DDA), the DIA strategy has the characteristics of high quantitative accuracy and high reproducibility; and the experimental method has broad applicability: up to 5000 proteins can be detected and quantified in one experiment [11, 12]. To the best of our

* Correspondence: wenhonglu16@163.com; guyq16@163.com
[1]National Health Commission Key Laboratory of Male Reproductive Health, National Research Institute for Family Planning, Beijing 100081, China
Full list of author information is available at the end of the article

knowledge, this technique has not previously been applied to the study of human cryopreserved sperm.

For these reasons, the aim of the current study is to compare the proteomic differences between fresh and cryopreserved human sperm, using DIA mass data. A further understanding the sperm proteins would be very helpful in explaining sperm cryoinjury and may establish biomarkers for sperm motility.

Methods

Ethics statement and sample collection

The study was approved by National Research Institute for Family Planning Ethics Committee on Human Subjects (2018018). Ejaculates were obtained from healthy semen donors attending the Human Sperm Bank, National Research Institute for Family Planning, in Beijing China. Informed consent was obtained from all the sperm donors involved in the study.

Study design and sample collection

Paired design was applied to this study. Every semen sample was divided into two parts: one for the cryopreserved group and the other for the fresh group. Our focus was the difference between the cryopreserved and fresh human sperm.

A total of 14 semen samples from 14 qualified healthy sperm donors were collected. The ages of the sperm donors were between 22 years and 29 years. One ejaculate was collected from these volunteers by masturbation after 3–5 days of sexual abstinence. Routine semen analyses were performed by Computer Aided Sperm Analysis (CASA)(HTM-IVOS, USA), according to the World Health Organization (WHO 2010) guidelines.

Among the whole sample of each group, 9 cryopreserved and fresh samples were used for proteomics analysis. Similar to the previous study [13], the 9 donors' ejaculates (each one divided into fresh and cryopreserved vials) were divided into 3 groups of 3. Then 5 for Western blot analysis.

Semen cryopreservation protocols

After complete liquefaction, 2 mL of each semen sample was divided into two parts: one for cryopreservation and the other placed in a 37 °C water bath as the control. Glycerol-egg-yolk-citrate (GEYC) was used as cryoprotectant containing 15% glycerol, 20% egg yolk, 1.3% glycine, 1.5% glucose, and 1.3% sodium citrate tribasic dehydrate, with a pH of 6.8–7.2. One volume of GEYC was added to two volumes of semen, drop by drop with swirling, and the mixture was incubated at 30–35 °C for 5 min. A slow sperm freezing method was performed according to the standardized programmable freezers (Kryo 360–1.7, Planner, United Kingdom) in our unit [12, 14]. Briefly, one volume of GEYC cryoprotectant was added to two volumes of semen, and the program was as follows: the samples tubes waerw cooled at 1.5 °C per minute from 20 °C to – 6 °C, at 6 °C per minute to – 100 °C, and at – 100 °C for 30 min, then the sample tubes were transferred to liquid nitrogen. After being preserved in the liquid nitrogen for a minimum of 2 days, a small portion (10 μL) of the frozen sample was thawed for sperm quality assessment.

Protein extraction and digestion

Protein extraction and digestion were performed as described previously [15]. The fresh and cryopreserved semen were centrifuged at 800 g for 10 min to remove seminal plasma, round cells and the cryoprotectant. Then, the sperm were washed three times with phosphate-buffered saline (PBS). Five hundred microliters of lysis buffer [8 M UREA, 100 mM Tris-HCl, pH 7.6, 1 mM PMSF (phenylmethylsulfonyl fluoride)(Roche, Germany)] was added to each sample. Then, the samples were sonicated(Sonics, USA) at 20 joules for 2 s × 10 at intervals of 15 s, and centrifuged at 18000 g for 15 min, after which the supernatant was extracted. Quantification was performed using the BCA method. The protein sample was frozen at – 80 °C. An aliquot of 20 μg was used for each sample to build the mixed and pooled library. Six samples and the pooled samples were subjected to enzymatic hydrolysis using a FASP (filter-aided sample preparation) enzymatic method.

Then, protein digestion was performed using the FASP protocol. In brief, protein (200 μg) was diluted with 50 mM dithiothreitol and incubated for 40 min at 56 °C. Further operation was carried out using the ultrafiltration tube method. The ultrafiltration tube was placed in a collection tube, and the protein sample was added to the ultrafiltration tube and centrifuged at 12000 g for 15 min. One hundred microliters of urea buffer containing 50 mM iodoacetamide was added to the ultrafiltration tube and it was then incubated for 20 min in the dark. The sample was washed twice by adding 100 μL urea buffer and centrifugede at 12000 g for 10 min to remove irrelevant substances. Then, 80 μL of 50 mM trypsin in NH_4HCO_3 was added to ultrafiltration tube, and the protein-to-enzyme ratio was 50:1. The samples were incubated at 37 °C for 16 h, and the released peptides were collected through centrifugation and directly determined by the protein concentration detection mode in the Nano-Drop instrument.

Spectral library generation

The samples (1 μg) were analyzed on an EASY-Nano-LC mass spectrometer (Thermo, USA). The peptides were separated using 0.1% formic acid, containing iRT standard peptide(Buffer A) and acetonitrile containing 0.1% formic acid(Buffer B), along a linear gradient from 3 to

32% at 300 nL/min for 120 min. The gradient of chromatographic separation was as follows: 3–7% buffer B for 0-3 min, 7–20% buffer B for 80 min,20–32% buffer B for 24 min, 32–90% buffer B for 1 min, and 100% buffer B for 120 min. For DDA, the source was operated by Orbitrap Fusion (Thermo Scientific, USA), at 2.1 kV. The DDA scheme included a full MS survey scan from m/z350 to m/z 1500 at a resolution of 60 k full-width half-maximum (FWHM)(at m/z 200) with automatic gain control(AGC) set to 4E5 (maximum injection time of 50 ms). The parameters of MS2 were as follows: 30 k FWHM (@ m/z 200), isolation window 1.6 Th, AGC set to 4e5 (maximum injection time of 50 ms). For, high-energy collision dissociation (HCD): MS2 Activation (collision energy: 35) was used, and dynamic exclusion was set to 40s.

For the generation of the spectral library, DDA data analysis was performed using Protein Discoverer 2.1 SP1(SEQUEST HT). The database is human proteins database from UniProt: "uniprot-organism-9606 + reviewed-yes.fasta, " and iRT peptide sequences were added to the database: (>Biognosys|iRT-Kit|Sequence_fusion LGGNEQVTRYILA GVENSKGTFIIDPGGVIRGTFIIDPAAVIRGAGSSEPVTG LDAKTPVISGGPYEYRVEATFGVDESNAKTPVITGAPYE YRDGLDAASYYAPVRADVTPADFSEWKLFLQFGAQGS SPFLK).

Raw data were analyzed according to the user guide of the software. The parameters were set as follows: the initial mass tolerance for precursor ions was: 10 ppm, and the mass tolerance for product ion spectra was 0.02 Da. Tryptic cleavage was selected, and the maximum allowable number of missing cleavage was 2. Carbamidomethyl of cysteine was set as the fixed modification, while oxidation of methionine and N terminal acetylation were set as variable modifiers. The identifications were filtered to satisfy an FDR of 1%, and the unique peptide number per protein was greater than one. Then, the result was used to build the DDA spectral library in Spectronaut Pulsar X(Biognosys, Switzerland). The library parameters used the default optimal parameter "GBS factory setting".

Protein identification and quantitation

For DIA, 2 μg peptides was taken from each sample and mixed with appropriate iRT standard peptides. Each sample was tested by DIA mass spectrometry for 2 h. The method consisted of a full MS1 scan at a resolution of 60 K from m/z 350 to m/z 1500, with AGC set to 4E5 (maximum injection time of 50 ms), followed by 46 DIA windows acquired at a resolution of 30 K FWHM with AGC set to 5e5 (maximum injection time of 55 ms); HCD: MS2 activation (collision energy: 35).

Finally, qualitative and quantitative analyses of DIA raw data were performed in Spectronaut Pulsar X. Database parameters were as follows: peptides FDR\ PSM FDR\ proteins FDR was 1%; at least three proteins were selected for each peptide, at most 6 optimal ion generation library spectra were selected, and iRT calibration $R^2 > 0.8$. The quantitative parameters were set as follows: the iTR standard used a nonlinear fit (local (non-linear) regression), the protein identification used a precursor Qvalue cutoff 0.01, the protein Qvalue cutoff of 0.01, the protein quantification used the peak area of sub-ions, and the average Intensity of at least three sub-ions was selected to quantify the protein. Protein quantification uses the ion peak area, and at least the average intensity quantification of three sub-ions is selected. Paired t-test was used as the analytical approach and *P*-value of 0.05 was set.

Bioinformatics analysis

All significantly differential proteins were used as input. The OmicsBean analysis tool [16] was used to retrieve the Gene Ontology Consortium categories, including: molecular function (MF), cellular component (CC) and biological process (BP). KEGG [17] pathway enrichment analysis was performed using the Kanehisa databases web service (https://www.kanehisa.jp/en/archive.html). The protein-protein interaction network (PPI) was constructed using the STRING [18] web service (http://www.string-db.org/).

Western blotting

According to our previous experience [19], the sperm protein samples were separated by 10% SDS polyacrylamide gel electrophoresis. The samples were then transferred to a polyvinylidene fluoride membranes, blocked with 2% (w/v) skim milk for 1 h, and incubated overnight with the primary antibody of glucose-6-phosphate isomerase (GPI), lactate dehydrogenase B (LDHB), alcohol dehydrogenase 5 (ADH5), and phosphoglycerate mutase 1 (PGAM1) (1:1000) (Abclone, China) at 4 °C temperature. After three washes with TBST, the membranes were incubated with horseradish peroxidase (HRP) in combination with anti-IgG for 1 h at room temperature (18–22 °C). Enhanced chemiluminescence revealed immunoreactivity. The relative signal intensity of protein bands was analyzed with Quantity One v.4.6.2.

Statistical analysis

Data are expressed as the mean ± SD and were analyzed with SPSS22.0 software (IBM, USA). Paired t-test was used as the analytical approach, and a *P*-value of 0.05 was set.

Results

Sperm motility

We aimed to assess the impact of cryopreservation on sperm motility (Table 1). Compared with fresh semen, a significant decrease in the percentage of progressive

Table 1 Characteristics of motility of fresh and post-thaw human sperm ($n = 14$) (Mean ± SD)

	Percentage of PR(%)	VAP (μm/s)	VSL (μm/s)	VCL (μm/s)
Fresh sperm	67.0 ± 7.5	42.4 ± 0.9	31.0 ± 1.7	65.2 ± 1.2
Post-thaw sperm	45.3 ± 2.51*	37.8 ± 2.4*	29 ± 0.5*	58.6 ± 5.8*

*: $P < 0.05$ compared with the Fresh group
PR progressive; *VAP* average path velocity; *VSL* straight line velocity; *VCL* curvilinear velocity.

sperm, and sperm motion parameters was observed in cryoperserved sperm, including average path velocity (VAP), straight line velocity (VSL), and curvilinear velocity (VCL).

Quantitative results of differential proteins

Compared with the spectral library, a total of 29,495 unique peptides and 5246 proteins were identified. Finally, 3790 proteins were quantitatively analyzed. Using the 1.5-fold or 0.67-fold change and the FDR-adjusted p-value of 0.05 as cutoffs, 174 (4.6%) significantly differential proteins were identified between fresh and cryopreserved sperm: 76 were increased and 98 were decreased in the cryopreserved group. The detail of the differential proteins due to cryopreservtaion are provided in the Additional file 1: Table S1.

Gene ontology enrichment

Enrichment analysis was performed based on the 174 significantly deregulated proteins. A total of 1544 biological processes(BPs), 275 cell components(CCs) and 261 molecular functions(MFs) were involved in the GO enrichment, and there were significant differences between the fresh and cryopreserved sperm($P < 0.05$). The number of differential proteins contained in each entry and its percentage of total differential protein are shown in Fig. 1. The detailed results of the GO enrichment are provided in Additional file 2: Table S2.

KEGG pathway and protein-protein interaction (PPI) network analysis

Pathway enrichment analysis was also performed by KEGG enrichment in order to identify the major biochemical pathways and signal transduction pathways. Several pathways were significantly disturbed in cryopreserved sperm, such as: ribosome, carbon metabolism and lysosome (Fig. 2). The details of the 16 pathways with significant differences are shown in Table 2. To show the main interactions and regulatory relationships of these proteins, the PPI network was constructed (Fig. 3).

According to the KEGG analysis, the results showed found that the metabolic pathways play an important role in cryopreservation (Fig. 2), including: propanoate metabolism, glyoxylate and dicarboxylate metabolism, glycolysi/gluconeogenesis, and pyruvate metabolism. Most of these pathways were down regulated in the cryopreserved sperm group (the green in the Fig. 3).

Validation of the glycolysis metabolic proteins

To further validate the outcome of the KEGG analysis, we used Western blotting to quantify the four dysregulated protein enzymes in glycolysis: GPI, LDHB, ADH5, and PGAM1.

These protein analysis results confirmed the previous genomic analysis of metabolomics, and the results confirmed the differential protein levels observed via 2DE (Fig. 4). The cryopreserved group had lower levels of

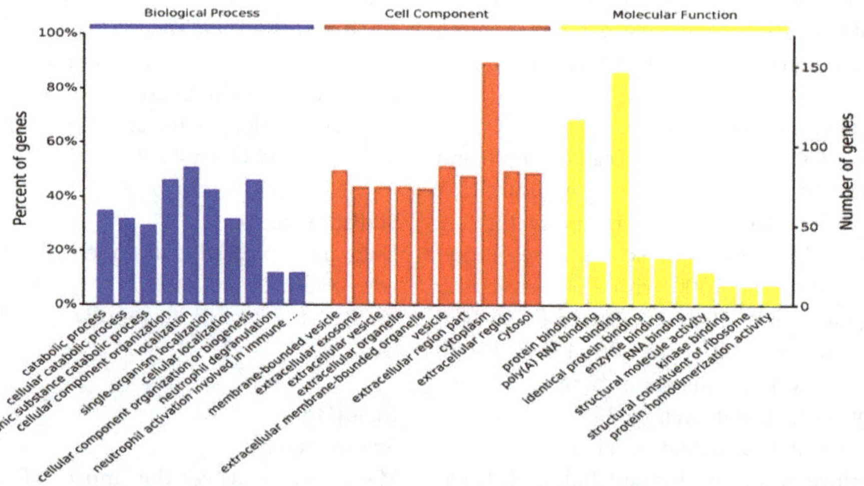

Fig. 1 Gene Ontology analysis classification and the enrichment result of differentially expressed proteins in the human freeze-thaw samples compared to the fresh group, in terms of Biological Process, Cell Component and Molecular Function

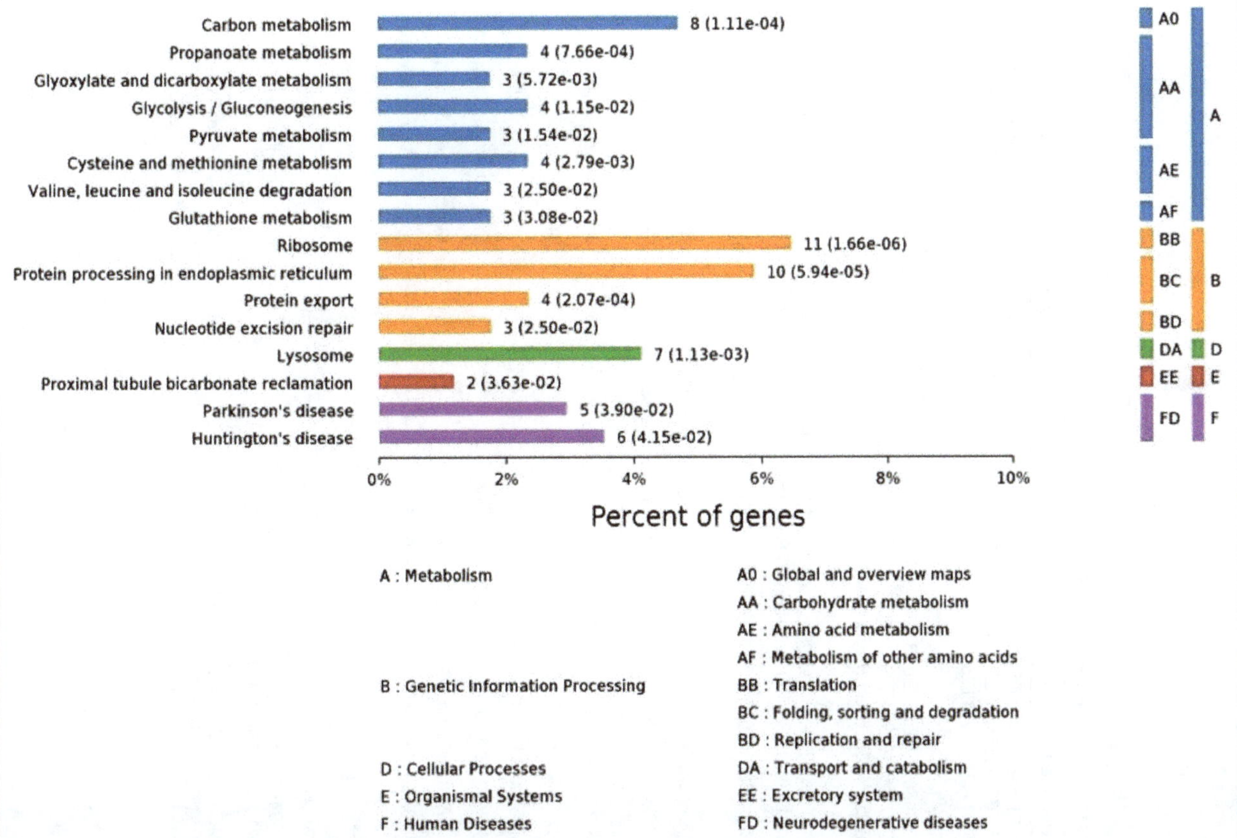

Fig. 2 Kyoto Encyclopedia of Genes and Genomes(KEGG) pathway enrichment analysis

GPI, LDHB, and PGAM1. and a higher level of ADH5 than the fresh sperm (Fig. 4).

Discussion

Worldwide, the percentage of male infertility ranges between 20 and 70% [20], and men with azoospermia or severe oligozoospermia will benefit from sperm cryopreservation. Furthermore, cryopreservation is a simple and effective technique for preserving fertility potential [4, 21]. However, after sperm cryopreservation, too many sperm lose their motility and fertility [5, 22]. Some sperm proteins have been recognized to be associated with sperm quality, and the loss of these proteins may be responsible for the decrease in fertility in sperm cryopreservation, such as: heat-shock protein 90 [23] and, Enolase1 (ENO1). However single protein bioresearch can only partly explain the cryodamage, and further study should be based on direct or indirect protein-protein interaction and mechanistic factors.

Proteomics technology has been identified as valuable tool for sperm [15, 24, 25]. Proteomic changes in human sperm as a result of cryoinjury have been reported previously. Wang et.al [13] found twenty-seven proteins that differed in abundance between fresh and cryopreserved sperm, by using two-dimensional polyacrylamide gel electrophoresis (2-DE) and mass spectrometry. However 2-DE has its limitations, including a low sensitivity of the densitometry analysis. Bogle et al. [26] used tandem mass tag (TMT) technology to identify potential proteomic changes at every stage of the cryopreservation process, but they did not compare fresh and cryopreserved sperm. Different from TMT, the DIA strategy has the characteristics of high quantitative accuracy and high reproducibility [11, 27]. Due to its global nature and enormous multiplexing capacity, DIA has been widely used in mechanistic studies and clinical biomarker screening in human reproduction for the enhanced protein coverage and analytical reproducibility [28]. In our study, a total of 174 significantly differential proteins were identified from 3790 quantitatively analyzed proteins, which is much more than previously reported discoveries [13, 26].

Improving upon previous studies on human cryopreserved sperm proteomics analysis [13, 26], our study performed KEGG analysis for the different proteins. KEGG is a frontier interdisciplinary subject based on life science and computer science. Bioinformatics analysis has been widely used as a powerful tool for data processing and prediction by employing various databases, and it has been widely used in the discovery of new biomarkers

Table 2 Detailed information of the Kyoto Encyclopedia of Genes and Genomes (KEGG) pathway enrichment results

<table>
<tr><th>Pathway Name</th><th>Pathway ID</th><th>P value</th><th>Genes: Name|Ratio(Cryopreservated/Fresh)</th><th>Count</th><th>Pop Hit</th><th>Class</th></tr>
<tr><td>Ribosome</td><td>hsa03010</td><td>1.66E-06</td><td>RPL10A|0.573336532743;RPS19|0.631553739412;RPS13|0.523487855699; RPL27|0.636693323276;RPS12|0.620311406135;RPS28|0.556462384813; MRPS7|1.61901451638;RPL30|0.585111111172;RPL26|0.525298518938; RPLP1|0.201692403302;RPS27|0.545857932715</td><td>11</td><td>138</td><td>Genetic Information Processing</td></tr>
<tr><td>Protein processing in endoplasmic reticulum</td><td>hsa04141</td><td>5.94E-05</td><td>CAPN1|0.483846314217;SEC63|1.64488179;NSFL1C|0.532234501825; RAD23B|0.544847606418;RAD23A|0.449570898437;SEC61A2|1.59938044965; SVIP|0.57175573788;SSR3|1.53947957741;SEC61G|12.6538069403; RBX1|0.63561326146</td><td>10</td><td>166</td><td>Genetic Information Processing</td></tr>
<tr><td>Carbon metabolism</td><td>hsa01200</td><td>1.11E-04</td><td>GPI|0.594470429855;MUT|1.64145141153;ALDH6A1|1.80998863199;MDH1|0.61379399419; ADH5|1.57385688652;GLUD1|1.60104289531;PGAM1|0.554594456772;PCCB|1.67972523554</td><td>8</td><td>113</td><td>Metabolism</td></tr>
<tr><td>Protein export</td><td>hsa03060</td><td>2.07E-04</td><td>SEC63|1.64488179;SEC61A2|1.59938044965;SEC61G|12.6538069403;IMMP1L|1.67051120115</td><td>4</td><td>23</td><td>Genetic Information Processing</td></tr>
<tr><td>Propanoate metabolism</td><td>hsa00640</td><td>7.66E-04</td><td>MUT|1.64145141153;ALDH6A1|1.80998863199;LDHB|0.606365006071;PCCB|1.67972523554</td><td>4</td><td>32</td><td>Metabolism</td></tr>
<tr><td>Lysosome</td><td>hsa04142</td><td>1.13E-03</td><td>CTSF|0.624627283152;GNS|0.637102261894;ARSA|0.494575557376;NAGA|0.650162388685; NPC2|0.426290016224;AGA|0.43725788109;CLTA|0.666776335796</td><td>7</td><td>123</td><td>Cellular Processes</td></tr>
<tr><td>Cysteine and methionine metabolism</td><td>hsa00270</td><td>2.79E-03</td><td>AHCY|0.597470127607;MDH1|0.61379399419;LDHB|0.606365006071;GSS|0.585813890146</td><td>4</td><td>45</td><td>Metabolism</td></tr>
<tr><td>Glyoxylate and dicarboxylate metabolism</td><td>hsa00630</td><td>5.72E-03</td><td>MUT|1.64145141153;MDH1|0.61379399419;PCCB|1.67972523554</td><td>3</td><td>28</td><td>Metabolism</td></tr>
<tr><td>Glycolysis / Gluconeogenesis</td><td>hsa00010</td><td>1.15E-02</td><td>GPI|0.594470429855;LDHB|0.606365006071;ADH5|1.57385688652;PGAM1|0.554594456772</td><td>4</td><td>67</td><td>Metabolism</td></tr>
<tr><td>Pyruvate metabolism</td><td>hsa00620</td><td>1.54E-02</td><td>MDH1|0.61379399419;LDHB|0.606365006071;ACYP1|0.490664299807</td><td>3</td><td>40</td><td>Metabolism</td></tr>
<tr><td>Valine, leucine and isoleucine degradation</td><td>hsa00280</td><td>2.50E-02</td><td>MUT|1.64145141153;ALDH6A1|1.80998863199;PCCB|1.67972523554</td><td>3</td><td>48</td><td>Metabolism</td></tr>
<tr><td>Nucleotide excision repair</td><td>hsa03420</td><td>2.50E-02</td><td>RAD23B|0.544847606418;RAD23A|0.449570898437;RBX1|0.63561326146</td><td>3</td><td>48</td><td>Genetic Information Processing</td></tr>
<tr><td>Glutathione metabolism</td><td>hsa00480</td><td>3.08E-02</td><td>GSS|0.585813890146;GGCT|0.573964558442;GSTK1|1.70055565858</td><td>3</td><td>52</td><td>Metabolism</td></tr>
<tr><td>Proximal tubule bicarbonate reclamation</td><td>hsa04964</td><td>3.63E-02</td><td>MDH1|0.61379399419;GLUD1|1.60104289531</td><td>2</td><td>23</td><td>Organismal Systems</td></tr>
<tr><td>Parkinson's disease</td><td>hsa05012</td><td>3.90E-02</td><td>ATP5F1|1.571159587;VDAC3|1.63594176768; UCHL1|0.613051768866;NDUFB8|1.71896191444;MT-ND3|1.54131079277</td><td>5</td><td>142</td><td>Human Diseases</td></tr>
<tr><td>Huntington's disease</td><td>hsa05016</td><td>4.15E-02</td><td>DCTN2|0.634124905506;ATP5F1|1.571159587;VDAC3|1.63594176768; CLTA|0.666776335796;AP2S1|4.07535354503;NDUFB8|1.71896191444</td><td>6</td><td>193</td><td>Human Diseases</td></tr>
</table>

The "Pop hit" is the total number of proteins in the pathway; the "Count "is the actually matched number

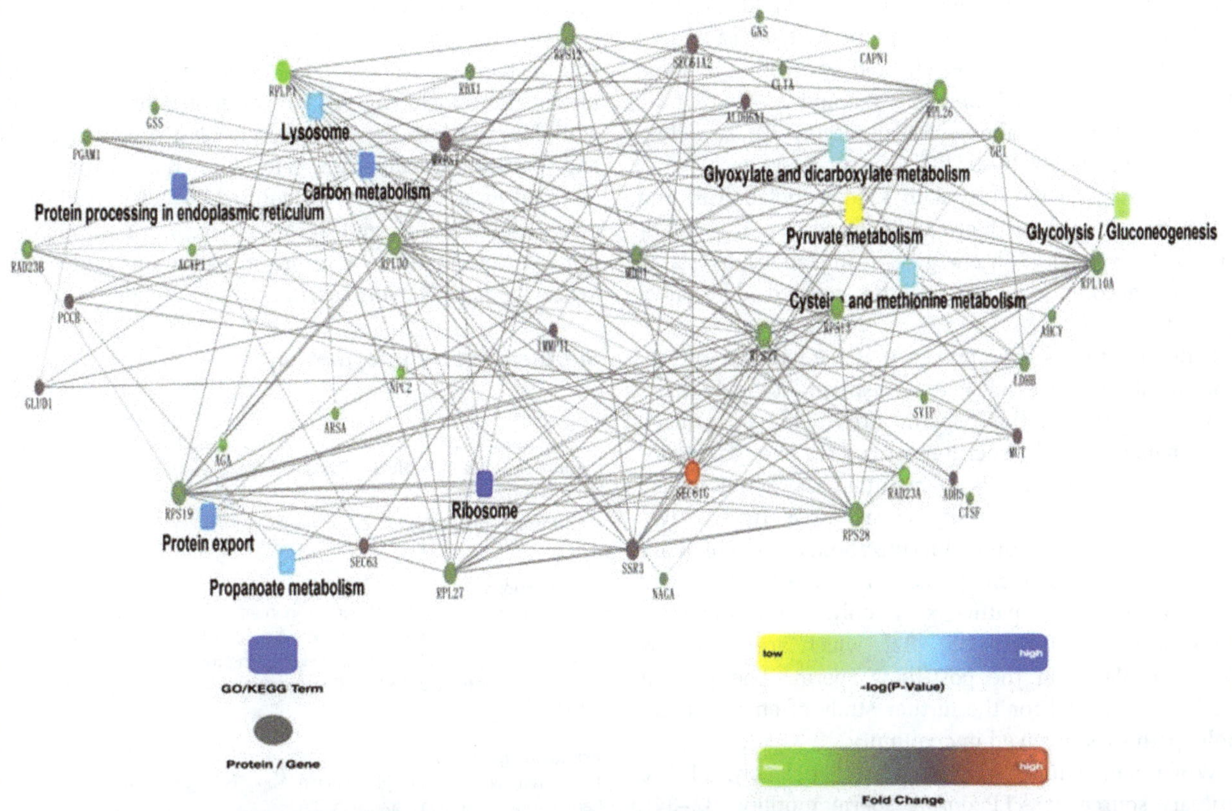

Fig. 3 Protein interaction network diagram (STRING)

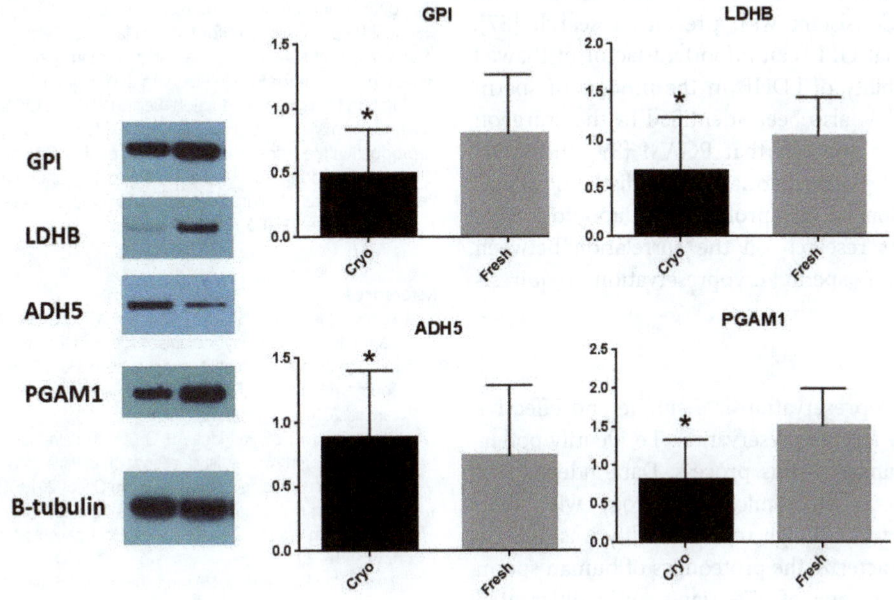

Fig. 4 Validation of the 2DE results by Western blot

and the study of new therapeutic targets [29, 30]. According to the KEGG analysis, the present study revealed that the metabolic pathways were affected by cryopreservation. This result confirmed previous research. Wang et al. found the decreased abundance of succinyl-CoA:3-ketoacid CoA transferase (OXCT1) in cryopreservated sperm, and this enzyme is involved in ketone metabolism and might be associated with glycolysis in sperm [13]. According to Bogle et al. [26], energy- and metabolism- related proteins account for 15% of the collated differential proteins.

Different studies have proven that the pathway of carbon metabolism is associated with sperm and male infertility [31]. In addition, sperm are highly specialized mammalian cells; the sperm must reserve enough adenosine triphosphate (ATP) to maintain the physiological processes, including motility, capacitation, hyperactivation, acrosome reaction and fertilization, all of which are highly energy dependent processes. The ATP is formed via two metabolic pathways: glycolysis and oxidative phosphorylation (OXPHOS) [32], which are extremely down regulated in the post-thaw sperm. The present study is beneficial for the further study of energy metabolic pathways involved in cryoinjury.

While many studies have reported that glycolysis is the primary source of ATP during sperm motility [32–34], OXPHOS is involved in maturation and differentiation [35]. Many study have also shown that sperm motility will significantly decrease in the process of cryopreservation and that ATP is extremely decrease in the post-thaw sperm [5, 36, 37]. Based on thede results, we focuesd the glycolysis pathway in future research. The four proteins related to glycolysis were identified by Western boltting. This study shows the a correlation between GPI and sperm motility. Consistent with previous research [37], our study show that GPI is an important factor of thawed sperm. The variability of LDHB in the process of sperm cryopreservation has also been identified in the sturgeon [38]. Early research suggests that PGAM [39] and ADH [40] is associated with spermatogenic distinction and affects the function of cell proliferation, apoptosis and migration. Further research on the correlation between PGAM1/ADH and sperm cryopreservation requiresis needed.

Conclusions

Human sperm cryopreservation is a simple and effective approach for male fertility preservation. To identify potential proteomic changes in this process, Data-independent acquisition (DIA), a proteomics technology with high quantitative accuracy and high reproducibility was used to quantitatively characterize the proteomics of human sperm cryopreservation. A total of 174 significantly differential proteins were identified between fresh and cryoperservated sperm: 98 were decreased and 76 were increased in the cryopreservation group. Bioinformatic analysis revealed that metabolic pathways play an important role in cryopreservation, including propanoate metabolism, glyoxylate and dicarboxylate metabolism, glycolysi/gluconeogenesis, and pyruvate metabolism. The four different proteins involved in glycolysis were identified by Western Blotting: GPI, LDHB, ADH5, and PGAM1. Our work will provide valuable information for future investigations and pathological studies involving sperm cryopreservation.

Supplementary information

Additional file 1: Table S1. The differential proteins due to cryopreservtaion.

Additional file 2: Table S2. The results of the GO enrichment.

Abbreviations

BP: Biological process; CC: Cellular component; DDA: Data-dependent acquisition; DIA: Data-independent acquisition; FWHM: Full-Width Half-Maximum; MF: Molecular function; PPI: Protein-protein interaction; VAP: Average path velocity; VCL: Curvilinear velocity; VSL: Straight line velocity

Acknowledgements

The authors wish to thank PhD. Guibin Wang, Beijing Proteome Research Center, forthe helpful assistance in DIA.

Authors' contributions

LLF and YQG conceived and supervised the study design. LLF, QA, KSZ and YL established the mass spectrometry workflow and performed the proteomic analysis. YT, XWW, JFX, FZ and YG analyzed proteomic data and performed bioinformatics analysis. WHL and XWL verify and interpretation all the data. LLF and YL drafted the manuscript. YQG, WHL, and XWL revised the manuscript. All authors have read and approved the manuscript.

Author details

[1]National Health Commission Key Laboratory of Male Reproductive Health, National Research Institute for Family Planning, Beijing 100081, China. [2]Department of Male Clinical Research/Human sperm bank, National Research Institute for Family Planning & WHO Collaborating Center for Research in Human Reproduction, Beijing 100081, China. [3]Graduate School of Peking Union Medical College, Beijing 100730, China. [4]Department of Reproductive Medicine, The Afliated Hospital of Qingdao University, Qingdao, Shandong 266000, People's Republic of China. [5]Institute of Pediatric Research, Children's Hospital of Soochow University, Suzhou, Jiangsu Province 215025, China.

References

1. Yogev L, Kleiman SE, Shabtai E, Botchan A, Paz G, Hauser R, Lehavi O, Yavetz H, Gamzu R. Long-term cryostorage of sperm in a human sperm bank does not damage progressive motility concentration. Hum Reprod. 2010;25(5):1097–103.
2. Tournaye H, Dohle GR, Barratt CL. Fertility preservation in men with cancer. Lancet. 2014;384(9950):1295–301.
3. Oktay K, Harvey BE, Partridge AH, Quinn GP, Reinecke J, Taylor HS, Wallace WH, Wang ET, Loren AW. Fertility Preservation in Patients With Cancer: ASCO Clinical Practice Guideline Update. J Clin Oncol. 2018;36(19):1994-2001.
4. Fu L, Zhang K, An Q, Zhou F, Lu W, Liang X, Gu Y. Low utilization of fertility preservation among Chinese male cancer patients. Int J Clin Exp Med. 2018; 11(9):9916–20.
5. Raad G, Lteif L, Lahoud R, Azoury J, Azoury J, Tanios J, Hazzouri M, Azoury J. Cryopreservation media differentially affect sperm motility, morphology and DNA integrity. Andrology. 2018;6(6):836-45.

6. Gomez-Torres MJ, Medrano L, Romero A, Fernandez-Colom PJ, Aizpurua J. Effectiveness of human spermatozoa biomarkers as indicators of structural damage during cryopreservation. Cryobiology. 2017;78:90–4.
7. Ribas-Maynou J, Fernandez-Encinas A, Garcia-Peiro A, Prada E, Abad C, Amengual MJ, Navarro J, Benet J. Human semen cryopreservation: a sperm DNA fragmentation study with alkaline and neutral comet assay. Andrology. 2014;2(1):83–7.
8. Kathrins M, Abhyankar N, Shoshany O, Liebermann J, Uhler M, Prins G, Niederberger C. Post-thaw recovery of rare or very low concentrations of cryopreserved human sperm. Fertil Steril. 2017;107(6):1300–4.
9. De Rose MB, Piccolomini MM, Belo ASS, Borges E, Jr., Filho FF: Proteomics in Human Reproduction. Protein and peptide letters 2018.
10. Cao X, Cui Y, Zhang X, Lou J, Zhou J, Bei H, Wei R. Proteomic profile of human spermatozoa in healthy and asthenozoospermic individuals. Reprod Biol Endocrinol. 2018;16(1):16.
11. Tsou CC, Avtonomov D, Larsen B, Tucholska M, Choi H, Gingras AC, Nesvizhskii AI. DIA-Umpire: comprehensive computational framework for data-independent acquisition proteomics. Nat Methods. 2015;**12**(3):258–64 257 p following 264.
12. Yang X, Guo Y, Cao XF, Jia YF, Wang XW, Xu JF, Zhou F, Li H, Liang XW, Lu WH, et al. Effect of cryopreservation on DNA methylation status of imprited genes in human sperm. J Reprod Medcine. 2015;24(5):402–8.
13. Wang S, Wang W, Xu Y, Tang M, Fang J, Sun H, Sun Y, Gu M, Liu Z, Zhang Z, et al. Proteomic characteristics of human sperm cryopreservation. Proteomics. 2014;14(2–3):298–310.
14. Hezavehei M, Sharafi M, Kouchesfahani HM, Henkel R, Agarwal A, Esmaeili V, Shahverdi A. Sperm cryopreservation: a review on current molecular cryobiology and advanced approaches. Reprod BioMed Online. 2018;37(3):327–39.
15. Wang G, Wu Y, Zhou T, Guo Y, Zheng B, Wang J, Bi Y, Liu F, Zhou Z, Guo X, et al. Mapping of the N-linked glycoproteome of human spermatozoa. J Proteome Res. 2013;12(12):5750–9.
16. Li F, Zhao D, Yang S, Wang J, Liu Q, Jin X, Wang W. ITRAQ-based proteomics analysis of Triptolide on human A549 lung adenocarcinoma cells. Cell Physiol Biochem. 2018;45(3):917–34.
17. Kanehisa M, Furumichi M, Tanabe M, Sato Y, Morishima K. KEGG: new perspectives on genomes, pathways, diseases and drugs. Nucleic Acids Res. 2017;45(D1):D353–d361.
18. Szklarczyk D, Franceschini A, Wyder S, Forslund K, Heller D, Huerta-Cepas J, Simonovic M, Roth A, Santos A, Tsafou KP, et al. STRING v10: protein-protein interaction networks, integrated over the tree of life. Nucleic Acids Res. 2015;43(Database issue):D447–52.
19. Liu Y, Wang J, Qin Y, Huang C, Archacki S, Ma J, Li D, Liu M. Identification of three mutations in the MVK gene in six patients associated with disseminated superficial actinic porokeratosis. Clinica Chimica Acta; Int J Clin Chem. 2016;**454**:124–9.
20. Agarwal A, Mulgund A, Hamada A, Chyatte MR. A unique view on male infertility around the globe. Reprod Biol Endocrinol. 2015;13:37.
21. Nahata L, Caltabellotta NM, Yeager ND, Lehmann V, Whiteside SL, O'Brien SH, Quinn GP, Gerhardt CA: Fertility perspectives and priorities among male adolescents and young adults in cancer survivorship. Pediatric blood & cancer 2018.
22. Isaac AV, Kumari S, Nair R, Urs DR, Salian SR, Kalthur G, Adiga SK, Manikkath J, Mutalik S, Sachdev D, et al. Supplementing zinc oxide nanoparticles to cryopreservation medium minimizes the freeze-thaw-induced damage to spermatozoa. Biochem Biophys Res Commun. 2017;494(3–4):656–62.
23. Cao WL, Wang YX, Xiang ZQ, Li Z. Cryopreservation-induced decrease in heat-shock protein 90 in human spermatozoa and its mechanism. Asian J Androl. 2003;5(1):43–6.
24. Li CJ, Wang D, Zhou X. Sperm proteome and reproductive technologies in mammals. Anim Reprod Sci. 2016;173:1–7.
25. Kosteria I, Anagnostopoulos AK, Kanaka-Gantenbein C, Chrousos GP, Tsangaris GT. The Use of Proteomics in Assisted Reproduction. In Vivo (Athens, Greece). 2017;31(3):267–83.
26. Bogle OA, Kumar K, Attardo-Parrinello C, Lewis SE, Estanyol JM, Ballesca JL, Oliva R. Identification of protein changes in human spermatozoa throughout the cryopreservation process. Andrology. 2017;5(1):10–22.
27. Muntel J, Xuan Y, Berger ST, Reiter L, Bachur R, Kentsis A, Steen H. Advancing urinary protein biomarker discovery by data-independent acquisition on a Quadrupole-Orbitrap mass spectrometer. J Proteome Res. 2015;14(11):4752–62.
28. Meyer JG, D'Souza AK, Sorensen DJ, Rardin MJ, Wolfe AJ, Gibson BW, Schilling B. Quantification of lysine acetylation and Succinylation stoichiometry in proteins using mass spectrometric data-independent acquisitions (SWATH). J Am Soc Mass Spectrom. 2016;27(11):1758–71.
29. Chen L, Lu D, Sun K, Xu Y, Hu P, Li X, Xu F. Identification of biomarkers associated with diagnosis and prognosis of colorectal cancer patients based on integrated bioinformatics analysis. Gene. 2019.
30. Zhang Y, Tang X, Pang Y, Huang L, Wang D, Yuan C, Hu X, Qu L. The Potential Mechanism of Bufadienolide-Like Chemicals on Breast Cancer via Bioinformatics Analysis. Cancers (Basel). 2019;11(1):91.
31. Singh K, Jaiswal D. One-carbon metabolism, spermatogenesis, and male infertility. Reprod Sci (Thousand Oaks, Calif). 2013;20(6):622–30.
32. du Plessis SS, Agarwal A, Mohanty G, van der Linde M. Oxidative phosphorylation versus glycolysis: what fuel do spermatozoa use? Asian J Androl. 2015;17(2):230–5.
33. Gibb Z, Aitken RJ. The impact of sperm metabolism during in vitro storage: the stallion as a model. Biomed Res Int. 2016;2016:9380609.
34. Hereng TH, Elgstoen KB, Cederkvist FH, Eide L, Jahnsen T, Skalhegg BS, Rosendal KR. Exogenous pyruvate accelerates glycolysis and promotes capacitation in human spermatozoa. Hum Reprod. 2011;26(12):3249–63.
35. Stendardi A, Focarelli R, Piomboni P, Palumberi D, Serafini F, Ferramosca A, Zara V. Evaluation of mitochondrial respiratory efficiency during in vitro capacitation of human spermatozoa. Int J Androl. 2011;34(3):247–55.
36. O'Connell M, McClure N, Lewis SE. The effects of cryopreservation on sperm morphology, motility and mitochondrial function. Hum Reprod. 2002;17(3):704–9.
37. Jiang XP, Wang SQ, Wang W, Xu Y, Xu Z, Tang JY, Sun HY, Wang ZJ, Zhang W. Enolase1 (ENO1) and glucose-6-phosphate isomerase (GPI) are good markers to predict human sperm freezability. Cryobiology. 2015;71(1):141–5.
38. Li P, Guo W, Yue H, Li C, Du H, Qiao X, Liu Z, Zhou Q, Wei Q. Variability in the protein profiles in spermatozoa of two sturgeon species. PLoS One. 2017;12(10):e0186003.
39. Zhang S, Zhao Y, Lei B, Li C, Mao X. PGAM1 is Involved in Spermatogenic Dysfunction and Affects Cell Proliferation, Apoptosis, and Migration. Reprod Sci (Thousand Oaks, Calif). 2015;**22**(10):1236–42.
40. Aly HA, El-Beshbishy HA, Banjar ZM. Mitochondrial dysfunction induced impairment of spermatogenesis in LPS-treated rats: modulatory role of lycopene. Eur J Pharmacol. 2012;677(1–3):31–8.

7

Sneeze and pop: A ruptured varicocele; analysis of literature, guided by a well-documented case-report

Daan J. Reesink[1*], Peter M. Huisman[2], Judith Wiltink[1], Arto E. Boeken Kruger[1] and Tycho M. T. W. Lock[3]

Abstract

Background: An acute scrotal hematoma, secondary to a spontaneous rupture of a varicocele is still a rare presentation in daily practice. However, multiple case reports have been reported. Sudden increase in abdominal pressure, resulting to an increased venous pressure can lead to a rupture of the varicocele. Literature search shows that due to uncertainty of the diagnosis, explorative surgery is often performed, sometimes resulting in unnecessary orchiectomies. The objective of this study was to determine classical clinical presentation of patients with a spontaneous rupture of a varicocele, determine the diagnostic procedure, and give an insight in the follow-up.

Case presentation: We present a case of a 24-year old male with acute scrotal swelling after sneezing. Subsequently, we carried out a systematic literature search to identify all eligible studies to determine classic clinical presentation of spontaneous ruptures of a varicocele.

Conclusion: The literature search shows that clinical presentation of idiopathic spontaneous scrotal hematomas is similar to testicular torsion, epididymo-orchitis, malignancy, or (incarcerated) inguinal hernia making differential diagnosis difficult. Especially when there has been increased abdominal pressure or strenuous activity preceding the symptoms, and the swelling is left sided, it should be included in the differential diagnosis for patient with acute inguinoscrotal swelling. Colour Doppler-Ultrasonography is recommended to distinguish between other causes of acute scrotum. The hematoma is usual self-limiting, justifying conservative treatment. Early surgical intervention is indicated with signs of ischaemia due to obstruction, infection of the hematoma, or uncertain diagnosis (i.e. malignancy). However, physicians should be cautious with direct exploration, as it led to unnecessary orchiectomy in 25% of patients. The hematoma can increase in size up to 3 months post-event, and it can take up to 15 months to completely resolve.

Keywords: Idiopathic spontaneous varicocele rupture, Spermatic cord hematoma, Hematocele

Background

A varicocele is present in about 15% of healthy males [1, 2]. A spontaneous rupture of a varicocele, resulting in an acute scrotal hematoma however, is a rare phenomenon. Sudden increase in abdominal pressure, resulting to an increased venous pressure can lead to a rupture of the varicocele. Symptoms can be similar to a torsion of the testis, torsion of appendix testis, epididymo-orchitis or malignancy. Imaging has shown to be challenging. We present a case of a 24-year old male with acute scrotal swelling.

* Correspondence: d.reesink@antoniusziekenhuis.nl
[1]Department of Urology, Tergooi Hospital Hilversum, Rijksstraatweg 1, 1261 AN Blaricum, The Netherlands
Full list of author information is available at the end of the article

A literature search on this topic during treatment of this patients resulted in the finding that due to uncertainty, explorative surgery is often performed, sometimes resulting in unnecessary orchiectomies. The aim of this study was to determine classical clinical presentation of patients with a spontaneous rupture of a varicocele, determine the diagnostic procedure and give an insight in the follow-up.

Case presentation

A 24-year old male was seen at the Emergency Department of our hospital with acute scrotal swelling on the left side, which started 5 days earlier. The symptoms started during a trip to Japan, where the patient had

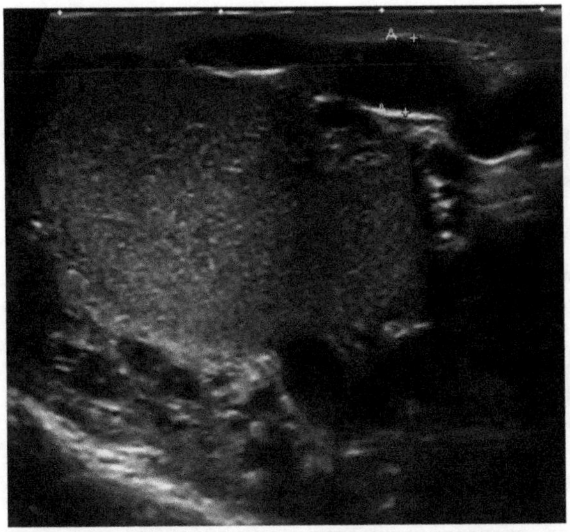

Fig. 1 Ultrasound of the left testis, 5 months prior to the ER visit, during a Valsalva Manoeuvre. A clear varicocele of 4.3 mm is visible (A-A)

multiple severe sneezes while walking outside. On examination, he had a large swelling of the left hemiscrotum. Except for a left sided varicocele (Fig. 1), which was diagnosed 6 months earlier in our hospital, the patient had no medical history. Blood-results were negative. Colour Doppler-Ultrasonography (CDU) showed the known varicocele, a normal vascularized left testis, and a swelling of low echogenicity of 39x29mm without blood flow, suiting a scrotal bleeding (Fig. 2). The hematoma was considered self-limiting, and spontaneous resorption was expected. However, after follow-up ultrasonography 2 months later, the swelling had increased in size (40x40mm) (Fig.3). The patient was referred to an academic hospital. A CT-scan of the abdomen showed a prominent vena spermatica on the left, without suspicion

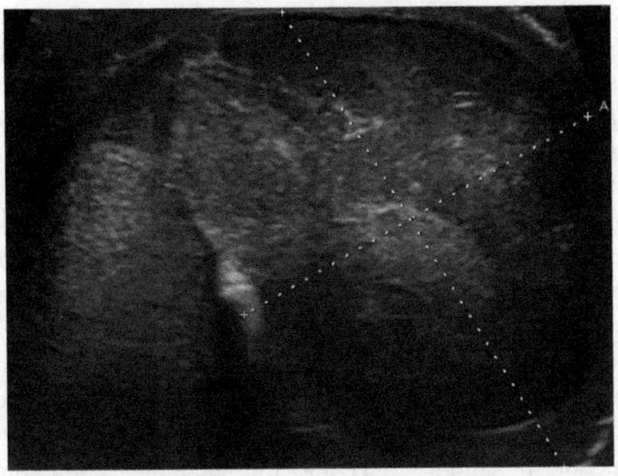

Fig. 2 Ultrasound of the same testis left, after presentation at the ER. Lateral of the testis, a large hypo echogenic, non-vascular mass of 39x29mm is visible

of an arteriovenous malformation. A 3D replica of the CT-scan, illustrating the size of the hematoma (Fig. 4).

Three months post-event, the hematoma even further increased in size to 50x37x30mm. Eventually, the patient underwent a microscopic inguinal varicocelectomy. After, the hematoma showed signs of reabsorption, decreasing in size to 38x24x21mm 4 months; 20x16x11mm 6 months; and to no residual hematoma eventually, 15 months post-event. The left testis itself did not differ in size at all follow-up points.

Discussion

An acute scrotal hematoma, secondary to a spontaneous rupture of a varicocele is still a very rare presentation in daily practice. However, multiple case reports have been reported.

Literature search

We carried out a systematic literature search for PubMed, EMBASE, and Cochrane Library, using Medical Subject Headings indexes, keyword searchers and publication types until May 2017. Additionally, the reference lists of included articles/case reports were also examined for potential studies. There was no language restriction, as long as all relevant info was present (in the abstract), and the abstract was in English. The following keywords were used in the search: varicocele rupture, or spermatic cord hematoma, or hematocele spermatic cord. The terms were separately searched or connected by the Boolean operators "AND" and "OR". We identified in our search 31 case reports. Differentiation could be made based on etiology into three major causes, i.e. idiopathic, spontaneous hematomas (18×) [3–20], (direct) traumatic (6×) [21–26], as a result of a coagulation disorder (4×) [27–30]. No abstract or not all necessary information was available in seven case reports. Since this article is on idiopathic, spontaneous hematoma's, only these case reports will be discussed. Results of the literature search are shown in Table 1.

Etiology

Idiopathic, spontaneous hematomas are thought to be the result of sudden increase of abdominal pressure transmitting to a varicocele. It's arbitrary whether abdominal trauma can lead to increased abdominal pressure, resulting in a ruptured varicocele [8]. A study of Shafik & Bedeir (1980). showed that patients with a left-sided varicocele develop an increased venous pressure during a Valsalva manoeuvre [31]. Various structures, (i.e. vein of the normal pampiniform plexus, a single varix or false aneurysm of the spermatic artery), have been identified as bleeding source. However, in the majority of cases the bleeding source at surgery cannot be identified [10].

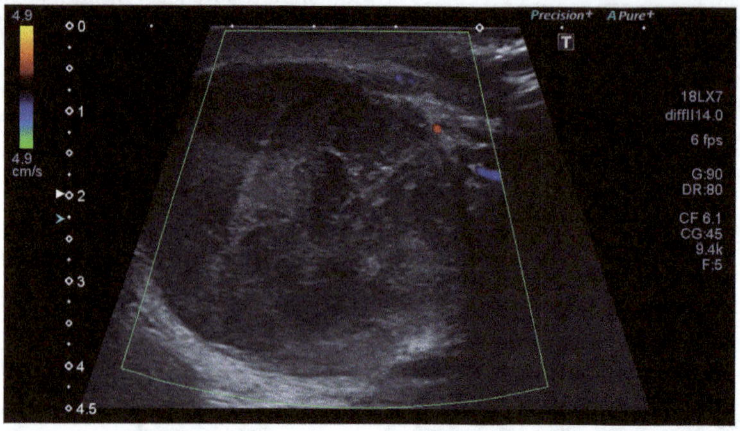

Fig. 3 Colour Doppler Ultrasound of the same testis left, 2 months after presentation. There is progression of the size of the mass to 40×40mm. The swelling is not demarcatable from the left testis. Although there is no vascular flow visible, due to the progression in size and the aspect of the swelling, a malignancy cannot be ruled out

Clinical presentation

Average age of presentation was 31 (±18) years, with the overall majority of males in their 20s at presentation. This makes distinction between possible testicular torsion, or malignancy difficult, since both affect mostly males between 15 and 35 [32]. Accurate differential diagnosis can possibly be facilitated by taking the patients history with emphasis on possible triggering events. Preceding events to the spontaneous scrotal hematoma in literature could all be narrowed down to increased abdominal pressure. Existing literature describes various activities preceding a spontaneous scrotal hematoma, reviewed in Table 1. Examples are pressure during defecation [4, 7, 9, 11], sexual intercourse [13], blunt abdominal trauma [5, 8, 14], heavy lifting [6], stretching in tight pants [15] or after fighter-pilot centrifuge training [19]. Another patient had a spontaneous hematoma after playing the saxophone [10]. After an inguinal hernia correction at 18 years, doctors had discouraged him from playing ever again. Although strict compliance of this advice, 35 years later he could not resist the urge to play. He presented himself at the ER an hour later. To our knowledge, a scrotal hematoma resulting from sneezing has never been described. When an unknown swelling is present in the scrotum, physicians should include the question whether any activities increasing abdominal pressure, or any strenuous activities, had preceded the swelling, when taking patients history.

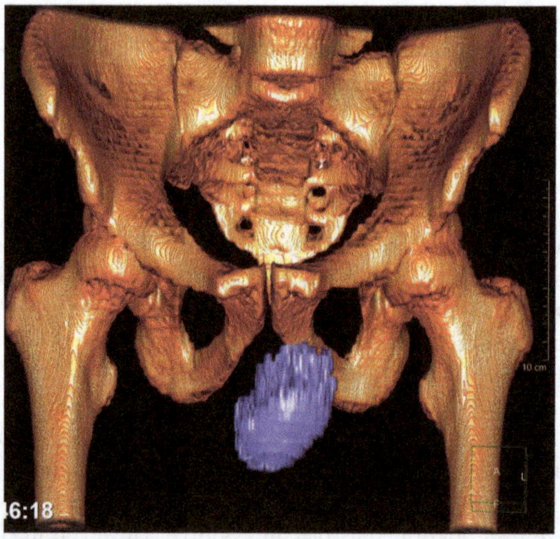

Fig. 4 Coronal 3D-replication of the CT images, illustrating the size of the hematoma

Reported clinical presentation of patients with a spontaneous ruptured varicocele is acute pain (83%), and acute (inguinal) scrotal swelling (100%), which could also be difficult to distinguish from testicular torsion, appendix testis torsion, or malignancy. Important to note is that patients with testicular cancer commonly present with a painless mass. Just 10 % of patients present with acute symptoms such as pain [33], so when pain is present malignancy becomes more unlikely. Ecchymosis can sometimes be seen after a few days (33%), but is rarely reported on. Unfortunately, none of the case reports reported on the cremaster reflex. With the exception of three cases, all spontaneous hematoma's (83%) were found on the left side, conform the higher incidence of left sided varicocele [2]. Varicoceles are more common on the left side due to a longer left testicular vein and congenital incompetence of the valves of the left testicular veins [34]. Other causes are entering of the left testicular vein on the left renal vein at a right angle, arching of the left testicular vein over the left testicular artery thereby compressing it (in some men), compression of the left testicular vein by the descending colon, or compression of the left renal vein between the superior mesenteric artery and the abdominal aorta (nutcracker effect) [35]. The question arises whether the right-sided cases therefore should be categorized as traumatic, even though their described etiology was different.

Table 1 Overview of case reports on idiopathic, spontaneous scrotal hematomas

Article/Case Report (year)	Age (years)	Preceding cause	Side (L/R)	Symptoms	Conservative or Treatment	Varicocele present?
Akay et al. (2015)	21	After marching	R	Pain, swelling, ecchymosis	Delayed exploration & orchiectomy due to ischaemia	
Aliabadi et al. (1987)	27	After defecation	L	Pain, swelling, ecchymosis	Exploration due to uncertain diagnosis	Yes
Bowman et al. (1998)	23	After football tackle	R	Pain, swelling, ecchymosis	Conservative.	
Chin et al. (2009)	33	After heavy lifting	L	Pain, swelling	Delayed exploration due to no improvement	Yes
Demir et al. (2010)	21	After defecation	L	Pain, swelling, ecchymosis	Conservative. Ligation after 3 weeks	Yes
Gordon et al. (1993)	22	After blunt abdominal trauma	L	Pain, swelling	Exploration due to uncertain diagnosis	Yes (History)
Kampel et al. (2015)	?	After centrifuge training	L	Pain, swelling	Conservative.	Yes
Kobayashi et al. (2006)	28	After defecation	L	Pain, swelling	Conservative. Ligation after 4 months	
Lindhorst et al. (2000)	53	After playing saxophone	L	Pain, swelling	Exploration due to suspected incarcerated inguinal hernia	Yes
Matsui et al. (2004)	69	After defecation	L	Pain, swelling	Conservative.	
Mirilas et al. (2010)	10	After skiing	L	Pain, swelling,	Exploration due to persisting pain	
Miyoshi et al. (1980)	22	?	L	Pain, swelling, ecchymosis	Exploration due to uncertain diagnosis.	
Nishiyama et al. (2005)	23	After sexual intercourse	L	Pain, swelling, ecchymosis	Conservative	Yes
Pepe et al. (2015)	16	After blunt abdominal trauma	L	Pain, swelling	Exploration due to persisting pain	
Ragozzino et al. (1993)	40	After stretching		Pain, swelling	Conservative	
Rolnick et al. (1965)	16	?	R	Pain, swelling, ecchymosis	Exploration & orchiectomy due to uncertain diagnosis	
Takezawa et al. (2011)	31	Secondary to nutcracker phenomena	L	Pain, swelling	Conservative	Yes
Vandana et al. (2015)	71	Unknown	L	Pain, swelling	Exploration & orchiectomy due to uncertain diagnosis	

L = Left, R = Right.? = Unknown. Symptoms with strikethrough indicates symptom not present

Diagnostics

Diagnosing a cause of acute scrotal pain and swelling can be difficult, and as stated the differential diagnosis should include conditions such as testicular torsion, malignancy, epididymo-orchitis, or (incarcerated) inguinal hernia [6, 14].

Blood analyses and coagulation tests could be performed to exclude any bleeding disorders. In one case, symptoms mimicked an epididymo-orchitis, due to leucocytosis [3]. No ultrasound was performed. The delay in treatment resulted in ischaemia due to obstruction, necrosis of the testis, and eventually orchiectomy.

CUD is the imaging modality of choice in evaluating patients who present with acute scrotal pain [35], especially in cases where testicular blood flow is of the essence. Gray-scale images are nonspecific for detecting testicular torsion. A distinction should be made between intra-testicular and extra-testicular hematomas, since intra-testicular hematomas can result in testicular infection or necrosis in 40% of patients without exploration [35]. A hematoma on CUD is shown as a heterogeneous, hypo-echogenic, non-vascular mass, which can be mistaken with a malignancy. CT-Abdomen or MRI can be used to diagnose arteriovenous malformations.

Imaging of the scrotum was performed in all but four cases [4, 10, 12, 16], where CUD was the mostly used modality. In all four cases without any imaging, exploration was performed, with one resulting in an orchiectomy due to suspected tumour [16].

Treatment

Surgical exploration is indicated when diagnosis is uncertain, or when a testicular torsion or ischaemia cannot be excluded, and orchiectomy can be performed when malignancy is highly expected, (or partial or a intraoperative biopsy). However, physicians should be cautious for unnecessary orchiectomy. When performing exploration, an inguinal approach is recommended, if malignancy is possible, to avoid scrotal violation. Additional arguments for exploration are possible future complications, i.e. testicular ischaemia due to obstruction of the hematoma on the funiculus [14], possible hematoma infection, or no regression in size of the hematoma. Eventually, microscopic ligation/embolisation of the varicocele can be performed [7, 9].

Overall, exploration was performed in ten patients (56%), indicating the lack of knowledge about idiopathic spontaneous hematomas of the scrotum. Direct exploration at presentation was performed in eight patients (44%). Reasons of direct exploration were uncertain diagnosis (63%) [4, 8, 12, 16, 18], suspected incarcerated inguinal hernia [10], or persisting pain [14, 20]. In the two patients, delayed exploration was performed due to no improvement of symptoms, or ischemia of the left testis [3, 6]. In 25% of patients, direct exploration resulted in orchiectomy [16, 18].

Present varicocele is usually diagnosed with imaging or surgical exploration after the forming of the hematoma. Besides the case report of Gordon et al. 1993 [8], this is the only known case report where the patient had a known untreated varicocele. However, there have been case reports without signs of a varicocele at exploration [4]. In eight case reports, a present varicocele was reported, after either CUD or during exploration. It is not known if special attention was given to possible varicoceles during US examination in all cases.

In general, the scrotal hematoma is considered self-limiting and should be treated conservatively. Symptoms can be treated with NSAID's, and RICE (rest, ice, compression and elevation of the scrotum).

In our patient, the hematoma increased in size up to 3 months post-event. Only after microscopic inguinal varicocelectomy the size of the hematoma started to decrease. It is unsure whether this is a result of the treatment or time. After 15 months, the hematoma was dissolved completely. It is important to inform the patient of the possible duration of completely reabsorption to avoid anxiety and unnecessary follow-up diagnostics.

Avoiding increased abdominal pressure for patients with known varicocele, to avoid spontaneous ruptures does not seem indicated. The scarcity of case reports, as a complication of a condition present in about 15% of males, shows its rarity. Recurrent hematomas have never been described.

Conclusion

An acute scrotal hematoma secondary to a spontaneous varicocele rupture is a rare phenomenon. A literature search on case reports shows that clinical presentation is often similar to testicular torsion, appendix testis torsion, or malignancy, making differential diagnosis difficult. Especially when there has been increased abdominal pressure or strenuous activity preceding the symptoms, and the swelling is left sided, it should be included in the differential diagnosis for patient with acute inguinoscrotal swelling. Colour Doppler-Ultrasonography is the golden standard to distinguish between other causes of acute scrotum. Early surgical intervention is justified with signs of ischaemia due to obstruction, infection of the hematoma, or uncertain diagnosis (i.e. malignancy). However, physicians should be cautious whereas direct exploration was performed in almost half the case reports, which led to unnecessary orchiectomy in 25% of patients. Otherwise, the hematoma is self-limiting, and conservative treatment is recommended. The hematoma can increase in size up to 3 months post-event, and it can take up to 15 months for the hematoma to completely resolve.

Abbreviations

CDU: Colour Doppler-Ultrasonography

Acknowledgements

Not applicable.

Authors' contributions

DJR was involved in literature search and acquisition of data. DJR, PMH and MTWTL contributed to data analysis and interpretation. DJR, PMH, JW, AEBK and MTWTL drafted the manuscript. All authors contributed substantial intellectual contributions and approved the final version of the manuscript.

Author details

[1]Department of Urology, Tergooi Hospital Hilversum, Rijksstraatweg 1, 1261 AN Blaricum, The Netherlands. [2]Department of Radiology, Tergooi Hospital, Rijksstraatweg 1, 1261 AN Blaricum, The Netherlands. [3]Department of Urology, University Medical Center Utrecht, Heidelberglaan 100, 3584 CX Utrecht, The Netherlands.

References

1. Kim ED, Lipshultz LI. Role of ultrasound in the assessment of male infertility. J Clin Ultrasound. 1996;24:437–53. https://doi.org/10.1002/(SICI)1097-0096(199610)24:8<437::AID-JCU4>3.0.CO;2-L.
2. Mehta AL, Dogra VS. Intratesticular varicocele. J Clin Ultrasound. 1998;26:49–51. https://doi.org/10.1111/j.1440-1673.2005.01445.x.
3. Akay S, Kaygisiz M, Oztas M, Turgut MS. Surgically Confirmed Intra- and Extratesticular Hematoma Clinically Mimicing Epididymo-Orchitis and Radiologically Mimicing Traumatic Torsion. Polish J Radiol. 2015;80:486–9. https://doi.org/10.12659/PJR.895138.
4. Aliabadi H, Cass AS. Nontraumatic rupture of varicocele. Urology. 1987;29:421–2 http://www.ncbi.nlm.nih.gov/pubmed/3564216.
5. Bowman JR, Anton M. Spermatic Cord Hematoma in a Collegiate Football Player: A Case Report. J Athl Train. 1998;33:65–68. 16558488.
6. Chin WN, Cadogan M, Wan R, Harrison L. Spontaneous rupture of a varicocoele. West Indian Med J. 2009;58:488–9.
7. Demir Ö, Temizkan AK. Spontaneous Rupture Of Varicocele Due To Strain-Defecation. Dokuz Eylül Üniversitesi Tıp Fakültesi Derg. 2010;24:33–6. https://doi.org/10.18614/DEUTFD.17052.
8. Gordon JN, Aldoroty RA, Stone NN. A spermatic cord hematoma secondary to varicocele rupture from blunt abdominal trauma: a case report and review. J Urol. 1993;149:602–3 http://www.ncbi.nlm.nih.gov/pubmed/8437276.
9. Kobayashi S, Machida T, Ishizaka K. A case of non-traumatic rupture of varicocele. Nihon Hinyokika Gakkai Zasshi. 2006;97:801–3 http://www.ncbi.nlm.nih.gov/pubmed/17025214.
10. Lindhorst E, Paolucci V. Saxophone spermatic cord hematoma. Am J Emerg Med. 2000;18:504–5. https://doi.org/10.1053/ajem.2000.7361.

11. Matsui Y, Utsunomiya N, Ichioka K, Ueda N, Yoshimura K, Terai A. Spontaneous rupture of varicocele testis associated with advanced pancreatic cancer. Int J Urol. 2004;11:1145–6. https://doi.org/10.1111/j.1442-2042.2004.00957.x.
12. Miyoshi N, Tokito T, Eto K, Arakawa M. Hematocele of the spermatic cord. Kurume Med J. 1980;27:93–5 http://www.ncbi.nlm.nih.gov/pubmed/7431816.
13. Nishiyama Y, Nagai A, Nasu Y, Watanabe M, Kusumi N, Monden K, et al. Varicocele rupture due to sexual intercourse. Int J Urol. 2005;12:585–7. https://doi.org/10.1111/j.1442-2042.2005.01096.x.
14. Pepe P, Bonaccorsi A, Candiano G, Pietropaolo F, Panella P, Pennisi M. Acute scrotum following traumatic spermatic cord hematoma: a case report and review. Urol case reports. 2015;3:35–6. https://doi.org/10.1016/j.eucr.2014.12.006.
15. Ragozzino MW. Stretcher's scrotum. N Engl J Med. 1993;328:815. https://doi.org/10.1056/NEJM199303183281120.
16. Rolnick D. Spontaneous hematoma of spermatic cord. Am J Surg 1965;109 April 1965:519–520. http://www.ncbi.nlm.nih.gov/pubmed/4006463.
17. Takezawa K, Nakazawa S, Yoneda S, Tanigawa G, Fujita K, Okumi M, et al. Renal autotransplantation for the treatment of nutcracker phenomenon which caused varicocele rupture: a case report. Hinyokika Kiyo. 2011;57:213–6 http://www.ncbi.nlm.nih.gov/pubmed/21646854.
18. Vandana G, Maruti D. Hematocele of the spermatic cord - A case report. Apollo Med. 2016;13:185–6. https://doi.org/10.1016/j.apme.2015.08.003.
19. Kampel L, Klang E, Winkler H, Gordon B, Frenkel-Nir Y, Shoam YE. Scrotal hematoma precipitated by centrifuge training in a fighter pilot with an asymptomatic varicocele. Aerosp Med Hum Perform. 2015;86:1063–5. https://doi.org/10.3357/AMHP.4338.2015.
20. Mirilas P, Mentessidou A, Argyris I, Petropoulos A. Hematoma of the spermatic cord in a child. Am Surg. 2010;76:E131–3. https://doi.org/10.1016/0002-9610(92)90118-B.
21. Redman JF, Rountree GA, Bissada NK. Injuries to scrotal contents by blunt trauma. Urology. 1976;7:190–1.
22. Shamsa A. Spermatic cord hematoma mimicking spermatic cord torsion in a neonate. Med J Islam Repub Iran. 2000;14:101–2. http://mjiri.iums.ac.ir/article-1-910-en.html.
23. Takasu A, Morita K, Kaneko N, Sakamoto T, Okada Y. Spermatic cord injury associated with blunt trauma. Am J Emerg Med. 2005;23:806–7. https://doi.org/10.1016/j.ajem.2005.02.053.
24. Teale TP. Case of Hematocele of the spermatic cord. Prov Med J Retrosp Med Sci. 1843;6:347–9 http://www.ncbi.nlm.nih.gov/pubmed/21380153.
25. Altarac S, Mareković Z, Kalauz N, Krhen I, Derezić D. Testicular trauma sustained during football. Acta Med Croatica. 1993;47:141–3 http://www.ncbi.nlm.nih.gov/pubmed/7509667.
26. Kumar S, Rao MS, Sharma SK, Raghu K, Datta BN. Traumatic organized hematoma of the spermatic cord. J Urol. 1981;126:275–6 http://www.ncbi.nlm.nih.gov/pubmed/7265381.
27. Crosse JE, Soderdahl DW, Schamber DT. "Acute scrotum" in Henoch-Schönlein syndrome. Urology. 1976;7:66–7 http://www.ncbi.nlm.nih.gov/pubmed/1246772.
28. Eyal I, Mizrachi S, Greif Z. Spermatic cord hematoma simulating torsion of testis in Henoch-Schönlein syndrome. Harefuah. 1989;116:260–1 http://www.ncbi.nlm.nih.gov/pubmed/2722078.
29. Handmaker H, Mehn WH. Hemorrhage into spermatic cord and testicle simulating incarcerated inguinal hernia. An unusual complication of anticoagulation therapy. IMJ Ill Med J. 1969;135:697–9 http://www.ncbi.nlm.nih.gov/pubmed/4182068.
30. McKenney MG, Fietsam R, Glover JL, Villalba M. Spermatic cord hematoma: case report and literature review. Am Surg. 1996;62:768–9 http://www.ncbi.nlm.nih.gov/pubmed/8751773.
31. Shafik A, Bedeir GA. Venous tension patterns in cord veins. I. In normal and varicocele individuals. J Urol. 1980;123:383–5 http://www.ncbi.nlm.nih.gov/pubmed/7359642.
32. Siegel RL, Miller KD, Jemal A. Cancer statistics, 2017. CA Cancer J Clin. 2017; 67:7–30. https://doi.org/10.3322/caac.21387.
33. Dogra VS, Gottlieb RH, Oka M, Rubens DJ. Sonography of the scrotum. Radiology. 2003;227:18–36. https://doi.org/10.1148/radiol.2271001744.
34. Gall H, Rudofsky G, Bähren W, Roth J, Altwein JE. Intravascular pressure measurements and phlebography of the renal vein: a contribution to the etiology of varicocele. Urologe A. 1987;26:325–30 http://www.ncbi.nlm.nih.gov/pubmed/3433597.
35. Dogra V, Bhatt S. Acute painful scrotum. Radiol Clin N Am. 2004;42:349–63. https://doi.org/10.1016/j.rcl.2003.12.002.

8

Analysis of the association between paternity and reoperation for urethral obstruction in adult hypospadias patients who underwent two-stage repair in childhood

Akihiro Kanematsu[1*], Shiro Tanaka[2], Takahiko Hashimoto[1], Michio Nojima[1] and Shingo Yamamoto[1]

Abstract

Background: The association between surgical outcome of hypospadias repair and long-term male reproductive function has not been documented. The purpose of this study was to clarify association between paternity in adult hypospadias patients and reoperation for urethral obstruction after two-stage repair during childhood.

Methods: Ninety hypospadias patients who underwent the same kind of two-stage repair in our institute by a single surgeon, were initially treated at < 18 years old, and who were ≥ 18 years old during the survey were included in the study. Present physical, social, and life status were evaluated by a mailed self-entry questionnaire, and clinical background and surgical outcome data were evaluated by medical records. National survey data of the general population were used as external control. The paternity rate of the patient groups was evaluated by Kaplan-Meier curve analysis and log-rank tests.

Results: Twenty-six patients (28.9%) underwent 43 reoperations after completion of the initial repair. Twelve patients were reoperated for obstructive complication (Study group) and were compared with 14 patients who were reoperated only for non-obstructive causes and 64 patients who were not reoperated as Study control group ($N = 78$). The Study group patients showed sexual intercourse rate and marriage rate not statistically different in comparison with the Study control, although marriage rate at 32.5 years old were lower than the general population ($p = 0.048$, z-test). None of the Study group achieved paternity, which showed a significant difference to the Study control ($p = 0.032$, log-rank test). The difference was also statistically significant in the analysis among the 31 married patients ($p = 0.012$, log-rank test). Patients reoperated for obstructive complication documented worsened Quality of Life score in the International Prostate Symptom Score (2.3 ± 2.0 vs. 1.4 ± 1.2, $p = 0.031$, t-test) and ejaculation problems (66.7% vs. 17.4%, $p = 0.003$, chi-square test).

Conclusions: History of reoperation for obstructive complication was associated with lower paternity rate in patients with hypospadias, presumably for multifactorial causes associated with marriage age and ejaculation problems. The present results may implicate importance of uncomplicated urethroplasty during childhood for achieving paternity, although it should be further tested in the future for larger groups of hypospadias patients.

Keywords: Epidemiology, Hypospadias, Paternity, Surgery, Urethral obstruction

* Correspondence: aqui@hyo-med.ac.jp
[1]Department of Urology, Hyogo College of Medicine, Mukogawacho 1-1, Nishinomiya, Hyogo 663-8501, Japan
Full list of author information is available at the end of the article

Background

Hypospadias is a defect in penile development. The natural history of mild hypospadias is unclear but could have a mostly benign course without treatment [1]. However, patients with more severe hypospadias undergo repair during infancy, in the hope that with corrected penis, the patient will subsequently have a normal reproductive function as a male. However, long-term consequences in patients with repaired hypospadias have been unclear.

Population based studies have reported decreased paternity in hypospadias patients, but precise disease and surgical background were not implicated in those studies [2, 3]. Several groups have recently conducted long-term follow-up studies, [4–9] and a Swedish group reported that sexual function and fertility of adult patients with hypospadias are equivalent to those of their age-matched controls but inferior in proximal type patients [7]. In our previous report, we introduced a survival analysis method for analyzing the outcome of patients with hypospadias operated at our institute. We also reported that patients with hypospadias in general had equivalent intercourse and marriage rates compared with the general population [10]. Our study also revealed that while sexual intercourse, marriage, and paternity occurred in serial order, overlap was scant in the factors associated with these three events. The intercourse rate was lower in patients with proximal hypospadias, and the marriage rate was lower in those without stable jobs. These were expected findings, but were statistically proven for the first time using multivariate survival analysis.

An unexpected finding in that study was the lower paternity rate in those who underwent reoperation after the initial repair. We did not analyze this finding further, because that study had included patients who had undergone diverse surgical procedures including two-stage repair, one-stage repair, and reoperative procedures after multiple repairs. Therefore, in this study, we analyzed the paternity data of our hypospadias patient cohort, exclusively limited to those who underwent the same initial two-stage repair operation in relation to surgical complications requiring reoperation. We hypothesized that reoperation for urethral obstruction after initial hypospadias repair could be related with decreased paternity, and aimed to clarify the association between them.

Methods

Subjects

Patients with hypospadias operated between 1973 and 1998 by a single surgeon at our institution were candidates for this study. During this period, no other surgeon performed hypospadias repairs at our institution. Two-stage repair was the preferred procedure. In the first stage, the chordee tissue surrounding the penile shaft was completely removed and glandular urethra was created by inverted preputial flap. In the second stage, the skin between glandular urethra and original meatus was tubularized using a method like the Johansson technique. This procedure was the mainstay for most hypospadias repairs for 25 years at our institution, with the exception of very mild glandular cases, for which, other techniques such as meatal advancement and glanuloplasty-incorporated procedures were performed [11].

Data collection

This study was approved by the Ethics Committee of the Hyogo college of Medicine (approval number 1147). We contacted the parents of the candidate patients by postal mail and asked them to forward a self-entry questionnaire and an informed consent form to the patients. In addition to the International Prostate Symptom Score (IPSS) [12] and the International Index of Erectile Function-5 (IIEF-5), [13] the survey included questions by Moriya et al., regarding the patients' educational and social history, sexual and marital experience, paternity, present complaints with respect to penile shape, hesitation before and after the first intercourse, and difficulties during intercourse and ejaculation, as described in the Additional file 2 [14]. History of additional surgery for hypospadias outside our institute was also obtained. Patients who had undergone a two-stage repair in our institute at < 18 years of age, were ≥ 18 years during the current survey, and had returned evaluable responses were included in the study. All study participants provided written informed consent. Those with documented sex development disorders, two with mixed gonadal dysgenesis and one with XX male, were excluded. As was done in our previous study, glandular and penile type hypospadias were compared with proximal type. Data of birth weight, gestational age at birth, hypospadias type, presence of undescended testes, and additional surgical procedures performed after repair completion were extracted from the patients' clinical records. National survey data of general population were used as external control to assess sexual intercourse and marriage rates, which were respectively defined as the percentage of the male population in the country that have had sexual intercourse and been married at least once [15].

Main outcome measures

Patients were initially divided into three groups, those with no reoperation and those reoperated for either non-obstructive or obstructive complications. Patients with a history of at least one reoperative procedure for obstructive causes were considered as reoperated for obstruction. Based on the findings described in the Additional file 1: Figure S1, patients having no reoperation and those reoperated only for non-obstructive cause were used as Study control group for the Study group of patients reoperated for obstructive causes (Additional file 1: Figure S1 and Fig. 1).

Statistical analyses

Kaplan–Meier curves were used for estimating rates of masturbation, heterosexual intercourse, marriage, and paternity. The intercourse and marriage rates were compared with the age-specific rates reported in a national survey of the general population, using z-tests with Kaplan–Meier estimates and their standard errors. Analyses for paternity were performed using the age at marriage of the patients with offspring, as the precise birth time of their children had not been asked in the questionnaire. The comparison between the subdivided groups was performed using a log-rank test on Kaplan–Meier curves, and comparison with General population was performed by z-tests, with $p < 0.05$ considered to be significant. Chi-square test and t-test were used to assess the differences between the groups. All statistical analyses were performed using JMP 9 software (SAS Institute Inc., Cary, NC, USA).

Results

Study population

Our initial pool consisted of 910 potential participants, with 392 (43.0%) questionnaires returned undelivered. Of the remaining 518 patients, 152 patients (28.4%) returned the completed questionnaires, as reported in our previous study [10]. Of these, 90 patients with a history of the same two-stage repair by the single surgeon [16] were included in this study (Fig. 1).

Development ladder of male sexual life

Development of male sexual activities is plotted in Fig. 2. Patients with hypospadias are known to experience sexual desire and begin masturbation during puberty similar to other males, [9, 14] which was a finding confirmed by our study cohort. The experience rates of both sexual intercourse and marriage also increased along with age. Consistent with the findings of our previous study, the rates were equivalent to the general population data derived from the national survey [10, 15]. Paternity rates also increased with participant age but did not equal marriage rates.

Classification and timing of reoperation

We classified reoperated participants based on whether the underlying urethral complication was obstructive or non-obstructive. In total, 26 patients (28.9%) underwent 43 reoperative procedures, of which 18, 24, and 1 were for obstructive, non-obstructive, and unknown causes, respectively (Table 1). The cumulative experience of reoperation after the initial repair completion is plotted in Fig. 3. The overall reoperation rate was < 20% at 2 years, as previously reported,(16) but continued to increase over the years. The timing of the first reoperation was similar between the patients operated for either obstructive ($n = 12$) or non-obstructive ($n = 14$) complications. The age of the last reoperation was 13.8 ± 8.2 y for those with obsructive complications, and 9.6 ± 5.5 y for those with non-obstructive complications ($p = 0.063$).

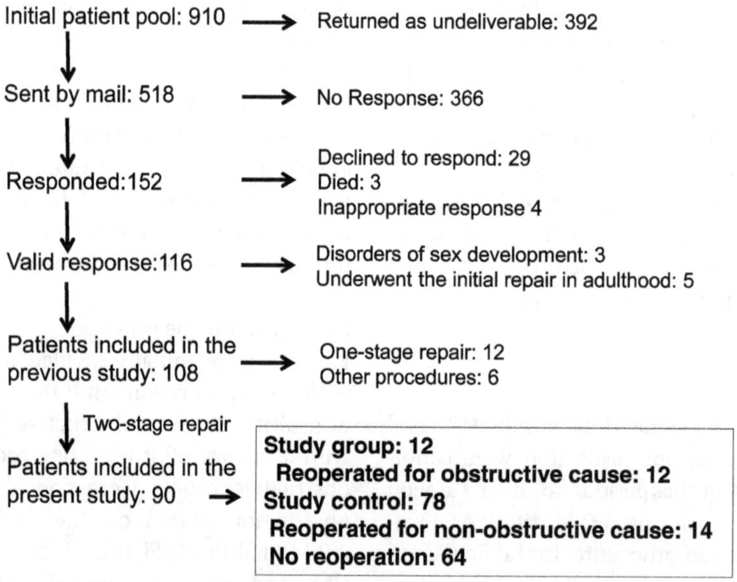

Fig. 1 A diagram showing selection of the study patients from the initial candidate pool

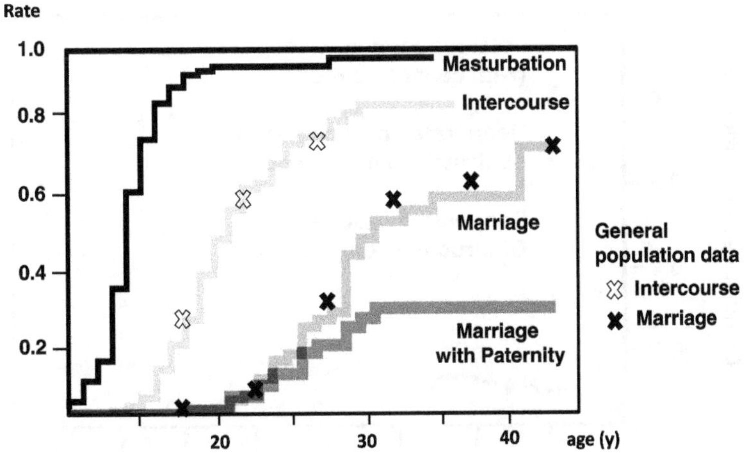

Fig. 2 Developmental ladder of male sexual activity in the study patients. Developmental ladder of male sexual activity in the study patients is demonstrated as Kaplan–Meier curves. Most of the patients experienced masturbation by the end of puberty. Intercourse and marriage rates of the general population as reported in the national survey are plotted by X. The intercourse and marriage rates were not statistically different to the control data (z-test) [10]. Paternity is plotted as date of marriage of the patients with offspring

Reoperation for obstructive complication is associated with a lower paternity rate

We, performed survival analysis of the patients. Those reoperated for obstructive causes were defined as Study group (n = 12). The non-reoperated cases ($n = 64$) along with the patients reoperated only for non-obstructive causes ($n = 14$) were grouped together as the Study control group ($n = 78$). The sexual intercourse rate was statistically equivalent between the Study group and the Study controls (Fig. 4a). However, in comparison with that in the General population, the age at marriage was equivalent in the Study controls, but significantly higher in the Study group at 32.5 years old (†: $p = 0.048$, z-test). Notably, no patients in the Study group had offspring. The difference was statistically significant both in the analyses among the total patients (Fig. 4c, $p = 0.032$ by log-rank test) and among the 31 married patients (Fig. 4d, $p = 0.012$ by log-rank test). The two cohorts of Study control group, patients without reoperation and patients reoperated only for non-obstructing complications showed similar curve in either analysis (Additional file 1: Figure S1A and B).

Table 1 Complication and time until reoperative procedures

Complication	Procedure	Case	Procedure	Post-operative time to procedure (mo)				
				Median	Min	Max	Mean	SD
Obstructive		12	18	41.5	3	120	86.2	41.5
Urethral stricture	Internal urethrotomy	7	12	44	3	120	44	42.9
	Urethral dilation	1	1	2	NA	NA	NA	NA
Meatal stenosis	Meatal cutback	2	2	15.5	3	28	NA	NA
Urethral dilatation	Reduction urethroplasty	3	3	96	17	252	NA	NA
Not obstructive		19[a]	24	30	6	190	76.7	75
Meatal regression	Meatoplasty	12	14	98	11	190	102.2	87.5
Fistula	Fistula closure	6	7	26	6	93	44.4	37.8
	Cutback to fistula	1	1	28	NA	NA	NA	NA
Recurrent bending	Chordectomy	1	1	18	NA	NA	NA	NA
	Repeat Urethroplasty		1	30	NA	NA	NA	NA
Unknown	Unknown	1	1	240	NA	NA	NA	NA
Total		26	43	41.5	3	332	82.2	41.5

[a] Including 5 cases who also had obstructive complications. One case had 1 fistula closure and 1 meatoplasty

SD Standard deviation

NA Not applicable

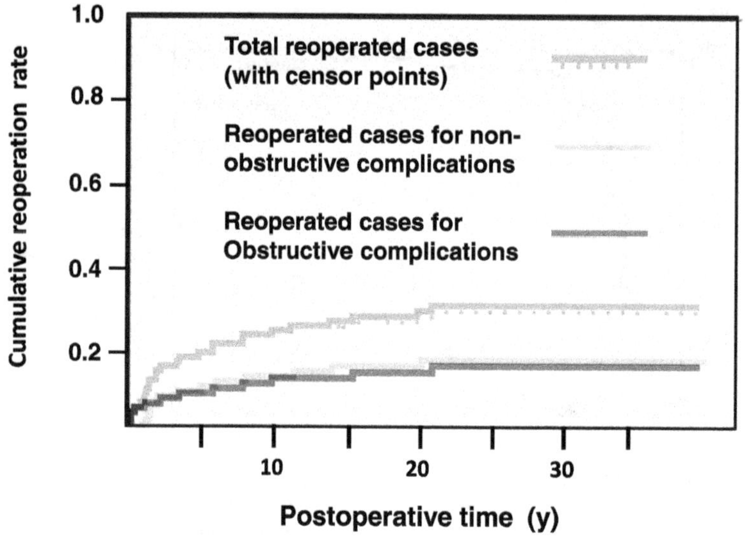

Fig. 3 Cumulative incidence of reoperation. Cumulative incidence of total reoperation ($n = 26$), reoperation for obstructive complications ($n = 12$), and reoperation for non-obstructive complications ($n = 14$) is plotted as Kaplan–Meier curves. Patients who had at least one procedure for obstructive causes were classified as reoperated for obstructive complications. For the patients undergoing multiple reoperations, event points were plotted as the date of first reoperation after the initial repair. Reoperative procedures decreased along with time but were performed for nearly 20 years postoperatively. The occurrence of reoperation was nearly identical between the patients operated for obstructive and non-obstructive complications

Clinical and social data of the patients stratified by presence and type of reoperation

Clinical and social data of the patients are listed in Table 2. While the gestational age at birth was lower in the Study group than in the Study controls, the birth weight was not significantly different. Interestingly, distribution of hypospadias type was similar among those who had reoperation and those who did not. No difference was noted in the rate of concomitant undescended testes either. The mean age at the time of survey and the follow-up time were significantly longer in the Study group than in the Study controls. Job status, intercourse rates, and marriage rates were equivalent between both groups. Although the Study group patients tended to marry older, hesitation before and after the first intercourse experience was not significantly higher than the Control.

Persistent difficulties in micturition and ejaculation in patients reoperated for urethral obstruction

Present symptoms of the patients were evaluated through a mailed questionnaire (Table 3). The IPSS-QOL score revealed impaired micturition status in the Study group compared with the Study controls. However, the difference between the two groups for the total IPSS as well as for each IPSS domain and subdomains (subdivided into either obstructive or non-obstructive symptoms) was not statistically significant. This may indicate that the impaired IPSS-QOL score may be related to micturition issues not expressed by specific IPSS questions.

The patients reported problems associated with sexuality by responding to IIEF-5 and questionnaires by Moriya et al.,[14] which included questions asking whether patients had problems with penile shape, sexual intercourse (i.e., if they had experienced any), and ejaculation. Patients were also asked whether they experienced any hesitation before and after their first intercourse experience. No statistically significant difference was noted in IIEF-5 Q1 nor in questions about penile shape and intercourse. The problem of bending was documented by 9/78 (11.5%) in control, and 1/11 (9.0%) in study ($P = 0.78$, not significant). It was problematic for sexual intercourse in only one patient in Control group. The main issue reported was that the patients had to squeeze the semen out during ejaculation, but none documented anejaculation. The only significant finding was that a higher proportion of the Study group had problems with ejaculation than that of the Study controls, specifically for weak or incomplete ejaculation (66.7% vs. 15.6%, $p = 0.0017$). Therefore, ejaculation difficulties were the only subjective problem significantly associated with a history of urethral reoperation for obstructive causes. These results may suggest that urethral obstruction have caused ejaculatory problems in the Study group patients.

Discussion

This study reports that reoperation for obstructive complications after the initial pediatric urethroplasty was associated with a decreased paternity rate in adult

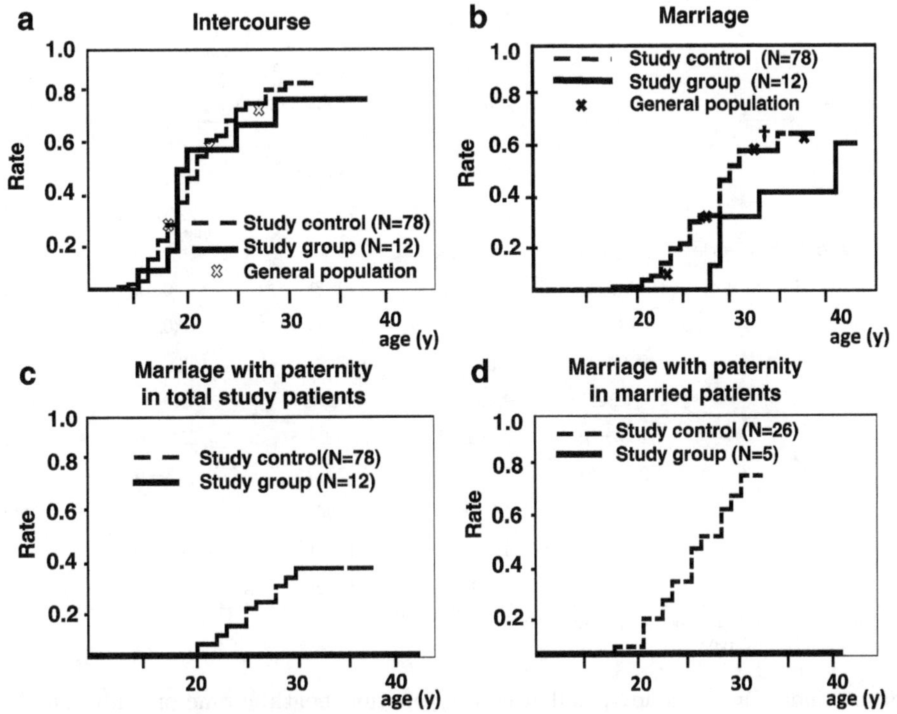

Fig. 4 The cumulative rate of sexual intercourse, marriage, and paternity. **a** and **b** The cumulative rate of sexual intercourse and marriage is shown, stratified as having been reoperated for obstructive complication (Study group) or others (Study controls), together with national survey data (General population, plotted by X). **a** No statistical difference was noted in the intercourse rate ($p = 0.76$) between the Study group and Study controls. There was no significant difference with the General population either. **b** The marriage rate of the Study group at 32.5 years old was significantly lower than that of the General population (†: $p = 0.048$, z-test). At 27.5 years old, the marriage rate of the General population and Study group was radically different, 36.7% vs. 0%, although *p*-values of the z-test could not be calculated because there was no event in the Study group before these time points. *P*-value for the difference in the marriage rate between the Study group and Study controls was not statistically significant in the log-rank test ($p = 0.13$). **c** and **d** No paternity was observed in patients reoperated for obstruction. Paternity rates were significantly lower in patients reoperated for obstruction in analysis of total patients (**c**, $p = 0.032$ by log-rank test) and in analysis of married patients (**d**, $p = 0.012$ by log-rank test)

hypospadias patients who had undergone a two-stage procedure at our institution. This type of study, linking a childhood surgical outcome with the adult potential for paternity, is scarce in literature.

This study was conducted as a sub-analysis of our previous report, which unexpectedly revealed that urethral reoperation was related to decreased paternity. Out of 108 patients in our earlier study, we selected out 90 patients who underwent a two-stage repair by a single surgeon from mild to severe type of hypospadias. Thus, we could analyze the surgical results without being confounded by differences in the surgical procedure. The two-stage repair was the mainstay for most of the hypospadias patients at the time. Among the 518 mailed patients with the exclusion of 80 cases in which operative procedure was not identified, 81.7% (358/438) underwent the same two-stage repair, which is equivalent to 83.3% (90/108) of the present and previous studies. This may indicate that our responders represent the total patient group treated during that period without significant selection bias with regard to the operation procedure.

We analyzed the type of reoperations the patients underwent and found that reoperations have been performed for more than 20 years after the initial repair. Such accumulation of reoperations in longer studies has also been reported by other authors [17]. This finding could explain why the final reoperation rate was as high as 28.9% in the surgeon's series who documented less than 10% reoperation rate in up to 5 years of follow-up [16]. The timing of urethrocutaneous fistula repair after the initial repair was relatively shorter than that of the other types of reoperation. The total fistula rate, 7.8% (7/90), was similar to the short-term result of the same surgeon's series, which reported a fistula rate of around 7.9–8.9% for all degrees of hypospadias [16]. Reoperations for other two major complications, urethral obstruction and meatal regression, typically occurred after a longer interval. Interestingly, in our patients, the complication rates between the proximal cases and the non-proximal cases were similar, presumably due to the uniformity of the procedure.

Table 2 Clinical and social data of the patients

		Total	Study Control			Study Group (Reoperated for obstruction)	P-value
			No reoperation	Reoperated No obstruction	Control Sum		
Number		90	64	14	78	12	
Gestational age at birth (weeks)		38.0 ± 3.1	38.3 ± 2.8	36.9 ± 3.1	38.2 ± 2.86	35.5 ± 5.1[a]	0.015
Birth weight (g)		2764 ± 783	2707 ± 812	2921 ± 733	2750.5 ± 760.5	2789 ± 863	0.88
Hypospadias type	Grandular and Penile	44 (0.49)	31 (0.48)	7 (0.50)	38(0.49)	6 (0.50)	1
	Proximal[b]	34 (0.38)	24 (0.38)	6 (0.43)	30(0.38)	4 (0.33)	
	Unknown	12 (0.13)	9 (0.14)	1 (0.07)	10(0.13)	2 (0.17)	
Undescended testis		9 (0.10)	7 (0.11)	1 (0.07)	8(0.10)	1 (0.08)	1
Operated age (y)		4.3 ± 2.9	4.6 ± 3.3	3.3 ± 1.6	4.3 ± 3.1	4.0 ± 1.7	0.74
Age at the time of survey (y)		28.7 ± 6.9	27.7 ± 8.1	27.5 ± 7..5	27.7 ± 6.4	34.8 ± 7.4[a]	0.0061
Follow up time (y)		24.3 ± 6.6	23.2 ± 5.9	24.2 ± 7.2	23.3 ± 6.1	30.8 ± 6.7[a]	0.0001
Stable job	n (rate)	57 (0.63)	42 (0.66)	7 (0.50)	49 (0.63)	8 (0.67)	1
Intercourse	n (rate)	77 (0.74)	43 (0.67)	8 (0.57)	51 (0.65)	9 (0.75)	0.74
Marriage	n (rate)	31 (0.34)	21 (0.33)	5 (0.36)	26 (0.33)	5 (0.42)	0.75

[a] Statistically significant compared with the Study control by t-test ($p < 0.05$)
[b] Proximal: Penoscrotal, Scrotal and Perineal Type

The most important finding in this study was that in a sharp contrast to that in the Study controls, paternity was absent in the Study group patients who were reoperated for obstructive complications of the urethra, despite the longer follow-up period and the higher age of the participants at the time of study. This is a novel finding, as paternity data in hypospadias patients have not previously been associated with a surgical outcome during childhood in the existing literature. While one relevant article from Sweden reported lower paternity in patients

Table 3 Questionnaire data of the patients

	Study Control			Study group (Reoperated for obstruction)	P-value
	No reoperation	Reoperated No obstruction	Control Sum		
Number	64	14	78	12	
IPSS total	3.5 ± 3.8	3.9 ± 4.5	3.6 ± 3.9	4.9 ± 5.6	0.31
IPSS-QOL	1.4 ± 1.2	1.4 ± 1.2	1.4 ± 1.2	2.3 ± 2.0	0.037[a]
IIEF-5 Q1	3.2 ± 0.9	3.6 ± 1.1	3.3 ± 0.9	3.3 ± 1.0	1
Married patients	21 (0.33)	5 (0.36)	26 (0.33)	5 (0.41)	0.75
Patients with paternity	10 (0.16)	3 (0.21)	13 (0.16)	0 (0.0)	0.2
IIEF-5 total (for married patients only)	20.6 ± 4.2	21.2 ± 2.3	20.7 ± 3.9	20.1 ± 2.9	0.75
Problems (Yes/Response (Rate))					
Penile shapes	33/64 (0.52)	9/14 (0.64)	42/78 (0.54)	5/11 (0.45)	1
Penile bending	7/64 (10.9)	2/14 (0.14)	9/78 (11.5)	1/11 (0.90)	0.78
Intercourse	13/49 (0.27)	0/8 (0.00)	13/57 (0.23)	4/9 (0.44)	0.22
Difficult intercourse for penile bending	1/45	0/8	1/53	0/9	1
Ejaculation	11/63 (0.17)	2/14 (0.14)	13/77 (0.17)	6/9 (0.67)	0.0042[b]
Weak or incomplete ejaculation	10/63 (0.16)	2/14 (0.14)	12/77 (0.16)	6/9 (0.67)	0.0017[b]
Hesitation for intercourse (Yes/Response (Rate))					
Before first intercourse	19/55 (0.35)	1/12 (0.08)	20/78 (0.30)	4/10 (0.40)	0.34
After first intercourse	10/44 (0.27)	0/8 (0.00)	10/52 (0.19)	3/8 (0.38)	0.48

[a] Statistically significant compared between Study group and control by t-test ($p < 0.05$)
[b] Statistically significant compared between Study group and control by Fischer' exact test ($p < 0.05$)

with proximal hypospadias, the surgical complications were not implicated as a cause, and the patients in that study had undergone diverse surgical procedures by multiple surgeons [7].

The cause of lower paternity in our Study group patients may be multifactorial. The z-test revealed that the marriage rate of the Study group at 32.5 years old was significantly lower than that of the General population, implying that these patients married later in life. We cannot infer whether reoperation for urethral obstruction delayed their marriage, either for psychological or physical reasons. Mureau et al. reported that, the later the patients underwent surgery, the greater were their inhibitions in seeking sexual contact and the later they made the first sexual contacts [18]. However, between the patients reoperated for obstructive or non-obstructive cause, the timing of the first and last reoperation was not statistically significant, nor was the age of first intercourse.

As another point, a later marriage may have reduced the child-bearing period, with presumably more aged partner that those who married earlier. There were 5 married patients in the study group, all of whom did not achieve paternity. Since we did not ask them whether they had attempted to have children, we cannot conclude whether they were infertile or simply elected to remain childless. It is plausible that urethral obstruction had an adverse effect on sperm emission, since the Study group documented difficulties with ejaculation at a rate significantly higher than the Study controls. Since 4 out of the 5 married Study group patients underwent only palliative surgery such as 3 internal urethrotomy and 1 urethral dilatation, they might still have had urethral obstruction persisting into adulthood. However, we lack the seminalysis, uroflow, and concrete penile shape data, which is a major limitation of our study, as we relied mainly on questionnaires to collect data. One interesting point is that, after exclusion of the patients reoperated for obstructive causes, the final paternity rate of the married patients in the Study controls reached nearly 80% on the Kaplan–Meier curve (Fig. 4d), which is equivalent to that of the general population at 83.3% [15]. We may thus infer that if there had been no obstructive pathology that required reoperation, the final paternity rate of hypospadias patients might have been closer to that of the general population.

Because this study is a sub-analysis of our previous study, it has the same kind of limitation as have been already documented in the earlier report. One drawback, inevitable in this type of study, was the limited response rate to the questionnaires, although our response rate at 28.4% was comparable to that in other similar studies [6, 14]. Limited response can cause selection bias, but we would like to note that there was no significant difference in background between the responders and non-responders with respect to hypospadias severity as reported in the previous study [15] and the type of initial repair procedure as described in this report. Another limitation is that the majority of the information regarding the present condition of the participants was obtained through a survey, and there is a lack of objective data, such as seminalysis or uroflowmetry. Since our data derive from limited number of patients, with 12 Study group patients without offsprings, of which only 5 were married, our findings should be further tested by future study by different groups and by ourselves. To overcome this drawback in such future studies, we may have to maintain a prospective follow-up protocol up to adulthood when we discharge our patients from outpatient visit today. Lastly, the data were obtained from patients who underwent a hypospadias repair surgery different from more recent procedures, and the patients were generally older at the time of initial repair than today. Over the last two decades, surgery for hypospadias correction has shifted to different types of one-stage repair, with the urethral plate as the preferred material compared to preputial skin used earlier [19, 20] and patients tend to be treated at a younger age. Although current repair like tubularized incised plate method may have better results than the procedures performed in this article, twenty to thirty year follow up should be needed to obtain final outcome, as described in this report.

Conclusions

The findings in this report may suggest that reoperation for urethral obstruction was associated with lower paternity, but because of the limited number of Study patients, it should be further tested by the future studies in larger groups of hypospadias patients. Nonetheless, the present results may implicate importance of uncomplicated urethroplasty during childhood for achieving paternity and may be a warning message from the past for current and future hypospadias surgeons.

Additional files

Additional file 1: Figure S1. The cumulative rate of paternity in reoperated patients with or without obstruction compared with patients without reoperation. A. and B.: Fig. 4c and d are repotted with Study control data subdivided into two cohorts, patients without reoperation and patients reoperated only for non-obstructing complications. Note that the two cohorts of the Study control show similar curve in either analysis. (PPTX 79 kb)

Additional file 2: Excerpts from Hypospadias-specific questionnaire (from Moriya et al. [14]). (DOCX 20 kb)

Abbreviations

IIEF-5: International Index of Erectile Function; IPSS: International Prostate Symptom Score; IPSS-QOL: IPSS Quality of Life Score

Acknowledgments
We thank Dr. Kimihiko Moriya for providing us the questionnaires. We acknowledge the contribution of late Dr. Fumihiko Ikoma, who performed the surgical procedures on the participants as described in this article.

Authors' contributions
AK designed the study, collected and analyzed data and prepared the manuscript. ST assisted and advised on statistical analyses. TH assisted in data collection. MN and SY have made major contribution in conception of the study, interpretation of data, and revision of the initial draft manuscript. All authors have read and approved the manuscript.

Author details
[1]Department of Urology, Hyogo College of Medicine, Mukogawacho 1-1, Nishinomiya, Hyogo 663-8501, Japan. [2]Department of Clinical Biostatistics, Graduate School of Medicine Kyoto University, Yoshida Konoecho, Sakyo, Kyoto 606-8501, Japan.

References

1. Schlomer B, Breyer B, Copp H, Baskin L, DiSandro M. Do adult men with untreated hypospadias have adverse outcomes? A pilot study using a social media advertised survey. J Pediatr Urol. 2014;10(4):672–9.
2. Schneuer FJ, Milne E, Jamieson SE, et al. Association between male genital anomalies and adult male reproductive disorders: a population-based data linkage study spanning more than 40 years. Lancet Child Adolesc Health. 2018;2(10):736–43.
3. Asklund C, Jensen TK, Main KM, Sobotka T, Skakkebaek NE, Jorgensen N. Semen quality, reproductive hormones and fertility of men operated for hypospadias. Int J Androl. 2010;33(1):80–7.
4. Rynja SP, de Jong TP, Bosch JL, de Kort LM. Functional, cosmetic and psychosexual results in adult men who underwent hypospadias correction in childhood. J Pediatr Urol. 2011;7(5):504–15.
5. Schonbucher VB, Landolt MA, Gobet R, Weber DM. Health-related quality of life and psychological adjustment of children and adolescents with hypospadias. J Pediatr. 2008;152(6):865–72.
6. Wang WW, Tu XA, Deng CH, Mo JC, Zhao L, Chen LW. Long-term sexual activity status and influencing factors in men after surgery for hypospadias. Asian J Androl. 2009;11(4):417–22.
7. Ortqvist L, Fossum M, Andersson M, Nordenstrom A, Frisen L, Holmdahl G, et al. Sexuality and fertility in men with hypospadias; improved outcome. Andrology. 2017;5(2):286–93.
8. Fraumann SA, Stephany HA, Clayton DB, Thomas JC, JCt P, Adams MC, et al. Long-term follow-up of children who underwent severe hypospadias repair using an online survey with validated questionnaires. J Pediatr Urol. 2014;10(3):446–50.
9. Vandendriessche S, Baeyens D, Van Hoecke E, Indekeu A, Hoebeke P. Body image and sexuality in adolescents after hypospadias surgery. J Pediatr Urol. 2010;6(1):54–9.
10. Kanematsu A, Higuchi Y, Tanaka S, Hashimoto T, Nojima M, Yamamoto S. Multivariate analysis of the factors associated with sexual intercourse, marriage, and paternity of hypospadias patients. J Sex Med. 2016;13(10):1488–95.
11. Duckett JW, Snyder HM 3rd. Meatal advancement and glanuloplasty hypospadias repair after 1,000 cases: avoidance of meatal stenosis and regression. J Urol. 1992;147(3):665–9.
12. Homma Y, Tsukamoto T, Yasuda K, Ozono S, Yoshida M, Shinji M. Linguistic validation of Japanese version of international prostate symptom score and BPH impact index. Nihon Hinyokika Gakkai Zasshi. 2002;93(6):669–80.
13. Marumo K, Murai M. Aging and erectile dysfunction: the role of aging and concomitant chronic illness. Int J Urol. 2001;8(8):S50–7.
14. Moriya K, Kakizaki H, Tanaka H, Furuno T, Higashiyama H, Sano H, et al. Long-term cosmetic and sexual outcome of hypospadias surgery: norm related study in adolescence. J Urol. 2006;176(4 Pt 2):1889–92 discussion 92–3.
15. A national survey on marriage and delivery. National Institute of Population and Social Security Research, 2010.
16. Schumacher S, Yabumoto H, Salge S, Shrestha G, Ikoma F. Surgical results of complete hypospadias repair in two stages. Int Urol Nephrol. 1997;29(3):333–40.
17. Spinoit AF, Poelaert F, Groen LA, Van Laecke E, Hoebeke P. Hypospadias repair at a tertiary care center: long-term followup is mandatory to determine the real complication rate. J Urol. 2013;189(6):2276–81.
18. Mureau MA, Slijper FM, van der Meulen JC, Verhulst FC, Slob AK. Psychosexual adjustment of men who underwent hypospadias repair: a norm-related study. J Urol. 1995;154(4):1351–5.
19. Baskin LS, Duckett JW, Ueoka K, Seibold J, Snyder HM 3rd. Changing concepts of hypospadias curvature lead to more onlay island flap procedures. J Urol. 1994;151(1):191–6.
20. Snodgrass W. Tubularized, incised plate urethroplasty for distal hypospadias. J Urol. 1994;151(2):464–5.

9

Comparison of Yang-Monti ileal ureter-bladder anastomosis versus Yang-Monti ileal ureter-ureteral anastomosis for the treatment of ureteral stenosis: A randomized controlled trial in a miniature pig model

Wang Zhenxing[1,2], Sun Zhaolin[3*], Yang Xiushu[3*], Luo Guangheng[3], Tian Ye[3], Shen Lei[4], Su Zhiyong[5] and Liu Hongming[6]

Abstract

Background: The aim of the present study was to establish an animal model of Yang-Monti ileal ureter-bladder anastomosis and Yang-Monti ileal ureter-ureteral anastomosis and compare the advantages and disadvantages of the two surgical methods.

Methods: Fourteen 12-month-old male Chinese miniature pigs weighing 21 ± 1.38 kg were randomly divided into two groups. Group A ($n = 7$) underwent end-to-end anastomosis of the left Yang-Monti ileal ureter, left ileal ureter and left lower ureter; group B (n = 7) underwent anastomosis of the left Yang-Monti ileal ureter, left ileal ureter and bladder. In both groups, the contralateral kidney was removed at 1 week postoperatively. The incision length and operation time of the two groups were compared. Changes in serum creatinine and urea nitrogen were observed preoperatively, and at 2, 6 and 12 weeks postoperatively. Venous pyelography and cystography were performed at 12 weeks postoperatively to determine the ureteral patency and vesicoureteral reflux. At 12 months postoperatively, urinary culture was performed, and the diameter and histological changes of the intestinal ureter were assessed.

(Continued on next page)

* Correspondence: 763920818@qq.com; 13985037039@139.com
[3]Department of Urology, Guizhou Provincial People's Hospital, No. 83 East Zhongshan Road, Guiyang 550002, Guizhou, China
Full list of author information is available at the end of the article

(Continued from previous page)

Results: Surgery was successfully completed in all 14 pigs. In group A, one pig died due to an anesthetic accident, and one pig died from a lung infection on postoperative day 4. In group B, one pig died from adhesive intestinal obstruction on postoperative day 7. The overall survival rate was 78.6%, and the 11 surviving pigs had no urinary or intestinal fistulae. Compared with group B, group A had a significantly longer surgical incision (30.86 ± 2.41 cm versus 26.71 ± 3.64 cm; $p = 0.01$) and shorter operation time (181.29 ± 15.10 min versus 157.71 ± 20.49 min; $p = 0.02$). The serum creatinine and urea nitrogen concentrations did not significantly differ between groups. All pigs had normal renal function pre- and postoperatively. There was no stenosis or obstruction on venous pyelography. The narrowest diameter of the ureter was significantly smaller in group B (5.90 ± 0.30 mm) than in group A (7.26 ± 1.06 mm; $p = 0.01$), but no contrast agent returned to the upper urinary tract in either group. *Escherichia coli* was detected on urine culture. In group A, one pig had obstruction of the ureteral ureter, while another had stenosis of the lower ureteral anastomosis. In group B, one pig had pelvic and intestinal ureteral dilatation; however, all anastomoses were patent. The ileal ureteral diameter was significantly larger in group A (9.40 ± 2.35 mm) than group B (6.62 ± 0.37 mm; $p = 0.02$). Two pigs in group A had separation of the transitional epithelium and columnar epithelial mucosa, with granulation tissue hyperplasia. The pigs with stenosis and obstruction had smooth fibrous tissue and smooth muscle of the anastomosis. In both groups, the two types of epithelial tissue were close together, and the intestinal villi were mildly atrophied and shortened.

Conclusions: An animal model of Yang-Monti ileal ureter-bladder anastomosis was successfully established. Compared with Yang-Monti ileal ureter-ureteral anastomosis, Yang-Monti ileal ureter-bladder anastomosis is simpler, more reliable, and results in fewer complications.

Keywords: Ureteral long stricture, Yang-Monti ileal ureter reconstruction, Ureter-bladder anastomosis, Ureter-ureteral anastomosis

Background

With the widespread development of urological endoscopic surgery, iatrogenic injury has become one of the most common causes of ureteral injury [1], and the incidence of long-term ureteral injury is increasing. The most serious complication of ureteroscopy is ureteral avulsion, with an incidence of 0.06–0.45% [2–5]. Most cases of lower ureteral avulsion are treated with ureteral bladder replantation. However, multiple operations cause adhesions and stenosis in the lower ureter, poor blood supply to the ureter, difficulty in healing postoperatively, scarring, and result in a ureter with a small diameter and thin wall, which is not conducive to anastomosis.

The Yang-Monti technique for ileal ureteral reconstruction is used in clinical practice and has good curative effects [6–8]. The characteristics of this method are that the alternative ureteral tube diameter is the same as that of the original ureter, the intestinal tube is short, the diameter of the replacement tube is small, and the intestinal tube is saved. In addition, the absorptive and secretive functions of the intestinal segment used in ureteral reconstruction are decreased because the absorbent surface area is limited and the mucous production is decreased, preventing occlusion of the lumen and postoperative metabolic abnormalities.

It remains controversial whether there is a need for an anti-reflux procedure in ureteral reconstruction. Some studies report that there is no need to establish an anti-reflux anastomosis, while others advocate the establishment of anti-reflux procedures [9–11]; furthermore, there is reportedly no difference in efficacy in accordance with the performance of an anti-reflux procedure [12]. In the non-anti-reflux procedure, the ileal ureter was implanted into the bladder directly. The operation is relatively simple and convenient, the operation time is short, and the incision is small. However, there may be a backflow of urine from the bladder to the replacement ureter or ipsilateral kidney, resulting in postoperative intestinal dilatation, ascending infection, pyelonephritis, hydronephrosis, and impaired renal function [13]. To reduce the incidence of such complications, anti-reflux anastomosis involves the insertion of a nipple structure at the ileal bladder junction [14], a proximal ileal wall tunnel anti-reflux procedure [15, 16], and an extra-urinary ureter tunnel extension (Lich-Gregoir method) [7, 12].

When the lower ureter is well preserved, the ileal ureter can be anastomosed to the lower ureter, but this may cause postoperative complications such as mucus obstruction and anastomotic stenosis. If the lower ureter cannot be anastomosed, the intestinal ureter needs to be re-implanted in the bladder to prevent reflux. This is achieved via Yang-Monti ileal ureter and bladder anastomosis or Yang-Monti ileal ureter and lower ureteral anastomosis [7]. We established animal models of the Yang-Monti ileal ureter and bladder anastomosis and the Yang-Monti ileal ureter and lower ureteral anastomosis to evaluate which method is more convenient to perform, and to compare the advantages and disadvantages of both methods.

Materials and methods

Materials

Fourteen 12-month-old male experimental Guizhou miniature pigs weighing 21 ± 1.38 kg were obtained from the Experimental Animal Center of Zunyi Medical College. The pigs were randomly numbered and divided into two groups using a computer program. Group A ($n = 7$) underwent anastomosis of the left Yang-Monti ileal ureter and the left lower ureter; group B ($n = 7$) underwent anastomosis of the left Yang-Monti ileal ureter and bladder. The contralateral kidney was removed from both groups at 1 week postoperatively to establish the two experimental animal models. The experiment was approved by the Medical Ethics Committee of Guizhou Provincial People's Hospital. All experimental procedures were conducted in accordance with local guidelines on the ethical use of animals and the Guide for the Care and Use of Laboratory Animals (National Institutes of Health, publication no. 85–23, revised 2011). Refinement refers to the improvement of conditions, the treatment of animals, and the improvement of animal welfare on the basis of scientific principles, or the improvement of experimental procedures and improvement of experimental techniques to avoid or alleviate the pain and nervousness of animals that are not related to the purpose of the experiment scientific method. The sample size was calculated based on a previous study [17] and the use of a formula. Although the present sample size was small, it was sufficient to identify statistically significant differences between the two groups.

Surgical procedures and postoperative treatment

Surgical steps

Group A

(1). Preoperative preparation: Animals were fasted for 24 h preoperatively and prevented from drinking water for 12 h preoperatively.

(2). Anesthesia: After being weighed, anesthesia was induced via an intraperitoneal injection of 3% pentobarbital sodium (Shanghai Xinya Pharmaceutical Co., Ltd.) at a dose rate of 30 mg/kg and an intravenous infusion of propofol (Sichuan Guorui Pharmaceutical Co., Ltd.) at a dose of 1–2 mg/kg. Anesthesia was maintained with an intravenous infusion of propofol at a dose of 1–2 mg/kg/h.

(3). Abdominal skin preparation: The skin was disinfected with 2.5% iodophor and the surgical area was draped with a sterile surgical towel. The skin was incised over the left rectus abdominis, and the subcutaneous tissue, muscle, and peritoneum were incised.

(4). Creation of a model of extensive ureteral injury: The left side of the colon was moved medially to reveal the left posterior peritoneum. The left posterior peritoneum was incised to enable the identification of the left ureter. The left ureter was cut at the renal pelvis, the lower ureter was preserved,. The middle and upper segments of the ureter were removed to create a model that replicated actual extensive ureteral injury.

(5). Selection of the intestinal segments: At a distance of 40 cm from the ileocecal junction, an ileal segment with an independent mesenteric blood supply was removed, and the surrounding tissues were protected with gauze.

(6). Restoration of intestinal continuity: The two cut ends of the intestine were thoroughly washed with physiological saline before being disinfected with 2.5% iodophor. The intestine was then anastomosed with 5–0 non-absorbable suture. The whole-layer was sutured first, and then the muscular layer was sutured to restore the continuity of the intestine and close the mesangial hole.

(7). Preparation of the intestinal ureter: The intestine was cut using a previously described method [17] (Fig. 1). The intestine was thoroughly cleaned and disinfected with saline and 2.5% iodophor before being cut into three 2-cm-long segments with independent and intact mesenteric vessels (Fig. 2a). A cross-section of the intestine was taken from the mesentery at the 6 o'clock position. The three intestinal segments were cut longitudinally (one was cut at the 9 o'clock position, one at the 12 o'clock position, and one at the 3 o'clock position) to create three rectangular sections of intestine (each of which was 4–6 cm long and 1.5 cm wide) (Fig. 2b). The adjacent intestinal pieces were sequentially sutured with an antibacterial micro-chord line (4–0) to form one rectangular piece of intestine with a length of 12–18 cm and a width of 2 cm (Fig. 2c). The piece of intestine was wrapped around a 30-cm-long F12 silica ureteral stent tube and sutured longitudinally with 5–0 absorbable suture (Johnson & Johnson) to form a long tubular structure to serve as a ureteral replacement segment (Fig. 2d).

(8). Reconstruction of the ureter and ureteral stump anastomosis: One end of the ureteral stent was placed in the renal pelvis, while the other end of the ureteral stent was inserted into the bladder through the native ureteral stump. A minimal incision was made in the apex of the bladder, and the stent tube was pulled out of the bladder to create a

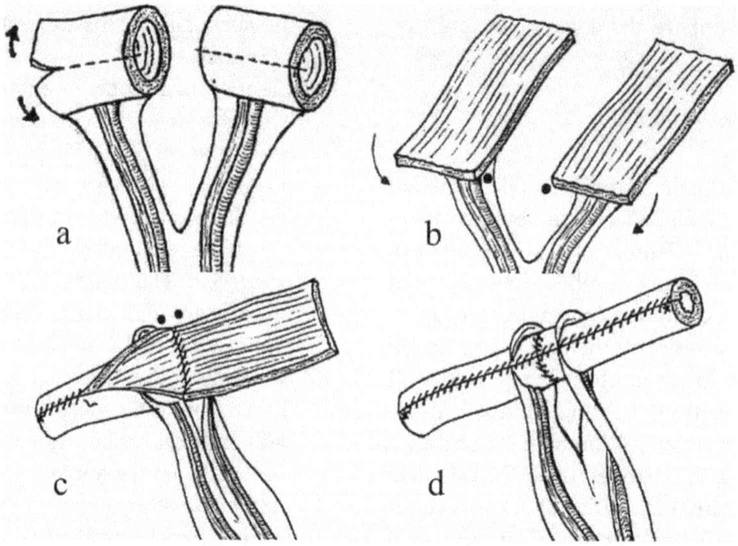

Fig. 1 Photographs showing the method used to obtain the intestinal segments. This figure is from reference [17]. **a** Two 2.5-cm-long adjacent ileal segments are isolated and detubularized through longitudinal incisions on one side, 0.5 cm from the mesentery implantation, and (**b**) two identical pediculated flaps are obtained. **c, d** These flaps are attached by the two short branches and the resulting flap is tubularized; a tube with two long branches separated by two mesenteric insertions is obtained

cystostomy. The bladder incision was sutured. The upper end of the reconstructed ureter was anastomosed to the native ureteral stump with 5–0 absorbable suture. The lower end of the reconstructed ureter was anastomosed to the remaining lower end of the native ureter (Fig. 2e).

(9). The distal end of the ureteral stent tube was placed under the skin of the left lower abdomen, and the incision was closed in a layered fashion.

Group B Steps (1)–(7) and (9) were the same as for group A.

(8) Anastomosis of the reconstructed ureter and the bladder stump: One end of the ureteral stent tube was placed in the renal pelvis, while the other end was placed in the bladder on the left side. A minimal incision was made in the apex of the bladder, and the stent tube was pulled out of the bladder to create a cystostomy. The bladder incision was sutured. The upper end of the reconstructed ureter was anastomosed to the native ureteral stump with 5–0 absorbable suture. The lower end of the reconstructed ureter was directly anastomosed to the bladder (Fig. 2f).

In both groups, the contralateral kidney and ureter were removed at 1 week postoperatively.

Postoperative treatment

All pigs were fasted for 24 h postoperatively before beginning a liquid diet on postoperative day 2. Normal feeding was recommenced 3–5 days after the initiation of the liquid diet. Pigs were administered a daily intramuscular injection of penicillin (1.5 ml/kg) and metronidazole (50 ml/day) for 5 days postoperatively. The ureteral stent tube was left in place for 4 weeks before being surgically removed. The pigs were anesthetized(3% pentobarbital sodium, 30 mg/kg) via intraperitoneal injection before the collection of tissues and organs for examination. After the specimens were collected, the pigs were euthanized via an intravenous injection of 3% pentobarbital sodium (100 mg/kg).

Observation indicators and data collection

The following data were collected for all pigs in both groups:

(1). Operation time and length of the surgical incision.

(2). Blood samples were taken to evaluate the serum creatinine and urea nitrogen concentrations preoperatively and at 2, 6, and 12 weeks postoperatively.

(3). Intravenous pyelography and cystography were performed at 12 weeks postoperatively to observe the ureteral patency and vesicoureteral reflux.

(4). Urine was collected from the bladder at 12 months postoperatively and cultured to check for the presence of urinary tract infection.

(5). Gross macroscopic observation and histological examination of the intestinal ureter were performed at 12 months postoperatively to evaluate the pathological changes of the anastomosis and intestinal ureter.

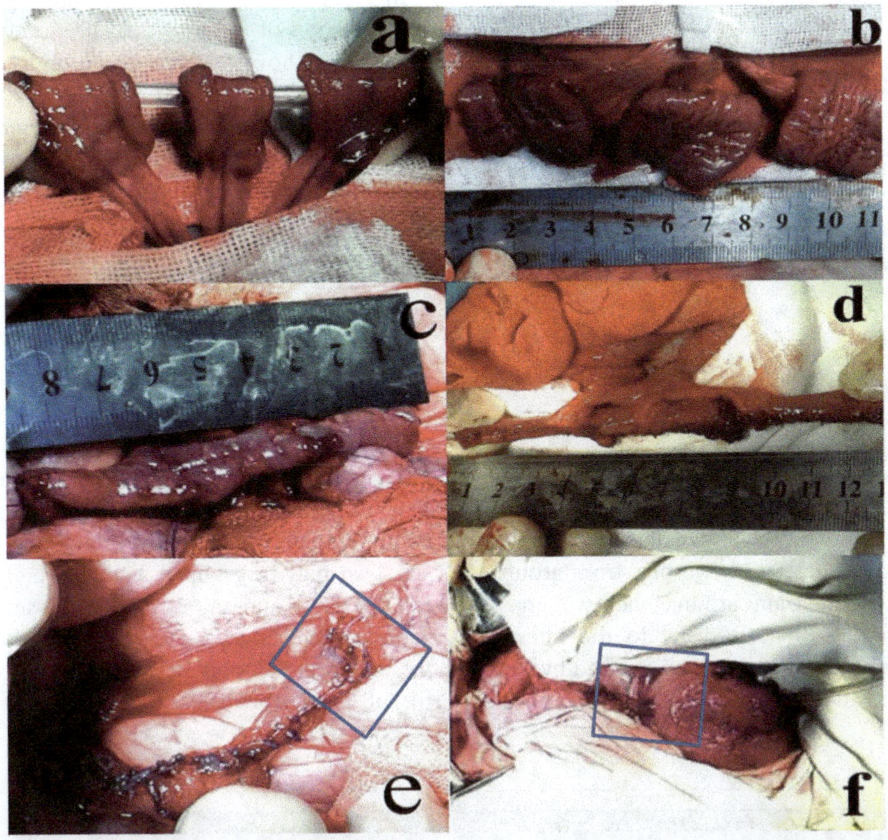

Fig. 2 Photographs showing the preparation of the intestinal segments used as replacement ureters. **a** The selection of each 2-cm-long segment with independent and complete mesenteric vessels. **b** Longitudinal incision of three segments of the intestine to form a three-section rectangular intestine. **c** Sequential suture of the adjacent intestine; the pieces are connected into a long rectangular intestine. **d** The intestinal segment is sutured to form a long tubular structure. **e** The inferior ureter is anastomosed to the lower part of the ureter (the anastomosis is marked with a blue rectangular frame). **f** Anastomosis of the intestinal ureter and bladder (the anastomosis is marked with a blue rectangular frame)

Statistical analysis

Animal grouping was designed in accordance with the principles of equilibrium, control, and repetition. All measurement data were expressed as the mean ± standard deviation. The *t*-test was used to compare data between the two groups. Differences were considered statistically significant at $p < 0.05$. Statistical analysis was performed using SPSS 24.0 software.

Results

The operation was successfully completed in all 14 miniature pigs. In group A, one pig died from an anesthetic accident, and another died from a lung infection on postoperative day 4. In group B, one pig died from adhesive intestinal obstruction on postoperative day 7. The overall survival rate was 78.6%, and the 11 surviving pigs had no urinary or intestinal fistulae. Compared with group B, group A had a significantly longer operation time ($p = 0.01$) and skin incision length ($p = 0.02$) (Table 1). The serum creatinine and urea nitrogen concentrations did not significantly differ between groups at any timepoint ($p > 0.05$). All pigs had normal renal function pre- and postoperatively (Table 2). Intravenous pyelography showed no stenosis or obstruction (Fig. 3a, b). The narrowest diameter of the ureter in group A was significantly larger than that in group B ($p = 0.01$) (Table 3). No contrast agent returned to the upper urinary tract in either group (Fig. 3c, d). *Escherichia coli* was detected in postoperative urine cultures from four pigs in group A and four pigs from group B.

Gross examination of the collected specimens revealed complete obstruction of the distal ends of the inferior

Table 1 Length of surgical incision and operation time ($\bar{x} \pm s$)

Groups	Numbers of samples	Surgical incision length (cm)	operation time (min)
Group A	7	30.86 ± 2.41	181.29 ± 15.10
Group B	7	26.71 ± 3.64	157.71 ± 20.49
P Value		0.01	0.02

Table 2 Serum creatinine and urea nitrogen values of each group before and after surgery ($\bar{x} \pm s$)

Groups	Time	Sample number	Cr (μmol/L)	BUN (mmol/L)
Group A				
	Before surgery	5	102.30 ± 27.60	5.67 ± 1.34
	2 weeks after surgery	5	113.80 ± 14.22	7.35 ± 3.63
	6 weeks after surgery	5	117.70 ± 30.09	6.01 ± 1.37
	12 weeks after surgery	5	102.00 ± 3.89	5.69 ± 0.91
Group B				
	Preoperative	6	101.10 ± 22.18	5.97 ± 1.07
	2 weeks after surgery	6	101.10 ± 5.53	6.24 ± 1.08
	6 weeks after surgery	6	102.10 ± 3.99	6.11 ± 1.08
	12 weeks after surgery	6	100.70 ± 15.19	6.35 ± 1.20

and lower ureters and narrowing of the other ends of the inferior and lower ureters in two pigs from group A. There was marked adhesion around the two anastomoses and obstructive stenosis distal to the intestinal ureter. The kidneys were atrophic with marked hydronephrosis and thin and transparent renal parenchyma (Fig. 4a).

In group B, one pig had moderate hydronephrosis and mild dilation of the intestinal ureter at 12 months postoperatively; however, the ileal ureter and anastomoses were patent (Fig. 4b). The rest of the pigs in group B had patent intestinal ureters and smooth anastomoses. The intestinal ureters were a reddish color, with a shape that was similar to that of the normal ureter. The intestinal ureters were slightly thicker than the normal ureters, and were surrounded by fibrous tissue and adipose tissue. There was continuous, intestinal mucosal atrophy on the surface of the intestinal ureters, with no signs of hydronephrosis.

The ileal ureteral diameter was significantly larger in group A than group B ($p = 0.02$) (Table 3).

Histological examination showed that two pigs in group A had separation between the transitional epithelium of the upper and lower ends of the ureters and the columnar epithelium, with granulation tissue hyperplasia. Two pigs in group A with ureteral obstruction had fibrous tissue and smooth muscle tissue hyperplasia and support stenosis at the anastomosis site (Fig. 5a, b). In the six surviving pigs in group B, the two types of epithelial tissue were close together in the ureteral ureters at both ends of the anastomosis (Fig. 5c, d). In both

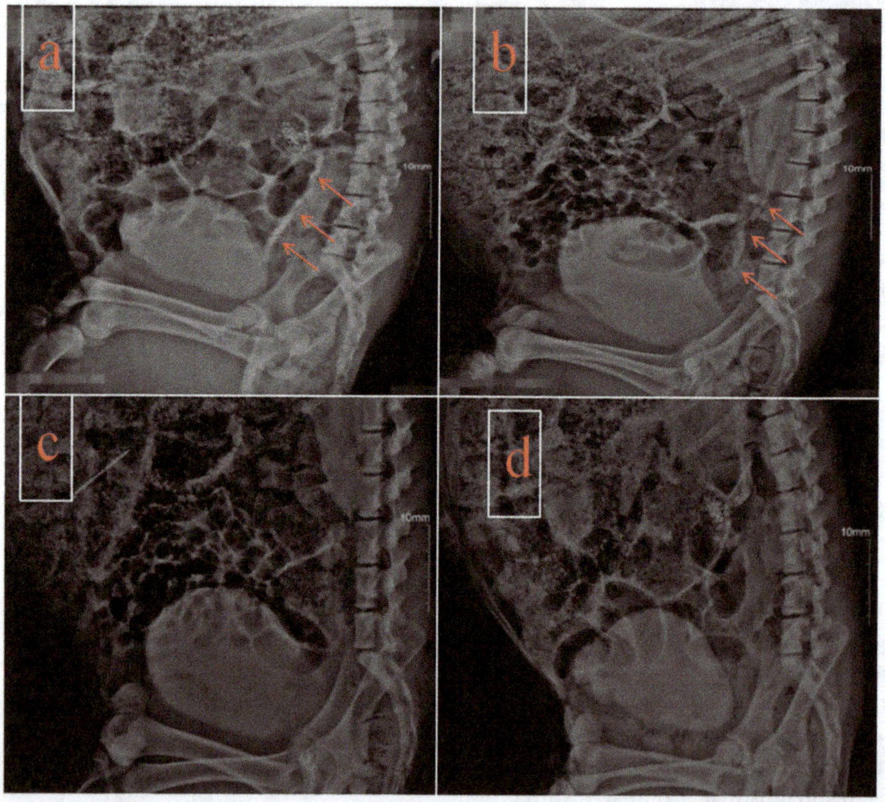

Fig. 3 Intravenous pyelography and cystography findings at 12 weeks postoperatively. **a** Intravenous pyelography of a pig in group B. **b** Intravenous pyelography of a pig in group A. The red arrow indicates the lack of stenosis and obstruction in both groups. **c** Cystography of a pig in group A. **d** Cystography of a pig in group B. There is no reflux of the contrast agent to the upper urinary tract

Table 3 Intestinal ureteral diameter ($\bar{x} \pm s$)

Groups	Number of samples	Intestinal ureteral diameter (mm)	
		Intravenous	pyelography
Group A	5	7.26 ± 1.06	9.40 ± 2.35
Group B	6	5.90 ± 0.30	6.62 ± 0.37
P value		0.01	0.02

groups, the replacement intestinal segments had shortened and atrophied villi compared with normal intestinal villi (Fig. 5e, f).

Discussion

In the present study, we successfully established an animal model of ileal ureter-bladder anastomosis and ileal ureter-ureteral anastomosis using the Yang-Monti technique. The serum creatinine and urea nitrogen concentrations did not significantly differ between the two groups at 2, 6, and 12 weeks postoperatively. The renal function was stable, with no postoperative renal dysfunction or failure.

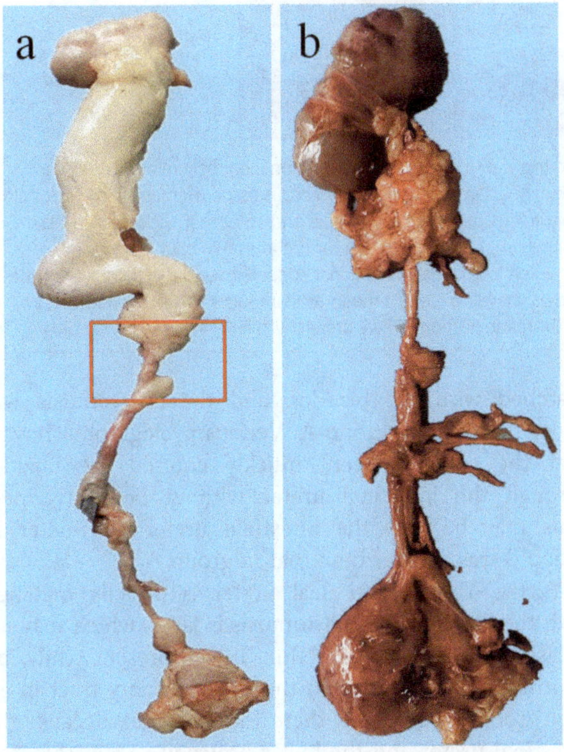

Fig. 4 Photographs showing the gross examination of the intestinal ureters collected at 12 months postoperatively. **a** Stenosis of the inferior ureter and the distal end of the ureter in a pig in group A. The stenosis is marked with a red rectangular frame. There is obvious expansion of the upper ureter and hydronephrosis; the renal parenchyma is thin, and the kidney is small. **b** In a pig from group B, the ileal ureter and anastomosis are unobstructed, with no hydronephrosis

The average operation time and length of the surgical incision in group A were significantly longer than in group B. This may be because the operational procedures in group B were relatively easier to perform than those in group A. In group A, the anastomosis between the intestinal ureter and the native ureter required the lower ureter to be fully freed. As the lower ureter is deeply located, the operational space available for the anastomosis was relatively small. In contrast, the intestinal ureter in group B was directly anastomosed to the bladder, and the lower segment of the ureter was not required. The bladder of the miniature pig is more easily recognized when it is full, and the apex wall, the two lateral walls, and the anterior and posterior walls of the bladder are not connected to the surrounding pelvic wall. As the position of the bladder in the pelvic cavity is not fixed, the bladder is movable and easier to find than the lower part of the ureter. Furthermore, it is easy to re-integrate the ureter and the left side of the bladder, and the operational space is large.

The most common complication of ileal ureteral surgery is urinary tract infection, which is related to bladder ileal reflux and intestinal mucus secretion; this complication is difficult to control and is often recurrent, eventually leading to hydronephrosis or multiple renal cortex abscesses and pyelonephritis [7, 18, 19]. Urine culture results show that the most frequently cultured organism is *E. coli*, followed by *Klebsiella pneumoniae* [12]. Yao et al. [20] performed short- and long-term observations of 60 patients with ileal ureters, and found abnormal changes in the urine (including a small amount of protein, white blood cells, pus balls, and intestinal mucus); however, only four patients had clinical symptoms of urinary tract infection, and the symptoms disappeared after treatment with antibiotics. Therefore, urinary changes do not necessarily indicate the presence of urinary tract infection, and antibiotic treatment is needed only when symptoms of acute infection occur [20]. The *E. coli* colonization seen in urine cultures in the present study is consistent with the literature. *E. coli* is a pathogenic pathogen of the intestine, and may move from the intestine to the urinary tract during surgery; no antibiotic treatment is required for such asymptomatic bacterial urinary infection.

The two methods used in ileal ureteral surgery and bladder anastomosis are non-anti-reflux and anti-reflux. In the non-anti-reflux procedure, the ileal ureter replaces the ureter directly after the bladder. The operation is relatively simple, the operation time is short, and the incision is small. However, there may be postoperative intravesical urine reflux to the replacement ureter or ipsilateral kidney, resulting in postoperative intestinal dilatation, ascending infection, pyelonephritis, hydronephrosis, and impaired renal function [13]. The

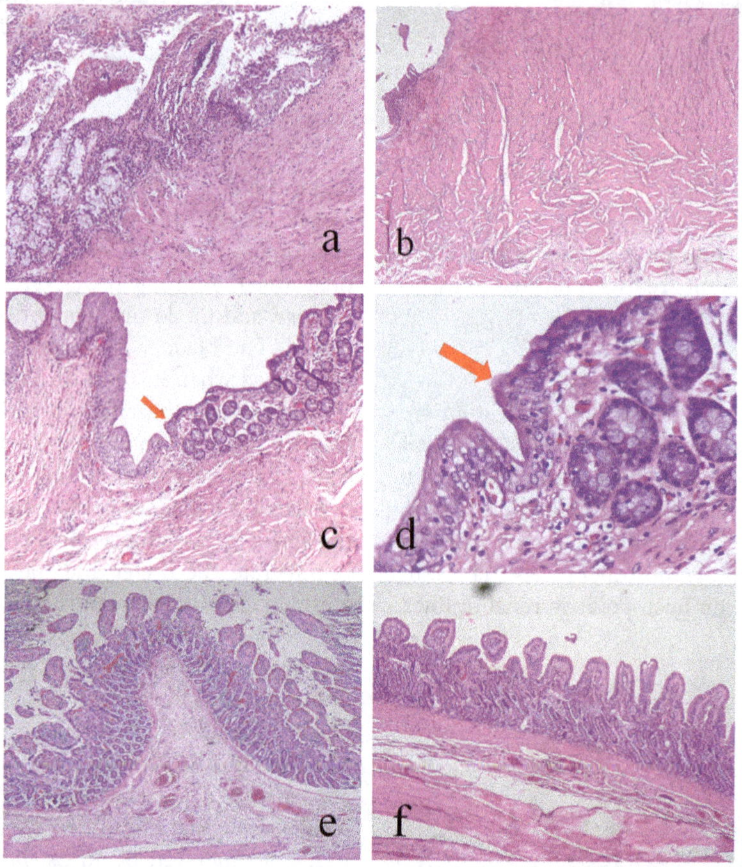

Fig. 5 Histological examination of the intestinal ureters at 12 months postoperatively. **a** In group A, the transitional epithelium and columnar epithelial mucosa are not close together, there is hyperplasia of the granulation tissue, lamina propria, and fibrous tissue (Hematoxylin-eosin stain (H-E); 100× magnification). **b** In group B, there is hyperplasia of the lamina propria, myometrial fibrous tissue, and smooth muscle, with hyaline degeneration (H-E; 40× magnification). **c** On the left side of the transitional epithelium and the right side of the intestinal epithelium,the two types of epithelial tissue were close together (H-E; 100× magnification). **d** On the left side of the transitional epithelium and the right side of the intestinal epithelium, there are transitional epithelial cells (marked with red arrows) crawling toward the intestinal mucosa and covering part of the intestinal mucosa (H-E; 400× magnification). **e** Normal intestinal villi (H-E; 40× magnification). **f** Ileal ureteral villi (H-E; 40× magnification)

incidences of such complications are reduced by the performance of anti-reflux anastomosis. In the present study, there was no stenosis obstruction observed in either group. However, the narrowest diameter of the intestinal ureter was significantly larger in group A than in group B.

On intraoperative measurement, the reconstructed intestinal ureteral diameter was still larger than the normal ureteral tube diameter. In group A, the ureter was cut longitudinally before the intestinal ureter and the lower ureter were anastomosed. Thus, the anastomosis is relatively small, the ileum is more stretched than the ureter, and the urine flows through the relatively narrow lower ureter after passing through the wide intestinal ureter. The urine flow rate is slowed, the stagnation time is long, and urine is retained in the intestinal ureter, which causes the intestinal ureter to expand; the indwelling endoscopic tube also causes postoperative expansion. In contrast, the intestinal ureter in group B was directly matched with the bladder, and the anastomosis was wider than that in group A. Venous pyelography showed that the contrast agent quickly entered the bladder through the intestinal ureter without being retained. This may be why the intestinal ureteral diameter in group B was smaller than that in group A.

As the Yang-Monti ileal ureter is directly matched with the bladder, the anastomosis is large, which may increase the likelihood of reflux. In the present study, no contrast agent returned to the upper urinary tract in either group. In group A, there was no reflux because the intestinal ureter and the lower ureter were anastomosed and the anti-reflux mechanism between the ureter and the bladder was retained. There was also no reflux in group B, even though the anastomosis of the intestinal ureter was large and directly opened to the bladder. The absence of reflux in group B may be because the intestinal ureteral diameter was close to that of the normal ureter, and the intestinal ureter had good elasticity and a long length. The ileum retains its peristaltic function after replacing the ureter, which is beneficial in preventing intravesical pressure [7, 12]. However, confirmation of this requires measurement of the intestinal ureter, renal pelvis, and intravesical pressure. Other possible reasons for the absence of reflux in group B are that the miniature pig has a short urethra, good bladder elasticity, and rapid urine emptying. Therefore, there is little need to establish an anti-reflux mechanism in the Yang-Monti ileal ureter in miniature pigs.

The intestinal epithelium is a single-layer columnar epithelium, while the urinary tract is a transitional epithelium. The examination of the intestinal tract after ileal ureter replacement showed that all of the anastomotic regions had unobstructed lumens, no epithelial proliferative changes in the junctional zone, and were located less than 1 cm from the adjacent junctional zone; this very short distance is covered by migration epithelial metaplasia [21]. In a previous study of ileal ureter reconstruction via the Yang-Monti method in rabbits, histological sections obtained 12 weeks postoperatively showed that stratified transitional epithelial cells had spread toward and covered part of the intestinal mucosa at the site of the anastomosis, and the intestinal mucosa on the inner surface of the ureter was obviously atrophied [22]. In another study in which ileal ureteral surgery was performed on miniature pigs, the columnar epithelium was still visible in the middle ileum at 3 years postoperatively; however, the villi were atrophied and some of the villi had become shorter and wider than normal [23]. In the present study, histological examination of the intestine and ureter was consistent with the findings of these previous studies. After the ileum was used to replace the ureter, its histological characteristics changed to adapt to the urinary environment. The transitional epithelium and the columnar epithelium were continuous and replaced the segmental columnar epithelium, indicating that the ileum that replaced the ureter maintained the shape and integrity of the epithelium, which may still have a mucosal barrier. Further experimental studies are needed to confirm whether the intestinal mucosal barrier changes in the urinary environment. In addition, after the ileum was used to replace the ureter, the intestinal mucosa shrank, the villi became shorter, and the absorption and secretion functions of the intestinal mucosa were correspondingly weakened. This may be related to the absence of obvious metabolic abnormalities and mucus secretion after Yang-Monti ileal ureteral reconstruction in the clinical setting, but requires confirmation in further studies of the absorption and secretion functions of intestinal mucosal epithelial cells.

In group A, the distal end of the inferior ureter and the lower end of the ureter were completely obstructed and stenotic, and there was marked hydronephrosis. In group B, one pig had hydronephrosis and mild dilation of the intestinal ureter, although the anastomosis was smooth. Histological examination showed that group A had hyperplasia of fibrous tissue and smooth muscle at the anastomosis site, suggesting the presence of stenosis or obstruction. In group A, the intestinal ureter was anastomosed with the lower ureter, which means that the lower ureter needed to be separated from the surrounding tissue. The thin ureteral wall may lead to poor blood supply in the lower ureter; thus, although there is good blood supply to the ileal ureter, there may be poor blood supply between the intestinal ureter and the lower ureter after anastomosis, resulting in fibrosis or scarring postoperatively. This may be why the incidence of stenosis or obstruction and hydronephrosis was higher in group A than in group B. In group B, the intestinal ureter was directly matched with the rich blood supply of the bladder, which limited the occurrence of postoperative stenosis or obstruction. Although there was no evidence of hydronephrosis and regurgitation on intravenous pyelography and cystography in group B, visual observation suggested the presence of hydronephrosis and mild dilation of the intestinal ureter. Furthermore, although the short-term imaging examination revealed no abnormal changes, the inguinal ureter may undergo compensatory changes over time after countering the persistent intravesical pressure.

Conclusions

We successfully established an animal model of Yang-Monti ileal ureteral reconstruction. Compared with the Yang-Monti ileal ureter-ureteral anastomosis, the Yang-Monti ileal ureter-bladder anastomosis is simpler, more reliable, and results in fewer complications.

Declarations

The work described herein is original research that has not been published previously and is not under consideration for publication elsewhere, in whole or in part. All authors of the manuscript have read and agreed to its content and are accountable for all aspects of the accuracy and integrity of the manuscript in accordance with The Basel Declaration, and all agree to the ethical guidelines of the International Council for Laboratory Animal Science and to the terms of the BioMed Central License Agreement and Open Data Policy.

Authors' contributions

ZW wrote the first draft of the manuscript. ZS, XY, GL, YT, LS, ZS and HL all reviewed the manuscript and were involved in its critical revision before submission. All authors read and approved the final manuscript.

Author details

[1]Basic Medical College, Guizhou Medical University, Guiyang 550004, China.
[2]Department of Urology, Guizhou Provincial People's Hospital affiliated to

Guizhou Medical University, Guiyang 550002, Guizhou, China. [3]Department of Urology, Guizhou Provincial People's Hospital, No. 83 East Zhongshan Road, Guiyang 550002, Guizhou, China. [4]Department of Surgical Operation Laboratory, Zunyi Medical University, No. 6 West Xuefu Road, Zunyi, Xinpu New District, China. [5]Department of Urology, Guizhou Medical University, No. 9 Beijing Road, Guiyang, Guizhou, China. [6]Department of Urology, Zunyi Medical University, No. 6 Xuefu West Road, Xinpu New District, Zunyi, Guizhou, China.

References

1. Chen XP, Tang JQ, Li XS, et al. A case report of ileal ureteral surgery for long-term ureteral defect and literature review. Chin J Clin. 2011;08:2410–3.
2. Al-Awadi K, Kehinde EO, Al-Hunayan A, et al. Iatrogenic ureteric injuries: incidence, aetiological factors and the effect of early management on subsequent outcome. Int Urol Nephrol. 2005;37(2):235–41.
3. Johnson DB, Pearle MS. Complicatiogs of ureteroscopy. Urol Clin Noth Am. 2004;31:157–71.
4. Wang Y, Ceng S, Zhong J, et al. Treatment of severe ureteral injury caused by ureteroscopy. Modern Prevent Med. 2009;26(4):2799.
5. Yin ZK, Wu XH, Tang W, et al. Analysis of prevention and treatment of ureteral fracture and avulsion with ureteroscopy in many hospitals in Chongqing. Chongqing Med. 2010;39(2):3059–62.
6. Maigaard T, Kirkeby HJ. Yang–Monti ileal ureter reconstruction. Scand J Urol. 2015;49(4):313.
7. Esmat M, Abdelaal A, Mostafa D. Application of Yang-Monti principle in ileal ureter substitution: is it a beneficial modification? Int Braz J Urol. 2012;38(6):779–87.
8. Ali-El-Dein B, El-Hefnawy AS, Shokeir AA, et al. 1063 bridging long ureteral defects using the Yang-Mobti principle: long-term follow-up. Eur Urol Suppl. 2011;10(2):328.
9. Bonfig R, Gerharz EW, Riedmiller H. Ileal ureteric replacement in complex reconstruction of the urinary tract. BJU Int. 2004;93:575–80.
10. Tanagho EA. A case against incorporation of bowel segments into the closed urinary system. J Urol. 1975;113:796–802.
11. Waldner M, Hertle L, Roth S. Ileal ureteral substitution in reconstructive urological surgery: is an antireflux procedure necessary? J Urol. 1999; 162:323–6.
12. Ali-el-Dein B, Ghoneim M. Bridging long ureteral defects using the Yang-Monti principle. J Urol. 2003;169(3):1074–7.
13. Xiong EQ, Jin XY, Song B, et al. Long-term follow-up of ileal ureteral surgery. Chin J Urol. 1996;17:249.
14. Shokeir AA, Ghoneim MA. Further experience with the modified ileal ureter. J Urol. 1995;154:45–8.
15. Xu YM, Jia Teng JL, Qian L, et al. Long-term efficacy of proximal anti-reflux technique in patients with ileal ureteral surgery. Chin J Urol. 2013;34(8):595–8.
16. Xu Y-M, Feng C, Kato H. Long-term outcome of ileal ureteric replacement with an iliopsoas muscle tunnel antirefluxing technique for the treatment of long-segment ureteric strictures. Reconstruct Urol. 2016;88:201–6.
17. Monti PR, de Carvalho JR, Arap S. The Monti procedure:applications and complications. Urology. 2000, May;55(5):616–21.
18. Fang WH. Treatment of 10 cases of ileal ureteral complications. J Anhui Med Univ. 2001;36(3):246.
19. Patel VR, Gosalbez R, Castellan M. Comparison between ureteral replacements using a transverse tubularized colonic tube or ileal ureter: experimental study in dogs. J Pediatr Surg. 2006;41:799–803.
20. Yao ZZ, Zhu YP, Zhang ZM, et al. Clinical analysis of 6 cases of free ileal segmental ureter. Journal of clinical surgery. 1995;3(5):261–2.
21. Cetinel B, Demirkesen O, Cetinel S. Et a1.The use of transversely tubularized bowel segment for segmental ureteral replacement. Urol Int. 2003;71(3): 246–50.
22. Wang XM. Experimental study on cutting ileal ileum to replace long segment defect of ureter. Wuhan: Southeast University; Dissertation, 2005.
23. Pabst R, Kamran D. Replacement of the ureter by an ileal loop. Quantitative aspects of long-term morphological alterations in minipigs. Br J Exp Pathol. 1983;64(3):293.

10

Experience with AMS 700 LGX penile prostheses for preserving penile length in Korea

Kang Sup Kim[1], Woong Jin Bae[2,3], Sae Woong Kim[2,3*] and Moo Yeon Lee[4*]

Abstract

Background: The purpose of this study was to report the outcomes of patients who underwent penile implantation with AMS 700 LGX inflatable penile prosthesis (IPP) in a single center by a single surgeon.

Methods: A total of 342 patients with erectile dysfunction who underwent AMS 700 LGX IPP implantation between October 2014 and April 2016 were included in this study. All patients were evaluated using the International Index of Erectile Function questionnaire preoperatively and at 3, 6, and 12 months postoperatively. We also investigated the mean stretched flaccid penile length before and after surgery as well as the complications related to and the mechanical reliability of the IPP.

Results: The questionnaire scores at 12 months were statistically significantly higher than the baseline scores. The mean stretched flaccid penile length was 11.1 ± 0.8 cm at baseline and was longer at 3 (11.9 ± 0.9 cm, $P < 0.001$), 6 (12.0 ± 0.9 cm, $P < 0.001$), and 12 (12.2 ± 0.7 cm, $P < 0.001$) postoperatively. There were no intraoperative or perioperative complications. However, one patient had infection and 10 patients developed mechanical failure during the follow-up duration.

Conclusions: The results of our study suggest that the AMS 700 LGX IPP could be used to prevent penile shortening in patients undergoing IPP implantation. Furthermore, erectile function and patient satisfaction were improved excellently.

Keywords: Erectile dysfunction, Penile prosthesis, Penile length

Background

Although oral phosphodiesterase type 5 inhibitors, vacuum erection devices, and intracavernosal vasoactive agent injection are the preferred therapies for erectile dysfunction (ED), penile prosthetic implants are regarded as effective, safe, and durable for patients who are refractory to medical treatment and/or prefer a more effective and permanent therapy. Since Scott et al. [1] first reported using an inflatable penile prosthesis (IPP) in five patients, IPPs have been used for successfully treating ED for many years. Constant device improvements have resulted in good functional outcomes, with a low complication rate and high patient satisfaction. Patient dissatisfaction with penile girth occurs rarely. The penile length could be increased with time owing to the length expansion of the IPP. With a larger erect penis, one can have a longer flaccid penile length. However, patient satisfaction regarding penile length during erection with the prosthesis has not been achieved in some patients. Therefore, if patients are dissatisfied with their penile length postoperatively, daily inflation of the penile prosthesis is recommended to produce corporal expansion, followed by surgical replacement with a longer cylinder [2].

The American Medical Service (AMS) 700 Ultrex (American Medical Service, Minneapolis, MN, USA) was developed in the 1990s to promote penile lengthening. However, mechanical failure and complications

* Correspondence: ksw1227@catholic.ac.kr; mylee@adamshospital.net
[2]Department of Urology, Seoul St. Mary's Hospital, College of Medicine, The Catholic University of Korea, 222, Banpo-daero, Seocho-gu, Seoul 06591, Republic of Korea
[4]Adams Urology Clinic, 513, Teheran-ro, Gangnam-gu, Seoul 06169, Republic of Korea
Full list of author information is available at the end of the article

occurred frequently; therefore, the use of this device was discontinued [3, 4]. AMS 700 LGX IPP (American Medical Service) was developed to overcome the mechanical problems of the AMS 700 Ultrex design to permit both penile girth and length expansion after IPP implantation. However, little has been reported about patient satisfaction postoperatively, especially with penile length, or the mechanical reliability or durability of this device, despite its widespread use by many andrologists [5].

Methods

This study was aimed at evaluating and reporting the results of the use of AMS 700 LGX for IPP implantation, including preservation of penile length, complications (such as infection, hemorrhage, mechanical failure, or voiding problems), and patient satisfaction after surgery.

IPP implantation is performed in patients to treat ED if they do not respond to conventional ED therapy, including failure of oral phosphodiesterase type 5 inhibitors with maximal-dose or intracavernosal injection therapy. Patients who underwent implantation with the AMS 700 LGX IPP at a single andrology center between October 2014 and April 2016 were included. We excluded patients who were undergoing repeat implantation operation or prosthesis implantation because of Peyronie's disease. Because ED treatment expenses, including IPP implantation procedures, are not covered by the Korean National Health Insurance program, the patient paid the related costs (operation and prosthesis fee and postoperative follow-up), and the type of penile prosthesis was selected by the patients and urologist together. Approximately 50% of the patients received AMS 700 LGX, 30% received AMS 700 CX, and 20% received AMS 700 CXR at the time of surgery (all from American Medical Service).

One andrologist (MYL) met all patients, gathered information on their medical history, and performed clinical and physical examinations. Data were obtained from the patients' medical records and interviews. The data included early and late postoperative morbidities, such as infection, mechanical malfunction, and other surgical complications. Patients answered the International Index of Erectile Function (IIEF) questionnaire before undergoing surgery. When patients visited the outpatient department, they completed the questionnaire in private before meeting with an andrologist. The IIEF is a self-administered instrument comprising domains related to sexual function such as erectile function, orgasmic function, sexual desire, satisfaction with intercourse, and overall satisfaction [6]. The severity of ED was measured using the IIEF erectile function domain scores: < 10, severe ED; 11–17, moderate ED; 18–25, mild ED; > 25, no ED. The stretched flaccid penile length and penile length with the IPP fully inflated were also measured before IPP implantation and at 1, 3, 6, and 12 months postoperatively. The penile length was measured from the pubopenile skin junction to the penile meatus, along the dorsal side of the penile shaft.

We obtained approval from our institutional ethical review board to perform this study, which was conducted in accordance with the principles of the Declaration of Helsinki. Informed consent was obtained from patients before the IPP procedure.

All statistical analyses were conducted using the SPSS statistical software (SPSS Inc., Chicago, IL, USA). Since this is a retrospective study, sample size calculation was not needed. The preoperative and postoperative IIEF scores and stretched flaccid penile length were compared using Student's t test. All data are presented as the mean ± standard deviation, and statistical significance was defined as $P < 0.05$.

Results

A total of 342 patients underwent implantation with the AMS 700 LGX IPP between October 2014 and April 2016. The mean age of the patients and ED period were 58.3 ± 9.2 and 4.3 ± 2.5 years, respectively. None of the patients had previously undergone IPP implantation. The indications for IPP implantation were vascular ED for 134 patients, diabetes mellitus for 130, and pelvic surgery such as radical prostatectomy or cystectomy for 48 (Table 1).

There were no perioperative or immediate postoperative complications. Transfusion and surgical revision were not required for any patients. Considering the long-term complications, one patient experienced infection at 3 months postoperatively and underwent IPP removal, and 10 patients experienced mechanical malfunction of the prosthesis.

The mean stretched flaccid penile length was 11.1 ± 0.8 cm at baseline and was longer at 3 months (11.9 ± 0.9 cm, $P < 0.001$), 6 months (12.0 ± 0.9 cm, $P < 0.001$)

Table 1 Patients' demographics

Characteristic	Mean ± SD or n (%)
Age (years)	58.3 ± 9.2
ED duration (years)	4.3 ± 2.5
Cause of ED	
Vascular insufficiency	134 (39.2)
Diabetes mellitus	130 (38.0)
Pelvic surgery	48 (14.0)
Others	30 (8.8)

ED Erectile dysfunction

and 12 months (12.2 ± 0.7 cm, P < 0.001) postoperatively. There was no significant difference in the stretched flaccid penile length between 6 and 12 months ($P = 0.31$). The mean and penile length with the IPP fully inflated was 11.8 ± 1.2 at baseline, 12.6 ± 1.0 at 3 months, 12.6 ± 1.1 at 6 months, and 12.7 ± 1.2 at 12 months. There was a statistically significant difference in penile length with the IPP fully inflated from baseline to 3, 6, and 12 months ($P < 0.001$). No statistical difference in penile length with the IPP fully inflated was noted between 6 and 12 months ($P = 0.14$) (Table 2).

Thirty-two of the 342 patients did not answer all of the questionnaires. Hence, 310 patients completed all of the questionnaires. We did not include this incomplete questionnaire in the present study. Table 3 presents the preoperative and postoperative IIEF scores of the patients in this study.

The total mean preoperative IIEF scores, IIEF erectile function domain scores, and IIEF satisfaction domain scores were 23.2 ± 2.9, 6.5 ± 2.5, and 6.4 ± 2.4, respectively. Postoperatively, the total IIEF scores were 41.8 ± 4.5, 55.3 ± 6.2, and 61.9 ± 9.5 at 3, 6, and 12 months, respectively (Fig. 1). The IIEF erectile domain scores were 15.2 ± 3.4, 20.5 ± 3.2, and 25.5 ± 3.9 at 3, 6, and 12 months, respectively (Fig. 2). Furthermore, the IIEF satisfaction domain scores were 12.8 ± 1.1, 14.5 ± 2.2, and 14.9 ± 4.5 at 3, 6, and 12 months, respectively (Fig. 3). Statistically significant improvements were observed for all postoperative total IIEF scores ($P < 0.05$), all postoperative IIEF erectile domain scores (P < 0.05), and all postoperative IIEF satisfaction domain scores (P < 0.05), compared with the preoperative scores (Table 3).

Discussion

IPP implantation is a well-known, established, and considerably satisfactory treatment option for ED. Although an IPP is regarded to have good mechanical reliability in the long term, patient satisfaction with penile length after surgery has not been achieved because of the patient's expectation in relation to the pre-implantation erect penis length. The causes of dissatisfaction with the penile length are long ED duration, obesity, in which there are added tissues in the prepubic area, and acquired penile disorder such as Peyronie's disease [7]. Deveci et al. [8] reported the stretched flaccid penile length before and after two- or three-piece IPP implantation in 56 patients. Although there were no statistically significant differences between the preoperative and postoperative penile lengths, 72% of the patients complained of a decrease in penile length after surgery. However, one study comparing the erect penile length after IPP implantation, through induced intracavernosal injection of vasoactive agents, with the length before surgery found that all 11 patients experienced a decrease in erect penile length, from 0.2 to 3.0 cm, after IPP implantation. Furthermore, 45.5% of the recipients reported that their subjective penile length shortened after surgery, and no patient thought that his postoperative penile length was longer than its preoperative length [9]. Henry et al. [10] prospectively assessed penile length measurements for 1 year after IPP implantation with the Coloplast Titan (Coloplast, Minneapolis, MN, USA), using an aggressive new length measurement technique to overcome reduced penile length. These patients underwent daily inflation of the IPP for 6 months and maximal inflation for 1–2 h daily for 6–12 months. Of these patients, 64.5% were satisfied with their penile length at 1 year and 74.2% of patients reported that their penile length increased. Because of the aggressive cylinder sizing and postoperative penile rehabilitation inflation protocol, all of the patients, except for two, experienced an increase (approximately 1 cm) in the stretched penile length. To prevent penile shortening, concomitant surgical interventions, such as a sliding technique, suprapubic lipectomy, suspensory ligament release, and ventral phalloplasty, have been developed and used [11, 12].

Although the exact mechanism of penile length shortening after IPP implantation has not been fully elucidated, incorrectly measuring the corporeal length during surgery and lack of glans tumescence after implantation might decrease the penile length [9]. Intraurethral alprostadil injection or oral phosphodiesterase type 5 inhibitors are used for enhancing the soft glans

Table 2 Preoperative and postoperative penile length of the patients

	Baseline	Postoperative			*P*-value[a]
		3 months	6 months	12 months	
Flaccid penile length	11.1 ± 0.8	11.9 ± 0.9	12.0 ± 0.9	12.2 ± 0.7	< 0.001
Penile length with the IPP fully inflated	11.8 ± 1.2	12.6 ± 1.0	12.6 ± 1.1	12.7 ± 1.2	< 0.001

[a]Baseline flaccid penile length, penile length with the IPP fully inflated, and all of the follow-up period (postoperative 3, 6, and 12 months) penile lengths were compared, and a statistical significance was observed

Table 3 Preoperative and postoperative IIEF scores of the patients

IIEF	Preoperative	Postoperative			*P*-value[a]
		3 months	6 months	12 months	
Total	23.2 ± 2.9	41.8 ± 4.5	55.3 ± 6.2	61.9 ± 9.5	< 0.05
Erectile function domain	6.5 ± 2.5	15.2 ± 3.4	20.5 ± 3.2	25.5 ± 3.9	< 0.05
Satisfaction domain	6.4 ± 2.4	12.8 ± 1.1	14.5 ± 2.2	14.9 ± 4.5	< 0.05

IIEF International Index of Erectile Function
[a]The preoperative IIEF scores and all of the follow-up period (postoperative 3, 6, and 12 months) scores were compared, and statistical significance was observed

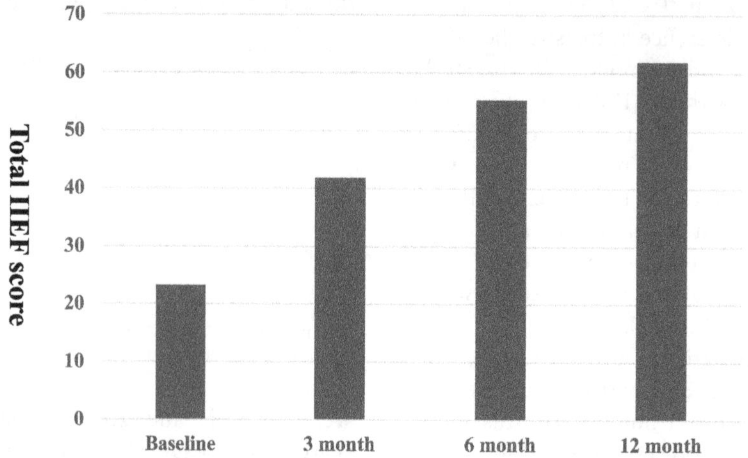

Fig. 1 Total IIEF score. Statistically significant difference was observed for baseline versus all postoperative parameters

after penile prosthesis implantation to increase the length of a shortened penis [13, 14].

In the 1990s, the AMS 700 Ultrex penile prosthesis was developed to prevent penile shortening and increase penile girth and length. Montague et al. [3] reported that 50 patients underwent implantation using the AMS 700 Ultrex. The penile length was increased by 1 cm in 12 patients, and in 28 patients, the postoperative penile length was the same as the intraoperative length expansion. However, because S-shaped deformities have occurred when using the AMS 700 Ultrex prosthesis and its durability is low, urologists have been discouraged from using this IPP. AMS 700 LGX, which allows both girth and length expansion of the cylinders with up to 20% elongation, was developed to overcome these disadvantages. Recently, one prospective study reported the mean penile length and recipient satisfaction after AMS 700 LGX implantation [5]. At 6 and 12 months, the stretched flaccid penile length was longer than the preoperative length. Six and 12 months postoperatively, the IIEF desired domain scores and overall satisfaction scores were statistically different from the preoperative scores. However, the mean Erectile Dysfunction Inventory of Treatment Satisfaction scores did not show significant improvement after implantation.

In the present study, at 6 and 12 months postoperatively, the stretched penile length was longer than the preoperative length. We confirmed that all postoperative total IIEF scores, postoperative IIEF erectile function domain scores, and postoperative satisfaction domain scores significantly improved, compared with the preoperative scores. Furthermore, complications such as infection, skin necrosis, and erosion occurred rarely. The mechanical malfunction rate was also very low, and no mechanical complications such as a cylinder aneurysm or S-shaped deformity occurred. Therefore, the AMS 700 LGX is an excellent IPP to preserve penile length in patients who are concerned about decreases in their original penile length and has a low rate of complications and mechanical malfunction.

The present study has several limitations. First, this is a retrospective study. Second, the IPP implantation

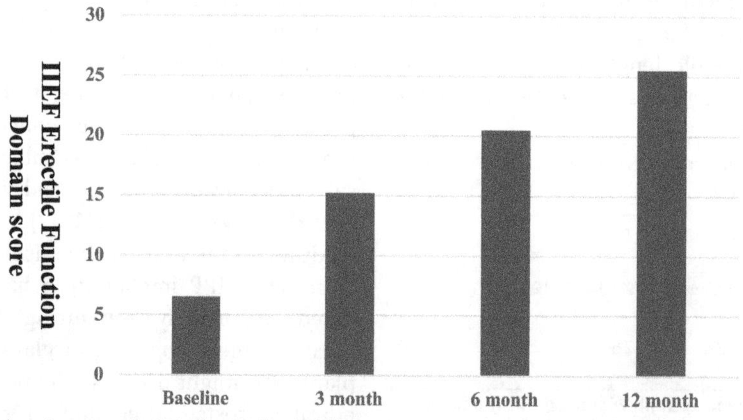

Fig. 2 IIEF erectile function domain scores. Statistically significant difference was observed for baseline versus all postoperative parameters

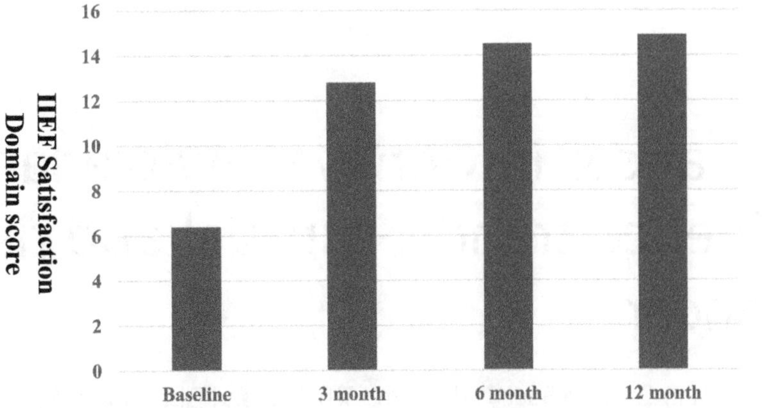

Fig. 3 IIEF satisfaction domain scores. Statistically significant difference was observed for baseline versus all postoperative parameters

procedures were performed by an andrologist who performs a high volume of these procedures; therefore, it is difficult to generalize our results to surgeons who are less experienced. Third, this study excluded patients with Peyronie's disease and corporal fibrosis as well as those who underwent a reoperation. A further study about the usefulness of AMS 700 LGX in patients with these conditions should be performed. Fourth, there are no validated questionnaires for evaluating erection and patient satisfaction with the IPP; hence, we used the IIEF to evaluate patients' satisfaction. Thus, an IPP-specific validated questionnaire should be developed in the future. Finally, we did not record the patients' weight, which could have resulted in some differences in the stretched flaccid penile lengths. Despite these limitations, our present study provides data on the outcomes of the use of and patient satisfaction with the AMS 700 LGX penile prosthesis in Korea for the first time.

Conclusions

We believe that the AMS 700 LGX is a safe and reliable prosthesis for patients with ED and is effective in preventing penile shortening in patients undergoing IPP implantation, with high patient satisfaction. A longer follow-up of these patients and a prospective study are mandatory to confirm these results.

Abbreviations

AMS: American Medical Service; ED: Erectile dysfunction; IIEF: International Index of Erectile Function; IPP: Inflatable penile prosthesis

Acknowledgements

This research was supported by the Bio & Medical Technology Development Program of the National Research Foundation (NRF) funded by the Ministry of Science & ICT(2018M3A9E8020861).

Authors' contributions

KSK, MYL, and SWK performed the research, analyzed the data, and wrote the paper. WJB analyzed and interpreted the data. MYL and SWK provided guidance and critically revised the paper. All authors read and approved the final manuscripts.

Author details

[1]Department of Urology, Incheon St. Mary's Hospital, College of Medicine, The Catholic University of Korea, 59, Dongsu-ro, Bupyeong-gu, Incheon 21431, Republic of Korea. [2]Department of Urology, Seoul St. Mary's Hospital, College of Medicine, The Catholic University of Korea, 222, Banpo-daero, Seocho-gu, Seoul 06591, Republic of Korea. [3]Catholic Integrative Medicine Research Institute, College of Medicine, The Catholic University of Korea, 222, Banpo-daero, Seocho-gu, Seoul 06591, Republic of Korea. [4]Adams Urology Clinic, 513, Teheran-ro, Gangnam-gu, Seoul 06169, Republic of Korea.

References

1. Scott FB, Bradley WE, Timm GW. Management of erectile impotence. Use of implantable inflatable prosthesis. Urology. 1973;2(1):80–2.
2. Montague DK, Angermeier KW. Future considerations: advances in the surgical management of erectile dysfunction. Int J Impot Res. 2000;12(Suppl 4):S140–3.
3. Montague DK, Lakin MM. Early experience with the controlled girth and length expanding cylinder of the American Medical Systems Ultrex penile prosthesis. J Urol. 1992;148(5):1444–6.
4. Wilson SK, Cleves MA, Delk JR 2nd. Ultrex cylinders: problems with uncontrolled lengthening (the S-shaped deformity). J Urol. 1996;155(1):135–7.
5. Negro CL, Paradiso M, Rocca A, Bardari F. Implantation of AMS 700 LGX penile prosthesis preserves penile length without the need for penile lengthening procedures. Asian J Androl. 2016;18(1):114–7.
6. Rosen RC, Riley A, Wagner G, Osterloh IH, Kirkpatrick J, Mishra A. The international index of erectile function (IIEF): a multidimensional scale for assessment of erectile dysfunction. Urology. 1997;49(6):822–30.
7. Montague DK. Penile prosthesis implantation: size matters. Eur Urol. 2007;51(4):887–8.
8. Deveci S, Martin D, Parker M, Mulhall JP. Penile length alterations following penile prosthesis surgery. Eur Urol. 2007;51(4):1128–31.
9. Wang R, Howard GE, Hoang A, Yuan JH, Lin HC, Dai YT. Prospective and long-term evaluation of erect penile length obtained with inflatable penile prosthesis to that induced by intracavernosal injection. Asian J Androl. 2009;11(4):411–5.
10. Henry GD, Carrion R, Jennermann C, Wang R. Prospective evaluation of postoperative penile rehabilitation: penile length/girth maintenance 1 year following Coloplast titan inflatable penile prosthesis. J Sex Med. 2015;12(5): 1298–304.
11. Lue TF, El-Sakka AI. Lengthening shortened penis caused by Peyronie's disease using circular venous grafting and daily stretching with a vacuum erection device. J Urol. 1999;161(4):1141–4.
12. Miranda-Sousa A, Keating M, Moreira S, Baker M, Carrion R. Concomitant ventral phalloplasty during penile implant surgery: a novel procedure that optimizes patient satisfaction and their perception of phallic length after penile implant surgery. J Sex Med. 2007;4(5):1494–9.
13. Benevides MD, Carson CC. Intraurethral application of alprostadil in patients with failed inflatable penile prosthesis. J Urol. 2000;163(3):785–7.
14. Mulhall JP, Jahoda A, Aviv N, Valenzuela R, Parker M. The impact of sildenafil citrate on sexual satisfaction profiles in men with a penile prosthesis in situ. BJU Int. 2004;93(1):97–9.

11

Testicular cancer in Geneva, Switzerland, 1970–2012: Incidence trends, survival and risk of second cancer

Robin Schaffar, Samaksha Pant, Christine Bouchardy, Hyma Schubert and Elisabetta Rapiti*

Abstract

Background: This paper describes the testicular cancer trends for incidence, survival, socio-economic status (SES) disparities and second cancer occurrence in Geneva, Switzerland, a high-risk population.

Methods: We included all testicular germ-cell tumors recorded in the population-based Geneva cancer registry during the period 1970–2012. Changes in incidence trends were assessed using Joinpoint regression to calculate the annual percentage change (APC). Overall and cancer-specific survivals (OS, CSS) were estimated by Kaplan Meyer methods. To evaluate the risk of a second cancer we calculated the Standardized Incidence Ratios (SIR) using the Geneva population incidence rates.

Results: The average annual testicular cancer rate was 7.32/100 000 men, with a non-significant increasing trend during the study period. The highest rates were observed among men younger than 39 years. Despite a trend toward earlier diagnosis, 14% of patients were diagnosed at a late stage. Patients with non-seminoma tumours and patients with low SES were more often diagnosed with an advanced stage. Both OS and CSS improved during the study period but with strong differences by age, stage, morphology and SES. The risk for developing a second cancer was more than doubled. This risk was particularly high for a contralateral testicular cancer, bladder cancer and pancreatic cancer.

Conclusions: Overall, there was no substantial increase in the incidence of testicular cancer in Geneva in recent decades, however the prognosis has improved. The high risk of developing a second cancer, the differences in stage at diagnosis and survival by SES, require enhanced awareness and surveillance by clinicians, patients and men in general.

Keywords: Testicular cancer, Second cancer, Trends, Incidence, Survival, Socio-economic status

Background

Testicular cancer is a rare cancer, with an annual incidence rate of 1.5 cases/100′000 men (world adjusted). In Western Caucasian populations in recent decades, there has been a sharp increase of the rate of this disease, and in Norway and Switzerland the rate went up to 12/100′000 [1]. The disease is more frequent in young men, aged less than 49 years. Hence, in 2012 in Switzerland the rate among men aged 15–39 years reached 20.9/100′000, representing the most prevalent cancer diagnosed in this age group [1].

* Correspondence: Elisabetta.Rapiti@unige.ch
Geneva Cancer Registry, Global Health Institute, University of Geneva, Geneva, Switzerland

Overall, in these countries has been observed an increase in the burden of the disease, also due to an important decrease in mortality rates following the advent of cisplatin-based chemotherapy [1, 2].

The disease has important physiological and psychological impacts on affected men and their families. Given their young age, issues of concern include not only recovery but also the consequences of both the disease and the treatment on sexuality and reproductive capacity.

There is a paucity of data regarding testicular cancer in Switzerland. The latest report from the Canton of Vaud showed one of the highest incidence rates in the world for the years 1974–1999, but with no clear upward trend since early 1990s [3–5].

The aim of this study is to provide an overall picture of testicular cancer in the high-risk canton of Geneva by studying the evolution for over 40 years of its incidence, prognosis, and occurrence of second cancers using population- based registry data.

Methods

Patients and data

We used data from the population-based Geneva Cancer Registry, which records information on all incident cases of malignant neoplasms occurring in the population of the canton (approximately 490′000 inhabitants) since 1970. Information collected by the registry includes patient's sociodemographic data, tumor data, in particular on the method of detection, histology, stage, treatment in the first 6 months after diagnosis, survival, and occurrence of second tumours. Data are systematically abstracted from hospital and laboratory records by trained tumour registrars. To collect missing clinical and therapeutic data, special questionnaires are sent out regularly to the private practitioners. Death certificates are consulted systematically.

From this database, we identified 624 men resident in the canton of Geneva who were diagnosed with a primary invasive testicular cancer between 1970 and 2012. Cases with non-germinal testicular cancer (24 lymphomas, two Sertoli cell carcinomas, seven Leydig cell tumors, and one leiomyosarcoma) were excluded.

Sociodemographic variables of interest for the study were age (≤29 years, 30–39 years, 40–49 year, 50+ years), place of birth (Switzerland, Europe, Other), socio-economic status (SES) categorized in three levels based on the patient's last occupation (low (manual employees, skilled and unskilled workers, including farmers), middle (non-manual employees and administrative staff), and high (professionals, executives, administrators, entrepreneurs)) and period of diagnosis (1970–1979, 1980–1989, 1990–1999, 2000–2012).

We considered the following variables to describe the tumour characteristics: method of detection (symptoms, fortuitous, routine check-up, autopsy or unknown); stage, categorized in four classes based on the pathologic tumor-node-metastasis (TNM) classification or, when absent, the clinical TNM classification; and morphology grouped in two classes: seminoma (International Classification of Diseases in Oncology version 10: 9060–9064 [6]) and non-seminoma (including embryonal carcinoma ICD-O 10: 9070, yolk sac tumor ICD-O 10: 9071, teratoma ICD-O 10: 9080, 9082, 9083, 9102, teratocarcinoma ICD-O 10: 9081, choriocarcinoma ICD-O 10: 9100, 9101, mixed germ-cell tumor ICD-O10: 9085).

The type of treatment received by the patients in the first 6 months after diagnosis was classified as surgery (yes vs. no), radiotherapy (yes vs. no) and chemotherapy (yes vs. no).

Statistical methods

We calculated the annual incidence rates per 100′000 men for 11 5-year-periods. We assessed trends in incidence rates using Joinpoint regression [7].

We compared patient, tumour and treatment characteristics by stage using $\chi 2$ (homogeneity and trend tests). Unknown categories were not included in the calculation of the $\chi 2$.

Person-years at risk of developing a second primary cancer (skin non-melanoma excluded) were calculated from the date of testicular cancer diagnosis to the date of the second cancer, date of death, date of departure or 31 December 2013, whichever came first. The expected number of cancer cases was calculated by multiplying the period-age and sex-specific cancer incidence rates of the Geneva population for the period 1970–2012 by the person-years stratified in 5-year intervals. The standardized incidence ratio (SIR) was defined as the ratio between the number of observed cases and the number of expected cases. We calculated SIRs by morphology, stage, treatment and second site of malignancy. A 2-tailed 95% confidence interval (CI) of the SIR was calculated assuming a Poisson distribution of the observed numbers [8].

The patients were followed for vital status from the date of diagnosis to the date of death, the date of departure from the Canton or 31 December 2013, whichever came first. Overall and testicular cancer- specific survival (OS and CSS, respectively) were estimated using the Kaplan Meier method and stratified by age at diagnosis, period of diagnosis, socio-economic status, stage and morphology. Survival differences were tested through log rank test. For the analyses on second primary cancer and survival, one case that was discovered at autopsy has been excluded (n = 589). Survival analyses were performed for the whole study period as well as for the most recent years (1990–2012).

Results

The final cohort comprised 590 patients diagnosed with testicular germ cell tumors between 1970 and 2012. Of these, 340 were diagnosed with seminoma and 250 with non-seminoma.

The incidence rate increased slightly during the period 1970–2012 (APC = 2.85; p = 0.134) but the trend was not statistically significant (Fig. 1). The trends by age group showed that the most substantial increase was observed in men aged 30–49 years (APC = 5.65, p = 0.197), and the highest incidence rate among patients aged 30–39 years (8.88/100′000) (Fig. 2).

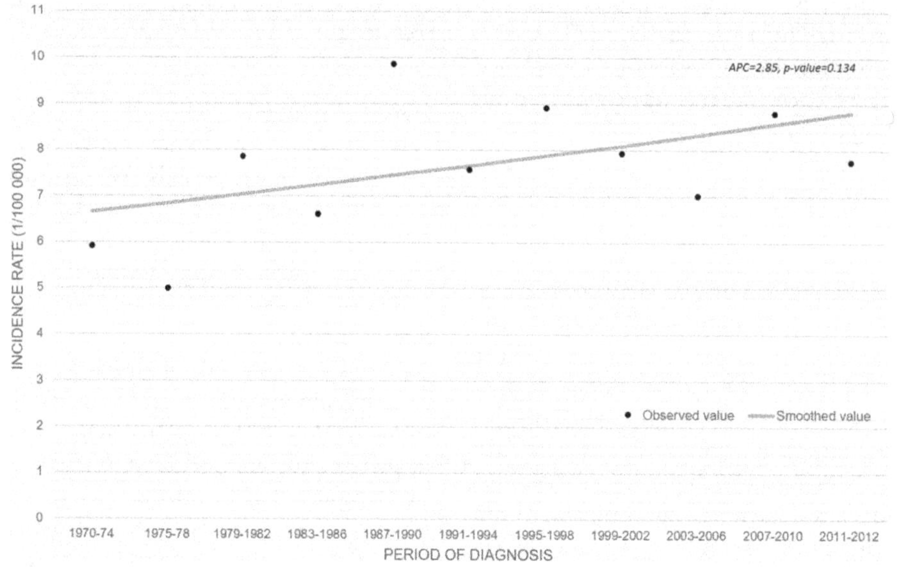

Fig. 1 Observed and smoothed incidence of germinal testicular cancer. 1970–2012

Table 1 shows the distribution of patient, tumor and treatment characteristics according to stage at diagnosis. During the study period, testicular cancer was diagnosed at an earlier stage: in 1970–1979 only 54% of all cancers were diagnosed at stage I while this proportion reached 72% in the period 2000–2012 (Chi2 test: $p = 0.038$, test for trend: p-value = 0.016). Lower SES was found to be associated with later stage at diagnosis: 21% of low SES men were diagnosed with stage III disease compared with 13 and 9% of the medium and high SES men, respectively (Chi2 test: $p = 0.034$, test for trend: p-value = 0.02). Regarding the morphology of the tumour, patients with non-seminoma were diagnosed with more advanced disease compared to seminoma (22, and 7.3% diagnosed at stage III respectively, p-value< 0.001). Radiotherapy was administered to 59.7 and 8.4% of patients with seminomas and non-seminomas, respectively. Chemotherapy was given to 17.4 and 54.4% of patients with seminomas and non-seminomas, respectively. Patients with an early stage at diagnosis were more likely to receive radiotherapy (72% at stage I vs. 5% at stage III; p-value = 0.001) and less likely to receive chemotherapy (29.7% at stage I vs. 36.4% at stage III, p = < 0.001). These results were also significant when the analysis was limited

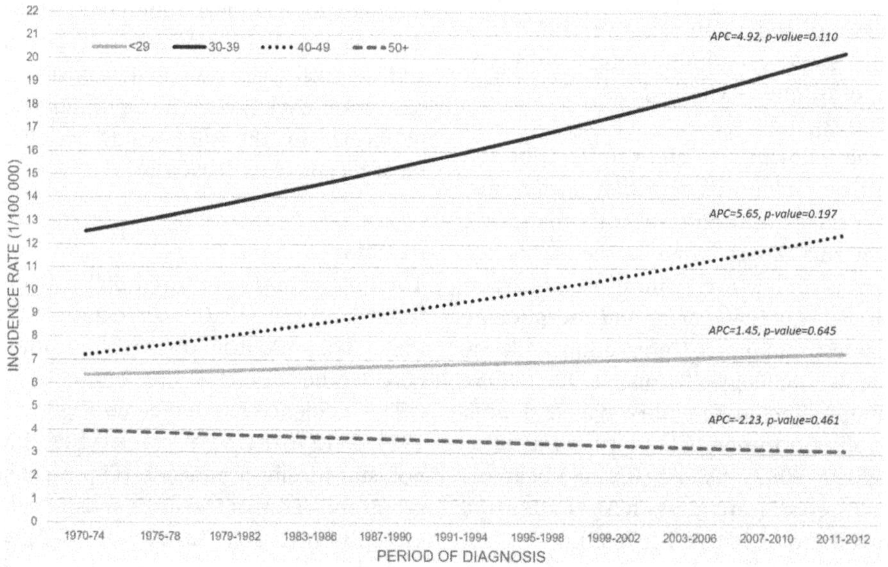

Fig. 2 Observed and smoothed incidence of germinal testicular cancer stratified by age groups. 1970–2012

Table 1 Socio-demographic, tumor and treatment characteristics according to clinical TNM among 590 men with TGCT. Geneva 1970–2012

	Stage I		Stage II		Stage III		Unknown	Total		*p*-value for Chi2 heterogeneity test[a]
	N	%	N	%	N	%	N	N	%	
Period										
1970–1979	39	54.2	21	29.2	12	16.7	11	83	100	0.038
1980–1989	74	59.7	32	25.8	18	14.5	9	133	100	
1990–1999	105	70	24	16	21	14	9	159	100	
2000–2012	153	71.8	32	15	28	13.2	2	215	100	
Age group										
≤ 29	116	62	39	20.9	32	17.1	13	200	100	0.089
30–39	144	73.1	28	14.2	25	12.7	9	206	100	
40–49	69	65.1	27	25.5	10	9.4	4	110	100	
50+	42	60.9	15	21.7	12	17.4	5	74	100	
Place of birth										
Switzerland	289	68	75	17.6	61	14.4	25	450	100	0.342
Europe	61	59.8	26	25.5	15	14.7	6	108	100	
Others	21	65.6	8	25	3	9.4	0	32	100	
Social class										
High	117	73.1	28	17.5	15	9.4	11	171	100	0.034
Medium	142	67.6	40	19	28	13.3	11	221	100	
Low	81	57.4	31	22	29	20.6	6	147	100	
Unknown	31	60.7	10	19.6	7	13.7	3	51	100	
Morphology										
Seminoma	245	74.5	60	18.2	24	7.3	11	340	100	<0.001
Non-seminoma	126	50.4	49	19.9	55	22	20	250	100	
Origin of diagnosis										
Symptoms	311	65.3	92	19.3	73	15.3	16	492	100	0.736
Fortuitous	31	73.8	7	16.7	4	9.5	1	43	100	
Check	8	66.7	3	25	1	8.3	0	12	100	
Autopsy							1	1	100	
Unknown	21	72.4	7	24.1	1	3.4	13	42	100	
Radiotherapy										
Seminoma										
No	94	70.7	22	16.5	17	12.8	4	137	100	0.007
Yes	151	77.0	38	19.4	7	3.6	7	203	100	
Non-seminoma										
No	122	57.6	39	18.4	51	24.1	17	229	100	0.001
Yes	4	22.2	10	55.6	4	22.2	3	21	100	
Chemotherapy										
Seminoma										
No	230	85.2	36	13.3	4	1.5	9	270	100	< 0.001
Yes	15	25.4	24	40.7	20	33.9	2	59	100	
Non-seminoma										
No	83	88.3	7	7.5	4	4.3	16	94	100	< 0.001
Yes	43	31.6	42	30.9	51	37.5	4	136	100	

[a]missing data are not considered for the chi2 test

to patients diagnosed in the most recent decades (1990–2013) (data not shown). Seven patients did not undergo surgery for their tumour. No association with stage at diagnosis was found for age and place of birth.

By the end of the study period, 106 deaths had occurred, 48 of which had testicular cancer as the underlying cause. The median follow-up was 10.9 years (range 0.06–42.4 years). Over the entire study period, the 10-year overall and cause-specific survival estimates were 88% (95% CI: 84–90) and 92% (95% CI: 89–94), respectively.

The 10-year survival trend for the whole study period, as well as survival stratified by age, SES, stage and morphology for the most recent years (1990–2012) are presented in Table 2. Both overall and cause specific survival improved significantly from the period 1970–1979 to 2000–2012 (from 65 to 94% for overall survival, p-value< 0.001; from 70 to 97% for cause-specific survival, p-value< 0.001). As the survival trend appeared to be stable from 1990 onwards, the results of survival by age, SES, stage and morphology were presented only for the more recent period.

Patients of low SES presented a lower specific survival compared with those from high social class (90, 95% CI: 79–95, vs. 98, 95% CI: 91–99) but the difference was not statistically significant (p-value = 0.078) for the period 1990–2012. It is however worth noting that when considering the whole period (1970–2012), SES was significantly associated with 10-year overall and specific survival SES (data not shown). We found a large difference in survival by stage at diagnosis, particularly for cancer-specific survival wherein men with stage I disease had a 10-year survival of 98% (95% CI: 96–100) while for men diagnosed with at stage III it was 81% (95% CI: 67–90) (p-value for log rank test< 0.001). Survival was higher for seminomas than non-seminomas for both overall and testicular cancer death (p-value for log-rank test< 0.001). Regarding morphology subtypes, patients with seminoma presented significantly higher survival rate (10-year overall survival: 96, 95%CI: 91–98; 10-year

Table 2 10-year overall and cancer-specific survival after a testicular cancer diagnosis. Geneva 1970–2012

	Overall			Specific		
	% surviving	95% CI	Log-rank	% surviving	95% CI	Log-rank
All patients	87%	[84–90]		92%	[89–94]	
By period						
1970–79	65%	[54–75]	< 0.001	70%	[59–79]	< 0.001
1980–89	86%	[78–91]		93%	[86–96]	
1990–99	94%	[88–97]		96%	[91–98]	
2000–12	94%	[87–97]		97%	[93–99]	
Patients diagnosed 1990–2012	94%	[90–96]		96%	[93–98]	
By age						
≤ 29	94%	[86–98]	0.015	96%	[90–99]	0.440
30–39	97%	[91–99]		98%	[94–100]	
40–49	94%	[83–98]		94%	[83–98]	
50+	83%	[61–93]		94%	[79–99]	
By social class						
High	94%	[85–98]	0.182	98%	[91–99]	0.078
Medium	97%	[91–99]		98%	[94–100]	
Low	88%	[77–94]		90%	[79–95]	
Unknown	91%	[65–98]		97%	[81–1.00]	
By stage						
I	96%	[92–98]	< 0.001	99%	[96–100]	< 0.001
II	93%	[74–98]		95%	[72–99]	
III	81%	[67–90]		81%	[67–90]	
Unknown	-	-		100%	-	
By morphology						
Seminoma	96%	[91–98]	0.014	98%	[94–100]	< 0.001
Non-seminoma	90%	[83–95]		93%	[87–96]	

specific survival: 99, 95% CI: 94–100) compared to non-seminoma tumours.

Among the 590 patients diagnosed with testicular cancer, 70 had had a second primary malignancy by the end of the follow-up period compared with 34.7 expected (SIR 2.02, 95% CI: 1.6–2.5, *p*-value = < 0.001) (Table 3). The risk for contralateral cancer of the testis was particularly high (SIR: 20.7, 95% CI: 11.9–33.7, *p*-value = < 0.001). The risk for pancreatic and bladder cancers was also increased (SIR 3.76, 95% CI: 0.8–11, *p*-value = 0.045 and SIR 3.98. 95% CI: 1.5–8.6, *p*-value = 0.005, respectively). The risk of pancreatic cancer was especially high for patients diagnosed with non-seminoma (SIR 9.8, 95% CI: 1.1–34, p- value = 0.018) and for those who had chemotherapy (SIR 13.0, 95% CI: 1.5–48.1, *p*-value = 0.011). The risk of bladder cancer was higher among patients with seminoma (SIR 4.4, 95% CI: 1.4–10.2, *p*-value = 0.006) and those treated with radiotherapy (SIR 5.1, 95% CI: 1.6–11.8, *p*-value = 0.004) (data not shown).

Discussion

This study shows that despite the high and increasing rate of testicular cancer in Switzerland overall, in Geneva the rate did not increase significantly between 1970 and 2012. However, there has been a clear trend towards earlier diagnosis and a significant improvement in survival in Geneva during this period, although differences by morphology and, to a lesser extent, by SES persist. The risk of developing a second cancer, particularly a contralateral testicular cancer, bladder or pancreatic cancer, is very high in these patients compared with the Geneva population.

A majority of Western countries have reported an increase in testicular cancer rates in recent decades [9, 10]. In Switzerland an increasing trend of testicular cancer has been observed over a period of 35 years with a growth of 1.4% every 2 years (95% CI: 0.7–2.0; p < 0.001). The increasing trend seems to be mainly driven, however, by cantons in the German speaking region which have higher incidence rates than those observed in the French speaking region, to which Geneva belongs [11]. In particular, the rates for the period 2011-2015was 12.1 (95% CI: 11.5–12.8) for the German speaking region and 8.9 (95% CI: 8.2—9.7) for the French speaking region. During the period 1970–2012, we observed only a not statistically significant slightly increasing trend, which was similar to that observed in the French-speaking canton of Vaud [4]. The authors of that study did not find an upward trend in testicular cancer rates during the period 1974–1999; they related their finding to the high testicular cancer rate already reached in the early 1990s [5].

Our results confirm that survival for testicular cancer has improved significantly since the 1970s, with 10- year cancer-specific survival now reaching 97%. This improvement can be ascribed to improvements in treatment, particularly with the advent of cisplatin and well defined management recommendations for the disease [12–14]. Survival rates are clearly associated with stage at diagnosis and morphology. In particular, patients in our study who were diagnosed at an advanced stage or with a non-seminoma cancer had a significantly worse survival, consistent with other studies [15].

Results about SES were not statistically significant and must be interpreted with caution. However, this study suggests that men with a low SES experience worse overall and cancer-specific survival in Geneva, despite obligatory health insurance which allows almost uniform access to healthcare and treatments [16]. SES inequalities observed in testicular cancer studies in England and Wales were attributed to differences in stage at diagnosis and access to treatment [17, 18]. In our study, men of low SES were more often diagnosed with an advanced stage, which could partially explain their lower survival and suggest delay in disease detection. Given the general consensus that routine screening of asymptomatic men, whether with palpation or biomarkers, is ineffective [12–14, 19], and that over 80% of our patients were diagnosed based on symptoms, it is important that both patients and clinicians have a high index of suspicion for this disease to avoid delay in diagnosis [14].

Because of their young age at diagnosis and the improving prognosis, men diagnosed with testicular cancer

Table 3 Standardized Incidence Ratios (SIR) for second primary cancer after a testicular cancer diagnosis according to site. Geneva 1970–2012

Localisation of the second cancer	Observed	Expected	SIR	95% CI	*p*-value
Controlateral testis	16	0.77	20.66	[11.9–33.7]	< 0.001
Pancreas	3	0.8	3.76	[0.8–11]	0.047
Bladder	6	1.51	3.98	[1.5–8.6]	0.005
Prostate	10	7.47	1.34	[0.6–2.5]	0.221
Stomach	2	0.93	2.15	[0.2–7.8]	0.239
Lung	6	5.4	1.2	[0.4–2.4]	0.385
All tumors (skin non-melanoma excluded)	70	34.73	2.02	[1.6–2.5]	< 0.001

are at increased risk of developing a second primary cancer during their lifetime. Compared with the Geneva population, our study population showed a doubling of their risk of a second cancer, especially of the contralateral testicular, pancreas or bladder. This is consistent with other reports. The increased risk of second primary cancers has been associated with the use of adjuvant therapies [20, 21]. We found an association between the use of radiotherapy and an excess risk of secondary bladder cancer, an infra-diaphragmatic site exposed to the radiotherapy field and between an excess of pancreatic cancer and treatment with chemotherapy, particularly in non-seminoma cancers. These findings align with those of other studies [21–24]. That said, the combined effect of both radiotherapy and chemotherapy on the risk of pancreatic cancer remains unclear. A previous study evaluating the risk of pancreatic cancer after treatment for Hodgkin's lymphoma suggested that patients who had both radiotherapy and > = 6 cycles of alkylating agents chemotherapy presented the highest risk [25]. Further studies should investigate if the same effect is observed for testicular cancers.

The risk of a second primary cancer for contralateral testicular cancer was extremely high and of the same order of magnitude as seen in other studies [21, 26–29]. Cryptorchidism, environmental exposures, epigenetic aberrations and genetic susceptibility are the suggested etiologic mechanisms for the development of this cancer [30]. The risk factors for a first testicular cancer can predispose for a second such cancer. However, in our study the risk of a second testicular cancer in patients who did not receive adjuvant therapies was the same as the risk for primary testicular cancer in the general population. This supports the theory that chemotherapy is a risk factor for the development of a second testicular cancer, contrasting the results of a study that found a reduced risk after chemotherapy with alkylating agents [31].

One limitation of our study is the relatively small number of cancer cases due to the rarity of testicular cancer and the small size of the population under study. Nevertheless, we included all of the 590 testicular cancer cases that occurred in the Geneva population over a 40-year period.

Another potential limitation is the possible lack of completeness of case ascertainment or lack of completeness of follow-up and treatment data. However, the accuracy of the Geneva cancer registry is rather high [32] in general and again as demonstrated in this study by the fact that only 1 case was discovered after death. Furthermore, the median time of follow-up was 11 years, cumulating in 7733 person-years of observation. Another marker of accuracy of the data is that all included cases were morphologically defined. Given the above, the findings are definitively generalizable to the overall patient population of Geneva, while caution should be used when trying to generalize them to other settings.

Conclusions

In contrast to the overall situation in Switzerland, there has been no significant increase in the incidence of testicular cancer in Geneva since 1970. At the same time, survival rates have been steadily improving. However, given the young age of patients affected, the very high risk of developing a second cancer, and the existence of strong inequalities in terms of stage at diagnosis and survival, heightened awareness of testicular cancer and its risks is vital, among both patients and clinicians, to promote early diagnosis and active surveillance of men diagnosed with this cancer.

Abbreviations

APC: Annual Percent Change; CI: Confidence Interval; CSS: Cause-Specific Survival; ICDO: International Classification of Diseases in Oncology; OS: Overall Survival; SES: Socio Economic Status; SIR: Standardised Incidence Ratio; TNM: Tumor-Node-Metastasis

Acknowledgements

The authors thank the staff of the Geneva Cancer Registry for their work and contribution.

Authors' contributions

ER, SP, CB, RS planned the study. HS collected the data. SP and ER carried out the literature review and prepared the draft of the paper. Data analysis was planned and implemented by RS and SP. ER, CB and RS provided input and feedback on the content data analysis and on the paper drafts. All authors read and approved the final manuscript.

References

1. Ferlay J, Ervik M, Lam F, Colombet M, Mery L, Piñeros M, Znaor A, Soerjomataram I, Bray F. Global Cancer Observatory: Cancer Today. Lyon: International Agency for Research on Cancer; 2018. Available from: https://gco.iarc.fr/today.
2. Tandstad T, Kollmannsberger CK, Roth BJ, Jeldres C, Gillessen S, Fizazi K, et al. Practice makes perfect: the rest of the story in testicular Cancer as a model curable neoplasm. J Clin Oncol. 2017 Nov;35(31):3525–8.
3. Levi F, Te VC, La Vecchia C. Testicular cancer trends in the Canton of Vaud, Switzerland, 1974-1987. Br J Cancer. 1990 Nov;62(5):871–3.
4. Levi F, Te V-C, Randimbison L, La Vecchia C. Trends in testicular cancer incidence in Vaud, Switzerland. Eur J Cancer Prev. 2003;12(4):347–9.
5. Levi F, Randimbison L, Te VC, Erler G, La Vecchia C. Risk of second cancer after testicular cancer in Vaud and Neuchâtel, Switzerland. Ann Oncol. 1999 Sep;10(9):1129–30.
6. ICD-10. International statistical classification of diseases and related health problems. Geneva: World Health Organization; 2011.
7. Kim HJ, Fay MP, Feuer EJ, Midthune DN. Permutation tests for joinpoint regression with applications to cancer rates. Stat Med. 2000 Feb;19(3):335–51.
8. Breslow NE, Day NE. Statistical methods in cancer research. Bd. 2: the design and analysis of cohort studies. Lyon: International Agency for Research on Cancer; 1987. p. 406. (IARC scientific publications)
9. Znaor A, Lortet-Tieulent J, Jemal A, Bray F. International variations and trends in testicular cancer incidence and mortality. Eur Urol. 2014 Jun;65(6):1095–106.
10. Nigam M, Aschebrook-Kilfoy B, Shikanov S, Eggener S. Increasing incidence of testicular cancer in the United States and Europe between 1992 and 2009. World J Urol. 2015 May;33(5):623–31.
11. Cancer data extracted from the Swiss national dataset managed by the Foundation National Institute for Cancer Epidemiology and Registration (NICER) [Internet]. [cited 2018 Jun 15]. Available from: Available from http://www.nicer.org/.
12. Souchon R, Hartmann M, Krege S, Lorch A, Mayer F, De Santis M, et al. Interdisciplinary evidence- based recommendations for the follow-up of

early stage seminomatous testicular germ cell cancer patients. Strahlenther Onkol. 2011 Mar;187(3):158–66.

13. Albers P, Albrecht W, Algaba F, Bokemeyer C, Cohn-Cedermark G, Fizazi K, et al. Guidelines on testicular Cancer: 2015 update. Eur Urol. 2015 Dec;68(6):1054–68.
14. Krege S, Beyer J, Souchon R, Albers P, Albrecht W, Algaba F, et al. European consensus conference on diagnosis and treatment of germ cell cancer: a report of the second meeting of the European germ cell Cancer consensus group (EGCCCG): part II. Eur Urol. 2008 Mar;53(3):497–513.
15. Sant M, Aareleid T, Artioli ME, Berrino F, Coebergh JW, Colonna M, et al. Ten-year survival and risk of relapse for testicular cancer: a EUROCARE high resolution study. Eur J Cancer. 2007 Feb;43(3):585–92.
16. OECD, WHO. OECD Reviews of Health Systems: Switzerland 2011 [Internet]. OECD Publishing; 2011 [cited 2018 Jun 15]. (OECD Reviews of Health Systems). Available from: https://read.oecd-ilibrary.org/social-issues-migration-health/oecd-reviews-of-health-systems-switzerland-2011_9789264120914-en.
17. Nur U, Rachet B, Mitry E, Cooper N, Coleman MP. Survival from testicular cancer in England and Wales up to 2001. Br J Cancer. 2008 Sep 23;99(Suppl 1):S80–2.
18. Woods LM, Rachet B, Coleman MP. Origins of socio-economic inequalities in cancer survival: a review. Ann Oncol. 2006 Jan;17(1):5–19.
19. Shaw J. Diagnosis and treatment of testicular cancer. Am Fam Physician. 2008;77(4):469–74.
20. Maroto P, Anguera G, Martin C. Long-term toxicity of the treatment for germ cell-cancer. A review. Crit Rev Oncol Hematol. 2018 Jan;121:62–7.
21. Travis LB, Fosså SD, Schonfeld SJ, McMaster ML, Lynch CF, Storm H, et al. Second cancers among 40 576 testicular Cancer patients: focus on long-term survivors. J Natl Cancer Inst. 2005;97(18):1354–65.
22. Kier MG, Hansen MK, Lauritsen J, Mortensen MS, Bandak M, Agerbaek M, et al. Second malignant neoplasms and cause of death in patients with germ cell Cancer: a Danish Nationwide cohort study. JAMA Oncol. 2016 Dec 1;2(12):1624–7.
23. Fung C, Fossa SD, Milano MT, Oldenburg J, Travis LB. Solid tumors after chemotherapy or surgery for testicular nonseminoma: a population-based study. J Clin Oncol. 2013 Oct 20;31(30):3807–14.
24. Hauptmann M, Børge Johannesen T, Gilbert ES, Stovall M, van Leeuwen FE, Rajaraman P, et al. Increased pancreatic cancer risk following radiotherapy for testicular cancer. Br J Cancer. 2016 Sep;115(7):901–8.
25. Dores GM, Curtis RE, van Leeuwen FE, Stovall M, Hall P, Lynch CF, et al. Pancreatic cancer risk after treatment of Hodgkin lymphoma. Ann Oncol. 2014 Oct;25(10):2073–9.
26. Osterlind A, Berthelsen JG, Abildgaard N, Hansen SO, Hjalgrim H, Johansen B, et al. Risk of bilateral testicular germ cell cancer in Denmark: 1960-1984. J Natl Cancer Inst. 1991 Oct 2;83(19):1391–5.
27. Fosså SD, Chen J, Schonfeld SJ, McGlynn KA, McMaster ML, Gail MH, et al. Risk of contralateral testicular cancer: a population-based study of 29,515 U. S. men. J Natl Cancer Inst. 2005;97(14):1056–66.
28. Andreassen KE, Grotmol T, Cvancarova MS, Johannesen TB, Fosså SD. Risk of metachronous contralateral testicular germ cell tumors: a population-based study of 7,102 Norwegian patients (1953-2007). Int J Cancer. 2011 Dec 15; 129(12):2867–74.
29. Travis LB, Curtis RE, Storm H, Hall P, Holowaty E, Van Leeuwen FE, et al. Risk of second malignant neoplasms among long-term survivors of testicular cancer. J Natl Cancer Inst. 1997;89(19):1429–39.
30. van der Zwan YG, Biermann K, Wolffenbuttel KP, Cools M, Looijenga LHJ. Gonadal maldevelopment as risk factor for germ cell cancer: towards a clinical decision model. Eur Urol. 2015 Apr;67(4):692–701.
31. van Leeuwen FE, Stiggelbout AM, van den Belt-Dusebout AW, Noyon R, Eliel MR, van Kerkhoff EH, et al. Second cancer risk following testicular cancer: a follow-up study of 1,909 patients. J Clin Oncol. 1993;11(3):415–24.
32. Forman D, Bray F, Brewster DH, Gombe Mbalawa C, Kohler B, Piñeros M, et al., editors. Cancer incidence in five continents. Lyon: International Agency for Research on Cancer; 2014.

12

Impact of case volume per year on flexible Ureteroscopy practice: An internet based survey

Omar Alhunaidi[1], Abdulrahman A. Ahmad[2], Ahmed R. EL-Nahas[1,3*], Bader Akroof[1], Ali Alamiri[1], Feras Al-Ajrawi[4], Abdullatif Al-Terki[1] and Mohamed El-Shazly[5]

Abstract

Background: To report current worldwide variation in techniques and clinical practice of flexible ureteroscopy (FURS) among endourologists of different case volumes per year.

Methods: Two invitations to complete an internet survey were emailed to Endourological Society members. Some of survey questions asked about indications of using FURS for renal and upper ureteral stones. Others were concerned with clinical practice of FURS (such as preoperative stenting, use of ureteral access sheath (UAS) and safety guidewire, technique of Laser lithotripsy and fragment retrieval, and post-FURS stenting. Responders were distributed into two groups; high-volume (> 100 cases/year) and low-volume surgeons (< 100 cases/year) and data were compared between both groups.

Results: Responses were received from 146 endourologists all over the world (62 high-volume and 84 low-volume). FURS for intrarenal stone > 20 mm was used by 61% of high-volume surgeons compared with 28.6% for low-volume ($P < 0.001$). Semirigid URS was used for upper ureteric stones in 68% among high-volume group and 82% in low-volume group ($P = 0.044$). UAS was used by 62% in low-volume group and 69% in high volume group ($P = 0.516$). Laser stone dusting was preferred by 63% in low-volume group versus 45% by high-volume ($P = 0.031$). More responders in low-volume group preferred to leave the stent for 6 weeks ($P = 0.042$).

Conclusions: The use of FURS for treating upper tract calculi has expanded by high volume endourologists to include large renal stones > 20 mm. Low-volume surgeons prefer to use semi-rigid URS for treatment of upper ureteral stones, to apply Laser stone dusting and maintain ureteral stents for longer periods.

Keywords: Flexible ureteroscopy, Survey, Stones, Ureteral access sheath, Flexible URS

Background

Treatment of upper urinary tract calculi has changed in recent years because of development of minimally invasive techniques such as flexible ureteroscopy (FURS) and miniaturized percutaneous nephrolithotomy (mini, ultra-mini and micro PCNL) [1]. Technological advances in FURS design (such as improved active tip deflection and digital image transfer), Laser lithotripsy techniques, advances in instruments as tipless baskets and ureteral access sheath (UAS) have resulted in increasing the utilization of FURS in treatment of renal and upper ureteric calculi. European Association of Urology (EAU) Guidelines recommended shock waves lithotripsy (SWL) and endourological for treatment of renal stones < 2 cm [2]. AUA guidelines recommended PCNL for treatment of large renal stones < 2 cm [3]. However, some experienced authors reported successful and safe use of FURS for treating larger stone burdens < 2 cm [4, 5].

The large variety of instruments used during FURS offered increased surgical efficiency, decreased frequency and severity of complications, and improved cost effectiveness. Many controversies in FURS indications, techniques and utilization of available instruments were addressed in previous surveys [6, 7]. However, the effect

* Correspondence: ar_el_nahas@yahoo.com
[1]Urology Department, Al-Amiri hospital, Kuwait City, Kuwait
[3]Urology and Nephrology Center, Mansoura University, Mansoura, Egypt
Full list of author information is available at the end of the article

of case volume per year on selection of certain indications, utilization of specific techniques and preference of instruments was reported in only one study that involved only European urologists [7]. High-volume URS cases per year was proved to result in better outcomes (such as shorter operative time, better stone free rates, shorter hospital stay, less need for retreatment, fewer and less severe complications) when compared with lower case-volume [8].

This study was conducted to report current worldwide variation in techniques and clinical practice of FURS among endourologists of different FURS workload per year.

Methods

Study design

An email invitation was sent to Endourological society members to answer an anonymous online survey in June 2017. A reminder email was sent after one month. The survey was conducted through SurveyMonkey® system and responses were collected over three months. By accepting the invitation to complete the online survey, all participants provided their informed consent to take part in the study. This study design did not require ethical approval because no patients were included.

Survey

The online questionnaire contained 14 questions (three questions asked about country, period of doing FURS and number of FURS per year, two asked about using FURS for upper ureteral and large renal stones and 9 questions were concerned with clinical practice of FURS (such as preoperative stenting and urine culture, use of ureteral access sheath (UAS) and safety guidewire, type of FURS (fiberoptic or digital), technique of Laser lithotripsy and fragment retrieval, post-FURS stenting indications and period).

Participants

Responders were divided into two groups based on number of cases per year, high-volume surgeon with > 100 case/year and low-volume surgeon < 100 case/year [6]. FURS technical details and practice were compared between the two groups.

Statistical analysis

Statistical analysis was performed using SPSS V20 software (USA). All variables were categorical and were expressed as numbers and percentages. Chi-square test was used to compare the difference between both groups. *P* Value < 0.05 was considered statistically significant.

Results

Participants

The survey was answered by 146 responders of 1204 (12%) Endourological society members from 40 countries. They represent all continents (50 from North America, 42 from Europe, 29 from Asia, 16 from South America and 9 from Africa).

Differences between high and low-volume Endourologists

Table 1 summarized the comparison between both groups. High-volume surgeons were practicing FURS for significantly longer periods than low-volume group ($P < 0.001$). FURS for intrarenal stones > 20 mm was used by 61.3% of high-volume group versus 28.6% of low-volume group ($P < 0.001$). Semi-Rigid ureteroscopy for upper ureteric stone was more frequently preferred by low-volume group (82%) in comparison with 68% in high-volume group ($P = 0.044$). Stone dusting was preferred by 63% by low-volume group versus 45% by high-volume ($P = 0.031$). Another significant difference was the period of post-URS stents as more responders in low-volume group preferred to leave the stent for 6 weeks ($P = 0.042$).

Similarities between high and low-volume Endourologists

Regardless of the case volume per year, most responders (96%) used FURS in non-stented ureters, 80% request preoperative urine culture, 76% were using semirigid URS for upper ureteric stones and 70% used a basket for retrieval of stone fragments after disintegration. Two third of responders routinely uses a safety guidewire and UAS during FURS (Table 1).

Discussion

The superior results of surgeons with higher volume URS cases in comparison with others with lower volume cases was attributed to increasing surgical experience of the treating team (endourologist, nurses and technicians) [8]. In the present study, we reported the effect of case-volume per year on clinical practice and preference of certain instruments and surgical techniques of FURS.

High-volume responders in the present survey performed significantly more FURS for renal calculi > 20 mm despite that EAU and American Urological Association (AUA) guidelines [2, 3] that recommended PCNL as the first line for this stone size. However, high-volume endourologists used their experience to reach efficient outcomes [5, 8]. Moreover, we observed an increase in the overall preference of FURS for large renal stones among all responders (42%) in comparison with the survey conducted by Dauw et al. who reported 11% [6]. This may be explained by the increased experience of FURS surgical techniques and advances in Laser lithotripsy technology.

Table 1 Comparison between high and low-volume groups

Variable	Low-volume (< 100 cases/year) 84 N. (%)	High-volume (> 100 cases/year) 62 N. (%)	*P* value	Total 146
Years of doing FURS			< 0.001	
< 5 Years	23 (27.4)	6 (9.7)		29 (20)
5–10 Years	28 (33.3)	12 (19.3)		40 (27.3)
> 10 Years	33 (39.3)	44 (71)		77 (52.7)
FURS for stones >2 cm:			< 0.001	
Yes	24 (28.6)	38 (61.3)		62 (42.5)
No	60 (71.4)	24 (38.7)		84 (57.5)
Semi-Rigid URS for Upper Ureteric Stones:			0.044	
Yes	69 (82)	42 (67.7)		111 (76)
No	15 (18)	20 (32.3)		35 (24)
Pre-FURS Ureteric stent			0.492	
Yes	4 (4.8)	2 (3.2)		6 (4)
No	80 (95.2)	60 (96.8)		140 (96)
Preoperative Urine Culture:			0.331	
Yes	65 (77.4)	52 (84)		117 (80)
No	19 (22.6)	10 (16)		29 (20)
Type of FURS:			0.287	
Digital	28 (33.3)	26 (42)		54 (37)
Fiberoptic	56 (66.7)	36 (58)		92 (63)
Use of Safety Guidewire:			0.312	
No	5 (6)	8 (13)		13 (9)
In some cases	22 (26)	17 (27.3)		39 (26.6)
In all cases	57 (68)	37 (59.7)		94 (64.4)
Ureteral Access Sheath			0.516	
Yes	52 (62)	43 (69.4)		95 (65)
No	3 (3.5)	3 (4.8)		6 (4.2)
In prestented cases	29 (34.5%)	16 (25.8)		45 (30.8)
Laser Lithotripsy			0.031	
Dusting	53 (63)	28 (45.2)		81 (55.5)
Fragmentation	31 (37)	34 (54.8)		65 (44.5)
Fragments retrieval			0.485	
No Retrieval	22 (26.2)	12 (19.4)		34 (23.3)
Basket	56 (66.7)	47 (75.8)		103 (70.5)
Forceps	6 (7.1)	3 (4.8)		9 (6.2)
Postoperative Stent			0.539	
All cases	49 (58.3)	33 (53.2)		82 (56.2)
Indicated cases	35 (41.7)	29 (46.8)		64 (43.8)
Period of stenting after ureteric injury:			0.042	
2 Weeks	12 (14.3)	12 (19.4)		24 (16.5)
4 weeks	52 (62)	45 (72.6)		97 (66.5)
6 weeks	20 (23.7)	5 (8)		25 (17)

The second important difference was the preference of semirigid URS for treatment of upper ureteric calculi. Although high-volume endourologists used semirigid URS less frequently than low-volume group (68% vs 82%, $P = 0.044$). However, a considerable number of endourologists in each group preferred semirigid URS for treatment of upper ureteric stones. This may be attributed to financial causes in some countries, less experience in using FURS by some urologists (especially in low-volume group) or choosing to start with semirigid URS and if stone fragments escaped to the kidney, FURS can be used to retrieve them. AUA guidelines recommended that a FURS should be available when performing URS for proximal ureteric calculi [3]. Galal et al. and Karadag et al. compared both techniques for treatment of proximal ureteric calculi and reported that FURS offered significantly better stone free rate ($P = 0.005$) but rigid URS had significantly shorter operative time (P = 0.005) and both had comparable complication rates [9, 10].

The third difference in this survey was utilization of Laser dusting of stones by more endourologists in low-volume group (63% vs 45%, $P = 0.031$). High-volume endourologists prefer fragmentation and stones retrieval to achieve immediate stone free status in most patients, while low-volume surgeons prefer dusting and leaving gravels for spontaneous passage. Dusting uses low energy, high-frequency and long pulse duration setting to fragment stones into fine powder and small fragments that are left for spontaneous passage [11]. The stone free rates for fragmentation and basket retrieval were significantly better than dusting, but operative time was shorter for dusting [12, 13].

The use of UAS with FURS has been a controversial issue in urological literature. Advantages of UAS include ease of multiple passages of the scope, rapid stone extraction, higher stone free rates, low intrarenal pressure during prolonged procedures [14, 15]. Other reports showed no advantages of UAS for stone free rate or operative time, while the incidence of complications was higher with UAS [16, 17]. In the present survey, the use of UAS was practiced by 62 and 69% of responders in group 1 and 2 respectively ($P = 0.516$). It is obvious that about two thirds of endourologists of different levels of case load believe that the advantages of UAS outweigh its disadvantages. A similar result was reported from a large European survey where 70.7% used UAS [7].

When asking about the use of a safety guidewire, 68% of group 1 and 60% of group 2 indicated that they used it in all cases. In the past, use of a safety guidewire was highly advised to allow smooth access to the pelvicalyceal system and facilitates ureteral stent placement in case of ureteral or collecting system injury [18]. A study by Western Endourological stone consortium showed that the risks for FURS damage were significantly decreased when using a safety guidewire [19]. Currently; and with increased use of UAS; there are some reports of FURS without a safety guidewire [20, 21]. In the present study, it was observed that 13% of high-volume surgeons did not use a safety guidewire compared to 6% of the other group. These rates are more than the reported 1.9% in the previous survey by Dauw et al. [6] and we think that it is expected to increase in future.

Another controversial issue is the placement of ureteric stent either before or after FURS. The present survey showed that the majority endourologists in both groups follow the AUA guidelines [3] in omitting ureteral stent placement prior to FURS. For post-FURS stenting, the AUA guidelines recommended ureteric stent placement in certain indications such as ureteral injury, ureteric stricture, large stone size, incomplete stone fragmentation, solitary kidney or impaired renal function [3]. However, in the present survey 58% of group 1 and 53% of group 2 placed a stent in all cases after FURS. These rates are comparable to previously reported 64% by Dauw et al. [6] and slightly more than the 44% reported in the European survey [7].

Low response rate (12%) in comparison with 20% in Dauw et al. survey among Endourology Society members [6] was the major limitation of the present study. However, responders represented all regions around the world. This survey included specific group of urologists who are interested in endourology as primary subspecialty. Therefore, the results cannot be extrapolated to general urologists. On the other hand, this study showed the differences in clinical practice of FURS among endourologists of low versus high-case volume. This is highly valuable to know the current controversies, agreement or disagreements with international guidelines. The future implications include conducting randomized controlled studies to compare the safety and efficacy of controversial issues involving FURS indications, instruments and clinical practice.

Conclusions

The use of FURS for treating upper tract calculi has expanded by high-volume endourologists to include large renal stones > 20 mm. Low-volume surgeons prefer to use semi-rigid URS for treatment of upper ureteral stones, to apply Laser stone dusting and maintain ureteral stents for longer periods. Ureteral access sheath is commonly used whatever the case-volume per year.

Abbreviations

AUA: American Urological Association; EAU: European Association of Urology; FURS: Flexible ureteroscopy; PCNL: Percutaneous nephrolithotomy; UAS: Ureteral access sheath; URS: Ureteroscopy

Acknowledgements

Not applicable.

Authors' contributions

OA: Design of the work, AAA: Acquisition of data and drafting the manuscript, ARE: Interpretation of data and drafting the manuscript, BA: Analysis of the data, AA: Acquisition and analysis of data, FA: Acquisition and analysis of data, AA: Revision of the manuscript, ME: Study conception. All authors read and approved the final manuscript.

Author details

[1]Urology Department, Al-Amiri hospital, Kuwait City, Kuwait. [2]Urology Department, Adan hospital, Hadiya, Kuwait. [3]Urology and Nephrology Center, Mansoura University, Mansoura, Egypt. [4]Urology Department, Al-Farwaniya hospital, Sabah Al Nasser, Kuwait. [5]Urology Department, Menoufia University, Al Minufya, Egypt.

References

1. De S, Autorino R, Kim FJ, Zargar H, Laydner H, Balsamo R, Torricelli FC, Di Palma C, Molina WR, Monga M, et al. Percutaneous nephrolithotomy versus retrograde intrarenal surgery: a systematic review and meta-analysis. Eur Urol. 2015;67(1):125–37.
2. Turk C, Petrik A, Sarica K, Seitz C, Skolarikos A, Straub M, Knoll T. EAU guidelines on interventional treatment for Urolithiasis. Eur Urol. 2016;69(3): 475–82.
3. Assimos D, Krambeck A, Miller NL, Monga M, Murad MH, Nelson CP, Pace KT, Pais VM Jr, Pearle MS, Preminger GM, et al. Surgical management of stones: American urological association/Endourological society guideline, PART II. J Urol. 2016;196(4):1161–9.
4. Bagley DH, Healy KA, Kleinmann N. Ureteroscopic treatment of larger renal calculi (>2 cm). Arab J Urol. 2012;10(3):296–300.
5. Aboumarzouk OM, Monga M, Kata SG, Traxer O, Somani BK. Flexible ureteroscopy and laser lithotripsy for stones >2 cm: a systematic review and meta-analysis. J Endourol. 2012;26(10):1257–63.
6. Dauw CA, Simeon L, Alruwaily AF, Sanguedolce F, Hollingsworth JM, Roberts WW, Faerber GJ, Wolf JS Jr, Ghani KR. Contemporary practice patterns of flexible Ureteroscopy for treating renal stones: results of a worldwide survey. J Endourol. 2015;29(11):1221–30.
7. Sanguedolce F, Liatsikos E, Verze P, Hruby S, Breda A, Beatty JD, Knoll T. EAU young academic urologists group ATN: use of flexible ureteroscopy in the clinical practice for the treatment of renal stones: results from a large European survey conducted by the EAU young academic urologists-working party on endourology and urolithiasis. Urolithiasis. 2014;42(4):329–34.
8. Kandasami SV, Mamoulakis C, El-Nahas AR, Averch T, Tuncay OL, Rawandale-Patil A, Cormio L, de la Rosette JJ, Group CUGS. Impact of case volume on outcomes of ureteroscopy for ureteral stones: the clinical research office of the endourological society ureteroscopy global study. Eur Urol. 2014;66(6): 1046–51.
9. Galal EM, Anwar AZ, El-Bab TK, Abdelhamid AM. Retrospective comparative study of rigid and flexible ureteroscopy for treatment of proximal ureteral stones. Int Braz J Urol. 2016;42(5):967–72.
10. Karadag MA, Demir A, Cecen K, Bagcioglu M, Kocaaslan R, Altunrende F. Flexible ureterorenoscopy versus semirigid ureteroscopy for the treatment of proximal ureteral stones: a retrospective comparative analysis of 124 patients. Urol J. 2014;11(5):1867–72.
11. Kronenberg P, Somani B. Advances in lasers for the treatment of stones-a systematic review. Curr Urol Rep. 2018;19(6):45.
12. Humphreys MR, Shah OD, Monga M, Chang YH, Krambeck AE, Sur RL, Miller NL, Knudsen BE, Eisner BH, Matlaga BR, et al. Dusting versus Basketing during Ureteroscopy-which technique is more efficacious? A prospective multicenter trial from the EDGE research consortium. J Urol. 2018;199(5): 1272–6.
13. El-Nahas AR, Almousawi S, Alqattan Y, Alqadri IM, Al-Shaiji TF, Al-Terki A. Dusting versus fragmentation for renal stones during flexible ureteroscopy. Arab J Urol. 2019;17(2):138–42.
14. Kourambas J, Byrne RR, Preminger GM. Does a ureteral access sheath facilitate ureteroscopy? J Urol. 2001;165(3):789–93.
15. Auge BK, Pietrow PK, Lallas CD, Raj GV, Santa-Cruz RW, Preminger GM. Ureteral access sheath provides protection against elevated renal pressures during routine flexible ureteroscopic stone manipulation. J Endourol. 2004; 18(1):33–6.
16. Traxer O, Wendt-Nordahl G, Sodha H, Rassweiler J, Meretyk S, Tefekli A, Coz F, de la Rosette JJ. Differences in renal stone treatment and outcomes for patients treated either with or without the support of a ureteral access sheath: the clinical research office of the endourological society ureteroscopy global study. World J Urol. 2015;33(12):2137–44.
17. Huang J, Zhao Z, AlSmadi JK, Liang X, Zhong F, Zeng T, Wu W, Deng T, Lai Y, Liu L, et al. Use of the ureteral access sheath during ureteroscopy: a systematic review and meta-analysis. PLoS One. 2018;13(2):e0193600.
18. Rodriguez-Monsalve Herrero M, Doizi S, Keller EX, De Coninck V, Traxer O. Retrograde intrarenal surgery: an expanding role in treatment of urolithiasis. Asian J Urol. 2018;5(4):264–73.
19. Taguchi K, Harper JD, Stoller ML, Duty BD, Sorensen MD, Sur RL, Usawachintachit M, Tzou DT, Wenzler DL, Isaacson D, et al. Identifying factors associated with need for flexible ureteroscope repair: a Western Endourology STone (WEST) research consortium prospective cohort study. Urolithiasis. 2018;46(6):559–66.
20. Dutta R, Vyas A, Landman J, Clayman RV. Death of the safety guidewire. J Endourol. 2016;30(9):941–4.
21. Ulvik O, Rennesund K, Gjengsto P, Wentzel-Larsen T, Ulvik NM. Ureteroscopy with and without safety guide wire: should the safety wire still be mandatory? J Endourol. 2013;27(10):1197–202.

13

Pure stress urinary incontinence: Analysis of prevalence, estimation of costs and financial impact

Emanuele Rubilotta[1*], Matteo Balzarro[1], Antonio D'Amico[1], Maria Angela Cerruto[1], Silvia Bassi[1], Chiara Bovo[2], Valerio Iacovelli[3], Daniele Bianchi[3], Walter Artibani[1] and Enrico Finazzi Agrò[3]

Abstract

Background: The prevalence of pure stress urinary incontinence (P-SUI) and the role of urodynamic investigation (UDI) prior to surgery for stress urinary incontinence (SUI) is debated. Since the exact prevalence of P-SUI is not clear, its clinical and economic impact is not well defined. The aims of this study were to evaluate the prevalence of P-SUI in a population of women who underwent UDI for urinary incontinence (UI), also assessing: 1) the correspondence between clinical diagnosis of P-SUI and urodynamic findings; 2) the analysis of costs in terms of UDI and eventually post-UDI avoided surgical procedures.

Methods: A single cohort of women who underwent UDI for UI between January 2012 and July 2016 was prospectively collected and retrospectively analyzed. Clinical P-SUI was defined by the strict criteria of the International Continence Society. For each patient, history, physical examination and UDI were collected. The correspondence between clinical and urodynamic findings of P-SUI was analyzed. The rate of clinical P-SUI changed after performing UDI and the number of unnecessary intervention after UDI were reported. A wide cost analysis of UDIs, and the amount of surgical procedures that were believed unnecessary after UDI was reported.

Results: Stress urinary incontinence was present in 323/544 (59.4%) patients. The prevalence of clinical P-SUI was 20.7% (67/323), while the prevalence of complicated SUI (C-SUI) was 79.3% (256/323). After UDI, diagnosis of P-SUI decreased to 18.3% (59/232). In 10.2% of cases (6/59) the scheduled middle urethral sling (MUS) was suppressed after the UDI results because 3/6 cases had detrusor overactivity and urge incontinence, in 2/6 cases SUI was treated with a conservative management, in 1/6 case an important voiding dysfunction was detected. Considering the national reimbursement in our country, the cost of each UDI was 296.5 euros and the total amount was 17,493.5 euros. So far the surgery-related savings covered 61.7–105.0% of the costs of total number of UDIs performed in the uncomplicated patients.

Conclusions: The prevalence of clinical P-SUI is relevant, involving about 20% of women with clinical SUI. Although the correspondence between clinical and urodynamic diagnosis was high, we demonstrated that UDI may help in some cases to avoid an inappropriate surgical treatment. Therefore, UDI prior to SUI surgery should be considered to achieve a correct diagnosis and a proper therapeutic strategy.

* Correspondence: emanuele.rubilotta@aovr.veneto.it
[1]Department of Urology, Azienda Ospedaliera Universitaria Integrata (AOUI), Piazzale Aristide Stefani, 1, 37126 Verona, Italy
Full list of author information is available at the end of the article

Background

Uncomplicated stress urinary incontinence (SUI), also called pure stress urinary incontinence (PSUI), and the role of urodynamic investigation (UDI) prior to surgery for SUI have been under debate in the last years [1–3].

Since the exact prevalence of P-SUI is not clear, its clinical and economic impact is even not well defined. It has been calculated that in women with uncomplicated SUI and a confirmatory preoperative basic office evaluation, from 13 to 33 millions of US dollars could be saved annually by not performing UDI test [4]. Nevertheless, other authors reported that savings obtained by not performing UDI in these patients seem to be moderate [5].

Considering the cost of a single UDI, it has been debated if it is useful in women with uncomplicated SUI prior to surgical correction. Few papers showed that an office evaluation is a sufficient work-up for women with uncomplicated SUI, since their incontinence surgery outcomes were not inferior if compared to women who underwent UDI [6, 7]. However, the correlation between real prevalence of uncomplicated SUI and costs of clinical evaluation, UDI and surgical treatment has never been systematically analysed.

The aim of our study was to evaluate the prevalence of clinical P-SUI in a population of women who underwent UDI for urinary incontinence (UI), assessing the correspondence between clinical diagnosis of P-SUI and urodynamic stress incontinence. Our secondary end-point was to analyze the costs of UDI in women with P-SUI, and the number of surgical procedures that were believed unnecessary after UDI, including related money savings.

Methods

A single cohort of women who underwent UDI for UI between January 2012 and July 2016 was prospectively collected and retrospectively analyzed. Data were obtained from an electronic database. Urodynamic tests were performed according to the Good Urodynamic Practice [7]. P-SUI was defined by the International Continence Society (ICS) criteria. All women with clinical P-SUI had no history of: (i) previous pelvic surgical treatments; (ii) pain; (iii) aematuria; (iiii) recurrent infections; (iiiii) voiding symptoms; (iiiiii) pelvic irradiation; (iiiiiii) suspected fistula. Inclusion criteria were: naive patients for SUI without pelvic organ prolapse.

All women underwent UDI and their data were assessed by a urologist skilled in UDI and female urology. For all the patients, the first evaluation was obtained in the outpatient clinic recording patient's history and physical exam. Though the history, the clinician assessed the prevalent type of incontinence and its duration, moreover urinalysis and urine culture were analyzed. The physical exam included abdominal, pelvic and vaginal examination, a stress test (with an ultrasound estimated bladder volume of 200 ml, and if negative with a bladder volume of 300 ml) and uroflowmetry with post-voiding residual volume [8]. Then, in case of sterile urine culture, a UDI was performed. Finally, the correspondence between clinical and urodynamic stress incontinence was evaluated.

UDI findings were compared with clinical data and the results were considered different when a UDI outcome was not correspondent to the pre-UDI expected clinical data. Clinical P-SUI was not confirmed when at least one of the following UDI observations was found: i) mixed urinary incontinence with predominant detrusor overactivity; ii) detrusor underactivity; iii) voiding dysfunction. Patients were considered to have a detrusor underactivity when Qmax was ≤12 ml/sec and Pdet/Qmax was ≤10 cmH2O [9]. Women were classified as having voiding dysfunction when Qmax was ≤12 ml/sec and Pdet/Qmax was ≥25 cmH2O [10, 11]. Depending on UDI results, surgical treatment options were discussed. Patients who had a change in the treatment strategy due to UDI results were recorded.

The exact cost of a single UDI was calculated with the support of the Clinical Management Department. The cost analysis included the human resources (one medical doctor and one nurse for each UDI) and all the materials used during the test. An additional economical evaluation was performed considering the National Health System reimbursement. Moreover, we calculated the total amount of expenses saved by not performing the scheduled surgical procedures of middle urethral sling (MUS) positioning, because they were believed unnecessary according to UDI results.

Results

Clinical SUI was diagnosed in 323/544 (59.4%) patients. Prevalence of clinical P-SUI was 20.7% (67/323), while prevalence of complicated SUI (C-SUI) was 79.3% (256/323).

After UDI, diagnosis of P-SUI decreased to 18.3% (59/323). In 11.9% (8/67) of patients diagnosis of clinical P-SUI was not confirmed due to the detection of predominant detrusor overactivity (3 cases), detrusor underactivity (4 cases), and voiding dysfunction (1 case).

In 8.96% of cases (6/67) the scheduled MUS was cancelled because of UDI results. In 3/6 patients detrusor overactivity and urge incontinence were detected, in 2/6 patients SUI was treated by pelvic floor rehabilitation, in 1/6 case an important voiding dysfunction was detected. Results are better shown in Fig. 1, which reports patients characteristics based on clinical and UDI diagnoses and details about surgical UI correction cancelled after UDI.

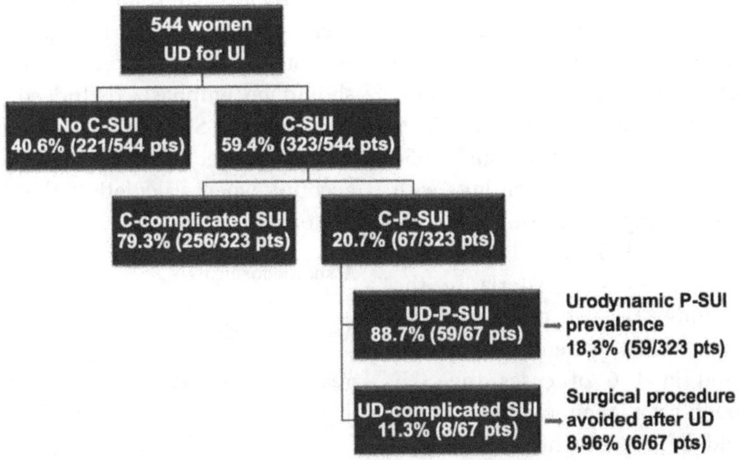

Fig. 1 Patients stratification based on clinical and urodynamic diagnoses, including their impact on surgical indications. (Legend: UDI: urodynamic investigation; UI, urinary incontinence; C-SUI: clinical stress urinary incontinence; P-SUI: pure stress urinary incontinence)

Being the Italian National Health System reimbursement for each UDI 296.5 €, the total cost for the 59 uncomplicated patients in our series was 17,493.5 €. If we consider a reimbursement by our National Health System ranging 1800–3073 € for each surgical procedure for female SUI (depending from the setting – Day Surgery or hospitalization for two or more days), the total amount saved thanks to UDI findings ranged 10,800–18,438 €. These savings cover 61.7–105.0% of the costs for total number of UDIs performed in the uncomplicated patients in our series.

Discussion

In the literature few data are available on P-SUI with a prevalence ranging from 5.2 to 36% [1, 2, 12, 13] (Table 1). In our series, prevalence was about 20%, aligned with the results reported by Jeong [13].

Some authors believe that the high prevalence of P-SUI could be secondary to restricted clinical skills [3]. For this reason, our lower rate might be related to a higher expertise in the field of urodynamics and female urology. Furthermore, this *know-how* could also explain the high correspondence between UDI findings and clinical data which is a relevant controversial topic in the literature (Table 1).

Some patients experienced a change in their therapeutic strategy after UDI, leading to a significant reduction of unnecessary surgical procedures (8.96%). Reversely, many women would have undergone an inappropriate surgical treatment (MUS) in case they did not perform UDI prior to surgery. Our results are aligned to those of Serati et al. who modified or cancelled the planned SUI surgery in 9.7 and 9.5% of cases, respectively [2].

In 2010, 260,000 MUS were implanted in the USA. If we consider a prevalence of clinical P-SUI of 20.7% (according to our study), we can therefore estimate that around 52,000 women underwent a MUS for P-SUI surgical correction [14]. Among these patients, almost 4659 (8.96%) might have undergone an unnecessary surgery if the UDI had not been administered before surgical treatment.

Thus, the issue of unnecessary surgical procedures seems to represent a major clinical and economic topic. Re-intervention rates related to voiding dysfunction or to mesh extrusion have been reported in 3.7% of cases [15]. Although with the limitations of this analysis, if we match such data with our results, an estimated number of 172 women may have experienced these complications due to an unnecessary surgical

Table 1 Pure stress urinary incontinence (P-SUI) prevalence, correspondence between clinical PSUI and urodynamic findings, and avoided surgery after urodynamic testing

	P-SUI prevalence	Correspondence	Avoided surgery
W. Agur et al., 2008	5.2%	–	–
S.J. Jeong et al., 2012 [13]	20.7%	79.1%	–
C.W. Nager et al., 2012 [1]	34%	43.2%	5.4%
M. Serati et al., 2015	36%	37.8%	9.5%
E. Rubilotta et al., 2019	20.7%	81.7%	8.96%

treatment. Moreover, considering the reported chronic pain rate of 4.1% after MUS, the estimated number of patients with this potential complication after an unnecessary surgery would be around 191. Considering literature data, 740 mesh removal procedures have been reported in peer-reviewed publications and 7654 meshes were removed in patients presenting with sling complications, thus leading to a total of 8394 complicated women after MUS [15]. Just in order to extend the analysis, if we apply our criteria to the population of the cited study [14], we confirmed the previously reported results: 1738 patients were supposed to have P-SUI and in 156 of cases the SUI surgical intervention could have been cancelled after UDI. These results would be even higher if we refer to the greater P-SUI prevalence reported by the other authors [1, 2].

In the light of these considerations, we believe that UDI may help in the clinical diagnostic process of all women presenting with SUI and not only in the complicated ones. Indeed, UDI might help to rule out unnecessary surgical treatments and their potential sequelae.

Cost analysis must contemplate both direct and indirect costs. The direct costs comprehend the total amount for a single UDI, for the surgical procedure, and for hospitalization. The negative externalities are those costs that occur in the complicated patients, including repeated UDI, use of devices, and potentially a new surgical treatment and hospitalization. Our estimated rate of unnecessary surgical treatment was 8.96%, meaning that without UDI these women would have had their insurance/health care to pay for their surgery without a confirmed indication. Nevertheless, insurance/health care would have paid even for the costs of the management of negative externalities.

In our study, we performed an analysis of the direct costs in a cohort of women with P-SUI. Analyzing the savings from the total number of UDIs performed in the uncomplicated patients in our series we found that costs of avoided surgical treatment covered the amount of money necessary for the UDIs. Regarding negative externalities, a complete cost evaluation should also include the potential legal actions due to complications after unnecessary interventions.

A limitation of our study may be related to the retrospective design, however all the data required were available for the analysis. A second limitation may be related to the different evaluations of the costs in diverse geographical areas.

Conclusions

The prevalence of clinical P-SUI is relevant, involving 1/5 of women with clinical SUI. The correspondence between clinical and urodynamic diagnosis is high. Nevertheless, in some patients an inappropriate treatment was avoided basing on urodynamic results. Although UDI involves an economic burden, its role should be emphasized. Indeed, according to our data, UDI prior to SUI surgery is useful to avoid unnecessary surgical procedures and this finding should be taken into account when calculating the real costs/savings about performing or not UDI.

Acknowledgements
None.

Authors' contributions
ER, MB designed the study, reviewed the literature and drafted the manuscript. SB, ADA, MAC participated in the design of the study, performed the procedures. CB performed the economic and statistical analysis. GV, PB participated in the study design and coordination. VI, DB participated in the study design and revised the manuscript. WA, EFA conceived of the study, participated in its design and coordination, supervised the draft. All authors read and approved the final manuscript.

Author details
[1]Department of Urology, Azienda Ospedaliera Universitaria Integrata (AOUI), Piazzale Aristide Stefani, 1, 37126 Verona, Italy. [2]Healthcare Department Administrator, Azienda Ospedaliera Universitaria Integrata (AOUI), Verona, Italy. [3]Department of Experimental Medicine and Surgery, Urology Unit, Tor Vergata University, Rome, Italy.

References

1. Nager CW, Brubaker L, Litman HJ, Zyczynski HM, Varner RE, Amundsen C, Sirls LT, Norton PA, Arisco AM, Chai TC, Zimmern P, Barber MD, Dandreo KJ, Menefee SA, Kenton K, Lowder J, Richter HE, Khandwala S, Nygaard I, Kraus SR, Johnson HW, Lemack GE, Mihova M, Albo ME, Mueller E, Sutkin G, Wilson TS, Hsu Y, Rozanski TA, Rickey LM, Rahn D, Tennstedt S, Kusek JW, Gormley EA, Urinary Incontinence Treatment Network. A randomized trial of urodynamic testing before stress-incontinence surgery. N Engl J Med. 2012; 366(21):1987–97.
2. Serati M, Topazio L, Bogani G, Costantini E, Pietropaolo A, Palleschi G, Carbone A, Soligo M, Del Popolo G, Li Marzi V, Salvatore S, Finazzi Agrò E. Urodynamics useless before surgery for female stress urinary incontinence: are you sure? Results from a multicenter single nation database. Neurourol Urodyn. 2016;35(7):809–12.
3. Van Leijsen SA, Kluivers KB, Mol BW, Broekhuis SR, Milani AL, Bongers MY, Aalders CI, Dietz V, Malmberg GG, Vierhout ME, Heesakkers JP. Can preoperative urodynamic investigation be omitted in women with stress urinary incontinence? A non-inferiority randomized controlled trial. Neurourol Urodyn. 2012;31(7):1118–23.
4. Norton PA, Nager CW, Brubaker L, Lemack GE, Sirls LT, Holley R, Chai TC, Kraus SR, Zyczynski H, Smith B, Stoddard A. Urinary incontinence treatment Network. The cost of preoperative urodynamics: a secondary analysis of the ValUE trial. Neurourol Urodyn. 2016;35(1):81–4 Epub 2014 Oct 18.
5. Finazzi Agrò E, Perugia C, Topazio L, Iacovelli V, Vespasiani G, Serati M. Urodynamic examinations performed before stress incontinence surgery in female patients: costs analysis in Italy. Neurourol Urodyn. 2016;35(issue S3): S51–2 Abstract n.52.
6. Serati M, Agrò EF. Urodynamics before surgery for stress urinary incontinence: the urodynamic examination is still one of the best friends of the surgeon and of patients with stress urinary incontinence. Eur Urol Focus. 2016;2(3):272–3.
7. Schafer W, Abrams P, Liao L, Mattiasson A, Pesce F, Spangberg A, Sterling AM, Zinner NR, van Kerrebroeck P. International continence society. Good urodynamic practices: uroflowmetry, filling cystometry, and pressure-flow studies. Neurourol Urodyn. 2002;21(3):261–74.
8. Guralnick ML, Fritel X, Tarcan T, Espuna M, Rosier PFWM. ICS-educational module: cough stress test in the evaluation of female urinary incontinence: introducing the ICS-uniform cough stress test. Neurourol Urodyn. 2018;37(5): 1849–55.
9. Gotoh M, Yoshikawa Y, Ohshima S. Pathophysiology and subjective symptoms in women with impaired bladder emptying. Int J Urol. 2006; 13(8):1053–7.

10. Defreitas GA, Zimmern PE, Lemack GE, Shariat SF. Refining diagnosis of anatomic female bladder outlet obstruction: comparison of pressure-flow study parameters in clinically obstructed women with those of normal controls. Urology. 2004;64(4):675–9 discussion 679-81.
11. Akikwala TV, Fleischman N, Nitti VW. Comparison of diagnostic criteria for female bladder outlet obstruction. J Urol. 2006;176(5):2093–7.
12. Agur W, Housami F, Drake M, Abrams P. Could the National Institute for health and clinical excellence guidelines on urodynamics in urinary incontinence put some women at risk of a bad outcome from stress incontinence surgery? BJU Int. 2009;103(5):635–9.
13. Jeong SJ, Kim HJ, Lee YJ, Lee JK, Lee BK, Choo YM, Oh JJ, Lee SC, Jeong CW, Yoon CY, Hong SK, Byun SS, Lee SE. Prevalence and clinical features of detrusor underactivity among elderly with lower urinary tract symptoms: a comparison between men and women. Korean J Urol. 2012;53(5):342–8.
14. Fabian G, Barcz E, Zwierzchowska A, Kociszewski J. Complications of sub-urethral sling procedures. Ginekol Pol. 2014;85:536–40.
15. Blaivas JG, Purohit RS, Benedon MS, Mekel G, Stern M, Billah M, Olugbade K, Bendavid R, Iakovlev V. Safety considerations for synthetic sling surgery. Nat Rev Urol. 2015;12(9):481–509.

14

Second-line treatment strategy for urothelial cancer patients who progress or are unfit for cisplatin therapy

Huitao Wang, Jianhe Liu*, Kewei Fang, Changxing Ke, Yongming Jiang, Guang Wang, Tongxin Yang, Tao Chen and Xin Shi

Abstract

Background: Second-line treatment for urothelial carcinoma (UC) patients is used if progression or failure after platinum-based chemotherapy occurs or if patients are cisplatin-unfit. However, there is still no widely accepted treatment strategy. We aimed to analyze the effectiveness and safety of second-line treatment strategies for UC patients.

Methods: The PubMed, Embase, and Cochrane databases were searched for randomized controlled trials (RCTs) that included UC patients who were cisplatin ineligible or unfit up to April 19, 2019. The primary outcomes were progression-free survival (PFS), overall survival (OS), and objective response rate (ORR).

Results: Thirteen trials that assessed 3502 UC patients were included. This study divided the network comparisons into three parts. The first part contained studies comparing taxanes and other interventions; the second part assessed investigator's choice chemotherapy (ICC)-related comparisons; and the third part assessed best support care (BSC). In the OS results of the first part, pembrolizumab (87.5%), ramucirumab plus docetaxel (74.6%), and atezolizumab (71.1%) had a relative advantage. Pembrolizumab also had advantages in ORR and severe adverse effect (SAE) results. Vinflunine and ramucirumab plus docetaxel had a relatively high surface under the cumulative ranking curve (SUCRA) rank by exploratory cluster analysis.

Conclusions: This study concluded that atezolizumab and pembrolizumab are superior to other treatments, mainly in OS results, but no treatment confers a significant advantage in PFS. Pembrolizumab still has relative advantages in ORR and SAE results compared to ICC. Due to limitations, more studies are necessary to confirm the conclusions.

Keywords: Urothelial carcinoma, Cisplatin-ineligible, Second-line, Meta-analysis

Introduction

Urothelial carcinoma (UC) is the most common cancer of the bladder and upper urinary tract and is invasive and lethal, especially in advanced and metastatic patients [1, 2]. Advanced UC (AUC) patients generally have a poor prognosis, and only a few patients survive more than 5 years [3]. Platinum-based first-line chemotherapy is a standard treatment for muscle-invasive UC (MIUC) and AUC patients and mainly includes gemcitabine plus cisplatin (GC) and methotrexate, vinblastine, doxorubicin, and cisplatin (MVAC) regimens [4, 5].

Although many patients have an initial objective response when they first receive platinum-based chemotherapy, some patients still have disease progression. For those patients, second-line treatment is then used [6, 7]. There is also a group of patients who are unfit for cisplatin treatment; the most common cause is renal insufficiency or neurological disease [8, 9]. For those patients, carboplatin-based treatment is usually applied. There are many types of second-line treatment for cisplatin-

* Correspondence: liujh1109@yeah.net
Department of Urology, The Second Affiliated Hospital of Kunming Medical University, No.374, Dianmian Avenue, Yunnan 650101, People's Republic of China

progression or unfit UC patients at present, including vinflunine, taxanes, checkpoint inhibitors, antiangiogenic therapy, etc. However, there is still no widely accepted treatment strategy.

Previous meta-analyses showed that immunotherapy can significantly improve UC patients' overall survival (OS) compared with chemotherapy, while antiangiogenic drugs combined with chemotherapy did not significantly improve patients' progression-free survival (PFS) and OS compared to chemotherapy alone. Taxanes and vinflunine treatment had similar effects but different side effects [10, 11]. A meta-analysis analyzed the efficacy of single and double chemotherapeutic drugs as second-line treatments. Although dual-drug combinations can improve the objective response rate (ORR) and PFS, they had no obvious benefit for OS [12]. This study will analyze the safety and effectiveness of second-line treatment strategies for UC patients with cisplatin progression or who are unfit for cisplatin by network meta-analysis to provide guidance for clinical treatment.

Methods

This network meta-analysis was reported in line with the preferred reporting items for systematic reviews and meta-analyses (PRISMA) and the PRISMA extension statement for network meta-analysis [13].

Data sources and searches

To identify studies for inclusion in this review, we searched the following public databases: PubMed, Embase, and the Cochrane Central Register of Controlled Trials up to April 19, 2019. The search terms used in the search strategy included ((((bladder OR intravesical OR urothelial OR urethral OR urothelium OR urinary)) AND (neoplasms OR cancer OR malignant OR carcinoma OR tumor)) AND (random* OR randomized OR randomised)) AND (cisplatin OR platin OR platinum OR carboplatin). Only English-language articles were considered. The search strategy is detailed in the supplementary materials (Additional file 4: Table S1). The references of related reviews were also checked to avoid omissions.

Study selection

Two authors independently selected the literature. In the case of any disagreements, a third author was introduced for discussion to reach a consensus. The inclusion criteria are as follows: 1, randomized controlled trials (RCTs); 2, studies that included UC patients who were cisplatin-resistant or unfit for cisplatin; 3, comparative studies on cytotoxicity therapy or immunotherapy; and 4, the outcome evaluation included one of the following: PFS, OS, and ORR. The exclusion criteria were as follows: 1, studies that compared the different doses or usage of the same drugs; and 2, studies that did not report one of the main outcomes (PFS, OS, or ORR). Conference abstracts, posters, and presentations of ongoing RCTs were also excluded because these brief reports do not contain detailed safety data.

Data extraction

Data extraction was performed at the study level but not at the individual level. The extraction contents included the following: author name, publication year, research location, sample size, age of patients, stage of disease, progression or unfit status after cisplatin, intervention treatment, control, outcome report, and follow-up period. The primary results included PFS, OS, and ORR results. The secondary results included severe adverse effects (SAEs) according to the National Cancer Institute (NCI) Common Terminology Criteria> = grade 3. The Cochrane Collaboration method, which includes seven specified domains, was used to assess the methodological quality of the included trials [14].

Data synthesis and statistical analysis

We used a frequentist framework, random-effects model for mixed multiple treatment comparisons. Network plots were produced for interventions and comparisons, and the node in each plot indicates the intervention regimen, while the line indicates each direct comparison [15]. We used odd ratios (ORs) and their 95% confidence intervals (Cls) to quantify the frequency of events results in the network meta-analysis, such as ORR and SAE results. Hazard ratios (HRs) and their 95% Cls were used to quantify the PFS and OS Cox regression results. The global inconsistency of the network analysis was evaluated by the fitness of the consistency model and the inconsistency model. Local inconsistency was assessed by the closed loops in the network for differences between direct and indirect comparisons. The surface under the cumulative ranking curve (SUCRA) probabilities were used to rank the treatments for each outcome [16]. Comparison-adjusted funnel plots were used to determine small-study effects in the analysis [17]. The SUCRA scores of all results were clustered by the average linkage clustering method to avoid the interference of individual deviation results on the overall results. A traditional meta-analysis was used to compare the interventions that could not be assessed by network meta-analysis. Data analyses were performed using STATA software (version 14.0; STATA Corporation, College Station, TX, USA).

Results

Literature search

The database searches yielded 1426 potentially relevant studies after the removal of duplications. A total of 1390 articles were excluded after screening the titles and abstracts. The full texts of the remaining 36 articles were assessed. Studies were excluded due to the following reasons: non-RCTs (9); conference abstracts (4); studies comparing the same intervention drugs (3); studies not analyzing cisplatin-progression or unfit patients (3); reviews (2); and duplicated publications (2) (Fig. 1). Finally, thirteen articles were included for further analysis [18–30].

In the included studies, 3502 cisplatin-progression or unfit UC patients were analyzed. The studies were all published after 2011. Two studies were located in the UK and France, while others were multicenter studies [22, 30]. All studies included AUC or metastatic UC patients. Two studies reported the results of the same population at different follow-up periods [18, 31], and this study combined the above two results (Table 1). All

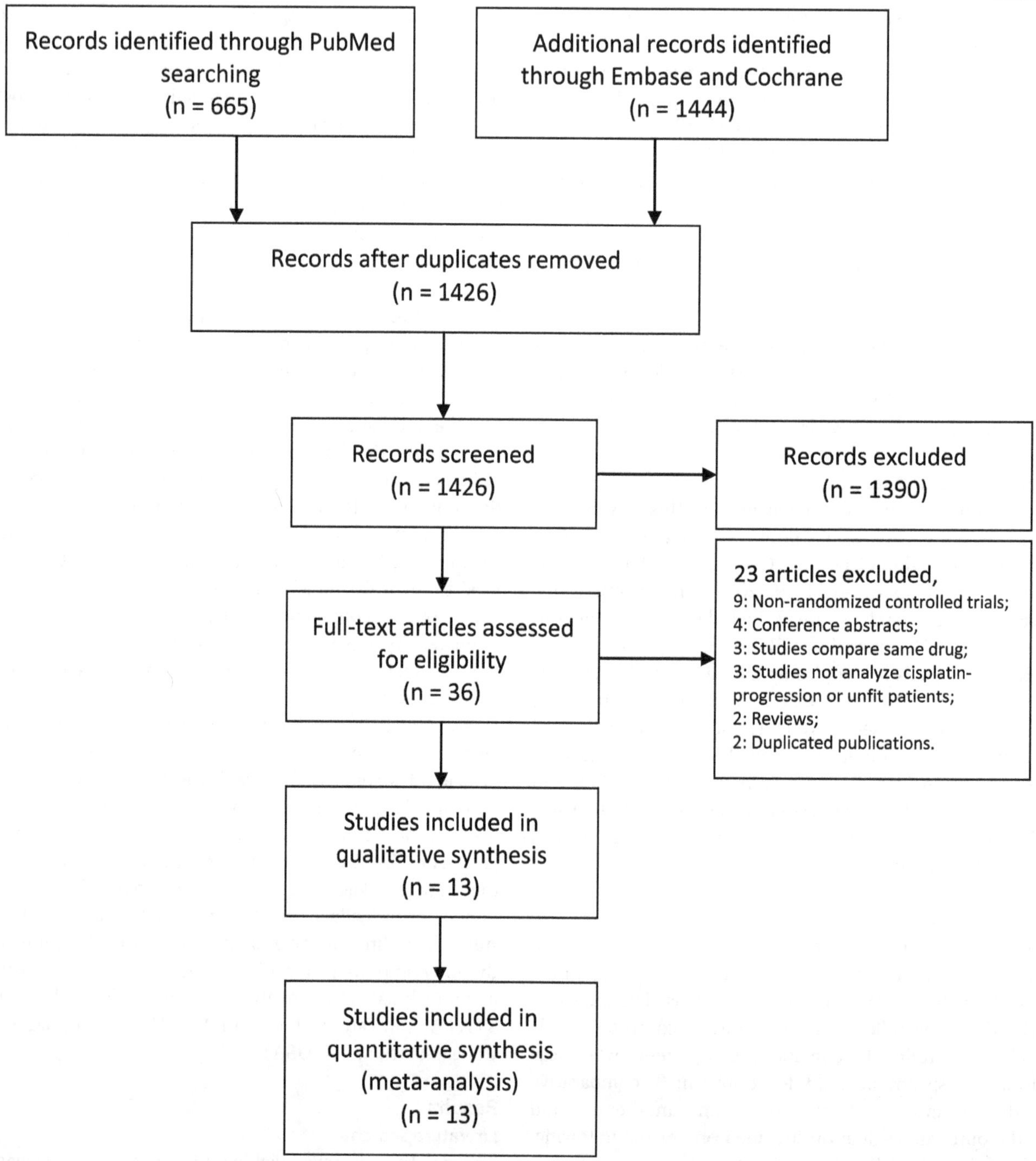

Fig. 1 Flow diagram of the study selection process

the studies were performed with a randomization design. Three studies were performed with a blindness design to reduce the impact of subjective awareness on the outcomes. Overall, the quality of the included studies was ideal (Fig. 2).

This study divided network comparisons into three parts. The first part contained studies comparing taxanes and other interventions, and the interventions included apatorsen plus docetaxel, icrucumab plus docetaxel, pazopanib, ramucirumab plus docetaxel, taxane, vandetanib plus docetaxel, and vinflunine. The second part contained studies comparing investigator's choice chemotherapy (ICC) and others, and interventions included atezolizumab, ICC, and pembrolizumab. The last part contained studies comparing best support care (BSC) and others, including personalized peptide vaccination (PPV) plus BSC, BSC, and vinflunine plus BSC. In the OS results, two ICC-related articles reported subgroup results according to different chemotherapy regimens [18, 20], so pembrolizumab and atezolizumab were also included in the OS results of the first part of the network analysis.

The first part of the taxane-related network analysis included PFS, OS, ORR and SAE results. Among the PFS results, there were six comparisons on taxane, among which the comparison of ramucirumab plus docetaxel and taxane was the most accurate (Fig. 3a). However, there were no significant differences among the network comparisons. Vinflunine and ramucirumab plus docetaxel ranked higher in the SUCRA results (Table 2).

Table 1 Characteristic of included studies

Author	Year	Location	Sample size	Title of research	Age[a]	Stage of disease	Reason of second-line therapy	Intervention	Control	Outcome	Follow-up[b]
Fradet Y [18] supplementa	2019	Multicentre	542	KEYNOTE-045	65(26–86)	Advanced	Progression	Pembrolizumab	ICC	OS;PFS; ORR;AE	Open
Rosenberg [19]	2018	Multicentre	200	Borealis-2	67(35–92)	Metastatic	Progression	Docetaxel plus Apatorsen	Docetaxel	OS;PFS; ORR;AE	Open
Powles T [20]	2018	Multicentre	931	IMvigor211	67(31–88)	Advanced or metastatic	Progression	Atezolizumab	ICC	OS;PFS; ORR;AE	Open
Petrylak DP [21]	2017	Multicentre	530	RANGE	66(32–86)	Advanced or metastatic	Progression	Docetaxel plus ramucirumab	Docetaxel placebo	PFS;ORR; AE	Open
Jones RJ [22]	2017	UK	131	NA	69(61–77)	Advanced or metastatic	Progression	Pazopanib	Paclitaxel	OS;PFS; AE;QOLS	Open
Bellmunt J [23]	2017	Multicentre	70	SECAVIN	63(35–80)	Advanced	Failure	Cabazitaxel	Vinflunine	ORR;PFS; OS	Open
Petrylak DP [24]	2016	Multicentre	148	NA	66(29–85)	Advanced or metastatic	Progression	Docetaxel plus ramucirumab	Docetaxel plus icrucumab	PFS;OS; ORR;SAE	Open
Santis MD [25]	2016	Multicentre	69	JASINT1	72(42–79)	Advanced	Unfit	Vinflunine; Gemcitabine	Vinflunine; Carboplatin	PFS;OS; SAE;ORR	25.9 M(24.3–26.5)
Noguchi M [26]	2015	Multicentre	80	NA	65(46–84)	Advanced	Progression	PPV plus BSC	BSC	PFS;OS; SAE	36 M
Bellmunt J [27]	2012	Multicentre	370	NA	NA	Advanced	Failure	Vinflunine;BSC	BSC	OS;PFS; ORR;SAE	21.5 M(16.7–25.3)
Choueiri TK [28]	2012	Multicentre	149	NA	NA	Advanced or metastatic	Progression	Docetaxel; vandetanib	Docetaxel; placebo	PFS;OS; SAE;ORR	Open
Santis MD [29]	2011	Multicentre	238	EORTC Study 30, 986	71(34–87)	Advanced	Unfit	Gemcitabine; carboplatin	Methotrexate; carboplatin; vinblastine	OS;PFS; ORR;SAE	Open
Culine Stephane [30]	2011	Frence	44	GETUG V01	76(48–86)	Advanced	Unfit	Gemcitabine	Gemcitabine; oxaliplatin	ORR;OS; SAE	Open

BSC Best support care, *ICC* investigator's choice chemotherapy, *NA* not available *PPV* personalized peptide vaccination
[a]Median (minimum-maximum)
[b]Open: follow-up until disease progress or patient death; M: months

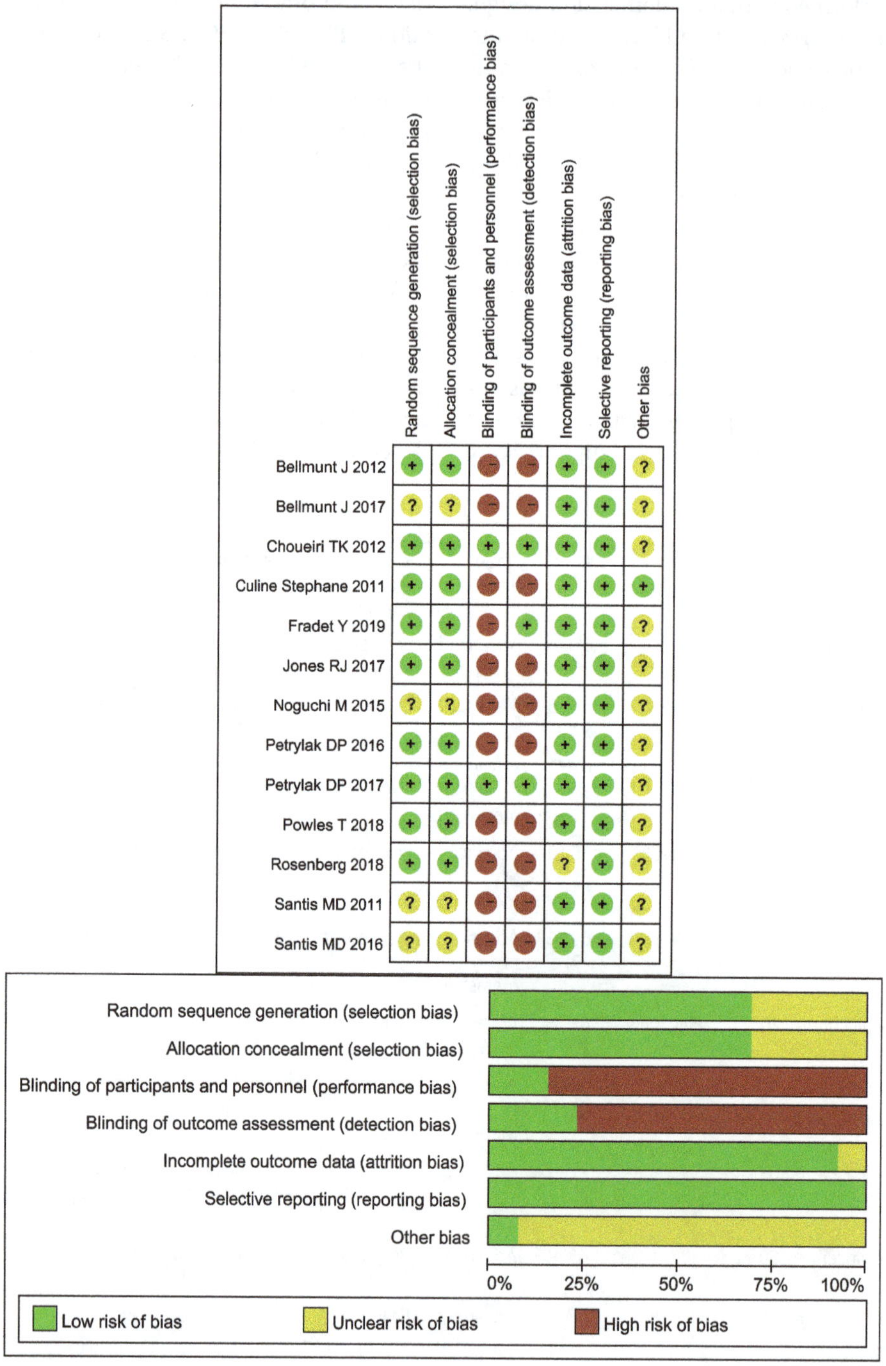

Fig. 2 Risk of bias of the included studies

In the OS results, there were eight comparisons on taxane, three on vinflunine, two on pembrolizumab and two on atezolizumab (Fig. 3b). In the consistency analysis, no local (Additional file 1: Figure S1) and global inconsistencies ($p = 0.2732$) were found. In network comparisons, atezolizumab was found to confer a significantly longer OS than pazopanib (ln HR: 0.49; 95% CI: 0.03, 0.95) and taxane (ln HR: 0.24; 95% CI: 0.03, 0.46). Pembrolizumab was significantly superior to pazopanib (ln HR:-0.61; 95% CI: − 1.07, − 0.15), taxane (ln HR: 0.36; 95% CI: 0.15, 0.57), and vandetanib plus taxane (ln HR: 0.55; 95% CI: 0.10, 1.01). Pembrolizumab (87.5%), ramucirumab plus docetaxel (74.6%), and atezolizumab (71.1%) had a relative advantage in the SUCRA results (Table 3). For the ORR results, there were six comparisons on taxane and a comparison between ramucirumab

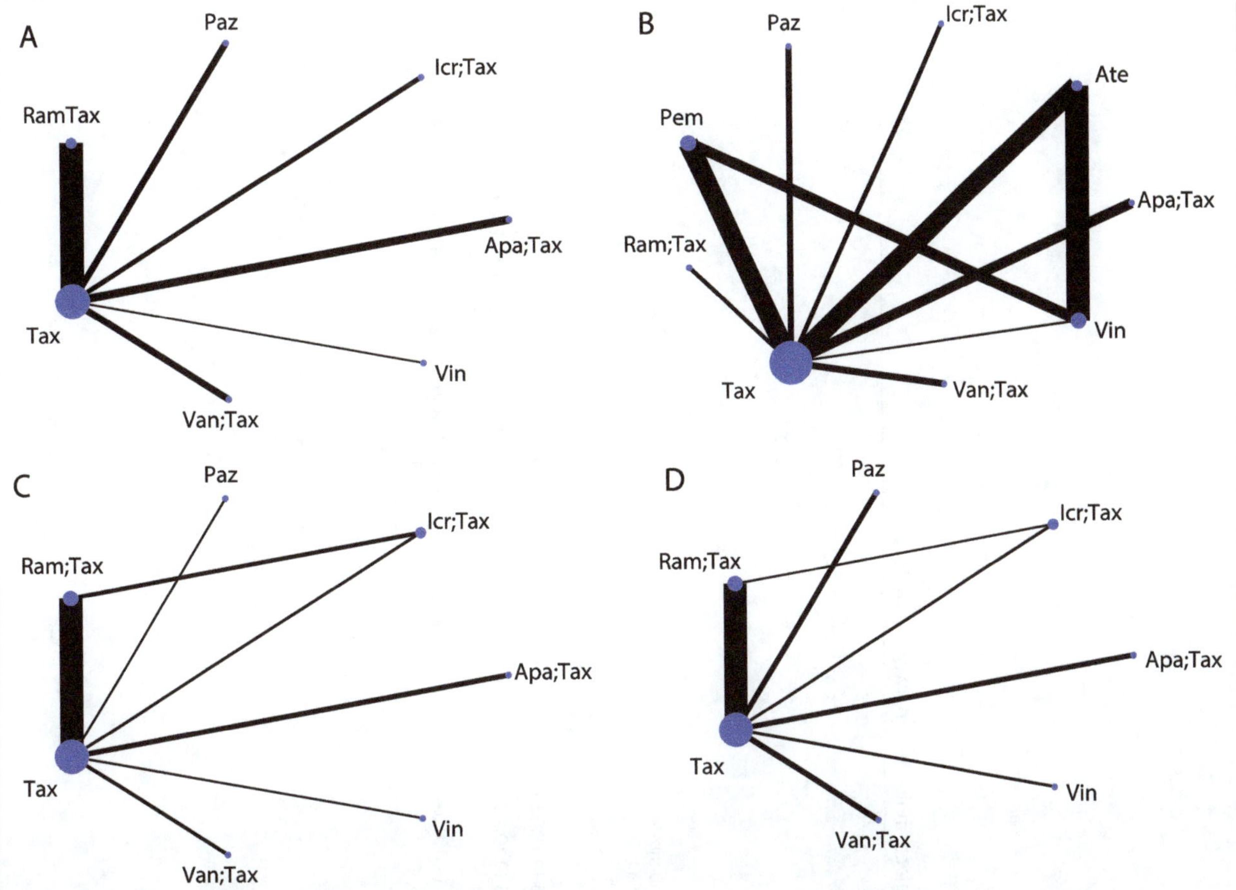

Fig. 3 First part: network comparisons of the interventions included in the analysis. A: PFS; B: OS; C: ORR; D: SAE. Abbreviations: Apa: apatorsen; Ate: atezolizumab; Icr: icrucumab; Paz: pazopanib; Pem: pembrolizumab; Ram: ramucirumab; Tax: taxane

Table 2 The league table for PFS estimates interventions according to their relative effects in first part network analysis

Apatorsen+Taxane (50.9%)[a]						
− 0.49 (− 1.90,0.93)	Vinflunine (79%)					
0.20 (− 1.09,1.49)	0.69 (− 0.73, 2.11)	Vandetanib+Taxane (36.3%)				
0.22 (−0.68,1.13)	0.71 (− 0.38, 1.80)	0.02 (− 0.90,0.94)	Taxane (31.7%)			
−0.35 (−1.47,0.77)	0.14 (− 1.13, 1.41)	− 0.55 (− 1.68,0.58)	−0.57 (− 1.23, 0.09)	Ramucirumab+Taxane (75.8%)		
0.31 (− 0.98,1.60)	0.80 (− 0.63, 2.22)	0.11 (− 1.19,1.41)	0.09 (− 0.83, 1.01)	0.66 (− 0.47,1.79)	Pazopanib (30.4%)	
0.08 (− 1.24,1.39)	0.56 (− 0.88, 2.01)	− 0.13 (− 1.45,1.20)	−0.15 (− 1.10, 0.80)	0.42 (− 0.73,1.58)	− 0.23 (− 1.56, 1.09)	Icrucumab+Taxane (45.9)

PFS Progression-free Survival
[a]The SUCRA probabilities are performed in brackets

Table 3 The league table for OS estimates interventions according to their relative effects in first part network analysis

Apatorsen+Taxane (66.6%)[a,b]								
− 0.02 (− 0.41,0.37)	Atezolizumab (71.1%)							
0.22 (−0.35,0.80)	0.24 (− 0.27,0.76)	Icrucumab+Taxane (36.3%)						
0.47 (−0.05,0.99)	**0.49 (0.03,0.95)**[b]	0.25 (−0.38,0.87)	Pazopanib (11.5%)					
−0.14 (− 0.53,0.25)	−0.12 (− 0.38,0.14)	−0.36 (− 0.88,0.15)	**− 0.61 (− 1.07,- 0.15)**	Pemborlizumab (87.5%)				
− 0.09 (− 0.67,0.50)	−0.07 (− 0.60,0.46)	−0.31 (− 0.99,0.37)	−0.56 (− 1.19,0.08)	0.05 (− 0.48,0.58)	Ramucirumab+Taxane (74.6%)			
0.22 (−0.10,0.55)	**0.24 (0.03,0.46)**	−0.00 (− 0.47,0.47)	−0.25 (− 0.66,0.16)	**0.36 (0.15,0.57)**	0.31 (− 0.18,0.80)	Taxane (31.6%)		
0.41 (−0.11,0.93)	0.43 (−0.02,0.89)	0.19 (− 0.43,0.81)	−0.06 (− 0.63,0.52)	**0.55 (0.10,1.01)**	0.50 (− 0.13,1.13)	0.19 (− 0.21, 0.59)	Vandetanib+Taxane (16.2%)	
0.07 (− 0.34,0.48)	0.09 (− 0.11,0.30)	−0.15 (− 0.68,0.38)	−0.40 (− 0.88,0.08)	0.21 (− 0.04,0.46)	0.16 (− 0.39,0.71)	−0.15 (− 0.40, 0.10)	−0.34 (− 0.82,0.13)	Vinflunine (54.6%)

OS Overall Survival
[a]The SUCRA probabilities are performed in brackets
[b]Bold font means significant different

plus docetaxel and icrucumab plus docetaxel (Fig. 3c). There were no local (Additional file 2: Figure S2) or global inconsistencies ($p = 0.4772$). Pazopanib had less ORR events compared to ramucirumab plus docetaxel (ln OR: -1.97; 95% CI: − 3.40, − 0.54) and vinflunine (ln OR: -2.27; 95% CI: − 4.32, − 0.21). Ramucirumab plus docetaxel had more events than taxane (ln OR: 0.76; 95% CI: 0.30,1.21). According to the SUCRA ranks, vinflunine (84.4%), ramucirumab plus docetaxel (82.4%), and apatorsen plus docetaxel (64.9%) have relative advantages (Table 4). There were no local (Additional file 3: Figure S3) or global inconsistencies ($p = 0.0878$) in the SAE results, and there were no significant differences in the network comparisons (Fig. 3d). Taxane had a relatively lower SAE frequency (79.8%) (Table 5). In addition to atezolizumab and pembrolizumab, exploratory cluster analysis showed that vinflunine and ramucirumab plus docetaxel had a relatively high SUCRA rank (Fig. 4). There were no small-study effects in the first part of the network analysis (Fig. 5).

The second part of the network analysis compared atezolizumab, pembrolizumab, and ICC (Fig. 6a-d). For the PFS results, there were no significant differences (Additional file 5: Table S2). For the OS results, atezolizumab (ln HR: 0.16; 95% CI: 0.01, 0.32) and pembrolizumab (ln HR: -0.36; 95% CI: − 0.55, − 0.16) were both superior to ICC (Additional file 6: Table S3). The ORR results showed that pembrolizumab is superior to atezolizumab (ln OR: -0.77; 95% CI: − 1.38, − 0.16) and ICC (ln OR: -0.77; 95% CI: − 1.25, − 0.29) (Additional file 7: Table S4). For the SAE results, pembrolizumab had a lower frequency of SAEs than atezolizumab (ln OR: 1.41; 95% CI: 0.91,1.90) and ICC (ln OR: 1.63; 95% CI: 1.21,2.04) (Additional file 8: Table S5). These results confirm the findings from the first part of the network analysis. Atezolizumab and pembrolizumab have advantages in OS. Pembrolizumab also has advantages in the ORR and SAE results. In the third part of the network analysis, BSC was evaluated as a control (Fig. 6e-g). No significant difference was found in either the PFS or OS results (Additional file 9: Table S6:Additional file 10: Table S7).

The interventions and comparisons that did not enter the network analysis were assessed by traditional meta-analysis. In only the ORR comparison between PPV plus BSC and BSC (OR: 25.85; 95% CI: 1.45, 461.43) was there a significant difference (Fig. 7). However, there was no objective response population in the BSC group in this study, so a large standard error value reduces the accuracy of the result.

Discussion

Platinum-based first-line chemotherapy is used to treat invasive-stage UC patients. When UC patients are cisplatin-ineligible or unfit, second-line treatment will be applied. However, the selection of second-line regimens in the clinic is still controversial. Conducting a comprehensive comparison among existing regimens and exploring more efficient and safe second-line treatments is still necessary. This work assessed the efficiency and safety of second-line therapy regimens for UC patients by network meta-analysis. The results showed that atezolizumab and pembrolizumab are superior to other treatments in only OS results, but no treatment confers a significant advantage in PFS results. Nevertheless, pembrolizumab still has relative advantages in ORR and SAE results. In addition to atezolizumab and pembrolizumab, exploratory cluster analysis showed that vinflunine and ramucirumab plus docetaxel had relatively high SUCRA ranks.

In a previous meta-analysis, immunotherapy, chemotherapy and antiangiogenesis were compared and analyzed. The results showed that immunotherapy, but not vinflunine, had more obvious benefits than taxanes regardless of PD-L1 status. Chemotherapy combined with vascular endothelial growth factor (VEGF) inhibitors did not significantly improve PFS or OS outcomes compared

Table 4 The league table for ORR estimates interventions according to their relative effects in first part network analysis

Apatorsen+Taxane (64.9%)[a]						
0.37 (− 1.08, 1.83)	Icrucumab+Taxane (46.8%)					
1.66 (−0.02,3.33)	1.29 (− 0.44,3.01)	Pazopanib (6%)				
−0.31 (−1.40, 0.77)	− 0.69 (− 1.72,0.35)	**−1.97 (− 3.40,- 0.54)**[b]	Ramucirumab+Taxane (82.4%)			
0.44 (− 0.54, 1.43)	0.07 (−1.00,1.14)	−1.22 (− 2.57,0.14)	**0.76 (0.30,1.21)**	Taxane (41.5%)		
0.93 (−0.60,2.46)	0.55 (−1.03,2.14)	−0.73 (−2.52,1.06)	1.24 (− 0.01,2.50)	0.49 (− 0.68, 1.65)	Vandetanib+Taxane (24%)	
− 0.61 (− 2.44, 1.22)	−0.98 (− 2.86,0.90)	**−2.27 (−4.32,- 0.21)**	−0.29 (− 1.91,1.32)	−1.05 (− 2.59, 0.50)	−1.54 (− 3.47,0.40)	Vinflunine (84.4%)

ORR Objective response rate
[a]The SUCRA probabilities are performed in brackets
[b]Bold font means significant different

Table 5 The league table for SAE estimates interventions according to their relative effects in first part network analysis

Apatoren+Taxane (49.6%)#						
−0.21 (−2.02,1.61)	Icrucumab+Taxane (38.5%)					
−0.25 (−2.00,1.51)	− 0.04 (− 1.85,1.77)	Pazopanib (36.7%)				
0.18 (−1.36,1.73)	0.39 (−0.98,1.76)	0.43 (−1.11, 1.97)	Ramucirumab+Taxane (59.7%)			
0.47 (−0.77,1.71)	0.68 (−0.64,2.00)	0.72 (− 0.52, 1.96)	0.29 (− 0.63,1.21)	Taxane (79.8%)		
−0.50 (−2.25,1.24)	− 0.29 (− 2.10,1.51)	−0.26 (− 2.00, 1.49)	−0.69 (− 2.22,0.85)	−0.98 (− 2.20, 0.25)	Vandetanib+Taxane (24.7%)	
0.24 (− 1.62,2.11)	0.45 (− 1.47,2.37)	0.49 (− 1.37, 2.35)	0.06 (− 1.61,1.73)	− 0.23 (− 1.62, 1.16)	0.75 (− 1.11,2.60)	Vinflunine (61.1%)

SAE Severe adverse effect
[a]The SUCRA probabilities are performed in brackets

to chemotherapy alone [10]. These findings are similar to our results. Among the network comparisons, there was no significant advantage of intervention in PFS results, and in OS results, immunotherapy had a relative advantage.

Immune checkpoint inhibitors are a research hotspot in anticancer treatment [32]. Programmed death receptor 1 (PD-1)/programmed death ligand 1 (PD-L1) is a pair of negative costimulatory factors that play a key role in the tumor immune escape mechanism. PD-L1 can be expressed in tumor microenvironment cells and can inhibit the activation of T cells through binding to PD-1, which also weakens the entire immune system of patients [33–35]. Immune checkpoint therapy prevents PD-1/PD-L1 binding in tumors and restores the cytotoxicity of T cells [36].

Atezolizumab is a monoclonal antibody that specifically binds to PD-L1 with few serious side effects [37]. Pembrolizumab is a highly selective and humanized IgG4-k homologous PD-1 monoclonal antibody that is approved by the Food and Drug Administration of the United States for first-line AUC treatment [38]. Immune checkpoint inhibitors block the PD-1/PD-L1 connection between tumor microenvironment cells and T cells and improve the patient's immune system. Compared with cytotoxic drugs, the OS of patients is significantly improved with this method. This improvement may be achieved through the regulation of the immune system. However, there was no difference in PFS, which may indicate the indirect effects of checkpoint inhibitors.

In one included study, subgroup analysis showed that PD-L1-combined positive scores with a cutoff between 1

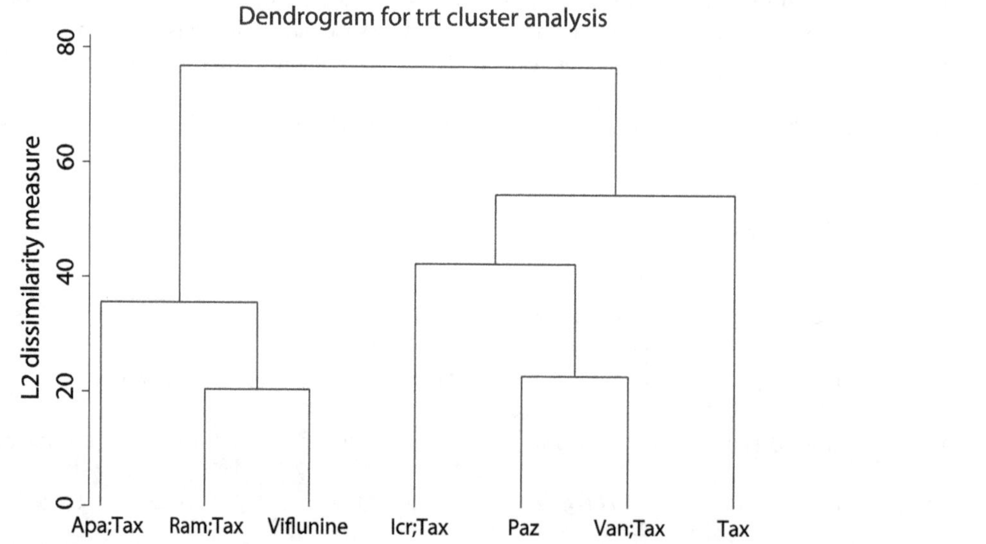

Fig. 4 Cluster analysis of the first part of the network analysis according to the SUCRA score. Abbreviations: Apa: apatorsen; Icr: icrucumab; Paz: pazopanib; Ram: ramucirumab; Tax: taxane

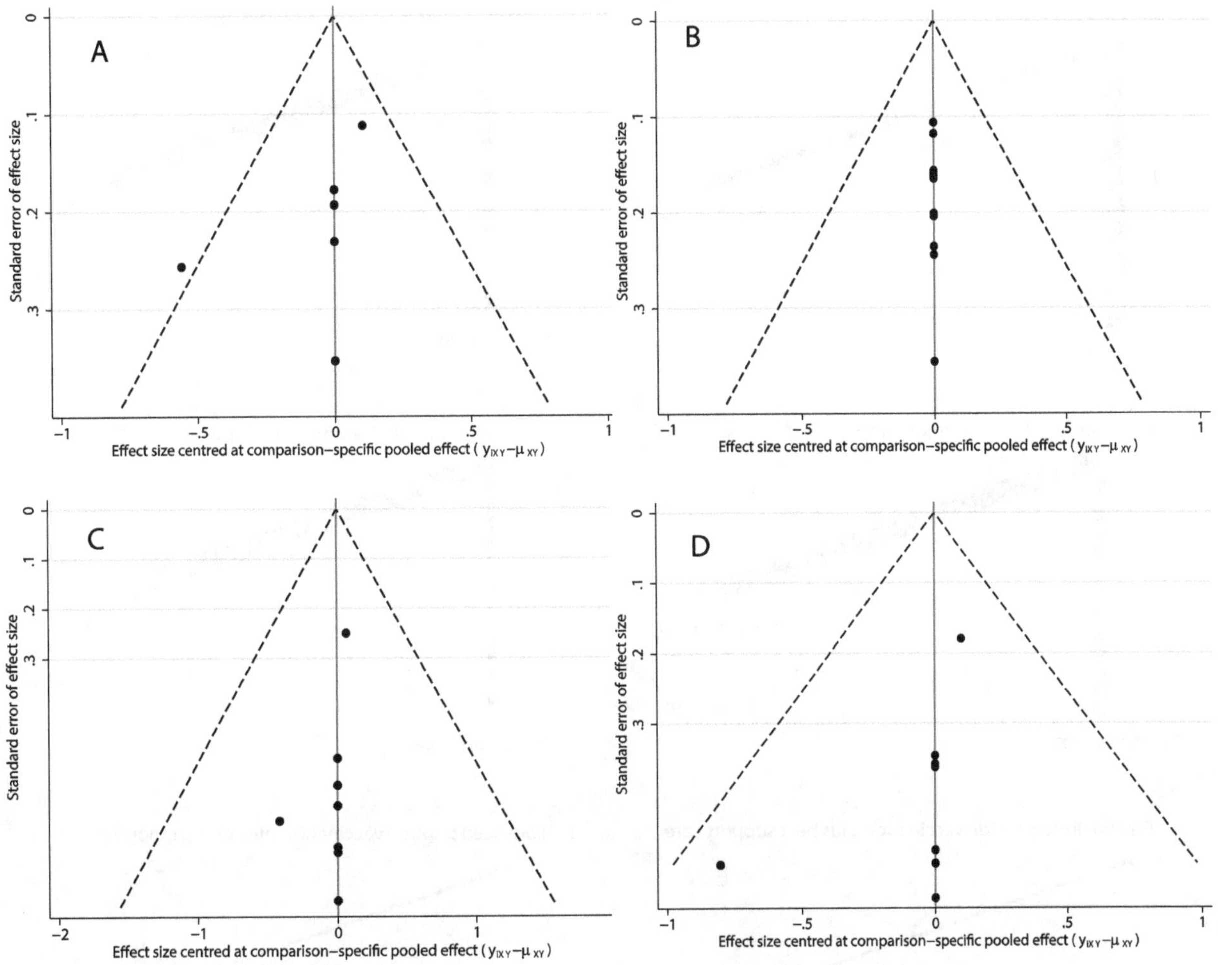

Fig. 5 Comparisons: adjusted funnel plots of the first part of the network meta-analysis. A: PFS; B: OS; C: ORR; D: SAE

and 10% could be predictive indicators that high positive-score patients have a longer OS period after checkpoint inhibitor application [31]. Unfortunately, there is still no PFS subgroup analysis report on the status of PD-L1 in this study. For other cancers, such as non-small cell lung cancer (NSCLC), an expression rate of PD-L1 greater than 50% can be used as reliable evidence for the use of immunological checkpoint drugs [39]. However, the IMvigor211 trial showed that in the PD-L1 expression rate in tumor-infiltrating immune cells in more than 5% of the population, atezolizumab did not provide significant benefits in patient survival [11, 20]. It is possible that the expression of PD-L1 in tumors or immune cells plays a more important role in guiding the application of PD-1 inhibitors than that of PD-L1 inhibitors. However, this view still needs further confirmation. Nonetheless, the above research also provides a research direction for individual treatment in clinical treatment.

PPV is also an individual treatment for patients with an improved immune system [26]. Up to four of the 31 human leukocyte antigen (HLA) vaccines were selected and applied according to the HLA type and host immunity before vaccination. However, in our research, PPV plus BSC is superior to BSC in only the ORR results but not the OS and PFS results. Nevertheless, this is still a novel attempt at individualized precise immunotherapy. Applying PPVs more conveniently and the quantity production of PPVs are the main issues.

Ramucirumab is an antagonist of VEGF. A previous meta-analysis suggested that its combination with docetaxel did not improve PFS and OS [10]. In our network comparison, ramucirumab plus docetaxel still has the advantage of a high SUCRA ranking, but there was no significant difference. However, ramucirumab had a better therapeutic effect in other tumors compared with UC, such as advanced gastric or esophagogastric junction adenocarcinoma and metastatic NSCLC [40–42]. In addition, antiangiogenic agents, such as icrucumab (targets vascular endothelial growth factor receptor 1, VEGFR1), pazopanib (VEGFR), and vandetanib (VEGFR3), also did not show obvious advantages.

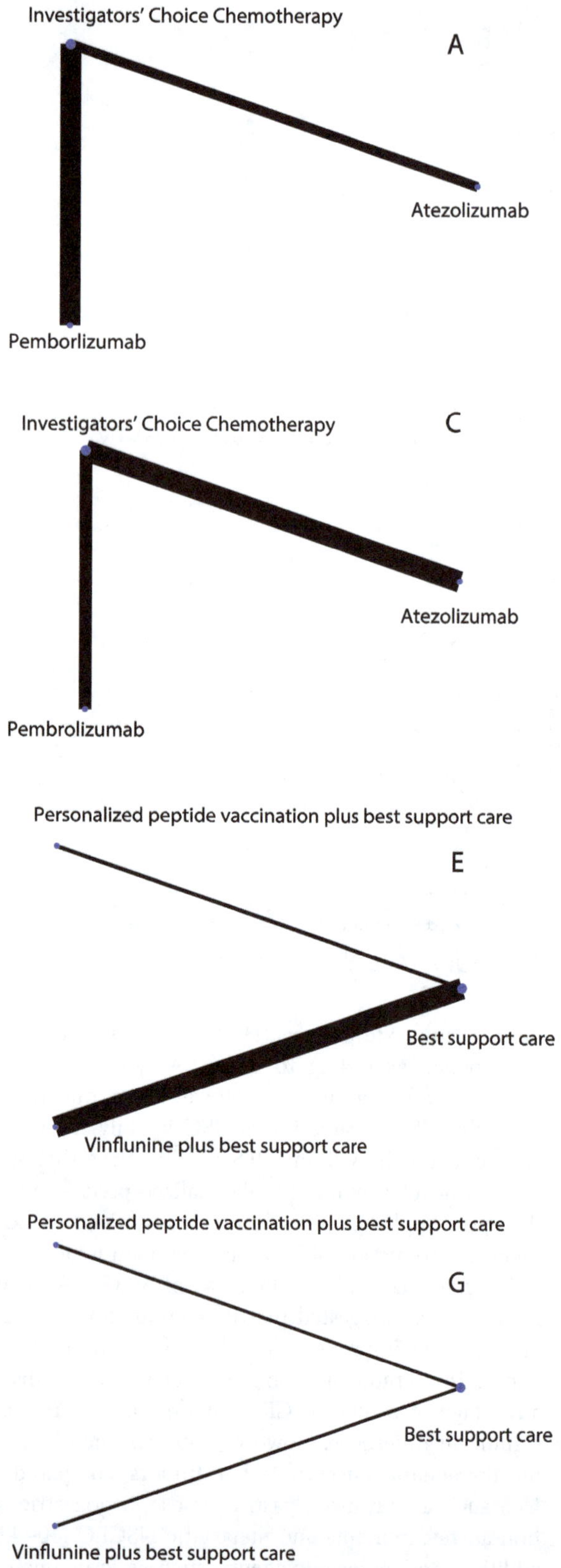

Fig. 6 Network comparisons for interventions included in the analysis. Second part of the network: A: PFS; B: OS; C: ORR; D: SAE. Third part of the network: E: PFS; F: OS; G: ORR

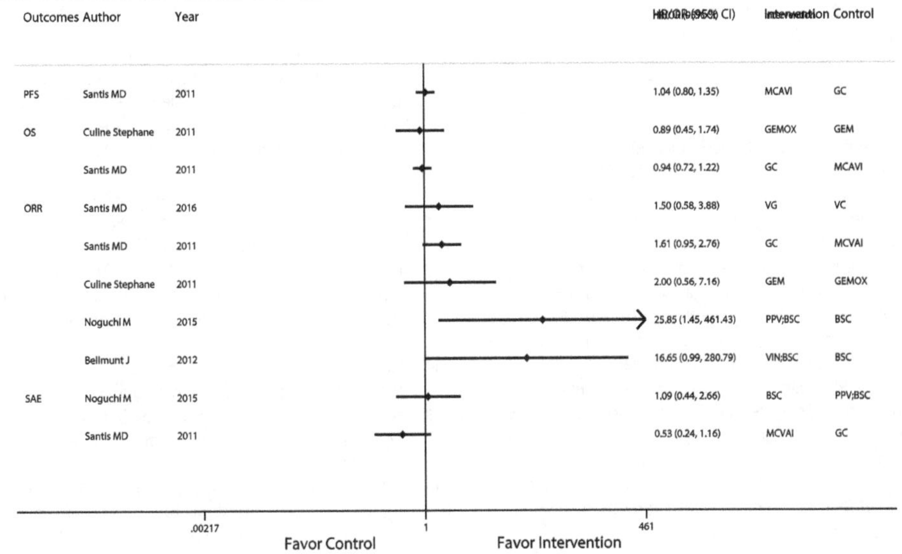

Fig. 7 Traditional meta-analysis of comparisons that were not included in the network meta-analysis. Abbreviations: BSC: Best support care; GC: Gemcitabine plus carboplatin; GEM: Gemcitabine; GEMOX: Gemcitabine plus oxaliplatin; MCAVI: Methotrexate plus carboplatin plus vinblastine; PPV: Personalized peptide vaccination; VC: Vinflunine plus Carboplatin; VG: Vinflunine plus Gemcitabine; VIN: Vinflunine

Antiangiogenesis therapy does not bring obvious survival benefits to UC patients, which indicates that blocking neovascularization does not affect the invasiveness of tumors. Likewise, systemic drug administration does not block the formation of neovascularization in UC, which has a relatively poor blood supply. At the superficial UC stage, intravesical perfusion can achieve a good therapeutic effect. Further research may not be limited to novel drug development but can improve effectiveness by changing the route of medication. For example, local urethral puncture injection with a cystoscope or even surface puncture injection under the guidance of radiography can efficiently reach the tumor microenvironment.

Limitation

Several limitations still exist. First, this study was conducted at the base trial level but not at the individual level. Second, the differences in patient characteristics between groups, such as between the cisplatin-ineligible and cisplatin-resistant patients, and the use of various ORR evaluation criteria are sources of heterogeneity in this study. Third, due to the absence of a common control, the network analysis was divided into three categories. Fourth, the impacts of drug dosage and the application period were not analyzed. Fifth, ICC and BSC interventions were selected for treatment according to the patients' condition and to investigate judgment, so heterogeneity exists. Sixth, taxanes were considered as one type drug in this study, including docetaxel, cabazitaxel, and paclitaxel. Seventh, this study will need to be updated when new drugs and clinical outcomes emerge.

Conclusions

At present, atezolizumab and pembrolizumab are superior to other treatments in only the OS results, but no treatment confers a significant advantage in PFS. Pembrolizumab still has relative advantages in ORR and SAE results compared to ICC.

Supplementary information

Additional file 1: Figure S1. Local inconsistency plot of loop-specific heterogeneity of the OS result in the first part of the network analysis.

Additional file 2: Figure S2. Local inconsistency plot of loop-specific heterogeneity of the ORR result in the first part of the network analysis.

Additional file 3: Figure S3. Local inconsistency plot of loop-specific heterogeneity of the SAE result in the first part of the network analysis.

Additional file 4: Table S1. The details of the search strategy in PubMed.

Additional file 5: Table S2. The league table for the PFS estimates of the interventions according to their relative effects in the second part of the network analysis.

Additional file 6: Table S3. The league table for the OS estimates of the interventions according to their relative effects in the second part of the network analysis.

Additional file 7: Table S4. The league table for the ORR estimates of the interventions according to their relative effects in second part network analysis.

Additional file 8: Table S5. The league table for the SAE estimates of the interventions according to their relative effects in the second part of the network analysis.

Additional file 9: Table S6. The league table for the PFS estimates of the interventions according to their relative effects in the third part of the network analysis.

Additional file 10: Table S7. The league table for the OS estimates of the interventions according to their relative effects in the third part of the network analysis.

Abbreviations

Apa: apatorsen; Ate: atezolizumab; AUC: advanced urothelial carcinoma; BSC: best support care; CIs: confidence intervals; GC: gemcitabine plus cisplatin; GEM: gemcitabine; GEMOX: gemcitabine plus oxaliplatin; HLA: human leukocyte antigen; HRs: hazard ratios; ICC: investigator's choice chemotherapy; Icr: icrucumab; MCAVI: methotrexate plus carboplatin plus vinblastine; MIUC: muscle-invasive urothelial carcinoma; MVAC: methotrexate, vinblastine, doxorubicin, and cisplatin; NCI: National Cancer Institute; NSCLC: non-small cell lung cancer; ORR: objective response rate; ORs: odd ratios; OS: overall survival; Paz: pazopanib; PD-1: programmed death receptor 1; PD-L1; programmed death ligand 1; Pem: pembrolizumab; PFS: progression-free survival; PPV: personalized peptide vaccination; PRISMA: preferred reporting items for systematic reviews and meta-analyses; Ram: ramucirumab; RCTs: randomized controlled trials; SAE: severe adverse effect; SUCRA: surface under the cumulative ranking curve; Tax: taxane; UC: urothelial carcinoma; VC: vinflunine plus carboplatin; VEGF: vascular endothelial growth factor; VEGFR: vascular endothelial growth factor receptor; VG: vinflunine plus gemcitabine; VIN: vinflunine

Acknowledgements

None.

Authors' contributions

Study concept and design: HW; Literature research: KF and CK; Data acquisition: YJ and TC; Data analysis: GW; Statistical analysis: XS and TY; Manuscript preparation: HW; Manuscript editing: JL; Manuscript review: JL. All authors have approved the manuscript and agree with its submission.

Authors' information

Department of Urology, The Second Affiliated Hospital of Kunming Medical University, Kunming, Yunnan, 650101, PR China.
Huitao Wang, Jianhe Liu, Kewei Fang, Changxing Ke, Yongming Jiang, Guang Wang, Tongxin Yang, Tao Chen, Xin Shi.

References

1. Lin T, Liu Z, Liu L, et al. Prospective evaluation of fluorescence in situ hybridization for diagnosing urothelial carcinoma. Oncol Lett. 2017;13(5): 3928–34.
2. Niegisch G, Gerullis H, Lin SW, et al. A real-world data study to evaluate treatment patterns, clinical characteristics and survival outcomes for first- and second-line treatment in locally advanced and metastatic Urothelial Cancer patients in Germany. J Cancer. 2018;9(8):1337–48.
3. Nakagawa T, Taguchi S, Kanatani A, et al. Oncologic outcome of Metastasectomy for Urothelial carcinoma: who is the best candidate? Ann Surg Oncol. 2017;24(9):2794–800.
4. Wu XJ, Zhi Y, He P, et al. Comparison of single agent versus combined chemotherapy in previously treated patients with advanced urothelial carcinoma: a meta-analysis. Onco Targets Ther. 2016;9:1535–43 PMCID: 4801158.
5. Hsieh MC, Huang CH, Chiang PH, Chen YY, Tang Y, Su YL. Tailored selection of first-line cisplatin-based chemotherapy in patients with metastatic urothelial carcinoma of bladder. J Cancer. 2016;7(10):1347–52 PMCID: 4934043.
6. Oing C, Rink M, Oechsle K, Seidel C, von Amsberg G, Bokemeyer C. Second line chemotherapy for advanced and metastatic Urothelial carcinoma: Vinflunine and beyond-a comprehensive review of the current literature. J Urol. 2016;195(2):254–63.
7. Zachos I, Konstantinopoulos PA, Tzortzis V, et al. Systemic therapy of metastatic bladder cancer in the molecular era: current status and future promise. Expert Opin Investig Drugs. 2010;19(7):875–87.
8. de Vos FY, de Wit R. Choosing chemotherapy in patients with advanced urothelial cell cancer who are unfit to receive cisplatin-based chemotherapy. Ther Adv Med Oncol. 2010;2(6):381–8.
9. Sella A, Kovel S. Combination of gemcitabine and carboplatin in urothelial cancer patients unfit for cisplatin due to impaired renal or cardiac function. Int Braz J Urol. 2012;38(1):49–56.
10. Ciccarese C, Iacovelli R, Bria E, et al. Second-line therapy for metastatic urothelial carcinoma: defining the best treatment option among immunotherapy, chemotherapy, and antiangiogenic targeted therapies. A systematic review and meta-analysis. Semin Oncol. 2019;46(1):65–72.
11. Di Nunno V, De Luca E, Buttigliero C, et al. Immune-checkpoint inhibitors in previously treated patients with advanced or metastatic urothelial carcinoma: a systematic review and meta-analysis. Crit Rev Oncol Hematol. 2018;129:124–32.
12. Raggi D, Miceli R, Sonpavde G, et al. Second-line single-agent versus doublet chemotherapy as salvage therapy for metastatic urothelial cancer: a systematic review and meta-analysis. Ann Oncol. 2016;27(1):49–61.
13. Hutton B, Salanti G, Caldwell DM, et al. The PRISMA extension statement for reporting of systematic reviews incorporating network meta-analyses of health care interventions: checklist and explanations. Ann Intern Med. 2015; 162(11):777–84.
14. Higgins JP, Altman DG, Gotzsche PC, et al. The Cochrane Collaboration's tool for assessing risk of bias in randomised trials. BMJ. 2011;343:d5928.
15. Greco T, Edefonti V, Biondi-Zoccai G, et al. A multilevel approach to network meta-analysis within a frequentist framework. Contemp Clin Trials. 2015;42:51–9.
16. Li D, Wang T, Shen S, et al. Effects of Fluroquinolones in newly diagnosed, sputum-positive tuberculosis therapy: a systematic review and network meta-analysis. PLoS One. 2015;10(12):e0145066.
17. Trinquart L, Chatellier G, Ravaud P. Adjustment for reporting bias in network meta-analysis of antidepressant trials. BMC Med Res Methodol. 2012;12:150.
18. Fradet Y, Bellmunt J, Vaughn DJ, et al. Randomized phase III KEYNOTE-045 trial of pembrolizumab versus paclitaxel, docetaxel, or vinflunine in recurrent advanced urothelial cancer: results of > 2 years of follow-up. Ann Oncol. 2019. https://doi.org/10.1093/annonc/mdz127 [Epub ahead of print].
19. Rosenberg JE, Hahn NM, Regan MM, et al. Apatorsen plus docetaxel versus docetaxel alone in platinum-resistant metastatic urothelial carcinoma (Borealis-2). Br J Cancer. 2018;118(11):1434–41.
20. Powles T, Duran I, van der Heijden MS, et al. Atezolizumab versus chemotherapy in patients with platinum-treated locally advanced or metastatic urothelial carcinoma (IMvigor211): a multicentre, open-label, phase 3 randomised controlled trial. Lancet. 2018;391(10122):748–57.
21. Petrylak DP, de Wit R, Chi KN, et al. Ramucirumab plus docetaxel versus placebo plus docetaxel in patients with locally advanced or metastatic urothelial carcinoma after platinum-based therapy (RANGE): a randomised, double-blind, phase 3 trial. Lancet. 2017;390(10109):2266–77.
22. Jones RJ, Hussain SA, Protheroe AS, et al. Randomized phase II study investigating Pazopanib versus weekly paclitaxel in relapsed or progressive Urothelial Cancer. J Clin Oncol. 2017;35(16):1770–7.
23. Bellmunt J, Kerst JM, Vazquez F, et al. A randomized phase II/III study of cabazitaxel versus vinflunine in metastatic or locally advanced transitional cell carcinoma of the urothelium (SECAVIN). Ann Oncol. 2017;28(7):1517–22.
24. Petrylak DP, Tagawa ST, Kohli M, et al. Docetaxel as Monotherapy or combined with Ramucirumab or Icrucumab in second-line treatment for locally advanced or metastatic Urothelial carcinoma: an open-label, three-arm, randomized controlled phase II trial. J Clin Oncol. 2016;34(13):1500–9.
25. De Santis M, Wiechno PJ, Bellmunt J, et al. Vinflunine-gemcitabine versus vinflunine-carboplatin as first-line chemotherapy in cisplatin-unfit patients with advanced urothelial carcinoma: results of an international randomized phase II trial (JASINT1). Ann Oncol. 2016;27(3):449–54.
26. Noguchi M, Matsumoto K, Uemura H, et al. An open-label, randomized phase II trial of personalized peptide vaccination in patients with bladder Cancer that progressed after platinum-based chemotherapy. Clin Cancer Res. 2016;22(1):54–60.
27. Bellmunt J, Fougeray R, Rosenberg JE, et al. Long-term survival results of a randomized phase III trial of vinflunine plus best supportive care versus best supportive care alone in advanced urothelial carcinoma patients after failure of platinum-based chemotherapy. Ann Oncol. 2013;24(6):1466–72.
28. Choueiri TK, Ross RW, Jacobus S, et al. Double-blind, randomized trial of docetaxel plus vandetanib versus docetaxel plus placebo in platinum-pretreated metastatic urothelial cancer. J Clin Oncol. 2012;30(5):507–12.
29. De Santis M, Bellmunt J, Mead G, et al. Randomized phase II/III trial assessing gemcitabine/carboplatin and methotrexate/carboplatin/vinblastine in patients with advanced urothelial cancer who are unfit for cisplatin-based chemotherapy: EORTC study 30986. J Clin Oncol. 2012;30(2):191–9.
30. Culine S, Flechon A, Guillot A, et al. Gemcitabine or gemcitabine plus oxaliplatin in the first-line treatment of patients with advanced transitional cell carcinoma of the urothelium unfit for cisplatin-based chemotherapy: a

randomized phase 2 study of the French genitourinary tumor group (GETUG V01). Eur Urol. 2011;60(6):1251–7.
31. Bellmunt J, de Wit R, Vaughn DJ, et al. Pembrolizumab as second-line therapy for advanced Urothelial carcinoma. N Engl J Med. 2017;376(11):1015–26.
32. Xu C, Chen YP, Du XJ, et al. Comparative safety of immune checkpoint inhibitors in cancer: systematic review and network meta-analysis. BMJ. 2018;363:k4226.
33. Sato M, Tamura R, Tamura H, et al. Analysis of tumor angiogenesis and immune microenvironment in non-functional pituitary endocrine tumors. J Clin Med. 2019;8(5):E695.
34. Jiang F, Yu W, Zeng F, et al. PD-1 high expression predicts lower local disease control in stage IV M0 nasopharyngeal carcinoma. BMC Cancer. 2019;19(1):503.
35. Incorvaia L, Badalamenti G, Rinaldi G, et al. Can the plasma PD-1 levels predict the presence and efficiency of tumor-infiltrating lymphocytes in patients with metastatic melanoma? Ther Adv Med Oncol. 2019;11: 1758835919848872.
36. Wei Y, Zhao Q, Gao Z, et al. The local immune landscape determines tumor PD-L1 heterogeneity and sensitivity to therapy. J Clin Invest. 2019;129(8):3347–60.
37. Yang S, Zhang Z, Wang Q. Emerging therapies for small cell lung cancer. J Hematol Oncol. 2019;12(1):47.
38. Yu SS, Dorff TB, Ballas LK, Sadeghi S, Skinner EC, Quinn DI. Immunotherapy in urothelial cancer, part 1: T-cell checkpoint inhibition in advanced or metastatic disease. Clin Adv Hematol Oncol. 2017;15(6):466–77.
39. Kim J, Cho J, Lee MH, Lim JH. Relative efficacy of checkpoint inhibitors for advanced NSCLC according to programmed death-Ligand-1 expression: a systematic review and network meta-analysis. Sci Rep. 2018;8(1):11738.
40. Yamaguchi K, Fujitani K, Nagashima F, et al. Ramucirumab for the treatment of metastatic gastric or gastroesophageal junction adenocarcinoma following disease progression on first-line platinum- or fluoropyrimidine-containing combination therapy in Japanese patients: a phase 2, open-label study. Gastric Cancer. 2018;21(6):1041–9.
41. Yoon HH, Bendell JC, Braiteh FS, et al. Ramucirumab combined with FOLFOX as front-line therapy for advanced esophageal, gastroesophageal junction, or gastric adenocarcinoma: a randomized, double-blind, multicenter phase II trial. Ann Oncol. 2016;27(12):2196–203.
42. Perol M, Ciuleanu TE, Arrieta O, et al. Quality of life results from the phase 3 REVEL randomized clinical trial of ramucirumab-plus-docetaxel versus placebo-plus-docetaxel in advanced/metastatic non-small cell lung cancer patients with progression after platinum-based chemotherapy. Lung Cancer. 2016;93:95–103.

15

Testicular epidermoid cysts: A reevaluation

Petra Anheuser[1,2*], J. Kranz[3], E. Stolle[4], D. Höflmayer[5], F. Büscheck[5], S. Mühlstädt[6], G. Lock[7] and K. P. Dieckmann[1,8]

Abstract

Background: Testicular epidermoid cysts (TECs) are rare benign testicular neoplasms. As TECs are rarely associated with germ cell tumours (GCTs), the understanding of biological behaviour and clinical management of TEC is unresolved.

Methods: We retrospectively searched the files of patients treated for testicular neoplasms and germ cell cancer in the time from 2000 to 2017. Those with TEC were subjected to closer review looking to clinical and histological features, and to results from imaging with ultrasonography (US), contrast enhanced sonography (CEUS) and magnetic resonance imaging (MRI).

Results: Among 589 patients undergoing surgery for testicular tumour, nine simple TECs were identified (1.5, 95% confidence intervals 0.53–2.50%). Median age was 26 years. Imaging revealed sharply demarcated roundish lesions with avascular central areas. Eight patients underwent testis-sparing excision with no recurrence ensuing. One had orchiectomy because of large size of the mass. Histologically, TECs consisted of cornifying squamous cell epithelium and no accompanying germ cell neoplasia in situ. Two additional cases (0.3% of all) required orchiectomy because these TECs were associated with ipsilateral GCT.

Conclusions: TEC is usually a benign lesion that can safely be diagnosed with US, CEUS and MRI due to its roundish shape and its avascular centre. Histologically, this TEC corresponds to the prepubertal-type teratoma unrelated to germ cell neoplasia in situ of the 2016 WHO classification. The other subtype of TEC that is associated with invasive GCT represents a teratoma of postpubertal-type. From a clinical point of view it could be easier to differentiate between a "simple TEC" which is benign (prepubertal type) and a "complex TEC" which is malignant because of its association with invasive GCT.

Keywords: Testicular neoplasm, Germ cell tumour, Epidermoid cyst, Testis sparing surgery, Scrotal sonography

Background

Testicular epidermoid cysts have been first reported in 1942 [1], but their histogenetic origin has been a matter of dispute ever since. Accordingly, clinical management has been a matter of controversy, likewise. In the recent WHO classification of 2016, testicular epidermoid cysts (TECs) are listed as teratoma of prepubertal type within the group of germ cell tumours unrelated to germ cell neoplasia in situ [2]. The ICD-O code 9084/0 denotes a benign behaviour of this neoplasm. However, TECs have also been documented as part of invasive testicular germ cell tumours (GCTs).Therefore it has been hypothesized that two different types of TECs exist, one a truly benign "simple" testicular EC and the other a "complex" TEC associated with GCT thus representing teratoma [4]. Due to the rarity of TECs there are only few systematic clinical evaluations available [4–6]. Most of the current knowledge is based on small clinical series and single case reports. To improve the over-all understanding of TECs we retrospectively reviewed our experience with simple TECs and with complex ECs.

* Correspondence: petra.anheuser@web.de
[1]Klinik für Urologie, Albertinen-Krankenhaus, Hamburg, Germany
[2]Urologische Klinik AK Wandsbek, Hamburg, Germany
Full list of author information is available at the end of the article

Methods

We retrospectively searched the files of all patients who underwent treatment for testicular neoplasms or germ cell cancer in the department of urology in Albertinen-Krankenhaus Hamburg in the time from January 2000 to March 2017. We looked into the histologies of the patients operated on testicular tumours and selected those with TEC for closer review. The relative incidence of TECs in relation to GCTs was determined by calculating proportions with 95% confidence intervals. Median age and side-localization of TECs were compared to findings in GCTs. Clinical and histopathological features as well as imaging findings of the TEC patients were tabulated and descriptively analysed. Ethical approval was given by the institutional ethical committee (Albertinen Ethikkommission: U3–2015).

Results

A total of 625 patients were identified during the 17 year time-span, of whom 589 underwent surgery for a testicular tumour. The remainder were comprised of extragonadal GCTs as well as relapsing patients or other patients receiving upfront chemotherapy. Among the surgical cases, nine patients were identified with simple TEC (1.5, 95% CI 0.53–2.50%) We also identified 2 patients (0.3, 95% CI 0–0.81%) with testicular epidermoid cysts in association with ipsilateral germ cell tumour ("complex TECs"). Median age of the patients with simple TEC was 26 years (range 11–34 years). Noteworthy: 2 patients were of prepubertal age and both were submitted to our department because of its status as testicular cancer unit. Otherwise the department does not offer pediatric services. Median age of the GCT patients was 36 years (interquartile range 31–45 years) which is not significantly different from the median age of TEC patients. The right side was afflicted in six patients (66.7, 95% CI 29.93–92.51%). In GCTs there was also a slight predominance of the right side (50.51, 95%CI 45.56–55.46%). Localization is not significantly different between the two groups because the confidence intervals are widely overlapping. The presenting symptom of the TECs was a palpable painless nodule in 8 cases. Remarkably, two patients reported extraordinarily long symptomatic intervals of 10 and 13 years, respectively. One TEC case was an incidental finding upon surgery for suspected spermatic cord torsion. The mean size of the lesions was 17.4 mm (ranging from 6 to 40 mm). Tests sparing surgery (TSS) was performed in 8 patients (Fig. 1a), only in the case with the 40 mm mass was an orchiectomy required. AFP and βHCG were negative in all cases. In three of the more recent cases, microRNA-371a-3p was measured in serum. Likewise, there was no elevation of this novel marker.

Regarding diagnostic procedures, all patients had scrotal ultrasound examination, 4 including contrast enhanced ultrasound (CEUS). Findings uniformly consisted of well demarcated roundish-shaped intratesticular lesions with a hyperechoic rim, no or little intralesional echogenicity and an acoustic shadowing on the posterior of the tumour. 5 patients had ring-shaped intralesional echogenicity corresponding to the onion-ring appearance (Fig. 1b). CEUS (all performed with 2.4 ml Sonovue, Bracco) demonstrated absence of contrast bubbles within the lesion indicating an avascular area (Fig. 1c, d). Scrotal magnetic resonance imaging (MRI) was available in 7 patients. Sharply demarcated bull-eyed intratesticular lesions were revealed in all cases with increased signal intensity at the rim of the lesions and no enhancement of the central area. T2-weighted imaging showed high intralesional signal intensity (Fig. 2a-d).

Histopathologically, all cases were classified as simple testicular epidermoid cysts with a surrounding fibrous membrane and layers of cornifying squamous epithelium as well as cell debris in the centre (Fig. 3a, b). No skin appendages and no GCNis were detected in any of these cases.

Follow-up is available in 7 patients with simple TEC. All of whom are well with no local recurrence after an average time-intervall of 6 years after surgery. One patient succumbed to cardiac failure, one was lost to follow-up.

Two patients had complex epidermoid cysts, one of whom was associated with embryonal carcinoma. The second patient had synchronous bilateral tumours with teratoma (80%) embryonal carcinoma (15%) and yolk sac tumour (5%) on the right side and a neuroendocrine tumour, GCNis and an epidermoid cyst on the left (Fig. 4). In both cases the preoperative imaging detected only a simple TEC (Fig. 5a, b). Consequently, both underwent TSS initially and even intraoperatively, the lesions were considered simple cysts. Only after histopathological detection of typical GCT in the surrounding tissue, orchiectomy was performed in a second session. The classic markers were elevated in the second patient (18 years) but this elevation was clearly related to the contralateral mixed nonseminomatous GCT. Both patients received cisplatin-based chemotherapy in addition to surgery and remained disease-free thereafter.

Discussion

Simple TEC is a rare but well-known lesion. As shown herein, TECs account for only 1.5% of all testicular neoplasms among post-pubertal men. This figure corresponds well with the 2.1% frequency reported previously [4, 5, 7] but it is clearly lower than the 10% relative incidence reported in a series from Taiwan [8]. Ethnic predisposition may account for that striking difference.

TECs have many clinical characteristics in common with GCT: Particularly clinical presentation with painless mass [9], the age predisposition of early adulthood and the preponderance of the right side. All these features were confirmed in our series. Reportedly, patients with TEC may have exceptionally long symptomatic intervals [10, 11]. Accordingly, two of our patients had noted a testicular nodule for as long as 10 and 13 years before surgery, respectively.

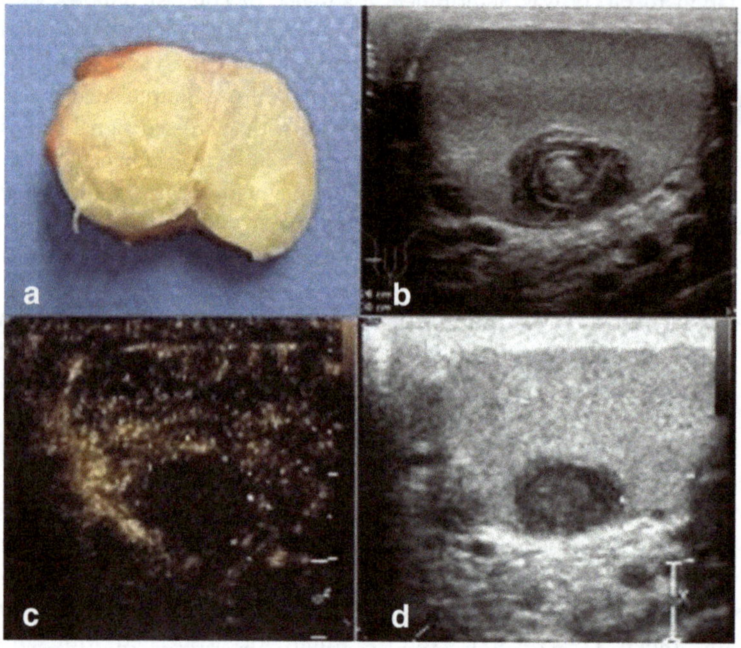

Fig. 1 **a** Surgical specimen of excised simple testicular epidermoid cyst. Largest diameter of cyst 1.2 cm. Note the sharply demarcated rim of cyst and the yellowish amorphic mass inside. At the external side of the rim small layer of normal testicular tissue (brownish). **b** B-mode sonography of testis harbouring epidermoid cyst. Note the typical onion ring shape of the cyst core. **c, d** Contrast enhanced ultrasonography (CEUS) of testis with simple epidermoid cyst. Dual display with B-mode scan (right side of figure) and CEUS imaging (left side of figure). Note the absence of contrast material (air bubbles) in the centre of the cyst, indicating avascular area

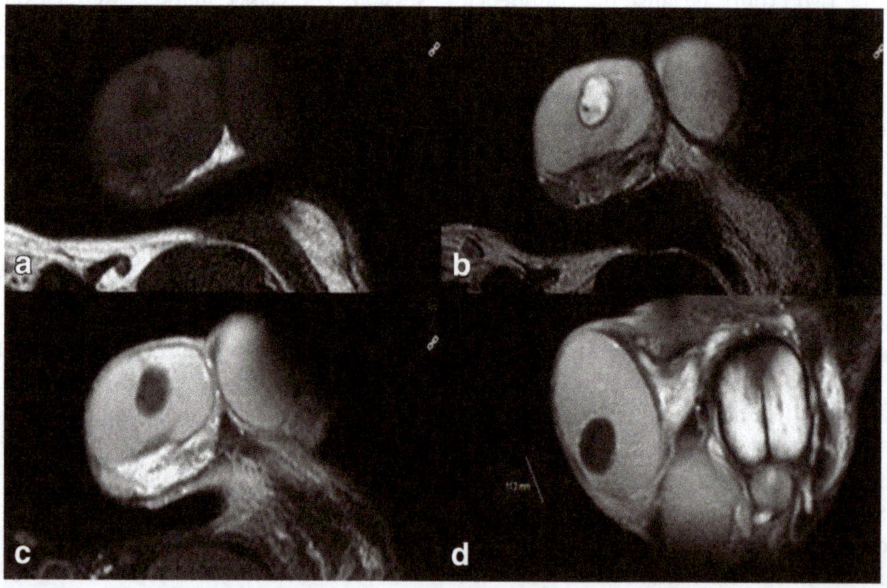

Fig. 2 Scrotal MRI of patient with simple testicular epidermoid cyst, 1.5 Tesla MRI, surface coil. **a** T1 weighted imaging showing cyst with lower signal intensity than testicular parenchyma. **b**. T2-weighted imaging: typical bull-eye appearance of epidermoid cyst. Note the high signal intensity within cyst core. **c** and **d**. T1-weighted imaging with application of gadolinium-based contrast material. Note signal enhancement in testicular parenchyma but not in the cyst core highlighting the avascular area within the cyst

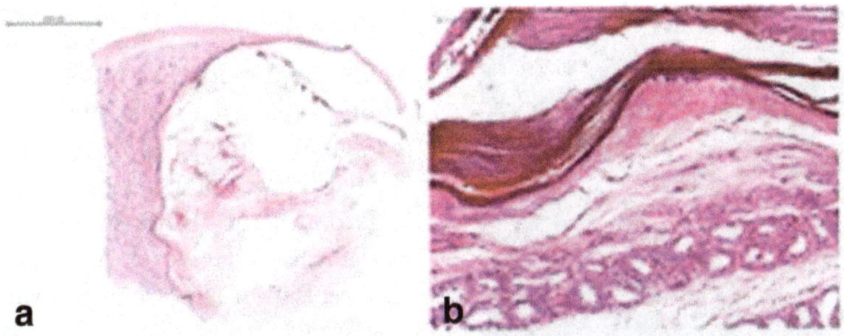

Fig. 3 **a** Histological section of surgical specimen with excised testicular epidermoid cyst. Note: Cyst lumen (right side of figure) with layers of cornifying squamous epithelium and cell debris. On the right side normal testicular parenchyma. The cyst is surrounded by a capsule of fibrous tissue. Magnification scale at the upper left side. Hematoxylin eosin stain. **b** Testicular parenchyma with seminiferous tubules. No germ cell neoplasia in situ. of surgical specimen with excised testicular epidermoid cyst, same patient, higher magnification, see scale at the upper left side. Note: Cyst lumen (upper side of picture) with layers of cornifying squamous epithelium and cell debris. Testicular parenchyma with seminiferous tubules. No germ cell neoplasia in situ. Some tubules with spermatogenesis. Haematoxylin eosin stain

Usually, the diagnosis can be safely made with B-mode scrotal ultrasound. The typical onion-ring phenomenon is present in about 60% of all cases [12, 13]. The cyst-like appearance and the roundish configuration are further typical findings of the present and previous series [8, 14, 15]. A more distinctive finding is the absence of vascularization of the cyst core documented with CCDS (colour-coded duplex sonography) and CEUS as shown in four of our cases and previously reported by others [16]. Scrotal MRI can likewise detect these morphologic features [17, 18]. The avascular nature of the cyst core is safely shown by the absence of signal enhancement after application of gadolinium-based contrast material [19–21]. This finding was confirmed in all 7 patients of our series undergoing MRI.

Local excision (TSS) is the treatment of choice for TEC as realized in 8 of our patients. Orchiectomy is exceptionally required in cases with a large mass and only little remaining testicular tissue. Accordingly, one of our cases underwent orchiectomy. Similar cases are reported [6, 11]. Recurrences after TSS have not yet been experienced until now and the same is true for 7 of our patients in whom follow-up is available.

Histopathological findings in our series fully accord with previous reports. The lesion typically consists of a well-defined cyst lined by a fibrous membrane and filled with layers of cornifying squamous epithelium and cell debris. No skin appendages are found in the cyst's lumen and no GCNis is present in the adjacent testicular parenchyma [22, 23].

The most striking finding of the present series is that simple TEC can obviously be mimicked by epidermoid cysts developing in association with full-blown GCT [24]. The association of TEC with ipsilateral GCT has been reported sporadically to date [3, 7, 25, 26]. The association of GCT with contralateral TEC has also been noted [27]. Urologic surgeons should be aware of the risk of concomitant GCT when conducting TSS of TEC. Therefore tumour marker measurements should be done preoperatively as is recommended for the examination of any scrotal mass [28]. As previously documented, the novel marker miR-371a-3p can

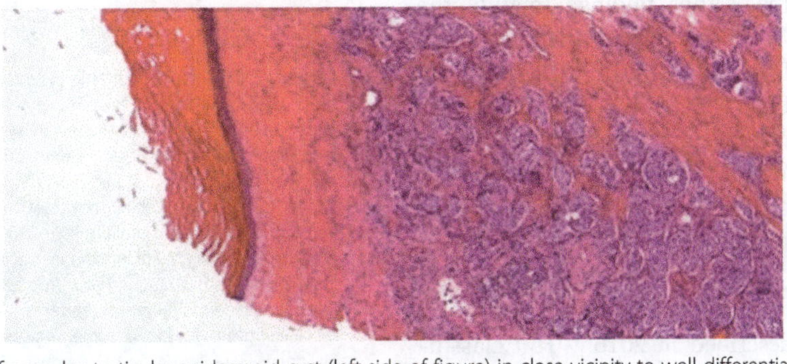

Fig. 4 Histological section of complex testicular epidermoid cyst (left side of figure) in close vicinity to well-differentiated neuroendocrine tumor in testicular tissue outside of cyst (right side of figure). 5x magnification, hematoxylin-eosin stain

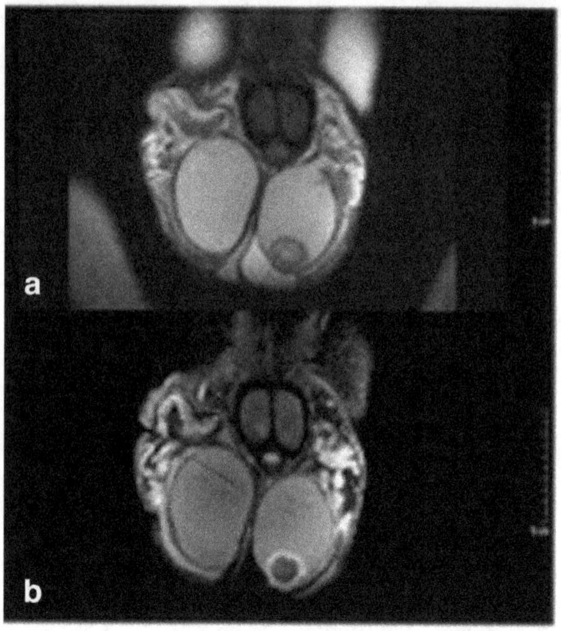

Fig. 5 a Patient (adult) with complex Testicular epidermoid cyst, scrotal MRI, 1.5 Tesla, surface coil, coronar section, T1 weighted imaging without contrast material: sharply demarcated roundish cystic lesion at the caudal pole of the left testis. **b** Patient (adult) with complex Testicular epidermoid cyst, scrotal MRI, 1.5 Tesla, surface coil, coronar section, Gadolinium contrast material: roundish intratesticular cyst at the caudal testicular pole. Note the signal enhancement in the rim region of the cyst, no uptake of contrast material in the cyst centre

substantially aid in diagnosing equivocal testicular masses [23]. Accordingly, miR371a-3p was elevated in both cases with complex TECs but not in the 3 cases with simple TEC. Frozen section examinations during TSS could be valuable for intraoperative assessment of the cyst [29, 30].

Since the first description of TEC by Dockerty and Priestly in 1942 [1] the histogenesis of the lesion remained poorly understood. Many clinical features, particularly age of predisposition, association with undescended testis and preponderance of the right side favour the origin from teratoma. Other findings (mainly the absence of GCNis and the very slow growth rate) argue against this theory. The WHO 2016 Classification System of Tumours defined TEC (and some other rare entities) as a specialized form of prepubertal-type teratoma that is unrelated to germ cell neoplasia in situ" [2] and that may occur in adulthood, too. Similarly, other prepubertal types of teratoma have been documented to sporadically occur in adult patients [31]. Thus, the simple TECs reported herein would represent teratomas of prepubertal type as described in 2016 WHO classification. The two cases with "complex TECs" reported herein would represent teratomas of postpubertal type (ICD-O 9080/3) according to the WHO classification with the "/3" coding for malignancy. This type of epidermoid cysts thus represents a specialised differentiation of teratoma analogous to the development of other benign structures within teratomas, e.g. hairs or teeth. The two types of TECs can be clearly differentiated with regard to the histogenesis according to the WHO classification. However, from a clinical point of view, this differentiation is not really advantageous. Therefore, it is suggested to define two distinct classes of TEC, clinically, the first representing the more common "simple TEC" without malignant features (i.e. without accompanying GCNis) and the second encompassing the "complex TEC" cases with accompanying GCT.

Conclusion

Testicular epidermoid cysts may occur in two different forms, the benign subtype, called "simple TEC", clinically, and the other subtype representing an epidermoid cyst that occurs in association with invasive germ cell tumours (GCNIS), called the "complex TEC", clinically. Urologic surgeons must be aware of the second type because conservative surgery would be inappropriate in these cases.

Acknowledgements
Not applicable.

Authors' contributions
AP: study design, data collection, manuscript writing, data analysis, management, revision management. KJ: data collection and analysis. SE: data collection and analysis. HD: data collection and analysis. BF: data collection and analysis. MS: data analysis. LG: data collection and conception. DKP: study design, data collection, supervison, management, revision management. All authors read and approved the final manuscript.

Author details
[1]Klinik für Urologie, Albertinen-Krankenhaus, Hamburg, Germany. [2]Urologische Klinik AK Wandsbek, Hamburg, Germany. [3]Klinik für Urologie und Kinderurologie, St.-Antonius Hospital, Eschweiler, Germany. [4]Institut für diagnostische und interventionelle Radiologie, Albertinen-Krankenhaus, Hamburg, Germany. [5]Institut für Pathologie, Universitätsklinikum Eppendorf, Universität Hamburg, Hamburg, Germany. [6]Universitätsklink und Poliklinik für Urologie, Martin-Luther-Universität, Halle-Wittenberg, Halle (Saale), Germany. [7]Klinik für Innere Medizin II, Albertinen-Krankenhaus, Hamburg, Germany. [8]Hodenzentrum Hamburg, Asklepios Klink Altona, Hamburg, Germany.

References

1. Dockerty MB, Priestly JT. Dermoid cysts of the testis. J Urol. 1942;48:392–400.
2. Moch H, Cubilla AL, Humphrey PA, Reuter VE, Ulbright TM. The 2016 WHO classification of Tumours of the urinary system and male genital organs-part a: renal, penile, and testicular Tumours. Eur Urol. 2016;70:93–105.
3. Huyghe E, Mazerolles C, Moran C, Khedis M, Khoury E, Nohra J, Soulie M, Plante P. Synchronous epidermoid cyst and mature teratoma of the testis: an unusual association. Urol Int. 2007;78:364–6.
4. Dieckmann KP, Loy V. Epidermoid cyst of the testis: a review of clinical and histogenetic considerations. Brit J Urol. 1994;73:436–41.
5. Price EBJ. Epidermoid cysts of the testis: a clinical and pathologic analysis of 69 cases from the testicular tumor registry. J Urol. 1969;102(6):708–13.
6. Deligne E, Houlgatte A, Best O, Camparo P, Denis E, Berlizot P. [Testicular epidermoid cyst: limits of conservative surgery. Report of 16 cases] [article in French]. Prog Urol. 2002;12:635–40.

7. Heidenreich A, Zumbe J, Vorreuther R, Klotz T, Vietsch H, Engelmann UH. Testikuläre Epidermiszyste: Orchiektomie oder Enukleationsresektion? Urologe A. 1996;35:1):1–5.
8. Meng E, Sun GH, Wu CJ, Chuang FP, Wu ST, Lee SS, Yu DS, Yen CY, Chen HI, Chang SY. Epidermoid cysts of the testes in Taiwanese men. Arch Androl. 2004;50(3):201–5.
9. Dieckmann KP, Becker T, Bauer HW. Testicular tumors: presentation and role of diagnostic delay. Urol Int. 1987;42:241–7.
10. Sut M, Thwaini A, Devlin B, Dooher M, Schattka F. Intratesticular epidermoid cyst: is radiological diagnosis enough? Cent European J Urol. 2011;64(4):228–9.
11. Park KK, Hyun CL, Kim SD, Kim YJ, Huh JS. The testis completely replaced by a huge epidermal cyst in an older man. World J Mens Health. 2015;33(2):117–20.
12. Day JM, Dyer RB. The onion ring sign. Abdom Imaging. 2015;40(6):2044–5.
13. Manning MA, Woodward PJ. Testicular epidermoid cysts: sonographic features with clinicopathologic correlation. J Ultrasound Med. 2010;29(5):831–7.
14. Bonkat G, Ruszat R, Forster T, Wyler S, Dogra VS, Bachmann A. [Benign space-occupying cysts in the testis. An overview][article in German]. Urologe A. 2007;46:1697–703.
15. Fu YT, Wang HH, Yang TH, Chang SY, Ma CP. Epidermoid cysts of the testis: diagnosis by ultrasonography and magnetic resonance imaging resulting in organ-preserving surgery. Br J Urol. 1996;78s:116–8.
16. Patel K, Sellars ME, Clarke JL, Sidhu PS. Features of testicular epidermoid cysts on contrast-enhanced sonography and real-time tissue elastography. J Ultrasound Med. 2012;31(1):115–22.
17. Dieckmann KP, Frey U, Lock G. Contemporary diagnostic work up of testicular germ cell tumours. Nat Rev Urol. 2013;10(12):703–12.
18. Cho JH, Chang JC, Park BH, Lee JG, Son CH. Sonographic and MR imaging findings of testicular epidermoid cysts. AJR Am J Roentgenol. 2002;178:743–8.
19. Pires-Gonçalves L, Silva C, Teixeira M, Costa-Dias S, Sousa-Mendes V. Testicular epidermoid cyst - ultrasound and MR typical findings with macroscopy correlation. Int Braz J Urol. 2011;37(4):534–5.
20. Tsili AC, Giannakis D, Sylakos A, Ntorkou A, Sofikitis N, Argyropoulou MI. MR imaging of scrotum. Magn Reson Imaging Clin N Am. 2014;22(2):217–38.
21. Cassidy FH, Ishioka KM, McMahon CJ, Chu P, Sakamoto K, Lee KS, Aganovic L. MR imaging of scrotal tumors and pseudotumors. Radiographics. 2010;30(3):665–83.
22. Reinberg Y, Manivel JC, Llerena J, Niehans G, Fraley EE. Epidermoid cyst (monodermal teratoma) of the testis. Br J Urol. 1990;66(6):648–51.
23. Loya AG, Said JW, Grant EG. Epidermoid cyst of the testis: radiologic-pathologic correlation. Radiographics. 2004;24(Suppl 1):S243–6.
24. Marko J, Wolfman DJ, Aubin AL, Sesterhenn IA. Testicular seminoma and its mimics. Radiographics. 2017;37(4):1085–98.
25. Johnson JW, Hodge EE, Radwin HM. Epidermoid cyst of testis: a case for orchiectomy. Urology. 1987;29(1):23–5.
26. Maizlin ZV, Belenky A, Baniel J, Gottlieb P, Sandbank J, Strauss S. Epidermoid cyst and teratoma of the testis: sonographic and histologic similarities. J Ultrasound Med. 2005;24:1403–9.
27. Stark L, Potratz D, Schäfer R, von Vietsch H. The synchronous appearance of multiple testicular epidermoid cysts and of a malignant mixed germinal tumor in the contralateral testis. [Article in German]. Urologe A. 1992;31(2):85–7.
28. Goldberg H, Klaassen Z, Chandrasekar T, Fleshner N, Hamilton RJ, Jewett MAS. Germ cell testicular tumors-contemporary diagnosis, staging and Management of Localized and Advanced disease. Urology. 2019;125:8–19.
29. Subik MK, Gordetsky J, Yao JL, di Sant'Agnese PA, Miyamoto H. Frozen section assessment in testicular and paratesticular lesions suspicious for malignancy: its role in preventing unnecessary orchiectomy. Hum Pathol. 2012;43(9):1514–9.
30. Matei DV, Vartolomei MD, Renne G, Tringali VM, Russo A, Bianchi R, Cozzi G, Bottero D, Musi G, Mazzarol G, et al. Reliability of frozen section examination in a large cohort of testicular masses: what did we learn? Clin Genitourin Cancer. 2017;15(4):e689–96.
31. Oosterhuis JW, Stoop JA, Rijlaarsdam MA, Biermann K, Smit VT, Hersmus R, Looijenga LH. Pediatric germ cell tumors presenting beyond childhood? Andrology. 2014;3:70–7.

16

Solitary fibrous tumor of the scrotum: A case report and review of the literature

Tsung-Hsin Chang[1,2], Marcelo Chen[1,2] and Chih-Chiao Lee[1,2*]

Abstract

Background: Solitary fibrous tumor (SFT) is a rare soft tissue tumor originally reported in the pleura. Although it has been reported in various extra-pleural sites, the occurrence of SFT in the scrotum is extremely rare. Herein, we present a 48-year-old man who had scrotal SFT. There are very few reported cases of genitourinary SFTs, this is only the fifth report of SFT of the scrotum in the English medical literature.

Case presentation: In this study, we report on a 48-year-old man who presented with a 5 × 8 cm scrotal mass between his testes. Physical examination revealed a 4.7 × 8.5 cm lobulated tumor mass located between his testicles. Surgical excision of the tumor with scrotal approach was done and pathology reported a SFT. The patient was alive without tumor recurrence or distant metastasis during ongoing follow-up for 9 months post-operatively..

Conclusion: Scrotal SFTs are very rare and only five cases have been reported in English literature to date. Treatment often involves surgical resection, and a definite diagnosis is made with the help of immunohistochemistry. The current general consensus for the management of SFTs is long-term follow-up after surgical excision of the tumor.

Keywords: Solitary fibrous tumor, Scrotum

Background

Solitary fibrous tumor (SFT) is a rare mesenchymal spindle cell neoplasm usually originating from the pleura. It was first described by Klemperer and Rabin in 1931 [1] and has since been reported in various extra-pleural sites. However, reports of urogenital SFTs are extremely rare and only a few cases of scrotal SFTs have been reported [2–9]. Treatment usually involves enucleation and excision of the tumor. Diagnosis is made with the help of immunohistopathological examinations. We hereby report the clinical and pathological characteristics of scrotal SFT.

Case presentation

A 48-year-old male presented with a slow-growing right scrotal mass for the past 2 years. This clearly-demarcated nodular mass was located over the middle-to-right side of the scrotum. The tumor had rapidly increased in size over the past 3 months, but there was no obvious pain or other symptoms. Physical examination revealed a 4.7 × 8.5 cm lobulated tumor mass located between his testicles, non adherent to the scrotum. It was freely movable with elastic consistency on palpation. The penis and testicles were normal in appearance. Testis tumor markers were all normal [alpha-fetoprotein (AFP) = 2.87 ng/mL, beta-human chorionic gonadotrophin (β-HCG) < 0.6 mIU/mL].

Scrotal ultrasonography showed a hypoechoic extra-testicular mass with clear contours and rich blood flow. Computed tomography (CT) showed a hypervascularized lobulated mass (4.7 × 8.5 cm) with contrast media enhancement in the midline of the scrotum (Fig. 1). He then underwent tumor excision via scrotal approach since the tumor did not seem originated from testicular or spermatic cord and the location of the tumor was superficial. A midline raphe incision was made and carry down to the tunica vaginalis. The tumor mass was not adherent to the surrounding tissues or testicles, it was a separated mass with clear margin that could be

* Correspondence: Keithchang0910@gmail.com
[1]Department of Urology, Mackay Memorial hospital, No.92, Sec. 2, Zhongshan N. Rd., Zhongshan Dist, 10449 Taipei City, Taiwan (Republic of China)
[2]Mackay Medical College, No.46, Sec. 3, Zhongzheng Rd., Sanzhi Dist, 252 New Taipei City, Taiwan (Republic of China)

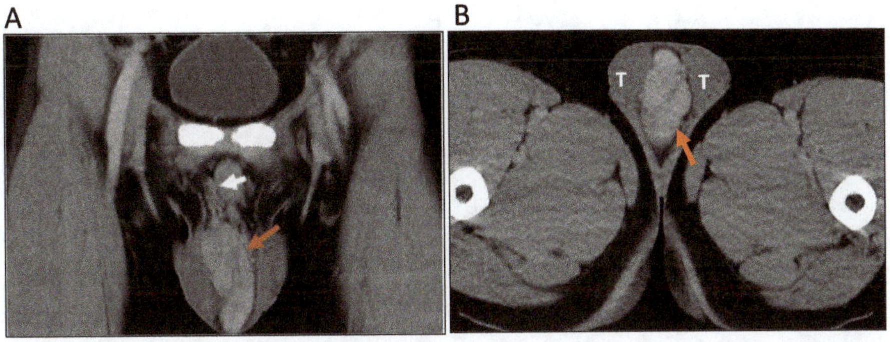

Fig. 1 CT image demonstrating. (**a**) A 4.7 × 8.5 × 3.5 cm tumor (red arrow) with vascular supply (white arrow) arising from the right spermatic cord. (**b**) An extra-testicular mass (red arrow) within the scrotum between the two testes (T)

easily dissected with blunt dissection method. The tumor was completely excised after ligating the main feeding vessels.

The resected specimen consisted of three lobulated and contiguous firm tumors, measuring 7.5 × 6.3 × 3.8 cm in size and weighing 76.5 g in total (Fig. 2a). Cut section of the tumor showed a well-defined, lobulated, whitish and firm tumor with some mucinous components (Fig. 2b). Microscopically, it was a hyper-cellular tumor with a vaguely fascicular growth pattern forming a patternless growth architecture (Fig. 3a) with minimal nulcear atypia rate and a mitotic count < 4 per 10 high power field. A few thin-walled, branching "staghorn appearance" vessels were also present in the tumor (Fig. 3b). The tumor cells had an ovoid to short spindle shape with indistinct borders and dispersed chromatin within vesicular nuclei. Immunohistochemically, the tumor cells were positive for STAT-6 (nuclear expression) (Fig. 4a) and CD34 (Fig. 4b), and negative for actin, desmin, CD117 and DOG-1. Based on the morphology and immunohistochemical studies, the diagnosis of SFT was made. The patient was alive without tumor recurrence or distant metastasis during ongoing follow-up for 9 months post-operatively with semi-annual CTs.

Discussion and conclusions

SFT is a soft tissue tumor which usually presents as a firm, grey-to-white colored, well-circumscribed solid mass. It was first reported by Klemperer and Rabin in 1931 in the pleura. Although the disease most commonly occurs in the pleura, extra-thoracic SFTs have been reported in many sites including the head and neck [10], intracranial and spinal cord meninges [11], eyes [12], thyroid [13], larynx [14], gastrointestinal system [15–17], genitourinary tract [18–20], pelvis [21] and soft tissue [22]. The most common extra-pleural locations are the meninges, followed by subcutaneous tissues of the lower limbs, the retroperitoneum, and the orbit [23]. Extra-pleural SFTs share similar histological features with pleural SFTs [23].

There are very few reported cases of genitourinary SFTs, and SFTs of the scrotum or para-testicular

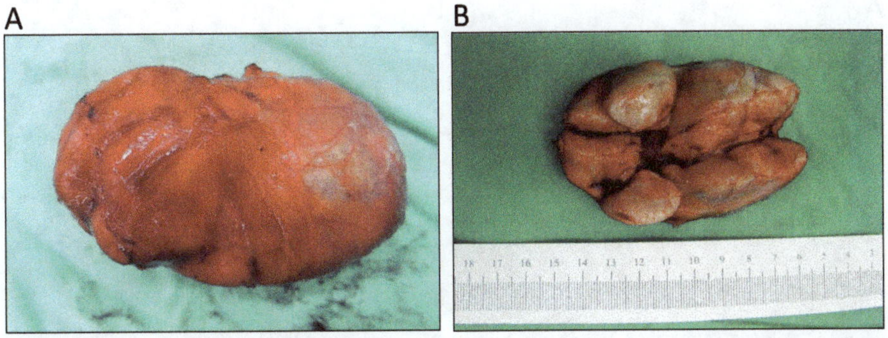

Fig. 2 Gross pictures. (**a**) Gross appearance of the tumor showed three connected tumor nodules encapsulated within a fibrous capsule. (**b**) The cut section of the tumor showed three well-defined, lobulated, whitish firm tumors, measuring 7.5 × 6.3 × 3.5 cm in total size. Some mucinous components can also be seen

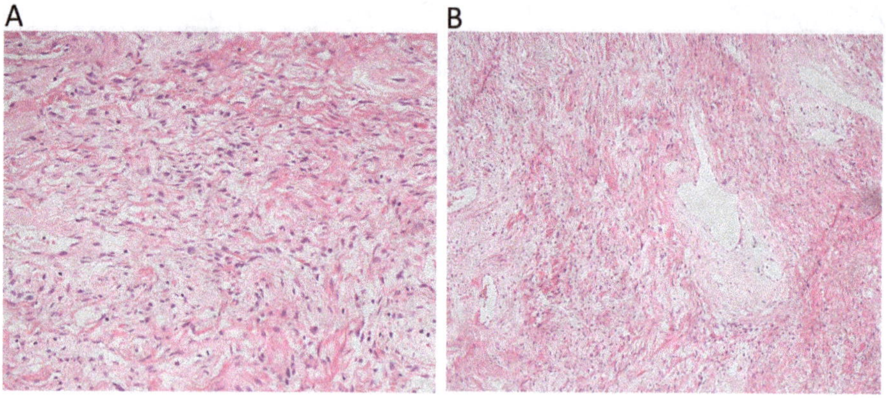

Fig. 3 Hematoxylin and eosin staining demonstrating. (**a**) spindle cells with a fascicular growth pattern forming a "patternless" growth architecture. (**b**) Thin-walled, branched "staghorn" configuration of vessels can be seen

SFTs are extremely rare (Table 1). This is only the fifth report of SFT of the scrotum in the English medical literature, and the only report with three documented connected nodules, which is different from the usual appearance of a SFT with a single solitary nodule.

The diagnosis of extra-pleural SFTs is challenging and relies on its clinical manifestations or imaging studies. Differential diagnosis of SFTs arising from para-testicles soft tissues can be challanging since it can show great similarity to those spindle cell fibroblastic associated tumors, such as angiomyolipomas, leimyoma, fibrosarcomas and gastrointestinal stromal tumors (GIST). Therefore, immunohistochemistry plays an important role in the diagnosis of SFTs. Traditionally, CD34 and BLC-2 have a high sensitivity for SFTs, and CD34 is only absent in 5 to 10% of typical SFTs [24]. BCL-2 is seen in almost all cases of SFTs [25, 26]. However, these traditional markers are not specific to SFTs, and they may also be present in many other mesenchymal tumors mimicking SFTs, which may lead to confusion and uncertainty in the diagnosis. In 2013, Chmelecki et al. [27] and Robinson et al. [28] reported that NAB2-STAT6, a new fusion gene expression present in the vast majority of SFTs, can be used as a unique molecular marker for the diagnosis of SFTs. Subsequent reports have demonstrated that the immunohistochemical nuclear expression of STAT6 in SFTs can distinguish SFTs from other histologic mimics, and that it can be used as a diagnostic tool [29–31]. Thus, in current clinical settings, the diagnosis of SFTs can be made if STAT6 nuclear expression, CD34 and BCL-2 are all strongly positive. NAB2-STAT6 fusion genetic tests may not be necessary for the diagnosis of SFTs under such circumstances.

SFTs are usually considered to follow a benign clinical course with a low potential of malignant change, and surgical excision of the lesion is usually

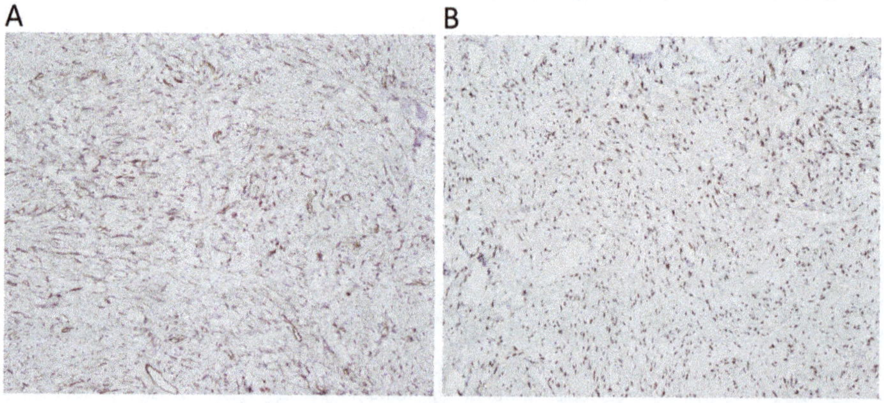

Fig. 4 Immunohistochemical features. (**a**) Positive nuclear expression of STAT6 in tumor cells. (**b**) Positive expression of CD34 in tumor cells

Table 1 Reported cases of paratesticular SFTs

Reference	Year	Age	Initial presentation	Location	Tumor size (cm)	Treatment	Recurrence/ Follow-up time	Immuno-histochemical features
Marquez MA et al. [2]	2001	67	Paratesticular mass	NA	9	Surgical excision	NA	CD34+, Vimentin+, Actin-, S100-, Keratin-
Garcia TM et al. [3]	2006	22	Pain	Left tunica vaginalis testis	3	Surgical excision with intraoperative biopsy	None/12 months	NA
Gutierrez-Diaz CM et al. [5]	2011	53	NA	Paratesticular	NA	NA	NA	CD34+, BCL-2 +, vimentin+
Lee GE et al. [4]	2011	61	Slow growing mass	Left scrotal sac	5 × 4	Surgical excision	NA/NA	CD34+
Barazani Y et al. [6]	2012	26	Painless firm mass	Left scrotum	6.1 × 5.5 × 4.3	Inguinal exploration	None/NA	CD34+, BCL-2 +, SMA -, Desmin-, S100-
Hu SB et al. [7]	2014	31	Left inguinoscrotal swelling	Left spermatic cord	3 × 2	Inguinal exploration	None/25 months	CD99+, Bcl-2+, Partial CD34+,, Focal S-100+, SMA+, CD68-
Zhou YH et al. [8]	2015	61	Slow growing mass	Left scrotum	4 × 4.5 × 5	Surgical excision (Inguinal)	None/6 months	CD34+, CD99+, Vimentin+, CD117, S100-, SMA-, Desmin-, CD68-
Zhao XY et al. [9]	2017	77	Painless mass	Left scrotum	11x9x8	Surgical excision	None/18 months	CD34+, CD99+, STAT6+

NA not available, *CD* cluster of differentiation, STAT6, activator of transcription 6

sufficient. There were no current consensus on how the surgical approach should be done. Since SFTs usually presents as a low-malignant potential tumor, both inguinal and scrotal approach for tumor exploration and excional had been reported. However, malignant pathology and behavior have been described in about 20% of SFTs [32]. The diagnosis of malignant SFT is based on pathologic examinations of histological features. The presence of hypercellularity, infiltrative margin growth, > 4 mitotic counts per 10 high-power fields and nuclear atypia have been reported to be histological malignant components [29, 32, 33]. In a multicenter study including 81 patients with surgically treated SFTs, patients with histologically malignant SFTs had higher local recurrence rates and higher incidence of metastasis [34]. Positive surgical margins, tumor size > 10 cm, and the presence of a high mitotic rate have been reported to be significantly correlated with a higher incidence of metastasis and worse overall survival.

In conclusion, SFT is a rare mesenchymal spindle cell neoplasm originally reported in the pleura, but it can be found in various sites throughout the body. Scrotal SFTs are very rare and only five cases have been reported to date. Treatment often involves surgical resection, and a definite diagnosis is made with the help of immunohistochemistry, especially the nuclear expression of STAT6. SFTs are often benign but there is a slight chance of malignancy. Patients with histologically malignant features may have worse prognosis. The current general consensus for the management of SFTs is long-term follow-up after surgical excision of the tumor. In our experience, we performed surgcial resection of the tumor via scrotal approach without additional interventions. 6-month follow-up with CT scan was conducted, we will continue the follow-up of this case to monitor long-term outcome of this rare disease.

Abbreviation
CT: Computed tomography; SFT: Solitary fibrous tumor

Acknowledgements
Not applicable.

Authors' contributions
THC made contributions to the acquisition of history, image and wrote the manuscript. CCL performed the treatment, and reviewed the manuscript to give clinical opinions. MC made supervision and helped reviewing the manuscript. All the authors read and approved the final manuscript.

References
1. Klemperer P, Coleman BR. Primary neoplasms of the pleura. A report of five cases. Am J Ind Med. 1992;22(1):1–31.
2. Márquez AM, Vicioso LR, Castro AL, Casals JS, Alcázar JR, Matilla AV. Paratesticular solitary fibrous tumor. J Archivos Espanoles de Urologia. 2001; 54(7):716–8.
3. García MT, Beltrán JA, Santolaya IG, Carrascosa VL, Tarín MP, CJDLJAedu S. Solitary fibrous tumor of the tunica vaginalis testis. Arch Esp Urol. 2006; 59(2):186–9.
4. Lee GE, Rha SE, Byun JY, Lee K, SWJJoUiM K. Paratesticular solitary fibrous tumor: a rare cause of a hypervascular extratesticular mass. J Ultrasound Med. 2011;30(2):279–81.
5. Ceballos MEG-D, Hernández-Solís A, Cruz-Ortiz H, González-Atencio Y, Cicero-Sabido RJCC. Solitary fibrous tumor: clinicopathological study of 16 cases. Modern Pathology : an official journal of the United States and Canadian Academy of Pathology, Inc. 2011;79:387–93.
6. Barazani Y, Tareen B. Rare case of paratesticular solitary fibrous tumour (lipomatous hemangiopericytoma). Can Urol Assoc J. 2012;6(3):E131–3.
7. Hu S, Yi L, Yang L, Wang Y. Solitary fibrous tumor of the spermatic cord: a case report and literature review. Exp Ther Med. 2015;9(1):55–8.

8. Zhou Y, Gong G, Tang Y, Tang J, Gan Y, YJljoc D. Pathology e: Paratesticular solitary fibrous tumor: a case report and review of literature. Int J Clin Exp Pathol. 2015;8(3):3358.
9. Zhao XY, Zeng M, Yang QY, Jing CP, Zhang Y. Scrotum solitary fibrous tumor: a case report and review of literature. Medicine (Baltimore). 2017; 96(48):e8854.
10. Smith SC, Gooding WE, Elkins M, Patel RM, Harms PW, McDaniel AS, Palanisamy N, Uram-Tuculescu C, Balzer BB, Lucas DR, et al. Solitary fibrous tumors of the head and neck: a multi-institutional Clinicopathologic study. Am J Surg Pathol. 2017;41(12):1642–56.
11. Bouvier C, Métellus P, de Paula AM, Vasiljevic A, Jouvet A, Guyotat J, Mokhtari K, Varlet P, Dufour H, Figarella-Branger DJBP. Solitary fibrous tumors and hemangiopericytomas of the meninges: overlapping pathological features and common prognostic factors suggest the same spectrum of tumors. J Brain Pathology. 2012;22(4):511–21.
12. Petrovic A, Oberic A, Moulin A, Hamedani M. Ocular adnexal (orbital) solitary fibrous tumor: nuclear STAT6 expression and literature review. Graefe's Arch Clin Exp Ophthalmol = Albrecht von Graefes Archiv fur klinische und experimentelle Ophthalmologie. 2015;253(9):1609–17.
13. Ghasemi-Rad M, Wang KY, Jain S, Lincoln CM. Solitary fibrous tumor of thyroid: a case report with review of literature. Clin Imaging. 2019;53:105–7.
14. Dotto JE, Ahrens W, Lesnik DJ, Kowalski D, Sasaki C, Flynn S. Solitary fibrous tumor of the larynx: a case report and review of the literature. Arch Pathol Lab Med. 2006;130(2):213–6.
15. Urabe M, Yamagata Y, Aikou S, Mori K, Yamashita H, Nomura S, Shibahara J, Fukayama M, Seto Y. Solitary fibrous tumor of the greater omentum, mimicking gastrointestinal stromal tumor of the small intestine: a case report. Int Surg. 2015;100(5):836–40.
16. Bratton L, Salloum R, Cao W, Huber AR. Solitary fibrous tumor of the sigmoid Colon masquerading as an adnexal neoplasm. Case Rep Pathol. 2016;2016:4182026.
17. D'Amico FE, Ruffolo C, Romano M, DID M, Sbaraglia M, Dei Tos AP, Garofalo T, Giordano A, Bassi I, Massani M. Rare neoplasm mimicking Neuoroendocrine pancreatic tumor: a case report of solitary fibrous tumor with review of the literature. Anticancer Res. 2017;37(6):3093–7.
18. Abeygunasekera AM, Ginige AP, Liyanage IS, Hareendra K. A solitary fibrous tumor of the kidney. J Cancer Res Ther. 2015;11(3):662.
19. Kouba E, Simper NB, Chen S, Williamson SR, Grignon DJ, Eble JN, MacLennan GT, Montironi R, Lopez-Beltran A, Osunkoya AO, et al. Solitary fibrous tumour of the genitourinary tract: a clinicopathological study of 11 cases and their association with the NAB2-STAT6 fusion gene. J Clin Pathol. 2017;70(6):508–14.
20. Prunty MC, Gaballah A, Ellis L, Murray KS. Solitary fibrous tumor of the pelvis involving the urinary bladder. Urology. 2018;117:27–30.
21. Fernandez A, Conrad M, Gill RM, Choi WT, Kumar V, Behr S. Solitary fibrous tumor in the abdomen and pelvis: a case series with radiological findings and treatment recommendations. Clin Imaging. 2018;48:48–54.
22. Nielsen GP, O'Connell JX, Dickersin GR, Rosenberg AE. Solitary fibrous tumor of soft tissue: a report of 15 cases, including 5 malignant examples with light microscopic, immunohistochemical, and ultrastructural data. Mod Pathol: an official journal of the United States and Canadian Academy of Pathology, Inc. 1997;10(10):1028–37.
23. Ronchi A, Cozzolino I, Zito Marino F, Accardo M, Montella M, Panarese I, Roccuzzo G, Toni G, Franco R, De Chiara A. Extrapleural solitary fibrous tumor: a distinct entity from pleural solitary fibrous tumor. An update on clinical, molecular and diagnostic features. Ann Diagn Pathol. 2018;34:142–50.
24. Chan JK. Solitary fibrous tumour--everywhere, and a diagnosis in vogue. Histopathology. 1997;31(6):568–76.
25. Chilosi M, Facchetti F, Dei Tos AP, Lestani M, Morassi ML, Martignoni G, Sorio C, Benedetti A, Morelli L, Doglioni C, et al. bcl-2 expression in pleural and extrapleural solitary fibrous tumours. J Pathol. 1997;181(4):362–7.
26. Suster S, Fisher C, Moran CA. Expression of bcl-2 oncoprotein in benign and malignant spindle cell tumors of soft tissue, skin, serosal surfaces, and gastrointestinal tract. Am J Surg Pathol. 1998;22(7):863–72.
27. Chmielecki J, Crago AM, Rosenberg M, O'Connor R, Walker SR, Ambrogio L, Auclair D, McKenna A, Heinrich MC, Frank DA, et al. Whole-exome sequencing identifies a recurrent NAB2-STAT6 fusion in solitary fibrous tumors. Nat Genet. 2013;45(2):131–2.
28. Robinson DR, Wu YM, Kalyana-Sundaram S, Cao X, Lonigro RJ, Sung YS, Chen CL, Zhang L, Wang R, Su F, et al. Identification of recurrent NAB2-STAT6 gene fusions in solitary fibrous tumor by integrative sequencing. Nat Genet. 2013;45(2):180–5.
29. Yoshida A, Tsuta K, Ohno M, Yoshida M, Narita Y, Kawai A, Asamura H, RJTAjosp K. STAT6 immunohistochemistry is helpful in the diagnosis of solitary fibrous tumors. Am J Surg Pathol. 2014;38(4):552–9.
30. Doyle LA, Vivero M, Fletcher CD, Mertens F, Hornick JLJMP. Nuclear expression of STAT6 distinguishes solitary fibrous tumor from histologic mimics. Mod Pathol. 2014;27(3):390.
31. Zhang X, Cheng H, Bao Y, Tang F, Wang Y. diagnostic value of STAT6 immunohistochemistry in solitary fibrous tumor/meningeal hemangiopericytoma. Zhonghua bing li xue za zhi = Chinese J Pathol. 2016;45(2):97–101.
32. Gold JS, Antonescu CR, Hajdu C, Ferrone CR, Hussain M, Lewis JJ, Brennan MF, Coit DG. Clinicopathologic correlates of solitary fibrous tumors. Cancer. 2002;94(4):1057–68.
33. England DM, Hochholzer L, McCarthy MJ. Localized benign and malignant fibrous tumors of the pleura. A clinicopathologic review of 223 cases. Am J Surg Pathol. 1989;13(8):640–58.
34. van Houdt WJ, Westerveld CM, Vrijenhoek JE, van Gorp J, van Coevorden F, Verhoef C, van Dalen T. Prognosis of solitary fibrous tumors: a multicenter study. Ann Surg Oncol. 2013;20(13):4090–5.

17

Bilateral adrenal hemorrhage after hip arthroplasty: An initially misdiagnosed case

Lei Wang[1,2], Xiao-fei Wang[1,2], Ying-chao Qin[3], Jia Chen[1,2], Cun-hai Shang[4], Guo-feng Sun[1,2] and Ning-chen Li[1,2,5*]

Abstract

Background: Bilateral adrenal hemorrhage (BAH) is a rare but potentially catastrophic condition. Its clinical manifestation is often non-specific and sometimes difficult to be diagnosed in time.

Case summary: A 57-year-old woman, who presented with severe fatigue, nausea and vomiting after left hip arthroplasty due to her femoral neck fracture in a local hospital, was transferred to our medical center. Laboratory results revealed significant hyponatremia, low serum cortisol and elevated serum ACTH. Computed tomography (CT) showed a bilateral adrenal mass, measured 3.6 × 2.7 cm on the left and 3.4 × 2.3 cm on the right. Further magnetic resonance imaging (MRI) confirmed the diagnosis of BAH. The patient was prescribed with oral prednisolone acetate, 5 mg, tid, and her condition improved gradually. Nine months after, the patient was in good condition with 5 mg prednisolone acetate per day. CT revealed a clearly shrunken adrenal mass compared with 9 months ago.

Conclusions: This case illustrates the difficulty in making the diagnosis of BAH with atypical presentation. Such cases necessitate greater alertness on the part of the clinician and require rapid diagnosis and prompt glucocorticoid replacement for better clinical outcomes.

Keywords: Bilateral adrenal hemorrhage, Arthroplasty, Stress, Anticoagulants, Glucocorticoid replacement, Case report

Background

Adrenal hemorrhage (AH) is a rare condition with a reported incidence of only 5 in 1,000,000 [1]. Bilateral adrenal hemorrhage (BAH) is extremely rare and comprises only 10% of all AH cases. However, BAH is potentially fatal, carrying a mortality rate of 15% [2]. BAH is reported to be associated with many issues such as trauma, surgery, infection, use of anticoagulants, antiphospholipid syndrome (APS), and heparin-induced thrombocytopenia (HIT), etc. Abdominal pain, fever, nausea, vomiting and hypotension are common but nonspecific symptoms of BAH. Most of the symptoms are manifestations of adrenal insufficiency and acute adrenal crisis [3].

* Correspondence: wjpurologycenter@sina.com
[1]Department of urology, Peking University Shougang Hospital, Peking University Health Science Center, Beijing 100144, China
[2]Peking University Wu Jieping Urology Center, Peking University Health Science Center, Beijing 100144, China
Full list of author information is available at the end of the article

In this study, we describe a rare case of BAH after hip arthroplasty in a 57-year-old female with left femoral neck fracture. The stress of trauma and surgery, including the use of enoxaparin after surgery, should be its inducing factors. With nonspecific manifestation, this case was misdiagnosed for the first 2 weeks and then achieved a good recovery with treatment consisting of glucocorticoid replacement.

Case presentation

A 57-year-old, previously healthy female suffered a serious car accident on May 3rd, 2018, which led to femoral neck fracture on her left side. Three days later, she underwent left hip arthroplasty in a local hospital. The patient was given enoxaparin (0.6 ml, ih. qd) for DVT prophylaxis on postoperative day (POD) one. The patient's postoperative recovery was uneventful until POD 8, when she complained of severe nausea and vomiting, accompanied by vague epigastric pain, ceased defecation, decreased appetite, generalized weakness and fever with a Tmax of 39 °C. No acute hypotensive episode or hypoglycemia was recorded.

"Bowel obstruction" was first considered, and the patient was transferred to the general surgery department on POD 10 for parenteral nutrition and intestinal obstruction-related treatment. Her vital signs included temperature 38.7 °C, heart rate 104, respiration 19, blood pressure 120/74 mmHg. The abnormal physical examination included mild abdominal distention, slight tenderness of the upper abdomen, and slightly active bowel sounds. Laboratory examination revealed hypernatremia (152 mmol/L, normal 135–145 mmol/L) and hypopotassemia (3.2 mmol/L, normal 3.5–5.5 mmol/L).

On POD 12, a computed tomography (CT) scan of the abdomen (Fig. 1) revealed a bilateral adrenal mass and a slightly enlarged spleen, but no signs of dilation or an air-fluid level within the intestine. However, the bilateral adrenal mass was thought to be adrenal adenoma and did not attract the properly deserved attention at that time. Consistent fluid resuscitation was given to correct low serum sodium and chlorine, and parenteral nutrition support was also given due to the patient's bad appetite and vomiting.

As the patient's condition did not improve significantly, she was transferred to our hospital on POD 25, with very poor appetite, severe fatigue, nausea, vomiting, and general malaise. The physical examination was unremarkable, and her vital signs included temperature 36.1 °C, heart rate 62, respiration18, blood pressure 120/65 mmHg. The laboratory values revealed significant hyponatremia (120 mmol/L), hypochloremia (88 mmol/L, normal 99–110 mmol/L), compensatory metabolic acidosis (pH 7.36, BB − 3.4 mmol/L), elevated AST (75 IU/L, normal 13–35 IU/L), a low serum cortisol of 1.9 μg/dL (normal 3.7–19.4 μg/dL), and a high serum ACTH of 313 ng/L (normal 7.2–63.3 ng/L). Blood potassium, glucose, hematocrit, creatinine, platelet count and coagulation profile were all normal. CT scan revealed a bilateral adrenal mass, measuring 3.6 × 2.7 cm on the left and 3.4 × 2.3 cm on the right (Fig. 2). Differential diagnosis included primary adrenal cancer or metastatic tumor. As no historical result could be offered, whether the adrenal mass was new-onset or had existed for a long period was not clear. Magnetic resonance imaging (MRI) was advised and confirmed the most likely diagnosis to be bilateral adrenal hemorrhage (Fig. 3).

Enoxaparin had been discontinued on admission, and the patient was started on oral prednisolone acetate, 5 mg, tid. Thereafter, the patient's condition improved gradually, her nausea and vomiting disappeared, and her appetite and physical power also recovered significantly. The patient was in normal serum cortisol level at the time of discharge. The dose of oral prednisolone acetate was decreased to 5 mg, bid. She was also told that oral steroids might not be discontinued in the rest of her life. Three months later, the patient was in good condition, and the dose of oral prednisolone acetate was decreased to 5 mg, qd. In the patient's latest follow-up 9 months after discharge, she still needed oral steroids replacement because of symptoms of adrenal insufficiency after complete withdrawal of the drug. MRI (Fig. 4) and CT (Fig. 5) images during her followup revealed a continuously shrunken adrenal mass compared with that during her hospitalization .

Discussion and conclusions

BAH is a rare but potentially catastrophic complication. The reported inducing factors include trauma, surgery, anticoagulants, infection, myocardial infarction, chronic

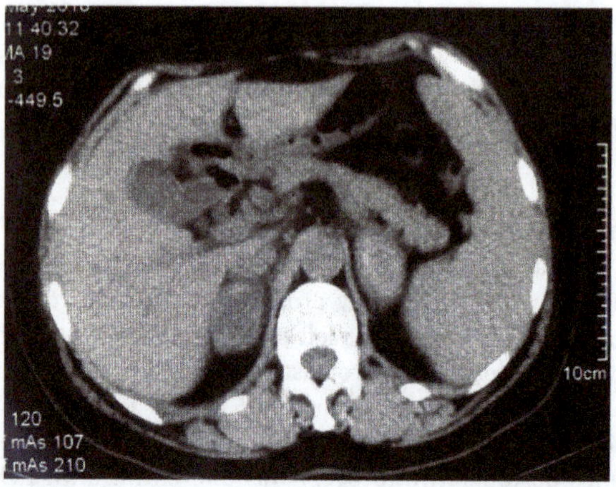

Fig. 1 Axial computed tomography scan abdominal (postoperative day 12) revealed a bilateral adrenal mass with mixed high density

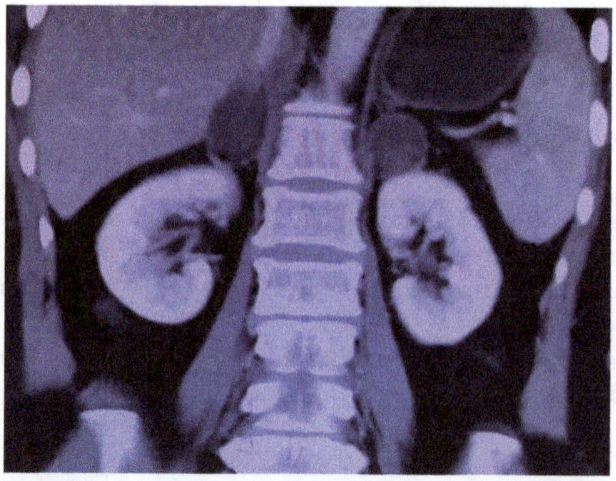

Fig. 2 Enhanced computed tomography (coronal section) on postoperative day 26 showed a bilateral adrenal mass, measured 3.6 × 2.7 × 4.8 cm on the left and 3.4 × 2.3 × 4.2 cm on the right, with enhancement only seen in peripheral area of the mass

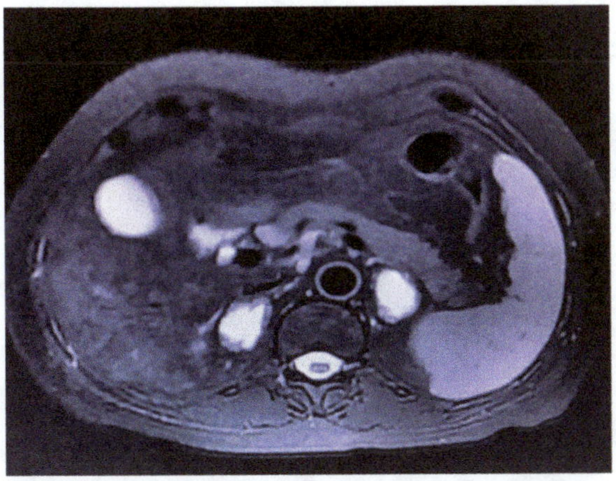

Fig. 3 Magnetic resonance imaging (axial section, T2 weighed) on postoperative day 33 displayed water signal intensity of long T2 in central regions of bilateral adrenal mass

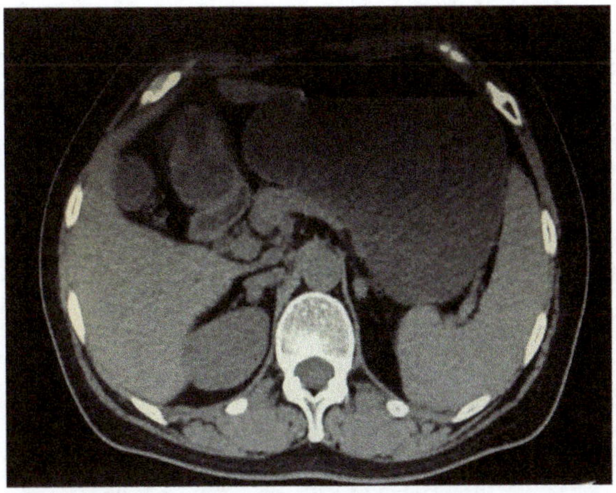

Fig. 5 CT scan (9 months after discharge) revealed a continuously shrunken adrenal mass, measured 1.4 × 0.9 cm on the left and 1.3 × 0.9 cm on the right, compared with 9 months ago

heart failure, APS, and HIT [4–8]. Cases without any of above risk factors have also been reported in previous literature [2, 3]. In this study, we report a rare such case in a middle-age female after hip arthroplasty. The most likely cause in this case is thought to be the use of enoxaparin, a common low-molecular-weight heparin used after surgery. Sharp stress from trauma and surgery is also considered to be a potential risk factor in this case. With the condition's nonspecific clinical manifestation, the patient did not receive a correct diagnosis and timely glucocorticoid replacement for 2 weeks after episode of adrenal crisis in a local hospital. However, the patient's recovery was rapid after BAH was diagnosed and oral prednisolone acetate was prescribed.

BAH after surgery is extremely rare. Mandanas S [9] had reviewed 36 such cases in the year of 2013. Herein, we made a further literature search and 12 additional cases published after the year of 2013 were summarized in Table 1 [6, 8–16]. The mechanism of AH has not been fully elucidated. Among potential mechanisms, the distinct vascular anatomy of the adrenal gland has been repeatedly mentioned [2, 7, 8]. The adrenal gland has an arterial network, and the blood flow is very fast. However, it only has a single vein, which leads to an abrupt transition of blood flow and renders the gland vulnerable to hemorrhage events. A sharp increase of arterial blood flow or a sudden thrombosis of the adrenal vein can all lead to AH. For example, stress-induced catecholamine increases adrenal blood flow, promotes platelet aggregation, and induces adrenal vein spasm, which results in the blood vessels being filled with a large amount of blood flow, the vascular wall being damaged and ruptured, and eventually leading to a bleeding. Other implicated factors include aging-related reduced capillary resistance in the adrenal vascular bed [15] and adrenal vein thrombosis in hypercoagulable states, such as antiphospholipid syndrome [7].

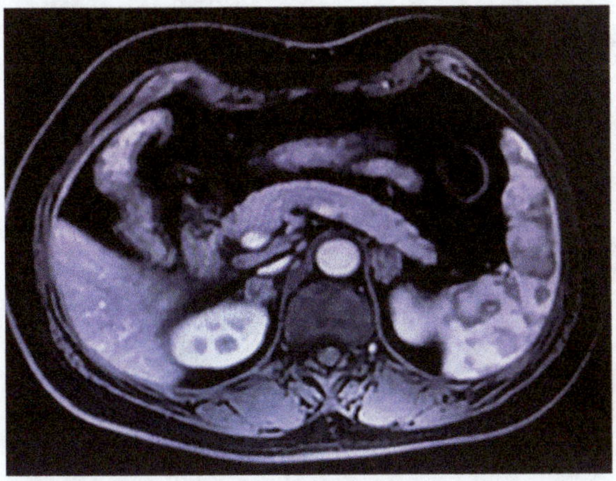

Fig. 4 Enhanced magnetic resonance imaging (postoperative day 140) revealed a clearly shrunken adrenal mass compared with 3 months ago

Heparin-induced-thrombocytopenia is thought to be another important factor. Though rare, AH has been reported repeatedly after the use of anticoagulants, including heparin, warfarin, dalteparin, doumadin, dabigatran, or enoxaparin [12, 17, 18]. K J Park [12] reviewed 16 cases of hip and knee arthroplasty patients who suffered from BAH. Anticoagulation prophylaxis was given in all of the cases as a routine modality to prevent deep venous thrombosis. Among them, HIT was identified as the cause of BAH after confirmatory HIT antibody tests in 7 cases. For our case, sharp stress from the femoral neck fracture and the subsequent hip arthroplasty surgery was a possible factor related to her BAH. We also postulate that the use of enoxaparin, whose relationship with BAH

Table 1 Summary of the literature on postoperative bilateral adrenal hemorrhage since 2013

No.	Year	Age	Gender	Procedure	DVT prophylaxis	POD	Symptoms	Lab. exams	Treatment	Outcome	Ref.
1	2013	52	F	Right hip arthroplasty	LMWH	9	Ap, hypotension, vomiting, weakness	Hyponatremia, hyperkalemia	Hydrocortisone fludrocortisone	Adrenal insufficiency, oral replacement	[9]
2	2014	67	M	Laparotomy, adhesiolysis	Not shown	4	Ap, confused, pyrexia	Hyponatraemia, hypocalcaemia hypermagnesaemia	Hydrocortisone	Long-term fludrocortisone	[10]
3	2014	48	F	Right partial nephrectomy	LMWH (for PE)	6	Syncope, hypotension, lethargy, fever	Thrombocytopenia, hyponatremia	Hydrocortisone	Adrenal insufficiency, oral replacement	[11]
4	2015	45	F	Chole-cystectomy	LMWH	9	Ap, fever, nausea, vomiting	Hyponatremia, thrombocytosis, antiphospholipid antibodies(+)	Fludrocortisone	well	[6]
5	2015	65	F	Total knee arthroplasty	LMWH enoxaparin	8	Vague, epigastric pain, lethargy, fever, nausea	Hyponatremia, hypokalemia	Hydrocortisone	well	[12]
6	2015	75	M	Total hip replacement	Warfarin	14	Watery diarrhoea, vomiting, hypotension	Hyponatremia, hyperkalemia	Hydrocortisone	Adrenal insufficiency, oral replacement	[13]
7	2015	48	F	Total knee arthroplasty	Aspirin LMWH	8	Ap, fever, hypotension	Thrombocytopenia, heparin platelet factor 4 antibody(+)	Steroids	Well	[14]
8	2016	93	F	Hemi-colectomy	Not shown	4	Ap, hypotension, syncope	hyponatremia, hypokalemia, heparin platelet factor 4 antibody(+)	Hydrocortisone	Stable, lifelong steroids	[15]
9	2017	76	F	Pancreaticoduodenectomy	Not shown	5	Ap, hypotension, nausea, vomiting	Hemoglobin drop, hyponatremia, hyperkalemia	Hydrocortisone	well	[16]
10	2018	65	F	Colectomy	LMWH	4	Fever, fatigue, lethargy, hypotension	Hyponatremia, hyperkalemia	Steroids	well	[8]
11	2018	72	M	Total colectomy	LMWH	5	Anorexia, lethargy, hypotension, fever	Hyponatremia; anticardiolipin antibodies(+)	Hydrocortisone	well	[8]
12	2019	57	F	Left hip arthroplasty	LMWH enoxaparin	8	Ap, fever, nausea, vomiting, weakness	Hyponatremia, hypochloremia, metabolic acidosis	Oral predni-solone acetate	Adrenal insufficiency, oral replacement	Our case

***DVT* Deep venous thrombosis, *POD* Postoperative day, *Lab.* Laboratory, *LMWH* Low-molecular-weight heparin, *Ap* Abdominal pain, *PE* Pulmonary embolism**

has only been reported once by K J Park [12] in 2015, could be a potential risk factor.

The clinical manifestation of BAH is often nonspecific and occurs as a result of hypocortisolism and hemorrhage, including symptoms such as abdominal pain, fever, nausea, vomiting, fatigue, weakness, confusion and hypotension. Acute adrenal insufficiency secondary to an adrenal hemorrhage, especially BAH, is severe and sometimes life-threatening. Thus, it requires prompt diagnosis and management to prevent death from primary adrenocortical insufficiency. In our case, the patient's clinical manifestation was nonspecific and confusing, which led to a misdiagnosis in the first 2 weeks in the local hospital.

Diagnosis of adrenal hemorrhage is challenge due to its low incidence, the vagueness of its signs and symptoms, and its nonspecific blood test abnormalities. As the patient is in condition of acute adrenal insufficiency, many abnormalities could be confirmed in biochemical tests, such as low cortisol, elevated ACTH, and sometimes hyponatremia and hyperkalemia [19]. Noncontrast abdominal CT is thought to be a standard diagnostic assessment but is sometimes difficult to interpret in the differential diagnosis, especially when the CT is performed after the acute hemorrhage phase. MRI of the adrenal glands has higher accuracy in differentiating adrenal hemorrhage and has advantages over conventional CT because it can easily distinguish adrenal hematoma from adjacent necrotic tissue and determine the onset time of hematoma.

Adrenal crisis due to hemorrhage is very dangerous. The mortality rate of BAH can reach 15% even after treatment. If the diagnosis or starting time of proper treatment is delayed, the mortality rate may be higher [16, 19]. Intravenous hydrocortisone and rapid fluids are recommended to be given as initial treatment. Hydrocortisone could be administered with a 100 mg bolus and then 200 mg per day by continuous intravenous infusion. As for resuscitating the patient with fluid, saline can be administered. Long-term patients may require lifelong steroid replacement. For our case, as the course of hypoadrenalism had lasted for 2 weeks and the patient had tolerated the condition to some extent, we only offered oral hormone supplementation, and the patient achieved a rapid recovery.

To the best of our knowledge, our BAH case is special with an initial misdiagnosis for up to 2 weeks. This case indicates that it's full of challenge in diagnosing a BAH with atypical clinical presentations. Such cases necessitate greater alertness on the part of the clinician and require rapid diagnosis and prompt glucocorticoid replacement for better clinical outcomes. Despite its rarity, due to its potentially fatal consequences, bilateral adrenal hemorrhage should be considered as a differential for acute deterioration of a patient's condition after surgery.

Abbreviations

ACTH: Adrenocorticotropic hormone; APS: Antiphospholipid syndrome; BAH: Bilateral adrenal hemorrhage; CT: Computed tomography; DVT: Deep venous thrombosis; HIT: Heparin-induced thrombocytopenia; MRI: Magnetic resonance imaging; POD: Postoperative day

Acknowledgements

No.

Authors' contributions

LW: Manuscript writing; XW: Data collection; CS: Image analysis; YQ, JC, GS: Patient treatment; NL: Manuscript Revision. All authors reviewed and approved the manuscript.

Author details

[1]Department of urology, Peking University Shougang Hospital, Peking University Health Science Center, Beijing 100144, China. [2]Peking University Wu Jieping Urology Center, Peking University Health Science Center, Beijing 100144, China. [3]Department of General Surgery, Shuangqiao Hospital in Chaoyang District, Beijing 100024, China. [4]Department of Medical Imaging, Peking University Shougang Hospital, Peking University Health Science Center, Beijing 100144, China. [5]Peking University Wu Jieping Urology Center, Peking University Shougang Hospital, 9# Jinyuanzhuang Road, Shijingshan District, Beijing 100144, China.

References

1. Arlt W, Allolio B. Adrenal insufficiency. Lancet. 2003;361:1881–93.
2. Fatima Z, Tariq U, Khan A, Sohail MS, Sheikh AB, Bhatti SI, et al. A rare case of bilateral adrenal hemorrhage. Cureus. 2018;10:e2830.
3. Dhawan N, Bodukam VK, Thakur K, Singh A, Jenkins D, Bahl J. Idiopathic bilateral adrenal hemorrhage in a 63-year-old male: a case report and review of the literature. Case Rep Urol. 2015;2015:503638.
4. Ketha S, Smithedajkul P, Vella A, Pruthi R, Wysokinski W, McBane R. Adrenal haemorrhage due to heparin-induced thrombocytopenia. Thromb Haemost. 2013;109:669–75.
5. Minami M, Muta T, Adachi M, Higuchi M, Aoki K, Ogawa R. Bilateral adrenal hemorrhage in a patient with antiphospholipid syndrome during chronic graft-versus-host disease. Intern Med. 2018;57:1439–44.
6. Dahan M, Lim C, Salloum C, Azoulay D. Spontaneous bilateral adrenal hemorrhage following cholecystectomy. Hepatobiliary Surg Nutr. 2016;5: 263–4.
7. Tormos LM, Schandl CA. The significance of adrenal hemorrhage: undiagnosed Waterhouse-Friderichsen syndrome, a case series. J Forensic Sci. 2013;58:1071–4.
8. Kolinioti A, Tsimaras M, Stravodimos G, Komporozos V. Acute adrenal insufficiency due to adrenal hemorrhage complicating colorectal surgery: report of two cases and correlation with the antiphospholipid antibody syndrome. Int J Surg Case Rep. 2018;51:90–4.
9. Mandanas S, Boudina M, Chrisoulidou A, Xinou K, Margaritidou E, Gerou S, Pazaitou-Panayiotou K. Acute adrenal insufficiency following arthroplasty: a case report and review of the literature. BMC Res Notes. 2013;6:370.
10. McNicol RE, Bradley A, Griffin J, Duncan G, Eriksen CA, Guthrie GJ. Post-operative bilateral adrenal haemorrhage: a case report. Int J Surg Case Rep. 2014;5:1145–7.
11. Winter AG, Ramasamy R. Bilateral adrenal hemorrhage due to heparin-induced thrombocytopenia following partial nephrectomy - a case report. F1000Res. 2014;3:24.
12. Park KJ, Bushmiaer M, Barnes CL. Bilateral adrenal hemorrhage in a total knee patient associated with enoxaparin usage. Arthroplast Today. 2015;1: 65–8.
13. Mudenha ET, Rathi M. Adrenal insufficiency due to the development of bilateral adrenal haemorrhage following hip replacement surgery. JRSM Open. 2015;6:2054270415609837.
14. Elshoury A, Khedr M, Abousayed MM, Mehdi S. Spontaneous heparin-induced thrombocytopenia presenting as bilateral adrenal hemorrhages and pulmonary embolism after total knee arthroplasty. Arthroplast Today. 2015;1:69–71.
15. Logaraj A, Tsang VH, Kabir S, Ip JC. Adrenal crisis secondary to bilateral adrenal hemorrhage after hemicolectomy. Endocrinol Diabetes Metab Case Rep. 2016;2016:16-0048.

16. Di Serafino M, Severino R, Coppola V, Gioioso M, Rocca R, Lisanti F, Scarano E. Nontraumatic adrenal hemorrhage: the adrenal stress. Radiol Case Rep. 2017;12:483–7.
17. McGowan-Smyth S. Bilateral adrenal haemorrhage leading to adrenal crisis. BMJ Case Rep. 2014;2014:bcr2014204225.
18. Best M, Palmer K, Jones QC, Wathen CG. Acute adrenal failure following anticoagulation with dabigatran after hip replacement and thrombolysis for massive pulmonary embolism. BMJ Case Rep. 2013;2013:bcr2012007334.
19. Bornstein SR, Allolio B, Arlt W, Barthel A, Don-Wauchope A, Hammer GD, et al. Diagnosis and treatment of primary adrenal insufficiency: an endocrine society clinical practice guideline. J Clin Endocrinol Metab. 2016; 101:364–89.

18

Prevalence and associated factors for dipstick microscopic hematuria in men

Karim Courtemanche, Peter Chan and Wassim Kassouf*

Abstract

Background: Microscopic hematuria is a common incidental finding on routine urinalysis. Although there are no clear recommendations to perform routine urinalysis, some studies have shown that up to 50% of general practitioners continue to perform annual routine urinalysis regardless of age or risk factors. The aim of this study was to identify associated factors and prevalence of dipstick microscopic hematuria in the general male population presenting to an annual public men's health fair.

Method: We conducted a retrospective analysis of prospectively collected data at an annual Men's Health fair from 2008 to 2013. Patient reported health questionnaires, basic physical exam including digital rectal exam, basic bloodwork and dipstick urinalysis data was examined.

Results: A total of 979 patients were reviewed. Of these, 850 provided a urine sample and were included in the final analysis. Seventy-three (8.6%) patients had positive hematuria on urinalysis. Average age in both groups was 55 years. Presence of microscopic hematuria was correlated with presence of diabetes and proteinuria with odds-ratio of 2.8 (1.3–5.8) and 2.9 (1.7–5.0) respectively on multivariate analysis. There was no significant correlation identified with age, hypertension, coronary artery disease, body-mass index, smoking, prostate specific antigen (PSA) or International Prostate Symptom Score (IPSS). Limitation of this study is the lack of follow-up and knowledge of subsequent investigations of patients.

Conclusion: Microscopic hematuria is a prevalent condition in the male population presenting to a health fair. The only factors associated with microscopic hematuria were diabetes and proteinuria. No association was found between hematuria and smoking, age, or lower urinary tract symptoms.

Keywords: Microscopic hematuria, Prevalence, Risk factors

Background

Many etiologies exist for microscopic hematuria such as infection, urolithiasis, benign prostate hyperplasia, malignancy, nephropathies or physiologic. About 3.6% of patients presenting with microscopic hematuria will present a urinary tract malignancy [1] but positive predictive value of microhematuria for malignancy is low and thus population screening has not been recommended [1–3]. The definition of microscopic hematuria is three or greater red-blood cells (RBC) per high power field on a properly collected microscopic urinalysis as per the American Urological Association guidelines [1] whereas the Canadian Urological Association guidelines require confirmation with a second microscopic urinalysis [4]. However, in clinical practice, microscopy is often not ordered or not performed by the laboratory. Several studies have confirmed that dipstick urinalysis has good specificity (65–95%) and sensitivity (91–100%) in detecting microhematuria; [5] rates of false positives and negatives are low and can be due to hemoglobinuria, myoglobinuria, ascorbic acid or reducing agents such as povidone.

Routine screening dipstick urinalysis is currently not recommended by any organization, including the Canadian Task Force on Preventive Health Care, as there is insufficient data to support this type of screening [6]. However, up to 50% of general practitioners perform a routine urinalysis on all their patients as part of annual health screening visits [7]. Microscopic hematuria (MH) is a common finding during routine urinalysis and leads to frequent referrals to urologists and nephrologists [8]. According to

* Correspondence: wassim.kassouf@muhc.mcgill.ca
Division of Urology, McGill University Health Center, 1001 Blvd Decarie, room E02.4366, Montreal, Quebec H4A 3J1, Canada

current guidelines, MH often prompts a workup of the lower and upper tracts with cystoscopy and abdominal imaging representing a significant cost to health care systems [4].

Our primary objective was to identify and describe factors associated with microscopic hematuria. We also report on the prevalence of MH in the male population presenting to a men's health fair.

Methods

Men who presented to an annual McGill University public men's health fair held in public venues in Montreal, Canada from 2008 to 2013 were included. Informed consents were obtained from all participants to permit anonymous analyses of collected data for educational and academic research purposes. All men who presented to this annual health fair were eligible for inclusion into the study. In addition to physical examination, patients were asked to complete a health questionnaire including socio-demographic data, medical history, medications, lifestyle (smoking, alcohol use and drugs), Metabolic Equivalent of Task scale (METs), Sexual Health Inventory for Men (SHIM), Androgen Deficiency in Aging Male (ADAM), Berlin questionnaire for obstructive sleep apnea (BQ), International Prostate Symptom Score (IPSS) and Overactive Bladder 8 (OAB8). Depending on their age, patients were offered prostate specific antigen (PSA), cholesterol panel and testosterone level testing. They also underwent a digital rectal exam and a dipstick urinalysis.

Patients who stated a previous history of hematuria or did not provide a urine sample were excluded from the final study population. Baseline characteristics were compared using t-tests for continuous variables and chi-square or Fisher exact for categorical variables depending on the number of patients in that particular analysis. Multivariate logistic regression was used to examine various factors and their association with microscopic hematuria and establish the odds-ratio of microhematuria on dipstick urinalysis. Where data was missing, analysis was done only with patients with complete records available. Missing data was primarily due to patients not answering specific questions on the questionnaire. Significant p values were set as two-tailed $p < 0.05$. Data was analyzed using SPSS version 17.

Results

Data was reviewed on 979 patients who presented to the men's health fair from 2008 to 2013; 850 provided a urine sample and had no history of previous hematuria and formed the basis of this report. Mean and median age of men was 54.7 and 55 respectively (range 20 to 87). Baseline demographics of the population are presented in Table 1 Mean body-mass index (BMI) was 27.6. Of 850 patients, 67 (7.9%) had diabetes mellitus (DM), 46 (5.4%) had coronary artery disease (CAD), 156 (18.4%) had hypertension (HTN) and 18 (2.1%) had a history of malignancy. From a urological aspect, 42 (4.9%) had a history of previous urological surgery, 42 (4.9%) had a history of urinary or urological infections and 41 (4.8%) had a history of stones.

Table 1 Demographics and comorbidities

Age in year (range)	55 (20–87)
Education Level	Grade 7 or lower: 3.1% (26)
	Some high school: 8.9% (76)
	High school graduate or CEGEP: 24.8% (211)
	Some University: 13.1% (111)
	University Graduate: 37.2% (316)
	Post-graduate studies: 11.4% (97)
Smoking history	Non-smoker: 67.9% (573)
	Smoker: 12.3% (104)
	Ex-smoker: 19.8% (167)
BMI (kg/m^2)	27.6 ± 5.0
Dipstick hematuria	Overall: 73 (8.6%)
	+: 41 (4.8%)
	++: 17 (2%)
	+++: 11 (1.3%)
	++++: 4 (0.5%)
Proteinuria	128 (15.1%)
Diabetes	67 (7.9%)
Hypertension	156 (18.4%)
Coronary artery disease	46 (5.4%)
PSA (ng/mL)	1.54 ± 1.74

Seventy-three (8.6%) patients demonstrated MH. There was no significant difference in rates of coronary artery disease, previous history of urolithiasis, malignancy, urological surgery, urological infections or hypertension between patients with and without MH. Smoking rates (present, past, ever) were similar in both groups (Table 2). Distribution of IPSS score categories was similar between both groups (6.1% vs 6.3% severe scores, $p = 0.825$). There was no difference between SHIM score categories ($p = 0.479$). On multivariable analysis, the only factors associated with MH were diabetes (OR 2.8, $p = 0.007$) and proteinuria (OR 2.9, $p = 0.0001$) (Table 3).

Discussion This study demonstrated that microscopic hematuria is prevalent in the male population and diabetes is the primary factor associated with increased risk of detecting MH on dipstick urinalysis.

Multiple studies evaluated the prevalence of microscopic hematuria with varying rates in a general screening population. Our observed prevalence of microscopic hematuria was 8.6% which is similar to other studies in

Table 2 Comparison of associated factors

Characteristic	No hematuria ($n = 777$)	Microhematuria ($n = 73$)	N	p
Age	54.7 (+/−12.9)	55.4 (+/−10.6)	850	0.669
Diabetes mellitus	7.1% (55)	16.4%(12)	850	0.005
Hypertension	18.3% (142)	19.2% (14)	850	0.849
Coronary artery disease	5.4% (42)	5.5% (4)	850	1.000
Malignancy	2.2% (17)	1.4% (1)	850	1.000
Urological surgery	4.8% (37)	6.8% (5)	850	0.431
History of urolithiasis	4.8% (37)	5.5% (4)	850	0.773
Urological infections	5.1% (40)	2.7% (2)	850	0.571
Smoking	12.4% (96)	11.3% (8)	844	0.778
Proteinuria	13.4% (104)	32.9% (24)	850	0.0001
IPSS category (mild, mod, severe)	Mild: 58% (407)	Mild: 61.9% (39)	765	0.825
	Moderate: 35.9% (252)	Moderate: 31.7% (20)		
	Severe: 6.1% (43)	Severe: 6.3% (4)		
OAB-q v8	39.6% (280)	34.3% (23)	774	0.434
SHIM	No ED: 48% (306)	No ED: 53.2% (33)	797	0.479
	Mild: 28.7% (183)	Mild: 27.4% (17)		
	Mild-Mod: 3.3% (85)	Mild-Mod: 8.1% (5)		
	Moderate: 6.1% (39)	Moderate: 9.7% (6)		
	Severe: 3.9% (25)	Severe: 1.6% (1)		
ADAM questionnaire positive	64.4% (482)	52.9% (37)	819	0.069
Metabolic syndrome	28.5% (142)	39.4% (13)	532	0.234
PSA > 4 ng/ml	7.3% (47)	7.5% (5)	715	0.950
BMI	< 25: 28.8% (220)	< 25: 26.0% (19)	837	0.688
	25–30: 45.5% (348)	25–30: 43.8% (32)		
	> 30: 25.7% (196)	> 30: 30.1% (22)		

men ranging from 2.5% [9] to 13% [10]. Previous studies have examined the risk factors of urinary tract malignancy diagnosed following workup of hematuria. Risk factors of malignancy identified in some of these studies were age, smoking, the presence of gross hematuria and positive cytology [11–13]. Kang et al. found in a screening study that male sex and diabetes increased the risk of finding underlying pathology on workup of MH [12]. None of the studies identified in our review of the literature analyzed factors associated with likelihood of detecting MH. In our study, a past medical history of diabetes increased the odds of hematuria by 2.8 times. Okada et al. showed that microscopic hematuria had little clinical significance in diabetic nephropathy and that creatinine doubling time or increase of serum creatinine was no different between patients with persistent MH or without MH [14]. Hematuria was also significantly associated with the presence of concomitant proteinuria with an odds ratio of 2.9, likely associated with the presence of diabetes. The increase risk of finding MH in diabetic patients especially in the context of proteinuria could be used to better counsel patients when these abnormal results are found.

Table 3 Multivariate logistic regression analysis of factors associated with microhematuria

Variable	OR	p
Diabetes	2.758 (1.312–5.799)	0.007
Hypertension	0.775 (0.383–1.568)	0.478
Coronary artery disease	0.965 (0.318–2.932)	0.951
Smoking	0.934 (0.427–2.045)	0.864
Proteinuria	2.882 (1.669–4.976)	0.0001
BMI ≥ 30	1.015 (0.966–1.068)	0.551
Age	0.998 (0.977–1.020)	0.857

How would the identification of factors associated with MH help counselling the patient? The yield of finding malignancy in patients with MH is very low. AUA meta-analysis found that the incidence of malignancy upon workup of asymptomatic MH was 3.3% when based on one positive urine sample [1]. According to current guidelines, MH prompts a workup of the lower and upper tracts with cystoscopy and abdominal imaging representing a significant cost to health care systems. [4] Further prospective studies are needed to evaluate whether the identification of factors associated with increased risk of MH may help stratifying patients who can obviate investigations with invasive procedures.

Some limitations exist in our study. All past medical history was self-reported by patients and may thus induce a bias. The population presenting to this health fair may not be representative of the general population as patients with specific concerns or who do not have regular medical follow-up may have been overrepresented. However, the prevalence of smoking and comorbidities such as hypertension, diabetes, and coronary artery disease was similar to rates in the general Canadian population [15, 16]. Furthermore, this was a single institution experience and this may limit generalizability of our findings. Another limitation is that the dipstick microhematuria was not confirmed with microscopy in this study. Several studies have confirmed that dipstick urinalysis has good specificity (65–95%) and sensitivity (91–100%) in detecting microhematuria [5, 17] but should still be confirmed with microscopy before ordering costly and invasive testing. Lastly and importantly, follow-up data was not available for our patient population to identify if these patients ultimately underwent full workup and their findings.

Conclusion

The prevalence of microhematuria in the general male population presenting to a public health fair was 8.6%, in keeping with other reported studies of prevalence of MH. Significant factors associated with MH were a history of diabetes and concomitant proteinuria.

Abbreviations

ADAM: Androgen Deficiency in Aging Male; BMI: Body-mass index; BQ: Berlin questionnaire; CAD: Coronary artery disease; DM: Diabetes mellitus; HTN: hypertension; IPSS: International prostate symptom score; METs: Metabolic equivalent of task scale; MH: Microscopic hematuria; OAB8: Overactive bladder 8; PSA: Prostate specific antigen; RBC: Red-blood cells; SHIM: Sexual Health Inventory for Men

Acknowledgements

Not applicable.

Authors' contributions

KC did the data entry, statistical analysis and interpretation of the data and was a major contributor in writing the manuscript. PC coordinated the collection of data from patients and contributed and approved the final manuscript. WK participated in the design of the study, reviewed the results and was a major contributor to writing the manuscript. All authors read and approved the final manuscript.

References

1. Davis R, Jones JS, Barocas DA, Castle EP, Lang EK, Leveillee RJ, Messing EM, Miller SD, Peterson AC, Turk TM, et al. Diagnosis, evaluation and follow-up of asymptomatic microhematuria (AMH) in adults: AUA guideline. J Urol. 2012;188(6 Suppl):2473–81.
2. Woolhandler S, Pels RJ, Bor DH, Himmelstein DU, Lawrence RS. Dipstick urinalysis screening of asymptomatic adults for urinary tract disorders. I. Hematuria and proteinuria. Jama. 1989;262(9):1214–9.
3. Hiatt RA, Ordonez JD. Dipstick urinalysis screening, asymptomatic microhematuria, and subsequent urological cancers in a population-based sample. Cancer Epidemiol Biomarkers Prev. 1994;3(5):439–43.
4. Wollin T, Laroche B, Psooy K. Canadian guidelines for the management of asymptomatic microscopic hematuria in adults. Can Urol Assoc J. 2009;3(1):77–80.
5. Thaller TR, Wang LP. Evaluation of asymptomatic microscopic hematuria in adults. Am Fam Physician. 1999;60(4):1143–1152, 1154.
6. Krogsboll LT. Guidelines for screening with urinary dipsticks differ substantially--a systematic review. Danish Med J. 2014;61(2):A4781.
7. Yafi FA, Aprikian AG, Tanguay S, Kassouf W. Patients with microscopic and gross hematuria: practice and referral patterns among primary care physicians in a universal health care system. Can Urol Assoc J. 2011;5(2):97–101.
8. Rao PK, Gao T, Pohl M, Jones JS. Dipstick pseudohematuria: unnecessary consultation and evaluation. J Urol. 2010;183(2):560–4.
9. Ritchie CD, Bevan EA, Collier SJ. Importance of occult haematuria found at screening. Br Med J (Clin Res Ed). 1986;292(6521):681–3.
10. Britton JP, Dowell AC, Whelan P. Dipstick haematuria and bladder cancer in men over 60: results of a community study. BMJ. 1989;299(6706):1010–2.
11. Cha EK, Tirsar LA, Schwentner C, Hennenlotter J, Christos PJ, Stenzl A, Mian C, Martini T, Pycha A, Shariat SF, et al. Accurate risk assessment of patients with asymptomatic hematuria for the presence of bladder cancer. World J Urol. 2012;30(6):847–52.
12. Kang M, Lee S, Jeong SJ, Hong SK, Byun SS, Lee SE, Jeong CW. Characteristics and significant predictors of detecting underlying diseases in adults with asymptomatic microscopic hematuria: a large case series of a Korean population. Int J Urol. 2015;22(4):389–93.
13. Loo RK, Lieberman SF, Slezak JM, Landa HM, Mariani AJ, Nicolaisen G, Aspera AM, Jacobsen SJ. Stratifying risk of urinary tract malignant tumors in patients with asymptomatic microscopic hematuria. Mayo Clin Proc. 2013;88(2):129–38.
14. Okada T, Nagao T, Matsumoto H, Nagaoka Y, Wada T, Nakao T. Clinical significance of microscopic haematuria in diabetic nephropathy in type 2 diabetes patients with overt proteinuria. Nephrol. 2013;18(8):563–8.
15. 2009 Tracking Heart Disease and Storke in Canada. 2016. http://www.phac-aspc.gc.ca/publicat/2009/cvd-avc/pdf/cvd-avs-2009-eng.pdf.
16. Robitaille C, Dai S, Waters C, Loukine L, Bancej C, Quach S, Ellison J, Campbell N, Tu K, Reimer K, et al. Diagnosed hypertension in Canada: incidence, prevalence and associated mortality. CMAJ. 2012;184(1):E49–56.
17. Matulewicz RS, DeLancey JO, Pavey E, Schaeffer EM, Popescu O, Meeks JJ. Dipstick urinalysis as a test for microhematuria and occult bladder Cancer. Bladder Cancer. 2017;3(1):45–9.

19

Langerhans cells in hypospadias: An analysis of Langerin (CD207) and HLA-DR on epidermal sheets and full thickness skin sections

Bernhard Haid[1,2*], Daniela Reider[3], Felix Nägele[4], Anne-Françoise Spinoit[5], Elisabeth Pechriggl[6], Nikolaus Romani[3], Helga Fritsch[4] and Josef Oswald[1]

Abstract

Background: Hypospadias are among the most common genital malformations. Langerhans Cells (LCs) play a pivotal role in HIV and HPV infection. The migration of LC precursors to skin coincides with the embryonic period of hypospadias development and genetic alterations leading to the formation of hypospadias impact the development of ectodermally derived tissues. We hypothesized that this might be associated with a difference in frequency or morphology of epidermal and dermal LCs in hypospadias patients.

Methods: A total of 43 patients from two centers were prospectively included into this study after parental consent and ethics approval. Epidermal and dermal sheets were prepared from skin samples of 26 patients with hypospadias, 13 patients without penile malformations and 4 patients with penile malformations other than hypospadias. Immunofluorescence staining of sheets was performed with anti-HLA-DR-FITC and anti-CD207/ Langerin-A594 antibodies. Skin sections from 11 patients without penile malformation and 11 patients with hypospadias were stained for Langerin. Frequencies as well as morphology and distribution of epidermal and dermal LCs on sheets and sections were microscopically evaluated. Cell counts were compared by unpaired t-tests.

Results: There was no difference in frequency of epidermal LCs, Neither on sheets (873 ± 61 vs. 940 ± 84LCs/mm^2, $p = 0.522$) nor on sections (32 ± 3 vs. 30 ± 2LCs/mm^2, $p = 0.697$). Likewise, the frequency of dermal LCs (5,9 ± 0,9 vs. 7.5 ± 1.3LCs/mm^2, $p = 0.329$) was comparable between patients with hypospadias and without penile malformation. No differences became apparent in subgroup analyses, comparing distal to proximal hypospadias ($p = 0.949$), younger and older boys ($p = 0.818$) or considering topical dihydrotestosterone treatment prior to surgery ($p = 0.08$). The morphology of the LCs was not different comparing hypospadias patients with boys without penile malformations.

Conclusions: LCs are present in similar frequencies and with a comparable morphology and distribution in patients with hypospadias as compared to children without penile malformations. This suggests that patients with hypospadias are not different from patients with normal penile development considering this particular compartment of their skin immunity.

Keywords: Langerhans cells, Hypospadias, Foreskin, HPV, HIV

* Correspondence: bernhard.haid@ordensklinikum.at
[1]Department of Pediatric Urology, Hospital of the Sisters of Charity, Ordensklinikum Linz, Seilerstätte 4, 4020 Linz, Austria
[2]Department of Urology, Ludwig Maximilians University, Marchioninistraße 15, 81367 Munich, Germany
Full list of author information is available at the end of the article

Background

Hypospadias affects 1 in 125–300 male births, representing the second most common genital malformation after undescended testes [1]. The malformation of the penis present in hypospadias, however, does not only involve the urethral opening being situated abnormally at the ventral side of the penis. All tissues including skin, notably on the ventral aspect of the penis, seem underdeveloped and altered in appearance. The events related to the formation of hypospadias happen in very early phases of the genital tubercle outgrow starting in gestational week 8; differentiation of the urethral epithelium is determined by mesenchymal signaling [2]. Thereby, not only the organogenesis of the urethra is defined but also prepuce morphogenesis and surface epithelia of ectodermal origin are influenced [3, 4].

Except concerning hormonal receptors, the repercussions of these early fetal events on other penile tissues have not yet been adequately investigated [3, 5].

Langerhans cells (LCs), the dendritic cells of epithelia, are dispersed in the epidermis as a dense network of immunologic gatekeepers, internalizing possible pathogenic antigens and presenting them to T-cells in draining lymph nodes, thereby initiating and regulating the specific immune response [6]. They are critically involved in human immunodeficiency virus (HIV) and human papillomavirus (HPV) infection [7, 8]. The typical hallmark of human LCs, as opposed to other dendritic cells, is the expression of Langerin (CD207), a C-type lectin serving as pathogen receptor and comprising the archetypical Birbeck granules [9]. LCs develop and seed the epithelial tissues already during embryogenesis, notably in the very

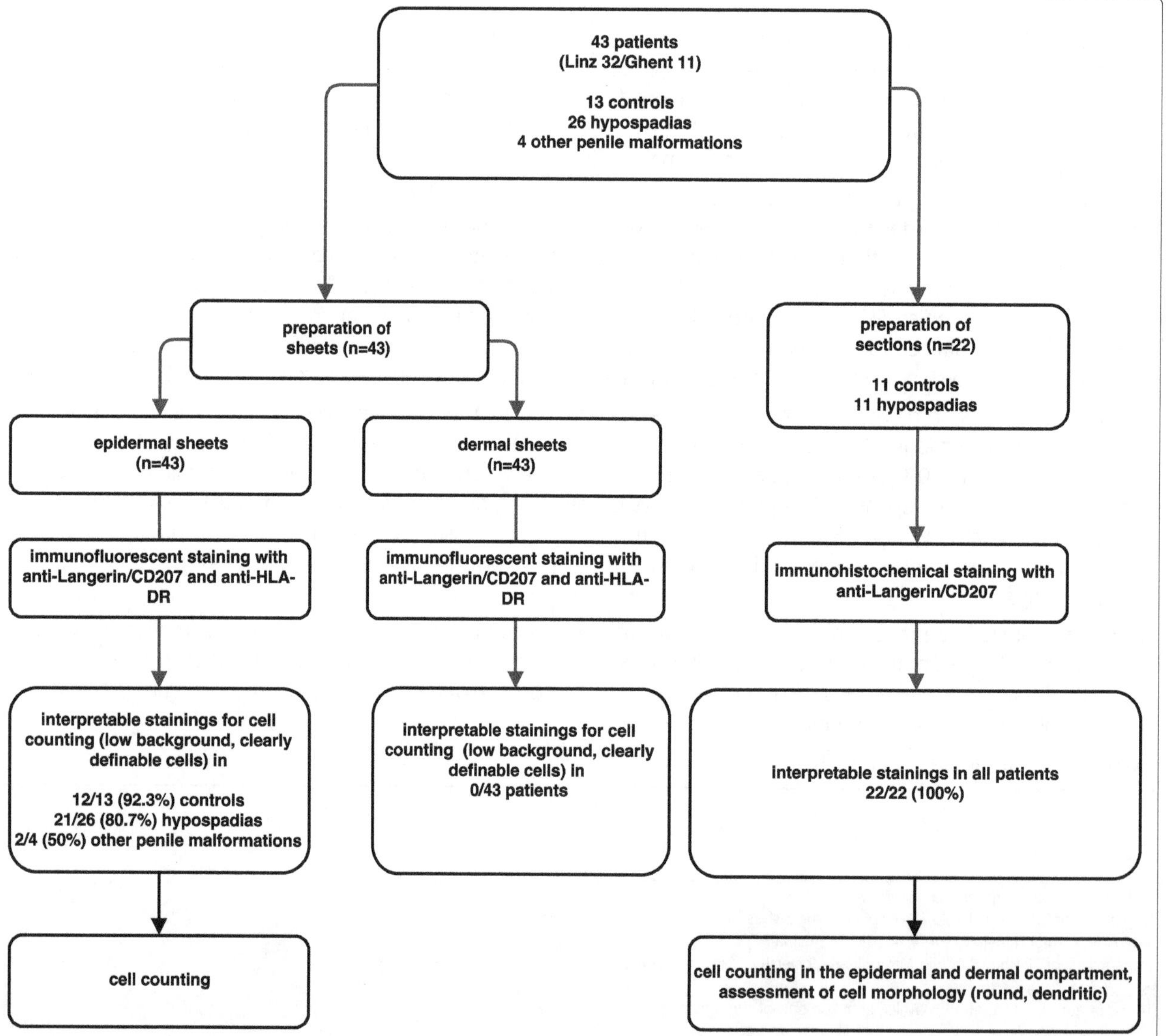

Fig. 1 Flowchart displaying the allocation of patients to the two methods and the respective staining protocols

Table 1 Patients characteristics

	all patients ($n = 43$)	Linz ($n = 32$)	Gent ($n = 11$)	p
age at surgery mean/median [months]	49 / 15	36 / 15	26 / 14	0.4[a]
no penile malformation (%)	13 (30.2%)	12 (37.5%)	1 (9.1%)	
hypospadias	26 (60.4%)	19 (59.4%)	7 (63.6%)	
distal hypospadias (% of all hypospadias)	16 (61.5%)	11 (57.9%)	5 (71.4%)	
proximal hypospadias (% of all hypospadias)	10 (38.5%)	8 (42.1)	2 (28.6%)	
thereof with preoperative androgen treatment (local DHT[b] for 6 weeks until 4 weeks before surgery)	7 (70%)	7 (87.5%)	0	
other penile malformations	4 (9.3%)	1 (3.1%)	3 (27.2%)	
buried penis	2 (50%)	0	2 (66.6%)	
epispadias	2 (50%)	1 (100%)	1 (33.3%)	

[a]students t-test [b] Dihydrotestosterone, applied twice daily

same period when later hypospadias are determined [10]. Differences in function of these specialized immune cells could implicate altered susceptibility to HIV or HPV.

Despite these important implications in the skin immune system, the presence or morphology of Langerhans Cells have never been investigated in patients with hypospadias up to now as to our knowledge.

We hypothesized that due to developmental differences in epithelial embryogenesis, the frequency or morphology and consequently also the function of epidermal and dermal LCs in patients with hypospadias might be altered in comparison to patients without a penile malformation.

Methods

The study protocol has been approved by the ethics committee of the Hospital of the Sisters of Charity (EK22/14). After informed consent of all parents a total of 43 patients (Linz/Ghent 32/11) were prospectively included.

During surgery, small pieces (7-10 mm^2) of whole preputial skin from lateral parts of the prepuce were obtained. Any sign of potential inflammation, for instance balanoposthitis or a clinical suspicion of Lichen Sclerosus as well as a history of balanoposthitis resulted in non-inclusion of the patient. In course of analyzing the samples, all section stainings were checked for histological signs of inflammation (dermal leucocyte infiltration) to subsequently exclude them in order to preclude a potential interference with our results. The preparation steps for the two different methods applied are detailed below. The allocation of specimens to the different methods is displayed in Fig. 1.

Patients' characteristics are presented in Table 1.

In patients with proximal hypospadias and a glans diameter of less than 14 mm, topical dihydrotestosterone 2.5% gel (Andractim®) was applied over a period of 6 weeks until 4 weeks prior to surgery twice daily.

Sheets

Immediately after harvesting, skin was freed from subepithelial fatty tissue and conserved in a sterile PBS/1%BSA (phosphate buffered saline / 1% bovine serum albumine) solution. At the latest 2 h thereafter, the skin was floated – dermal side down – on 0.5 M ammoniumthiocyanate

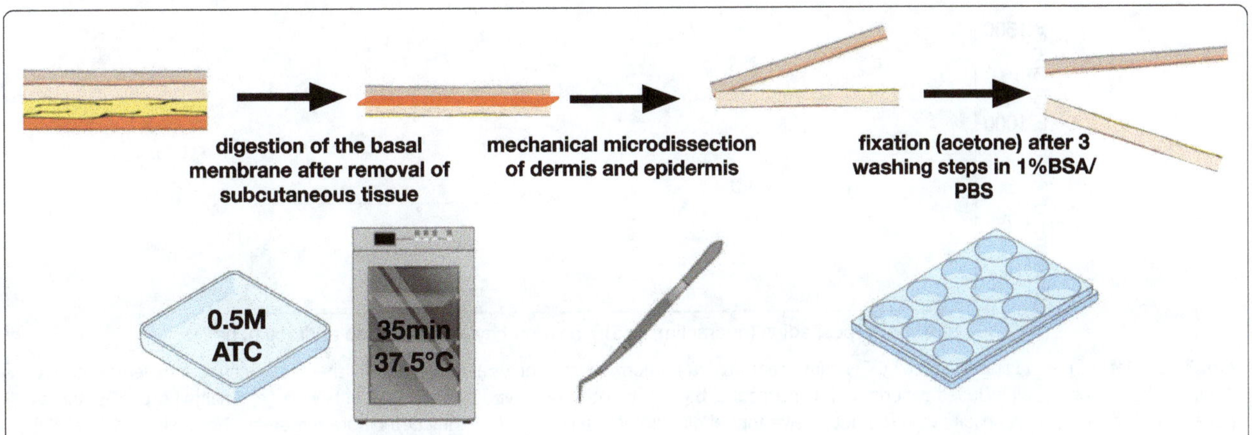

Fig. 2 Schematic display of epidermal / dermal sheet preparation technique from human full skin. ATC, ammoniumthiocyanate

solution for 35 min at 37 °C. The epidermis was then peeled off the dermis using microsurgical instruments. After fixation (synthesis grade acetone, 20 min at room temperature) and three washing steps using PBS/1%BSA, the dermal and epidermal sheets were cut into small pieces (4-5 mm^2), frozen in a drop of PBS/1%BSA and stored at − 20 °C [11]. A detailed protocol of sheet preparation is provided in Fig. 2.

After thawing, epidermal as well as dermal sheets were incubated with an unconjugated primary antibody (anti-human CD207/Langerin; clone MB22-9F5, mouse IgG1, Miltenyi Biotec, Bergisch Gladbach, Germany) for 1 h at 37 °C, followed by three 10-min washing steps. Subsequently the sheets were incubated with a fluorochrome-coupled secondary antibody (Alexa-Fluor 594-conjugated, isotype-specific goat anti-mouse IgG1, Invitrogen/Thermo-Fisher) for 1 h at 37 °C, again followed by three 10-min washing steps. The staining sequence was extended by incubating the sheets with an excess concentration of mouse IgG (100 μg/ml)) to quench residual free binding sites of the preceding anti-mouse Ig antibodies. Finally, sheets were incubated with

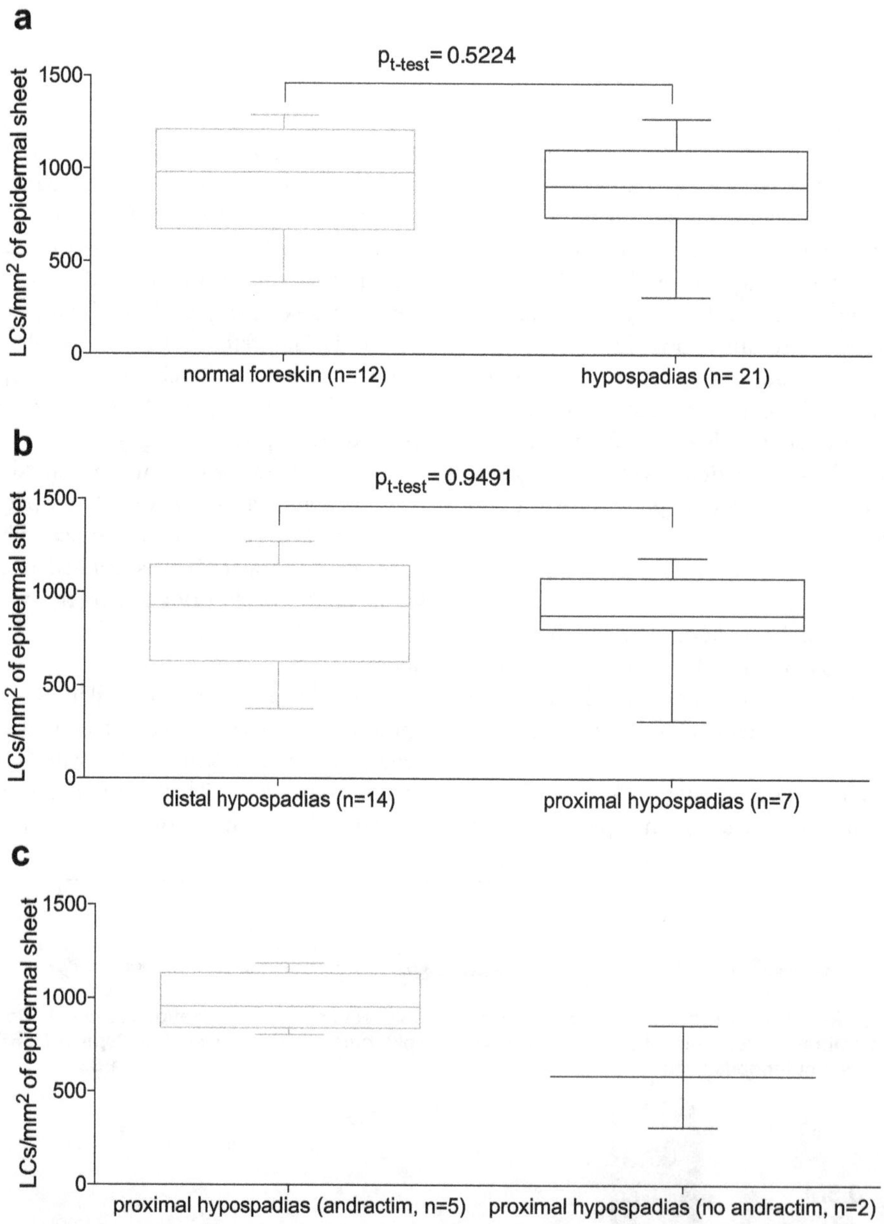

Fig. 3 Box-plots of mean Langerhans cell (LC) counts per mm^2 on immunofluorescence stained epidermal sheets comparing **a** patients without penile malformations to all included patients with hypospadias, **b** patients with distal hypospadias to patients with proximal hypospadias, and **c** patients with proximal hypospadias who did not receive topical dihydrotestosterone (DHT, andractim) before surgery to those who did receive 6 weeks of DHT until 4 weeks prior to surgery. Error bars represent min-max

anti-human HLA-DR (clone L243, mouse IgG2a, BioLegend) followed by Alexa-Fluor 488-conjugated, isotype-specific goat anti-mouse IgG2a, Invitrogen/Thermo-Fisher) for 1 hour each at 37 °C. For nuclear staining, dermal sheets were incubated in DAPI dilactate (Invitrogen® / Molecular Probes). For each antibody, an isotype control staining was performed to exclude unspecific staining results. Immunolabeled specimens were mounted in Vectashield mounting medium (Vector Laboratories, Burlingame, CA) and analyzed on a conventional fluorescence microscope (Olympus BX60).

Only when an unequivocal epidermal keratinocyte structure ("cobblestone pattern") could be seen in transmission light, stainings were considered valid. Due to the thickness of the dermal part of the sheets, reproducible cell counting in the dermis was not possible using sheets and conventional fluorescence microscopy.

On every epidermal sheet, HLA-DR+ and langerin+ cells cells were counted in 12 high power fields (40× objective lens magnification). Density of cells/mm^2 was calculated by means of a calibrated micrometer slide.

Sections

Immediately after harvesting, full skin of 22 patients (Fig. 1) was fixed in 4% formaldehyde (2–4 h) and then immersed in paraffin blocks for conservation and transport. 5 µm whole skin sections were prepared on a rotation microtome and mounted on SuperFrost® Plus slides. The sections were stained using anti-human CD207/Langerin (clone 929F3.01 undiluted hybridoma cell supernatant, rat IgG2a, gift of Dr. S. Saeland and Dendritics, Lyon, France) followed by immunohistochemical labeling (Ventana universal secondary antibody, biotinylated IgG anti-goat/mouse/rat; Ventana ultra view DAB-MAP detection kit) using a standardized, automatized staining technique (DAP-MAP IHC discovery research standard protocol, Ventana, Roche®).

LCs were counted in 4 epidermal and 4 dermal fields that were placed randomly measuring 100x100µm/section and patient. Counting and measuring was performed using the Image J Software (National Institute of Health, Bethesda, ML, USA).

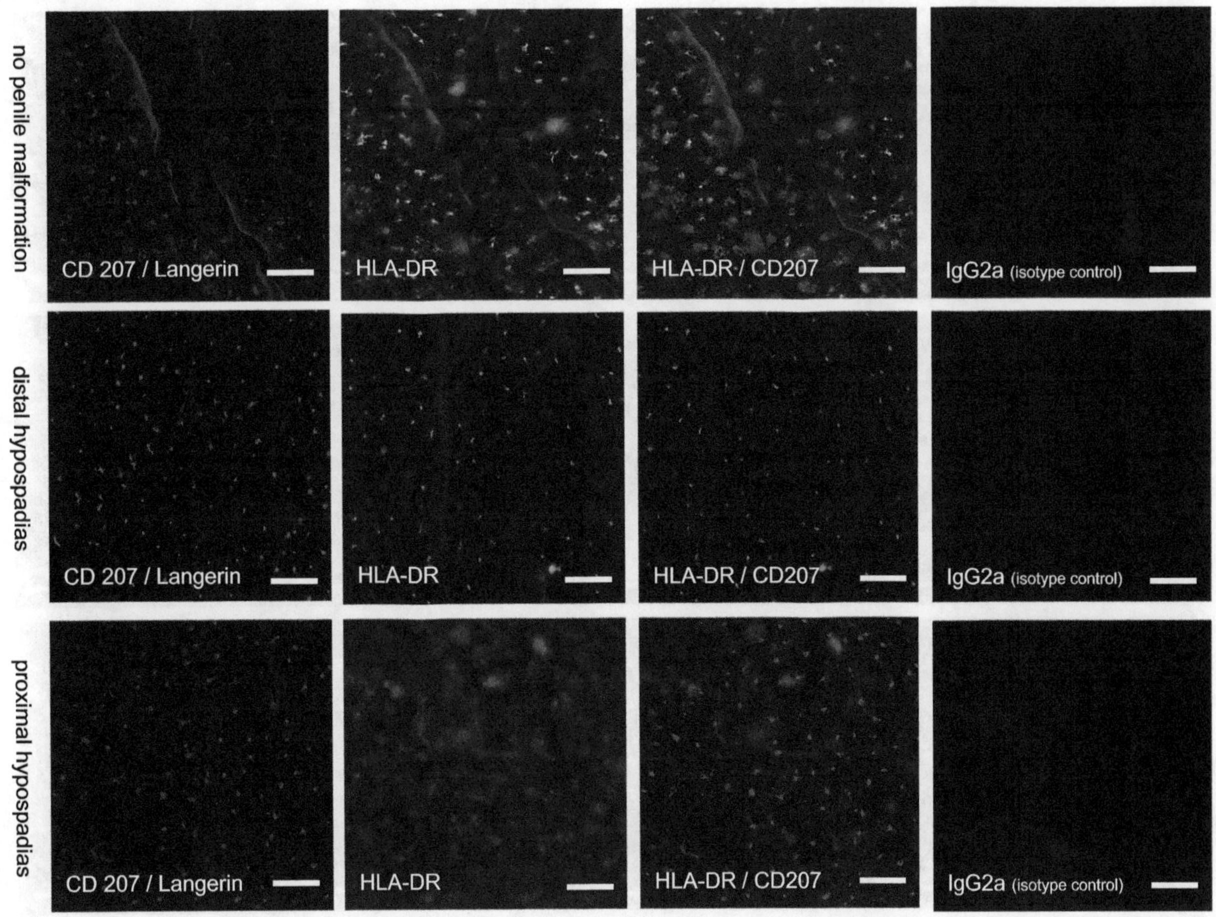

Fig. 4 Immunofluorescence stainings with anti-HLA DR and anti-CD207 / Langerin as well as IgG2 isotype controls of epidermal sheets. Scale bar represents 60 µm

LC morphology was classified into round and dendritic shaped and documented alongside cell counting, specifying the relative proportions of round and dendritic shaped LCs.

Statistics

Cell counts for epidermal and dermal LCs on sheets as well as on sections were compared by unpaired t-tests. The cut-off for the alpha error was defined as < 0.05, for multiple testing a Bonferroni correction was applied. Data analysis and figure design was performed using Prism 6.0 (Graphpad Software, Inc., San Diego, CA, USA).

Results

Sheets

Interpretable staining without signs of inflammation (dermal leucocyte infiltration) could be achieved in samples from 12 patients (92.3% of all included patients) without penile malformations, 14 (87.5%) with distal hypospadias, 7 (70%) with proximal hypospadias, one with buried penis (50%) and one with epispadias (50%) translating into a total of 81.4% of all epidermal sheets prepared being amenable for analysis. HLA-DR/CD207 double positive cells were considered LCs.

The mean frequency of epidermal HLA-DR/CD207 double positive cells per mm^2 accounted to 873.4 ± 61.6 in patients with hypospadias ($n = 21$) as compared to 940.2 ± 84.2 in patients without penile malformation ($n = 12$, $p = 0.522$, t-test). There was no significant difference in LC frequency between distal and proximal hypospadias (876.2 ± 78.7, $n = 14$, distal vs. 867.6 ± 105.5, $n = 7$ proximal, $p = 0.9491$). Comparing patients with proximal hypospadias who had received topical dihydrotestosterone prior to surgery to those who had not, we found no significant difference in epidermal LC density (585.5 ± 273.1, $n = 2$ vs. 980.4 ± 68.9, $n = 5$, $p = 0.0857$). The morphology of the epidermal LCs was the same in all samples Figs. 3 and 4.

Stainings of the dermal sheets revealed single Langerin-positive cells, however, due to background staining reliable and reproducible cell counting on these sheets was not

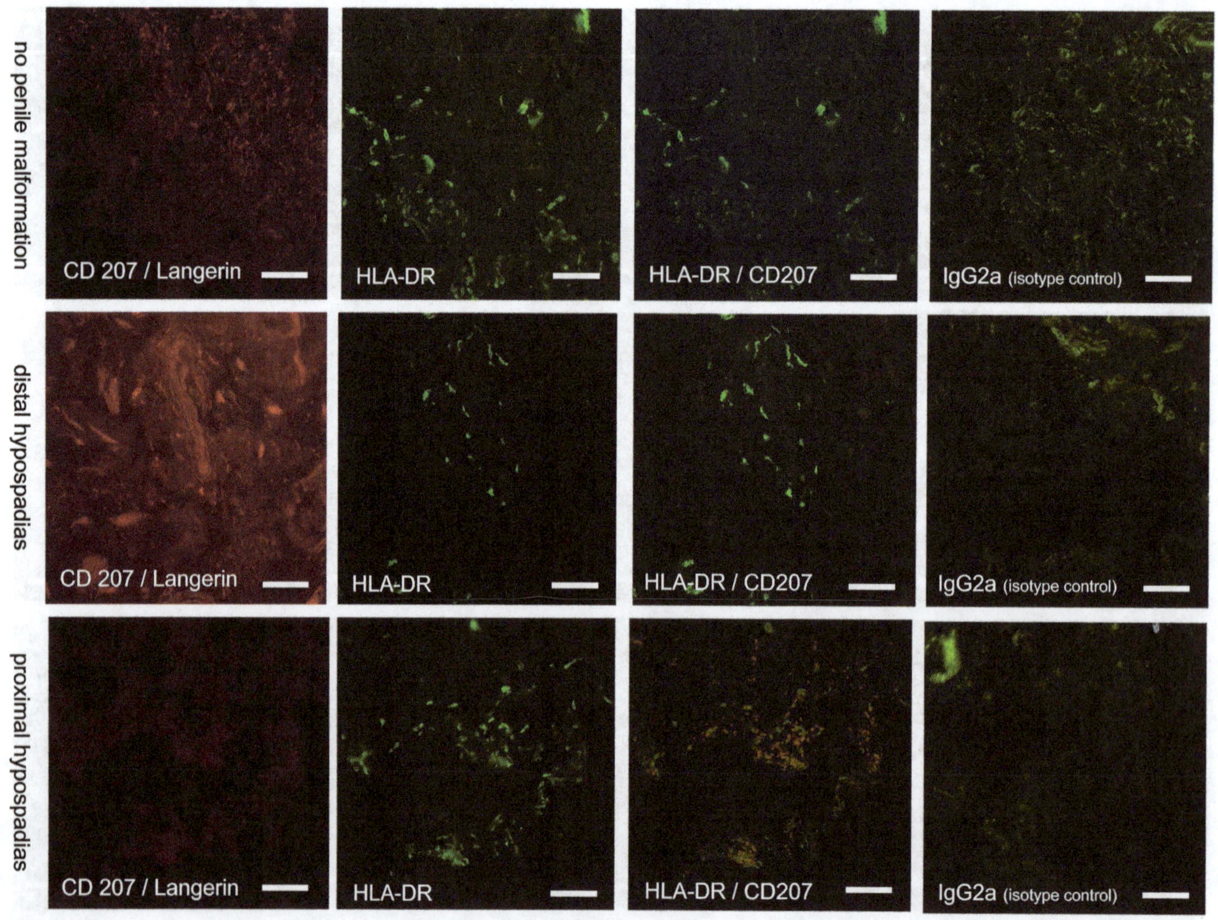

Fig. 5 Immunofluorescence stainings with anti-HLA DR and anti-CD207 / Langerin as well as IgG2 isotype controls of dermal sheets. Note that none of the HLA-DR+ cells depicted co-expresses Langerin. Scale bar represents 60 μm

possible with the available microscopic facilities. Figure 5 provides immunofluorescent images showing the dermal sheet staining.

The morphology of the epidermal LCs was comparable in all samples. Most epidermal LCs were dendritically shaped, however, some (10–15%) were rounded. No conspicuous and consistent differences could be detected in comparison with LCs from healthy foreskin. While most epidermal HLA-DR-positive cells were also Langerin positive, on some sheets we found areas with intermingled HLA-DR single positive cells. Sample images of single Langerhans cells and their morphology, as defined for this project, are shown in Fig. 6.

LC frequency accounted to 930.3 ± 65.61 ($n = 14$) in patients < 1 year of age, 1028 ± 80.26 ($n = 7$) in patients between 1 and 3 and 907.0 ± 75.65, (n = 14) in patients over 3 years of age ($p = 0.818$ < 1 vs. > 3 years of age) Fig. 7.

The patient with buried penis had a mean LC count of 880.3/mm^2. In the single interpretable staining of a patient with epispadias we found 1055.79 LCs/mm^2.

Sections

On all stained sections ($n = 22$, 11 hypospadias, 11 patients without penile malformation), clearly evaluable staining results were achieved. Dermal as well as epidermal LC

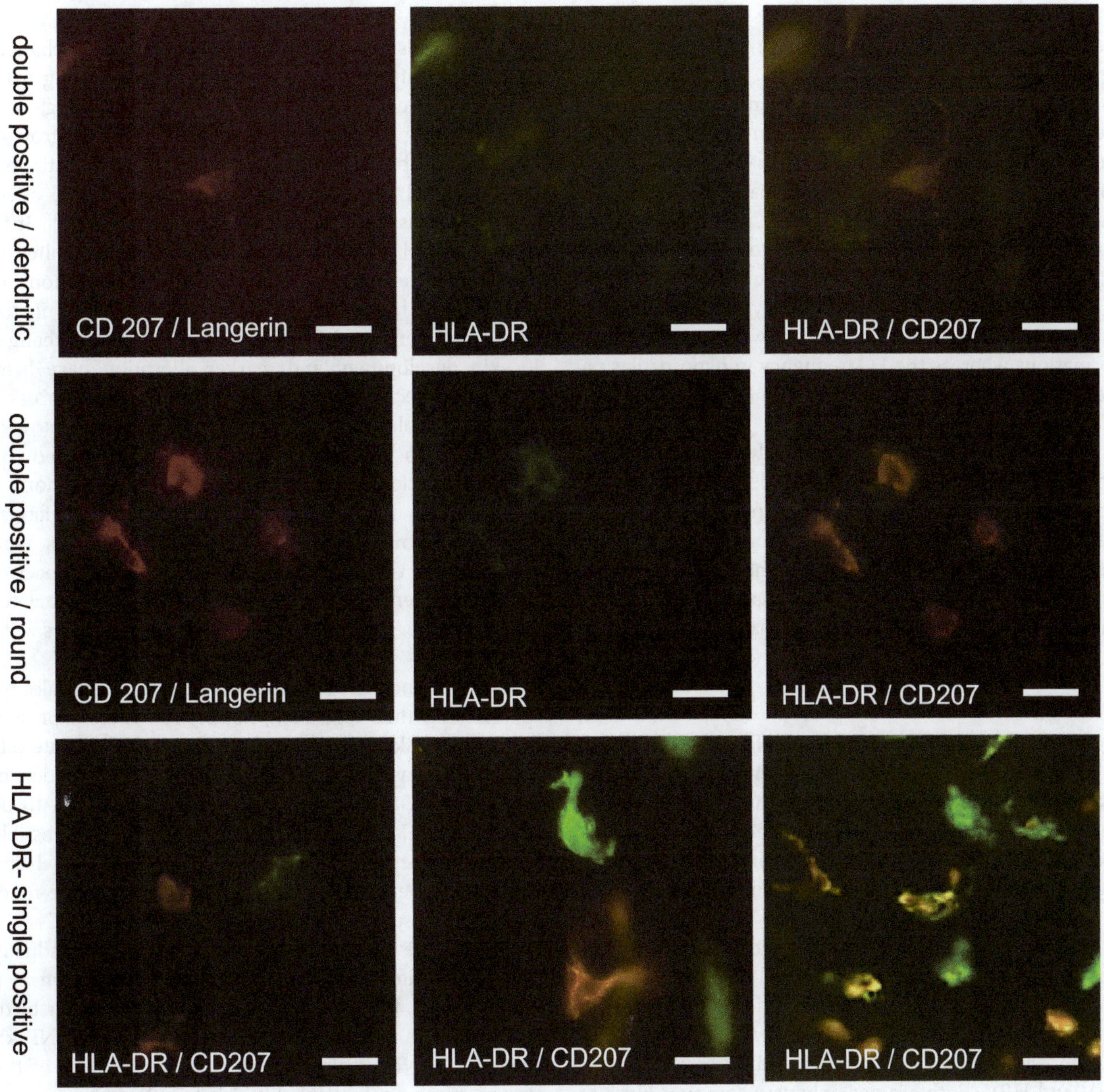

Fig. 6 Morphology of epidermal LCs (dendritic, round). Note rare examples of HLA-DR single positive epidermal cells. Scale bar represents 10 μm

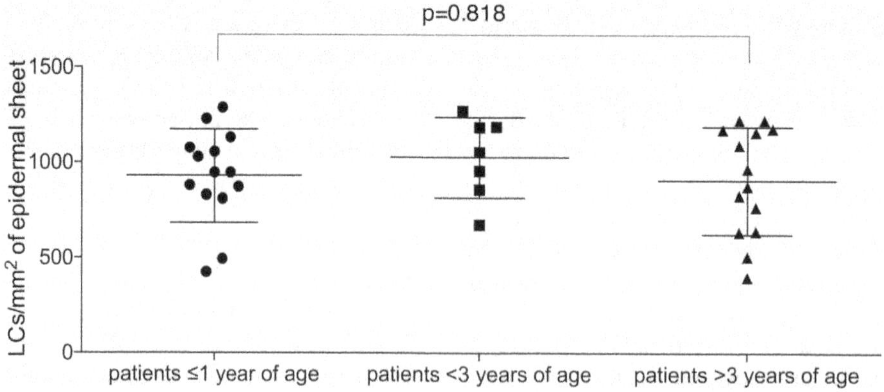

Fig. 7 Dot-plots of LC frequency of patients aged ≤1 year, between 1 and 3 years and < 3 years. Lines represent mean with standard deviation

density was assessed. CD207-positive cells were considered LCs.

In the epidermis, we found a mean of 31.8 ± 2.7 LCs per mm^2 ($n = 11$) in samples from patients without penile malformation as compared to 30.5 ± 1.9 ($n = 11$) in samples from patients with hypospadias ($p = 0.697$). In patients with distal hypospadias the LC frequency was similar as compared to those with proximal hypospadias (28.2 ± 2.1, $n = 7$ vs. 34.4 ± 3.1, $n = 4$, $p = 0.13$).

In the dermis a mean LC frequency per mm^2 of 5.9 ± 0.9, n = 11 was assessed in patients without penile malformations whereas the LC frequency in hypospadias patients accounted to 7.5 ± 1.3, n = 11 ($p = 0.329$) Figs. 8 and 9.

Morphology was comparatively analyzed on samples of about 100 LCs each in epidermis and dermis. 8.4% of all epidermal LCs were round as compared to 91.6% with a dendritic appearance. In contrast, virtually all (99.1%) dermal CD207/Langerin+ cells had a round shape. There was no difference in the proportion of shapes of LCs comparing patients with and without penile malformations.

Discussion

By thorough evaluation using two different methods our data demonstrate that LCs are present in patients with hypospadias in the same frequency and morphology as in foreskin from children without penile malformation. Consequently, we assume that their ontogeny is not disturbed and we hypothesize their immunological function is preserved in hypospadias patients.

The relevance of this finding – negative data – becomes apparent in view of the altered (fore) skin embryology and the changes to skin function in hypospadias patients as well as when considering the role of LCs in the foreskin in sexually transmitted diseases, notably HIV and HPV. Both are not only very common but also associated with a massive burden of morbidity.

Hypospadias are linked to early embryological changes at time of outgrow of the genital tubercle starting from gestational week 8, when mesenchymal signaling, notably involving FGF, which is required for the outgrow of the genital tubercle, determines epithelial differentiation. Mesenchymal FGF signaling has been shown to affect ectodermal as well as endodermal epithelia [4]. In a murine model, ectodermal deletion of FGFR2 resulted in the most severe hypospadias with major alterations to the foreskin, highlighting a major role of FGFR2 in the developing genital surface epithelia [3]. Various changes in skin development and marker allocation have been shown to occur as a consequence [2, 12]. Foreskin derived fibroblasts from children with hypospadias react differently to endocrine stimuli, possibly based on genetic variation in these subjects [13]. Furthermore, a subcutaneous muscle layer, termed the "dartos fascia" has been shown to be disorganized in patients with hypospadias [14]. This evidence highlights the impact of early fetal events during the outgrow of the genital tubercle on the development of penile skin in boys with hypospadias.

Androgen and estrogen receptors as well as molecules responsible for their regulation, notably ZEB1, are expressed differently in skin of hypospadias patients [5, 15]. Interestingly, ZEB1 has also been implicated in the regulation of the fate of CD8$^+$ T-cells [16] and has been shown to be relevant in LC maturation [17]. This points at a possible relationship between androgen receptor regulation being involved in the embryology of hypospadias and the functioning of the specific immune system – including LCs.

LCs acquire their typical immunophenotye gradually during fetal life and after birth. It has been shown in a mouse model, that Langerin is expressed only after birth [18]. Another prototypical marker of LCs, the NF-κB activator RANK, is already expressed by the end of the second trimester in adult like levels [19]. LC precursor cells, however, are present in the dermis as early as

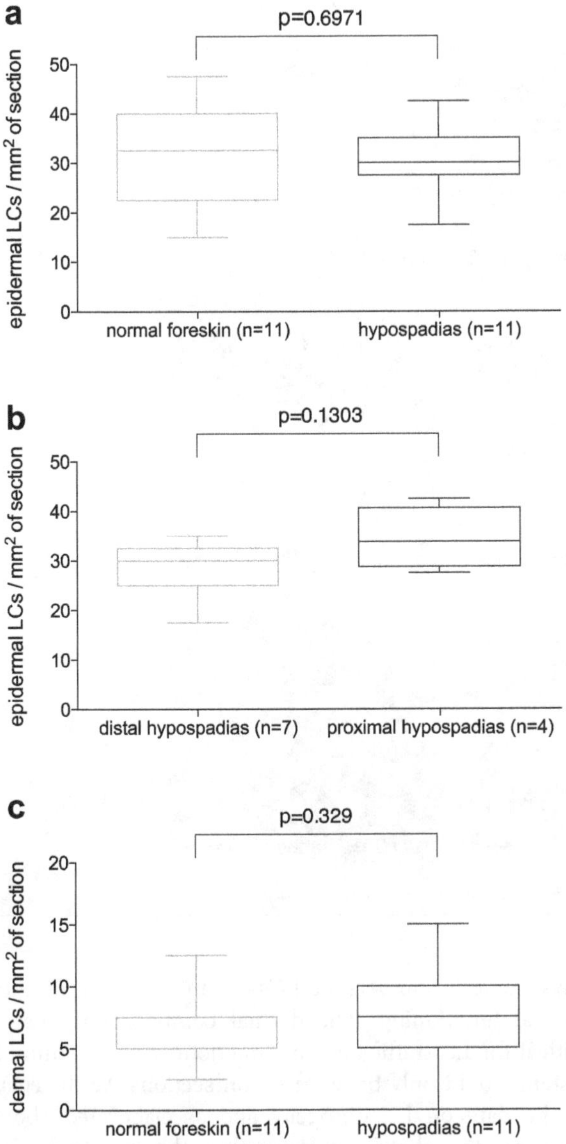

Fig. 8 Box-plots of mean Langerhans cell (LC) counts per mm^2 on immunohistochemically stained full skin sections comparing **a** patients without penile malformations to all included patients with hypospadias, **b** patients with distal hypospadias to patients with proximal hypospadias, and **c** dermal LC counts per mm^2 in patients without penile malformations to all included patients with hypospadias. Error bars represent min-max

gestational week 9–14 [20]. This matches the timeframe, when – at the level of the genital tubercle – changes become effective that ultimately lead to the formation of hypospadias [1]. Consequently, finding a frequency of LCs unchanged compared to patients without penile malformation, might be interpreted as evidence for an unhindered colonization of the penile skin with immune precursor cells in early fetal life. Our findings would suggest that the penile skin epithelium might be less affected by the underlying genetic changes, at least with regard to the skin-resident Langerhans cells.

LC frequency in human foreskin as well as in the glandular epithelia has been assessed multiply, notably in connection with HIV research. The LC frequency in vaginal and foreskin epithelium was found to be high, comparable to our results. Also, an age related difference in LC frequency in foreskin epidermis has been described [21]. In our study, we could not observe different LC frequency dependent on patients' age.

LCs are critically involved in HIV infection, with the removal of the foreskin leading to a reduced probability of female to male transmission from 2.49 to 1.18% [7, 22]. Independent from LC frequency also the polarity of exposition was found to modify the probability of infection with the inner foreskin being more susceptible to HIV infection [23]. Our findings might be interpreted as indirect evidence that males affected by hypospadias carry the same risk of HIV infection compared to those who have no genital malformation. However, lacking a direct proof this remains hypothetical but fits the lack of reports about excess HIV infection rates in hypospadias patients. Removal of foreskin during hypospadias surgery implies the same relative protection in hypospadias patients as compared to others.

HPV infects basal epithelial cells [24]. The presence of foreskin is related to the likelihood of transmission from men to women as well as the likelihood of persistence of infection [25]. Unlike in HIV infection, LCs play a critical role in modifying the response of the immune system to the HPV infection. The presence of T regulatory cells – presumably a result of lacking co-stimulation by LCs - in HPV associated cervical cancer lesions has been shown to probably be associated to worse outcomes [26]. Furthermore LCs are critically involved in rendering T-cells unresponsive and thereby allowing for HPV progression [8]. Penile cancer is relatively rare and often associated with HPV. Additionally, a role in the inhibition of cutaneous carcinogenesis has been attributed to LCs in a murine model for squamous cell cancer [27].

Like for HIV, our finding of an unchanged frequency of LCs in hypospadias patients points at a risk of HPV infection similar to that of a non-hypospadias population, however, without direct proof.

Preoperative hormonal treatment is commonly used, mainly for proximal hypospadias to increase glandular diameter and penile girth in order to prevent postoperative complications. It has been shown in an animal model, that androgen stimulation induces topical inflammation, what could be relevant to LC activation and migration [28]. The lag time between androgen application and surgery in our patients was at least 4 weeks whereas there was no "testosterone holiday" in the abovementioned animal model. Furthermore, we used topical

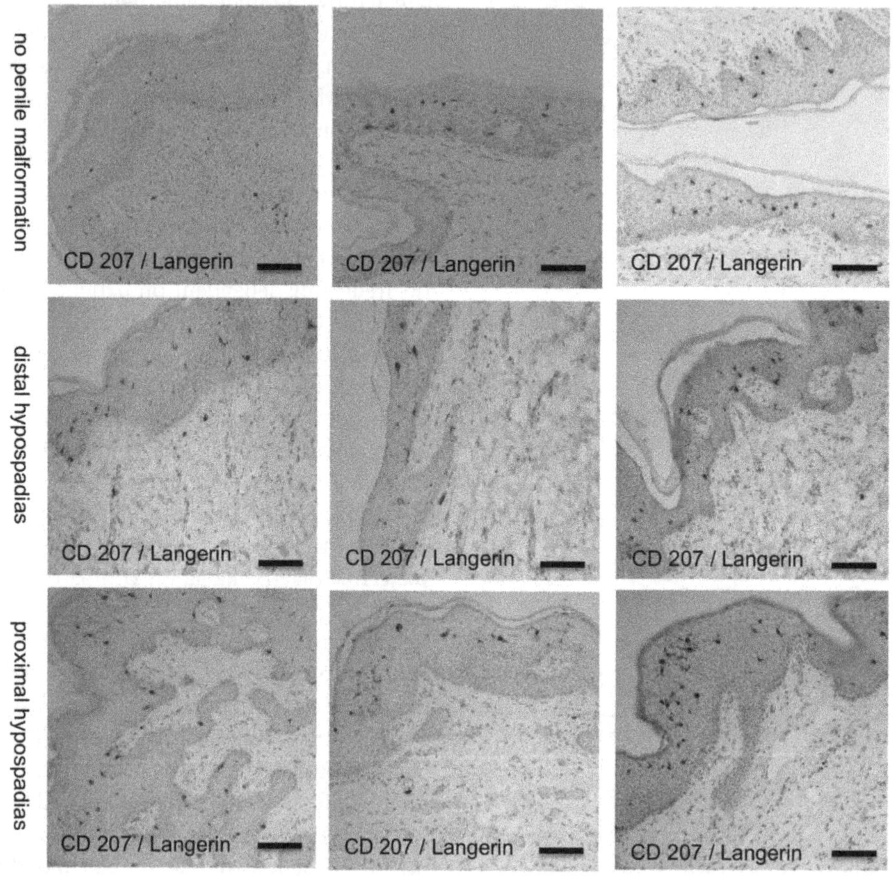

Fig. 9 Immunohistochemically stained full skin sections with anti-Langerin (929F3.01). Scale bar represents 100 μm

dihydrotestosterone whereas in the cited study, intramuscular testosterone was applied. In our patient cohort, 5/7 proximal hypospadias received a preoperative topical treatment with dihydrotestosterone ointment. As there was no difference in LC frequency, we conclude that preoperative androgen application – with a "testosterone holiday" of 4 weeks and topical administration – does not prompt LC migration by a topical inflammatory response.

Studying potential repercussions of embryological events in human tissues implicates a number of limitations. Prenatal sampling of skin is unprecedented in humans; such research would require an animal model, as to our ends also for genital malformations. We are limited to describing the state of LCs after birth, however, we cannot draw any conclusions on whether the ontogeny and the colonization of skin by these cells during embryological developments is as normal as their appearance in our samples. Moreover and most importantly, the lack of a functional evaluation of the LCs, e.g. by induction of inflammation prior to tissue sampling, that is not possible due to ethical concerns, limits the scope of our study. We therefore rely on the presence of physiological numbers of LCs as an indicator of their normal functioning. The dermal compartment, that is critical for LC traffic and the functioning of the immune system, could only be assessed on sections. With regard to the data on LC ontogeny and as elaborated above, however, the choice to investigate the frequency and anatomy of LCs after birth by sheet and section analysis seemed an important and logical step. In case of a disrupted embryological colonization, changes were to be expected [18].

In view of these limitations, the conclusions made herein are limited to a snap-reading of physiological LC frequency. With these findings relying on a meticulous sampling excluding any bias and two different methods for analysis (sheets and sections), however, the data itself seem undisputable. Furthermore this is the first report in literature to assess LCs in children with penile malformations.

For future research, refined techniques such as multicolour-flow-cytometry of skin cell suspensions or single-cell-transcriptome-analyses may reveal peculiarities of the immune system in the skin of hypospadias patients [29, 30]. Furthermore, animal models with inducted penile malformations, as for example FGF10 of

FGFR2 knockout mice could help shedding more light onto LC ontogeny, postnatal animal models could address the question of LC functionality [31, 32].

Conclusions

Langerhans cells are present in the foreskin of hypospadias patients in a normal frequency and morphology compared to patients without penile malformation. This might suggest that patients with hypospadias are not different from patients with normal penile development considering their specific skin immunity, at least considering the epidermal compartment. Functional aspects as well as the dendritic cell subset composition of the dermis remain to be studied.

Abbreviations

A488: Alexa Fluorochrome 488 (green); A594: Alexa Fluorochrome 594 (red); BSA: bovine serum albumine; CD: cluster of differentiation; DAPI: 4',6-Diamidin-2-phenylindol (blue); HIV: Human Immunodeficiency Virus; HLA: Human Leucocyte Antigen; HPV: Human Papilloma Virus; ICH: Immunohistochemistry; LC: Langerhans Cell; PBS: phosphate buffered saline

Acknowledgements

The authors would like to thank the staff of the Laboratory for Langerhans Cell Research at the Department for Dermatology and Venereology and at the histopathological laboratory at the Section for Clinical and functional Anatomy, both at the Medical University Innsbruck, Austria for their patient support. Furthermore we would like to thank Dr. Becker, Dr. Koen and Dr. Berger for their help with patient recruitment and sample acquisition during hypospadias surgery at the Department for Pediatric Urology, Ordensklinikum Linz, Hospital of the Sisters of Charity.
Part of this data have been presented at the Annual Conference of the European Association of Urology (EAU) 2018 and therefore the abstract is published in European Urology Supplements. The Abstract published does not exceed the word limit of 400:
Haid B, Reider D, Spinoit AF, Nägele F, Pechriggl E, Romani N, Oswald J. Is the skin immune system compromised in patients with hypospadias? Eur Urol Suppl 2018;17:e995.

Authors' contributions

BH, NR and JO drafted the study protocol, NR, HF and JO supervised the manuscript drafting and the whole experimental work. BH wrote the manuscript. BH presented the project to the ethics committee, BH and AFS retrieved all samples and prepared epidermal and dermal sheets. DR performed the laboratory analysis of all sheets including immunofluorescent staining and cell counting. FN and EP performed the sections staining and preparation, FN and BH did the cell counting on sections. All authors read, edited and approved the manuscript including all figures.

Author details

[1]Department of Pediatric Urology, Hospital of the Sisters of Charity, Ordensklinikum Linz, Seilerstätte 4, 4020 Linz, Austria. [2]Department of Urology, Ludwig Maximilians University, Marchioninistraße 15, 81367 Munich, Germany. [3]Department for Dermatology and Venereology, Medical University Innsbruck, Anichstraße 35, 6020 Innsbruck, Austria. [4]Section for clinical and functional Anatomy, Medical University Innsbruck, Müllerstraße 59, 6020 Innsbruck, Austria. [5]Department of Urology, University Clinic Gent, Corneel Heymanslaan 10, 9000 Gent, Belgium. [6]Department of Plastic, Reconstructive and Aesthetic Surgery, Medical University Innsbruck, Innerkoflerstraße 1, Innsbruck, Austria.

References

1. Bouty A, Ayers KL, Pask A, Heloury Y, Sinclair AH. The genetic and environmental factors underlying hypospadias. Sex Dev. 2015;9:239–59.
2. Kurzrock EA, Baskin LS, Li Y, Cunha GR. Epithelial-mesenchymal interactions in development of the mouse fetal genital tubercle. Cells Tissues Organs. 1999;164:125–30.
3. Gredler ML, Seifert AW, Cohn MJ. Tissue-specific roles of fgfr2 in development of the external genitalia. Development. 2015;142:2203–12.
4. Harada M, Omori A, Nakahara C, Nakagata N, Akita K, Yamada G. Tissue-specific roles of FGF signaling in external genitalia development. Dev Dyn. 2015;244:759–73.
5. Qiao L, Tasian GE, Zhang H, Cao M, Ferretti M, Cunha GR, et al. Androgen receptor is overexpressed in boys with severe hypospadias, and ZEB1 regulates androgen receptor expression in human foreskin cells. Pediatr Res. 2012;71:393–8.
6. Steinman RM. Dendritic cells: understanding immunogenicity. Eur J Immunol. 2007;37(Suppl 1):S53–60.
7. Ganor Y, Bomsel M. HIV-1 transmission in the male genital tract. Am J Reprod Immunol. 2011;65:284–91.
8. Woodham AW, Yan L, Skeate JG, van der Veen D, Brand HE, Wong MK, et al. T cell ignorance is bliss: T cells are not tolerized by langerhans cells presenting human papillomavirus antigens in the absence of costimulation. Papillomavirus Res. 2016;2:21–30.
9. Valladeau J, Ravel O, Dezutter-Dambuyant C, Moore K, Kleijmeer M, Liu Y, et al. Langerin, a novel c-type lectin specific to langerhans cells, is an endocytic receptor that induces the formation of birbeck granules. Immunity. 2000;12:71–81.
10. Schuster C, Vaculik C, Fiala C, Meindl S, Brandt O, Imhof M, et al. HLA-DR+ leukocytes acquire CD1 antigens in embryonic and fetal human skin and contain functional antigen-presenting cells. J Exp Med. 2009;206:169–81.
11. Ober-Blöbaum JL, Ortner D, Haid B, Brand A, Tripp C, et al. Monitoring skin dendritic cells in steady state and inflammation by immunofluorescence microscopy and flow cytometry. In: Inflammation methods and protocols. New York: Springer Science and Business Media; 2017. p. 37–53.
12. Pechriggl EJ, Bitsche M, Blumer MJF, Fritsch H. The male urethra: spatiotemporal distribution of molecular markers during early development. Ann Anat. 2013;195:260–71.
13. Qin X-Y, Sone H, Kojima Y, Mizuno K, Ueoka K, Muroya K, et al. Individual variation of the genetic response to bisphenol a in human foreskin fibroblast cells derived from cryptorchidism and hypospadias patients. PLoS One. 2012;7:e52756.
14. Spinoit A-F, Van Praet C, Groen L-A, Van Laecke E, Praet M, Hoebeke P. Congenital penile pathology is associated with abnormal development of the dartos muscle: a prospective study in a large cohort of children undergoing primary penile surgery at a tertiary referral center. J Urol. 2014.
15. Qiao L, Tasian GE, Zhang H, Cunha GR, Baskin L. ZEB1 is estrogen responsive in vitro in human foreskin cells and is over expressed in penile skin in patients with severe hypospadias. J Urol. 2011;185:1888–93.
16. Guan T, Dominguez CX, Amezquita RA, Laidlaw BJ, Cheng J, Henao-Mejia J, et al. ZEB1, ZEB2, and the mir-200 family form a counterregulatory network to regulate CD8+T cell fates. J Exp Med. 2018.
17. Konradi S, Yasmin N, Haslwanter D, Weber M, Gesslbauer B, Sixt M, et al. Langerhans cell maturation is accompanied by induction of n-cadherin and the transcriptional regulators of epithelial-mesenchymal transition ZEB1/2. Eur J Immunol. 2014;44:553–60.
18. Tripp CH, Chang-Rodriguez S, Stoitzner P, Holzmann S, Stössel H, Douillard P, et al. Ontogeny of langerin/CD207 expression in the epidermis of mice. J Invest Dermatol. 2004;122:670–2.
19. Schöppl A, Botta A, Prior M, Akgün J, Schuster C, Elbe-Bürger A. Langerhans cell precursors acquire RANK/CD265 in prenatal human skin. Acta Histochem. 2015;117:425–30.
20. Schuster C, Mildner M, Mairhofer M, Bauer W, Fiala C, Prior M, et al. Human embryonic epidermis contains a diverse langerhans cell precursor pool. Development. 2014;141:807–15.
21. Hussain LA, Lehner T. Comparative investigation of langerhans' cells and potential receptors for HIV in oral, genitourinary and rectal epithelia. Immunology. 1995;85:475–84.
22. Tobian AAR, Serwadda D, Quinn TC, Kigozi G, Gravitt PE, Laeyendecker O, et al. Male circumcision for the prevention of HSV-2 and HPV infections and syphilis. N Engl J Med. 2009;360:1298–309.
23. Ganor Y, Zhou Z, Tudor D, Schmitt A, Vacher-Lavenu M-C, Gibault L, et al. Within 1 h, HIV-1 uses viral synapses to enter efficiently the inner, but not outer, foreskin mucosa and engages langerhans-t cell conjugates. Mucosal Immunol. 2010;3:506–22.

24. Raff AB, Woodham AW, Raff LM, Skeate JG, Yan L, Da Silva DM, et al. The evolving field of human papillomavirus receptor research: a review of binding and entry. J Virol. 2013;87:6062–72.
25. Grabowski MK, Kong X, Gray RH, Serwadda D, Kigozi G, Gravitt PE, et al. Partner human papillomavirus viral load and incident human papillomavirus detection in heterosexual couples. J Infect Dis. 2016;213:948–56.
26. van Esch EMG, van Poelgeest MIE, Trimbos JBMZ, Fleuren GJ, Jordanova ES, van der Burg SH. Intraepithelial macrophage infiltration is related to a high number of regulatory T cells and promotes a progressive course of hpv-induced vulvar neoplasia. Int J Cancer. 2015;136:E85–94.
27. Ortner D, Tripp CH, Komenda K, Dubrac S, Zelger B, Hermann M, et al. Langerhans cells and NK cells cooperate in the inhibition of chemical skin carcinogenesis. Oncoimmunology. 2017;6:e1260215.
28. Hofer MD, Cheng EY, Bury MI, Xu W, Hong SJ, Kaplan WE, et al. Androgen supplementation in rats increases the inflammatory response and prolongs urethral healing. Urology. 2015;85:691–7.
29. Alcántara-Hernández M, Leylek R, Wagar LE, Engleman EG, Keler T, Marinkovich MP, et al. High-Dimensional phenotypic mapping of human dendritic cells reveals interindividual variation and tissue specialization. Immunity. 2017;47:1037–1050.e6.
30. Villani A-C, Satija R, Reynolds G, Sarkizova S, Shekhar K, Fletcher J, et al. Single-cell rna-seq reveals new types of human blood dendritic cells, monocytes, and progenitors. Science 2017;356: 6335, eaah4573.
31. Petiot A, Petiot A, Perriton CL, Dickson C, Cohn MJ. Development of the mammalian urethra is controlled by Fgfr2-IIIb. Development. 2005;132:2441–50.
32. Ober-Blöbaum JL, Ortner D, Haid B, Brand A, Tripp C, Clausen BE, et al. Monitoring skin dendritic cells in steady state and inflammation by immunofluorescence microscopy and flow Cytometry. Methods Mol. Biol. New York, NY: Springer New York; 2017;1559:37–52.

20

Assessing somatization in urologic chronic pelvic pain syndrome

C. S. North[1,2*], B. A. Hong[3], H. H. Lai[4] and D. H. Alpers[5]

Abstract

Background: This study examined the prevalence of somatization disorder in Urological Chronic Pelvic Pain Syndrome (UCPPS) and the utility of two self-report symptom screening tools for assessment of somatization in patients with UCPPS.

Methods: The study sample included 65 patients with UCPPS who enrolled in the Multidisciplinary Approach to the Study of Chronic Pelvic Pain (MAPP) Study at Washington University. Patients completed the PolySymptomatic PolySyndromic Questionnaire (PSPS-Q) ($n = 64$) and the Patient Health Questionnaire-15 Somatic Symptom Severity Scale (PHQ-15) ($n = 50$). Review of patient medical records found that only 47% ($n = 30$) contained sufficient documentation to assess Perley-Guze criteria for somatization disorder.

Results: Few (only 6.5%) of the UCPPS sample met Perley-Guze criteria for definite somatization disorder. Perley-Guze somatization disorder was predicted by definite PSPS-Q somatization with at least 75% sensitivity and specificity. Perley-Guze somatization disorder was predicted by severe (> 15) PHQ-15 threshold that had > 90% sensitivity and specificity but was met by only 16% of patients. The moderate (> 10) PHQ-15 threshold had higher sensitivity (100%) but lower specificity (52%) and was met by 52% of the sample.

Conclusions: The PHQ-15 is brief, but it measures symptoms constituting only one dimension of somatization. The PSPS-Q uniquely captures two conceptual dimensions inherent in the definition of somatization disorder, both number of symptoms and symptom distribution across multiple organ systems, with relevance for UCPPS as a syndrome that is not just a collection of urological symptoms but a broader syndrome with symptoms extending beyond the urological system.

Keywords: Interstitial cystitis, Urological chronic pelvic pain syndrome, Chronic prostatitis, Somatization disorder, Symptom screening, Psychiatric diagnosis, Polysymptomatic, Polysyndromic, Somatoform, Psychoform

Introduction

Urological chronic pelvic pain syndrome (UCPPS), which includes interstitial cystitis/bladder pain syndrome (IC/BPS) and chronic prostatitis/chronic pelvic pain syndrome (CP/CPPS), is a symptom-based syndrome without objective testing or diagnostic biomarkers. UCPPS is diagnosed only through assessment of symptoms and symptom patterns reported by patients with this disorder. Bothersome symptoms characterizing UCPPS include not only the core urological symptoms of pelvic pain and urinary frequency/urgency but also an auxiliary halo of non-urologic pain (e.g., abdominal pain) and other symptoms extending beyond the urological system (e.g., nausea, dizziness, or palpitations) [3, 6, 16, 17].

To avoid unnecessary medical tests, procedures, and surgeries, it is important to sort out symptoms of somatoform disorders from medical illness, but this task has historically proven difficult for both psychiatrists and non-psychiatric physicians. Like many other functional disorders, UCPPS has many symptoms in common with somatization disorder, and patients diagnosed with UCPPS may include some patients who have somatoform disorders. In the current version of American diagnostic criteria for psychiatric disorders, the *Diagnostic and Statistical Manual of*

* Correspondence: carol.north@utsouthwestern.edu
[1]The Altshuler Center for Education & Research at Metrocare Services, The University of Texas Southwestern Medical Center, 1250 Mockingbird Lane, Suite 330, Dallas, TX 75247-4914, USA
[2]Department of Psychiatry, The University of Texas Southwestern Medical Center, 5323 Harry Hines Blvd., Suite NE5.102, Dallas, TX 75390-9070, USA
Full list of author information is available at the end of the article

Mental Disorders, 5th edition (*DSM-5*), [2] the previous diagnostic section on somatoform disorders was replaced with a section covering somatic symptom and related disorders; the former diagnosis of somatization disorder has been replaced by somatic symptom disorder, which does not require specified numbers of symptoms across organ systems or symptoms that are "medically unexplained."

Some patients with UCPPS report not just symptoms confined to the definition of the syndrome but also multiple symptoms across multiple organ systems. One-fourth of patients with UCPPS have been observed to have this pattern of symptoms distributed widely across organ systems [16, 17]. This symptom presentation has been termed "polysymptomatic, polysyndromic", [17, 21] and it is reminiscent of the classic presentation of somatization disorder. Somatization disorder has historically been well known to psychiatrists and other physicians as a chronic disorder defined by the presentation of multiple symptoms distributed across many organ systems. To represent somatization disorder, the symptoms had to be determined to have no medically explainable etiology. Like UCPPS, somatization disorder requires documentation of characteristic symptoms and symptom patterns reported by patients, because there are no objective tests for biomarkers to identify the disorder. For many years, these two symptom-based syndromes may have coexisted without recognition of the overlap between them.

The diagnosis of somatization disorder (under the name Briquet's syndrome) has historically been made using criteria that were first established by Perley and Guze [23] and formally validated in 1972 [7]. The Perley-Guze criteria are recognized as the original, well-validated, and most comprehensive criteria for this diagnosis [7, 21, 23, 29]. The original Perley-Guze criteria continue to be accepted as valid for diagnosis of somatization disorder, regarded by some experts as superior to (and somewhat more stringent than) the most recently established criteria [1] for the disorder [21]. The Perley-Guze criteria remain meaningful today because psychiatrists and non-psychiatric physicians still need to understand the clinical significance of the symptoms their patients report. Although the Perley-Guze criteria have no relevance for making a *DSM-5* diagnosis of somatic symptom disorder, their utility for sorting out symptoms and symptom patterns is still important.

Various somatic symptom measures have been developed and used in different populations and settings for assessment of somatic symptoms and somatization syndromes. The PolySymptomatic PolySyndromic Questionnaire (PSPS-Q) developed by Lai et al. [17] has been used in UCPPS research to identify not only the large numbers of somatic symptoms reported by these patients but also their distribution across multiple organ systems that are characteristic of somatoform disorders. The PSPS-Q was conceptually derived from the Perley-Guze criteria. The Patient Health Questionnaire-15 Somatic Symptom Severity Scale (PHQ-15, 13] has also been used to assess somatization symptoms in patients with UCPPS.

The purpose of this study was to examine the prevalence of somatization disorder in UCPPS using the Perley-Guze criteria and to compare two self-report symptom screening tools—the PSPS-Q and the PHQ-15 to assist the evaluation of UCPPS. Its findings should be of interest to many psychiatrists, urologists, and primary care physicians who need to evaluate the medical symptoms in their patients.

Methods

A sample of 65 patients with UCPPS was recruited from consecutive patients presenting to the Washington University urology clinic in the early years of the Multidisciplinary Approach to the Study of Chronic Pelvic Pain (MAPP) project at one site. Study inclusion criteria were 1) age $\geq$ 18 years, 2) report of an unpleasant sensation of pain, pressure, or discomfort perceived by the patient to involve the bladder and/or pelvic region and associated with lower urinary tract symptoms, e.g., urgency, for most of the time during the most recent 3 months, and 3) symptoms were not explained by another identifiable urological cause. Exclusion criteria were active urinary tract infection, cancer, urethral stricture, neurological disease, fistula, radiation cystitis, cyclophosphamide cystitis, urinary tuberculosis, or open bladder surgery. These inclusion and exclusion criteria were adapted from the MAPP Research Network working definition of UCPPS [18]. Approval for this study was obtained from the Institutional Review Board of Washington University, and written informed consent was provided by all patients at the time of their enrollment into the study.

Data for this study were collected between March 2010 and October 2012. As part of the MAPP study, participants provided information on demographics, symptom duration; ratings of their pain; frequency and urgency on 0–10 numeric ratings scales; Interstitial Cystitis Symptom and Problem Indexes [22]; the Genitourinary Pain Index [4]; the Complex Medical Symptoms Inventory to assess symptoms of irritable bowel syndrome (IBS) or fibromyalgia [28]; and a whole body map to characterize the location and distribution of pain in the past week [15]. A full list of data collected from the MAPP Epidemiology and Phenotyping Study has previously been described [18].

The Washington University electronic outpatient medical records of the patients in this sample were reviewed by an expert psychiatric diagnostician (C.S.N.), a urologist (H.H.L.), and an experienced medical/clinical psychologist (B.A.H.) to formally assess Perley-Guze criteria for somatization disorder. These 3 clinicians from different areas of expertise provided multidisciplinary consensus through interactive discussion of each patient's medical history in the clinical records. A definite diagnosis requires ≥25 symptoms in ≥9 symptom categories, but probable diagnosis (requiring ≥20 symptoms in ≥9 symptom categories) has been utilized historically to include histories strongly suggestive of somatization disorder but not quite meeting sufficient numbers of symptoms [7, 23]. The probable diagnosis option was formalized for use in suboptimal circumstances affording insufficient data for complete assessment—such as the current study in which investigators were unable to obtain data through collection of clinical information directly from patients over long periods of time.

At the baseline clinic visit, demographic information was recorded and the patients completed the PSPS-Q and the PHQ-15. The PSPS-Q is a self-report symptom questionnaire assessing 59 somatic symptoms across 10 symptom categories, derived from the 59-item yes/no Perley-Guze symptom checklist and also requiring ≥25 symptoms distributed among ≥9 of 10 possible symptom categories [20]. Only symptoms considered by the patient to represent "a lot of trouble" are counted as Perley-Guze symptoms. The PSPS-Q, unlike the original Perley-Guze criteria historically used in clinical practice and research, does not exclude medically unexplained symptoms. The symptom count/symptom group scoring algorithm used for determining the original Perley-Guze criteria was applied for scoring the PSPS-Q data. Because the 4 menstrual symptoms comprising 1 of the 10 Perley-Guze symptom groups do not apply to men, the PSPS-Q scoring threshold for men was reduced to ≥21 symptoms in ≥8 categories for definite somatization and to ≥16 symptoms in ≥8 categories for probable somatization.

The PHQ-15 is a self-report symptom questionnaire derived from the Patient Health Questionnaire that consists of 15 items scored from 0 ("not bothered at all") to 2 ("bothered a lot"), with scores of 5, 10, and 15 respectively representing mild, moderate, and severe somatization. The PHQ-15 has demonstrated validity and reliability and is widely used for screening and monitoring somatization and somatic symptom severity in clinical practice and research [12–14, 25]. The moderate PHQ-15 threshold score of ≥10 has been demonstrated to detect patients with medically unexplained physical symptoms with 30% sensitivity and 93% specificity, and with positive predictive and negative predictive values (PPV and NPV) of .40 and .89 respectively [5].

The PSPS-Q was completed by 64 patients and the PHQ-15 was completed by 50 of these patients. Probable and definite self-report PSPS-Q somatization were not associated with non-completion of the PHQ-15.

Statistical analysis

Data analysis for this study was conducted using SAS version 9.4 (SAS Institute, Cary, NC). Descriptive findings are represented as counts with proportions and means with standard deviations (SD). Comparisons of numerical variables with a dichotomous variable for sex used Wilcoxon two-sample rank sum tests (PROC NPAR1WAY WILCOXON in SAS) using t approximations with a continuity correction of 0.5. Dichotomous variables generated by different forms of assessment were compared through tests of sensitivity, specificity, PPV, and NPV, as well as with chi-square tests.

Results

The 64 patients with PSPS-Q data and medical record review was 48% male, 86% non-Hispanic white, 6% Hispanic, and 8% other race/ethnicity. The sample had a mean (SD) age of 46.8 (16.1) years. The mean (SD) duration of UCPPS symptoms was 10.2 (12.0) years. IBS was present in 30%, fibromyalgia in 8%, and chronic fatigue syndrome in 13%. Mean (SD) ratings on a scale of 1–10 were 4.9 (2.4) for pain, 4.8 (2.8) for frequency, and 5.0 (2.6) for urgency. The mean (SD) genitourinary pain index total score was 24.2 (9.6). The mean (SD) Interstitial Cystitis Symptom and Problem Indexes were 9.5 (5.2) and 8.2 (4.6) respectively. The mean (SD) number of body sites outside the pelvis that had pain was 3.8 (3.6) (of a maximum of 42 sites). Of the 34 female patients (52% of the sample), all had the clinical diagnosis of interstitial cystitis/bladder pain syndrome (IC/BPS). Of the 31 male patients (48% of the sample), 28 had the clinical diagnosis of chronic prostatitis/chronic pelvic pain syndrome (CP/CPPS), and 3 had the dual diagnoses of IC/BPS and CP/CPPS.

The medical records of more than one-half of the patients (53%, 34/64) were found to contain insufficient documentation (largely because of a lack of medical records by primary care providers and clinicians of other disciplines) to allow the identification of patterns of multiple somatoform symptoms across multiple organ systems; thus, the medical records of only 30 patients could be used to assess Perley-Guze criteria for somatization disorder.

Somatization disorder was uncommon in this UCPPS sample: only 2 patients (6.5%) met definite Perley-Guze criteria based on medical record review. Two additional patients (6.5%) met probable Perley-Guze criteria. All 4 of these patients were female.

The mean (SD) number of somatic symptoms on the self-report PSPS-Q was 14.9 (11.2) and the mean (SD) number of symptom groups was 6.4 (3.0). Men and women did not differ on numbers of PSPS-Q symptoms or symptom groups. One-third (33%, 21/64) of the sample met the threshold for at least probable PSPS-Q somatization, including 17/64 (27%) with definite PSPS-Q somatization. Insufficient medical record documentation was not associated with number of symptoms or positive symptom groups reported on the PSPS-Q.

Among the 30 patients with sufficient medical records, 11 (37%) met the probable PSPS-Q somatization threshold, including 8 (27%) who met the definite threshold. Medical record review found that 38% of the 8 patients meeting the definite PSPS-Q threshold met Perley-Guze criteria for somatization disorder (2 probable, 1 definite). The fourth patient meeting (definite) Perley-Guze criteria for somatization disorder by medical record review was not forthcoming on the PSPS-Q, reporting only 2 symptoms in 1 symptom group.

Table 1 presents data for prediction of definite and probable Perley-Guze somatization disorder criteria by medical record review from definite and probable PSPS-Q somatization. The definite PSPS-Q threshold was significantly associated by chi-square test with probable Perley-Guze somatization disorder, which it detected with sensitivity and specificity levels of at least 75% and positive predictive value of 38%.

The mean (SD) PHQ-15 score was 8.7 (4.4), representing a mild-to-moderate level of somatization; 42% (21/50) scored at or above the moderate threshold of 10 and 10% (5/50) scored at or above the severe threshold of 15. PHQ-15 scores were higher for women than for men (mean = 10.3, mean = 4.7 vs. mean = 6.7, SD = 2.9; $z = 2.86$, $p = .004$. Insufficient medical record documentation was not associated with PHQ-15 scores.

Table 2 presents results for prediction of definite Perley-Guze somatization disorder by medical record review from PHQ-15 thresholds representing mild, moderate, and severe somatization. (Because the 2 patients with probable but not definite somatization disorder by medical record review did not complete the PHQ-15, prediction of probable somatization disorder by the PHQ-15 was not possible.) The moderate PHQ-15 threshold ≥ 10 identified 52% of the sample and predicted definite Perley-Guze somatization disorder with 100% sensitivity but only 52% specificity and a PPV of only 15%, not meeting statistical significance by chi-square test. A severe PHQ-15 score ≥ 15, however, identified just 16% of the sample, and this threshold significantly predicted definite Perley-Guze somatization disorder by chi-square test with at least 90% for both sensitivity and specificity, and with a PPV of 50%. Half (2 of the 4) of the patients with a severe PHQ-15 score ≥ 15 had definite Perley-Guze somatization disorder by medical record review.

Table 1 Definite and probable PSPS prediction of definite and probable Perley-Guze somatization disorder by medical record review ($n = 30$)

	Sensitivity	Specificity	PPV	NPV	p
Predicting definite Perley-Guze somatization disorder by medical record review (7% of the sample)					
Definite PSPS (27% positive)	50%	75%	13%	95%	.469
Probable PSPS (37% positive)	50%	64%	9%	95%	1.000
Predicting probable Perley-Guze somatization disorder by medical record review (13% of the sample)					
Definite PSPS (27% positive)	75%	81%	38%	95%	.048
Probable PSPS (37% positive)	75%	69%	27%	95%	.126

PPV positive predictive value, *NPV* negative predictive value, *PSPS* polysymptomatic, polysyndromic, *PSPS-Q* PSPS Questionnaire

Table 2 PHQ-15 prediction of definite Perley-Guze somatization disorder by medical record review ($n = 25$)

	Sensitivity	Specificity	PPV	NPV	p
PHQ-15 threshold					
5 (92% positive)	100%	9%	9%	100%	.664
10 (52% positive)	100%	52%	15%	100%	.480
15 (16% positive)	100%	91%	50%	100%	.020

PPV positive predictive value, *NPV* negative predictive value

Discussion

This study examined and compared data from a 59-item self-report symptom questionnaire (PSPS-Q) and a 15-item self-report screening questionnaire (PHQ-15) with medical record review to assess Perley-Guze criteria for somatization disorder in a sample of patients with UCPPS. Medical record review by 3 experts confirmed that 6.5% of the patients with UCPPS had definite and another 6.5% had probable or definite somatization disorder. Thus, it was uncommon for UCPPS patients to meet definite Perley-Guze criteria for somatization disorder (only 6.5%). This frequency is similar to the 1–6% point prevalence of somatization disorder in primary care patients reported by a recent systematic review that identified, from a total of 992 publications, 32 studies from 24 countries involving > 70,00 patients [9]. Self-reported PSPS-Q somatization (both probable and definite thresholds) had higher sensitivity and specificity for prediction of probable than for definite Perley-Guze somatization disorder verified by medical record review.

Perley-Guze somatization disorder verified by medical record review was predicted by both self-reported questionnaires. Probable Perley-Guze somatization disorder was predicted by PSPS-Q definite somatization with at least 75% sensitivity and specificity, and by moderate (threshold ≥ 10) PHQ-15 scores with higher sensitivity (100%) but lower specificity (52%). These two comparisons were not completely comparable, however, because the PSPS-Q comparison included patients with both definite ($n = 2$) and probable ($n = 2$) Perley-Guze somatization disorder but the PHQ-15 comparison could not include the 2 probable Perley-Guze somatization disorder cases who did not complete the PHQ-15. Neither definite nor probable PSPS-Q somatization were significantly associated with moderate or higher PHQ-15 scores. The prediction of definite Perley-Guze somatization disorder by the PHQ-15 was statistically significant using a higher PHQ-15 threshold (≥15, representing severe somatization), with > 90% sensitivity as well as specificity. Using the severe PHQ-15 threshold also substantially reduced the patient pool under consideration to 16% of all patients versus 52% selected by the moderate PHQ-15 threshold. In summary, the PSPS-Q had greater sensitivity but lower specificity than the moderate PHQ-15 threshold that has been previously reported for identifying somatization disorder, and a higher (severe) PHQ-15 somatization threshold performed better than the PHQ-15 moderate somatization threshold for prediction of Perley-Guze somatization disorder.

A limitation to attempting to assess somatization disorder criteria by any self-report questionnaire is that patients cannot be expected to determine whether their own symptoms are medically explained or unexplained. For this reason, self-report symptom questionnaires cannot be used to diagnose somatization disorder [17, 21]. Two patient reporting behaviors further limit self-report questionnaires: 1) patients with somatization disorder do not report all their symptoms at once, focusing their medical complaints on or even limiting them to the organ system of the specialist, which necessitates collection of symptoms across different visits and to different medical specialists [19, 20]; 2) these patients may provide medically plausible but incorrect explanations for their symptoms and may even attribute their symptoms to medical disorders they do not have [11, 19].

Limitations of this study include the small sample selected in a treatment setting and investigated at a single site from a specialty service at an academic institution that may not be representative of other samples and settings. Verification of diagnoses of somatization disorder through medical record review was not possible for more than half of the patients in this study because the available patient records were limited to one or very few visits to a limited set of providers, likely resulting in substantial underestimation. The small sample size coupled with low numbers of patients meeting Perley-Guze criteria for somatization disorder by medical record review resulted in low power to detect subgroup differences; regardless, analyses in this study suggested patterns of association of symptom measures with the diagnosis of somatization disorder which deserve further study with larger samples in settings with more complete medical records.

Not only has the traditional means of assessing diagnostic criteria through medical record review been lost with the evolution to current medical record systems, but the diagnosis of somatization disorder itself has been lost from established diagnostic criteria in *DSM-5*. This loss is still controversial, and somatization disorder is recognized as one of the few validated psychiatric disorders, consistently included in previous versions of the manual (and remains part of the International Classification of Diseases system). This diagnosis was replaced in *DSM-5* with somatic symptom disorder, an unvalidated syndrome that is overly broad and inappropriately inclusive of patients with nonpathological distress attributable to medical illness [8, 10, 24, 26, 27].

Identifying patients with polysymptomatic, polysyndromic symptom-reporting patterns characteristic of somatization disorder in patient populations with UCPPS is of clinical importance because their medical outcomes are distinctly worse than those of other patients. These patients may require different clinical interventions, to avoid unnecessary medical tests, procedures, and surgeries. The prevalence of somatization disorder in UCPPS is unknown despite attempts to estimate it using various symptom measures and methods.

Without the time-honored tools historically used to identify somatization syndromes through detailed medical records and longitudinal assessment of patients' evolving symptoms, other means of identifying patterns of somatization are needed. The PSPS-Q or the PHQ-15 might be useful for identifying polysymptomatic, polysyndromic presentations by completing a screening tool in the pre-appointment waiting area to systematically address symptoms outside the urinary system that are not the focus of the brief clinical history gathered by urologists. This information might prompt urologists to collect additional history to identify patterns of multiple symptoms distributed across multiple organ systems that is characteristic of somatization disorder.

An advantage of the PHQ-15 over the PSPS-Q is that it is less burdensome to complete, with only 15 items compared to 59 in the PSPS-Q. However, the PSPS-Q uniquely captures two conceptual dimensions inherent in the definition of somatization disorder rather than one: it not only counts the number of symptoms, but it also assesses the extent of symptom distribution across multiple organ systems that is integral to the conceptualization and diagnosis of somatization disorder. Consideration not just of number of symptoms but also their distribution across organ systems has relevance for the appreciation of UCPPS as a syndrome that is not just a collection of urological symptoms but a broader syndrome with symptoms extending beyond the urological system.

Although the self-report PSPS-Q does not exclude medically unexplained symptoms, the Perley-Guze symptom algorithm has been found to retain its validity even without this exclusion [29]. Brief symptom measures with as few as 15 items cannot be expected to assess both the volume of symptoms and their distribution throughout the organ systems that is provided with the 59 symptom items of the PSPS-Q.

Conclusions

The PHQ-15 is brief, but it measures symptoms constituting only one dimension of somatization. The PSPS-Q uniquely captures two conceptual dimensions inherent in the definition of somatization disorder, both number of symptoms and symptom distribution across multiple organ systems, with relevance for UCPPS as a syndrome that is not just a collection of urological symptoms but a broader syndrome with symptoms extending beyond the urological system. Few UCPPS patients (only 6.5%) met definite Perley-Guze criteria for somatization disorder by medical record review, but the PSPS-Q identified somatization in 27% of the sample and the PHQ-15 severe threshold identified somatization in 16%.

Abbreviations

CP/CPPS: Chronic prostatitis/chronic pelvic pain syndrome; DSM-5: Diagnostic and Statistical Manual of Mental Disorders, 5th edition; IBS: Irritable bowel syndrome; IC/BPS: Interstitial cystitis/bladder pain syndrome; MAPP: Multidisciplinary Approach to the Study of Chronic Pelvic Pain; NPV: Negative predictive value; PHQ-15: Patient Health Questionnaire-15 Somatic Symptom Severity Scale; PPV: Positive predictive value; PSPS-Q: PolySymptomatic PolySyndromic Questionnaire; SD: Standard deviation; UCPPS: Urological Chronic Pelvic Pain Syndrome

Acknowledgements

We thank the MAPP Research Network for review of the manuscript for this article for scientific accuracy.

Authors' contributions

All authors of this article participated in the design of the study, data analysis and interpretation, and writing of the manuscript. All of the authors read and approved the final manuscript.

Author details

[1]The Altshuler Center for Education & Research at Metrocare Services, The University of Texas Southwestern Medical Center, 1250 Mockingbird Lane, Suite 330, Dallas, TX 75247-4914, USA. [2]Department of Psychiatry, The University of Texas Southwestern Medical Center, 5323 Harry Hines Blvd., Suite NE5.102, Dallas, TX 75390-9070, USA. [3]Department of Psychiatry, School of Medicine, Washington University School of Medicine, St. Louis, MO, USA. [4]Departments of Surgery and Anesthesiology, Division of Urologic Surgery, Washington University School of Medicine, St. Louis, MO 63110, USA. [5]Department of Internal Medicine, Division of Gastroenterology, Washington University School of Medicine, St. Louis, MO 63110, USA.

References

1. American Psychiatric Association. Diagnostic and Statistical Manual of Mental Disorders, 4th Text Revision edition. Washington, DC: American Psychiatric Association; 2000.
2. American Psychiatric Association. Diagnostic and Statistical Manual for Mental Disorders. 5th ed. Washington, DC: American Psychiatric Association; 2013.
3. Clauw DJ, Schmidt M, Radulovic D, Singer A, Katz P, Bresette J. The relationship between fibromyalgia and interstitial cystitis. J Psychiatr Res. 1997;31(1):125–31.
4. Clemens JQ, Calhoun EA, Litwin MS, McNaughton-Collins M, Kusek JW, Crowley EM, Landis JR. Validation of a modified National Institutes of Health chronic prostatitis symptom index to assess genitourinary pain in both men and women. Urology. 2009;74(5):983–7 quiz.
5. den Boeft M, van der Wouden JC, Rydell-Lexmond TR, de Wit NJ, van der Horst HE, Numans ME. Identifying patients with medically unexplained physical symptoms in electronic medical records in primary care: a validation study. BMC Fam Pract. 2014;15:109.
6. Erickson DR, Morgan KC, Ordille S, Keay SK, Xie SX. Nonbladder related symptoms in patients with interstitial cystitis. J Urol. 2001;166(2):557–61.
7. Feighner JP, Robins E, Guze SB, Woodruff RA, Winokur G, Muñoz R. Diagnostic criteria for use in psychiatric research. Arch Gen Psychiatry. 1972; 26:57–62.
8. Frances A, Chapman S. DSM-5 somatic symptom disorder mislabels medical illness as mental disorder. Aust N Z J Psychiatry. 2013;47(5):483–4.
9. Haller H, Cramer H, Lauche R, Dobos G. Somatoform disorders and medically unexplained symptoms in primary care. Dtsch Arztebl Int. 2015; 112(16):279–87.
10. Hauser W, Wolfe F. The somatic symptom disorder in DSM 5 risks mislabelling people with major medical diseases as mentally ill. J Psychosom Res. 2013;75(6):586–7.
11. Hiller W, Rief W, Brahler E. Somatization in the population: from mild bodily misperceptions to disabling symptoms. Soc Psychiatry Psychiatr Epidemiol. 2006;41(9):704–12.
12. Kocalevent RD, Hinz A, Brahler E. Standardization of a screening instrument (PHQ-15) for somatization syndromes in the general population. BMC Psychiatry. 2013;13:91.
13. Kroenke K, Spitzer RL, Williams JB. The PHQ-15: validity of a new measure for evaluating the severity of somatic symptoms. Psychosom Med. 2002; 64(2):258–66.
14. Kroenke K, Spitzer RL, Williams JB, Lowe B. The patient health questionnaire somatic, anxiety, and depressive symptom scales: a systematic review. Gen Hosp Psychiatry. 2010;32(4):345–59.
15. Lai HH, Jemielita T, Sutcliffe S, Bradley CS, Naliboff B, Williams DA, Gereau RW, Kreder K, Clemens JQ, Rodriguez LV, Krieger JN, Farrar JT, Robinson N, Landis JR. Characterization of whole body pain in urological chronic pelvic pain syndrome at baseline: a MAPP research network study. J Urol. 2017; 198(3):622–31.
16. Lai HH, North CS, Andriole GL, Cupps L, Song D, Ness TJ, Hong BA. Urological symptoms in a subset of patients with urological chronic pelvic pain syndrome and a polysymptomatic, polysyndromic pattern of presentation. J Urol. 2013;191(6):1802–7.
17. Lai HH, North CS, Andriole GL, Sayuk GS, Hong BA. Polysymptomatic, polysyndromic presentation of patients with urological chronic pelvic pain syndrome. J Urol. 2012;187(6):2106–12.
18. Landis JR, Williams DA, Lucia MS, Clauw DJ, Naliboff BD, Robinson NA, van BA, Sutcliffe S, Schaeffer AJ, Rodriguez LV, Mayer EA, Lai HH, Krieger JN, Kreder KJ, Afari N, Andriole GL, Bradley CS, Griffith JW, Klumpp DJ, Hong BA, Lutgendorf SK, Buchwald D, Yang CC, Mackey S, Pontari MA, Hanno P, Kusek JW, Mullins C, Clemens JQ. The MAPP research network: design, patient characterization and operations. BMC Urol. 2014;14:58.
19. Martin RL. Problems in the diagnosis of somatization disorder: effects on research and clinical practice. Psychiatr Ann. 1988;18:357–62.
20. Murphy GE. The clinical management of hysteria. J Am Med Assoc. 1982; 247(18):2559–64.
21. North CS, Yutzy SH. Somatization disorder. In: In Goodwin and Guze's psychiatric diagnosis. 7th ed. Oxford: Oxford University Press; 2018. p. 207–26.
22. O'Leary MP, Sant GR, Fowler FJ Jr, Whitmore KE, Spolarich-Kroll J. The interstitial cystitis symptom index and problem index. Urology. 1997;49(5A Suppl):58–63.
23. Perley MJ, Guze SB. Hysteria--the stability and usefulness of clinical criteria. N Engl J Med. 1962;266(9):421–6.
24. Rief W. A commentary on: somatic symptom disorder: an important change in DSM. J Psychosom Res. 2013;75(6):584.
25. van Ravesteijn H, Wittkampf K, Lucassen P, van de Lisdonk E, van den Hoogen H, van Weert H, Huijser J, Schene A, van Weel C, Speckens A. Detecting somatoform disorders in primary care with the PHQ-15. Ann Fam Med. 2009;7(3):232–8.
26. Wakefield JC. DSM-5, psychiatric epidemiology and the false positives problem. Epidemiol Psychiatr Sci. 2015;24(3):188–96.
27. Wakefield JC. Diagnostic issues and controversies in DSM-5: return of the false positives problem. Annu Rev Clin Psychol. 2016;12:105–32.
28. Williams DA, Schilling S. Advances in the assessment of fibromyalgia. Rheum Dis Clin N Am. 2009;35(2):339–57.
29. Woodruff R. Hysteria: an evaluation of objective diagnostic criteria by the study of women with chronic medical illness. Br J Psychiatry. 1968;114(514): 1115–9.

21

Paroxetine in the treatment of premature ejaculation

Dong Zhang, Yue Cheng, Kerong Wu, Qi Ma, Junhui Jiang and Zejun Yan*

Abstract

Background: Paroxetine is one of the selective serotonin reuptake inhibitors (SSRIs) used in the treatment of premature ejaculation (PE). However, this use is not approved in many countries. The purpose of this systematic review and meta-analysis is to review the efficacy and safety of paroxetine for PE patients.

Methods: We searched relevant randomized, controlled trials through May 2018, using PubMed, Embase and Cochrane Central Register. The main endpoint included intra-vaginal ejaculatory latency time (IELT) and side effects in the treatment of PE. Cochrane Collaboration's Revman software, version 5.3, was used for statistical analysis.

Results: Out of 493 unique articles, a total of 19 randomized, controlled trials (RCTs) were reviewed. Quite a few RCTs were considered to have unclear risk of bias because of limited information. Pooled outcomes suggested that paroxetine was more effective than placebo, fluoxetine and escitalopram at increasing IELT (all $p < 0.05$). However, there existed a high level of heterogeneity in the paroxetine vs. fluoxetine groups and the paroxetine vs. placebo groups. Comparing paroxetine with tramadol, sertraline, phosphodiesterase 5 inhibitors (PDE5Is), local lidocaine gel, behaviour therapy or dapoxetine, we found that the increase in IELT was not statistically significant between groups. Paroxetine combined with tadalafil or behaviour therapy was more efficacious than paroxetine alone (all $p < 0.05$). Although the side effects in the combination group were more common than in the paroxetine alone group, the most common adverse events, such as nausea, muscle soreness, palpitation and flushing, were mild and tolerable. The main limitations of this systematic review and meta-analysis were the different definitions of PE and short follow-up times.

Conclusions: According to this systematic review and meta-analysis, paroxetine provided better efficacy than placebo, fluoxetine and escitalopram in the treatment of PE, with well-tolerated side effects. The combination group had better efficacy than the paroxetine alone group.

Keywords: Premature ejaculation, Paroxetine, Meta-analysis, Systematic review

* Correspondence: 35485787@qq.com
Department of Urology & Nephrology, Ningbo First Hospital, The affiliated hospital of ZheJiang University, 59, Liuting Street, Ningbo, Zhejiang, China

Background

Premature ejaculation (PE) is recognized as one of the most common diseases of sexual dysfunction, affecting approximately 20–30% of men [1]. It has been proved that PE can influence the quality of intercourse, resulting in distress and anxiety and even impacting the relationships between partners [2]. While the aetiology of PE remains controversial,it is increasingly becoming recognized that [3–5] psychological problems, somatic disorders and/or neurobiological disturbances, and polymorphisms of the serotonin transporter or its promoters frequently co-occur in the same individual. However, other potential aetiologic factors [6–10], including depression,erectile dysfunction,metabolic syndrome,chronic prostatitis and thyroid dysfunction, have been definitely established as causative in PE.

According to the new International Society for Sexual Medicine (ISSM) guidelines [11], PE is defined as "ejaculation that always occurs after less than 1 minute of vaginal penetration from the first sexual experience (lifelong PE), or a clinically significant and bothersome reduction in latency time, often ≤3 minutes (acquired PE),and the inability to delay ejaculation on all or nearly all vaginal penetrations,and negative personal consequences, such as distress, frustration and/or the avoidance of sexual intimacy." Therefore, we use intravaginal ejaculatory latency time (IELT) to evaluate the endpoint of PE.

Over the past few decades, many feasible therapies have been explored by andrologists, such as selective serotonin reuptake inhibitors (SSRIs), topical anaesthetics, tricyclic antidepressants, PDE5Is, α-receptor blockers and surgery. Although, many of them have been reported to be useful for PE with well-tolerated side effects, none of them has been approved by the FDA (Food and Drug Administration) except for dapoxetine. Paroxetine is one of the SSRIs, which increase the amount of 5-hydroxytryptamine (5-HT) in postsynaptic membrane receptors and thus delay ejaculation. Although it is not approved by the FDA, it has the advantage of lower dropouts and cost, with almost identical effects to dapoxetine [12, 13]. Recently, there have been numerous high-quality randomized, controlled trials (RCTs) comparing paroxetine with other therapeutic options for the treatment of PE. To our knowledge, this study is the first meta-analysis to report on the efficacy and safety of paroxetine in the treatment of PE. The purpose of this systematic review and meta-analysis is to review the efficacy and safety of paroxetine for PE patients.

Methods

Inclusion and exclusion criteria

The study inclusion criteria were diagnosis of PE but not erectile dysfunction, a stable relationship with the same sexual partner, and RCTs comparing paroxetine with other medical therapies for PE.

The study exclusion criteria were diabetes, hepatic or renal impairments, urogenital diseases, patients with ejaculation dysfunction, quasi-randomized trials, non-randomized trials, observational studies, case reports, and abstracts and letters.

Literature search and data sources

We used subject terms (MeSH) including "premature ejaculation" and "paroxetine" with their free words to search for relevant clinical trials through May 2018 in PubMed, Embase and Cochrane Central Register. The complete search used for PubMed was (premature ejaculation [MeSH terms] OR premature ejaculation [Text word]) AND (paroxetine [MeSH terms] OR paroxetine [Text word]). The primary research process was to find the whole articles that were relevant to paroxetine and other drugs for PE. Then, the eligible RCT articles were collected based on our criteria. All of the processes were independently completed by two authors. Consensus was reached by discussion if there was any disagreement. We tried our best to contact the corresponding authors if data were missing.

Data extraction

One reviewer read the articles and compiled notes of the authors, date of publication, drugs and dosage, number of participants, clinical effects, side effects and PE types. All numerical data were then checked by the other reviewer.

Quality assessment and statistical analysis

According to the Cochrane risk of bias tool [14] (including bias of selection, performance, detection, attrition, reporting, and other), we could define each item as low risk or unclear or high risk, finally devising a risk of bias summary graph. Two reviewers complete the quality assessment of each study. We used Review Manager software, version 5.3 (Cochrane Collaboration, Oxford, United Kingdom), to analyse dichotomous and continuous data on side effects and IELT, respectively. A fixed or the random effect model was applied for meta-analysis according to the value of heterogeneity, which was assessed by the Mantel-Haenszel chi-square test and I^2 statistic. If the p value was < 0.1 and $I^2 > 50\%$, it was suggested that the heterogeneity was unacceptable, and sensitivity analysis should be performed. We used the mean difference (MD) to compare the IELT and relative risk (RR) to compare side effects between the different groups. Funnel plots were used to assess the publication bias if more than 10 RCTs were included in a comparison. A p value less than 0.05 was considered to indicate statistical significance. The confidence interval was established at 95%.

Results

Description of studies

Search results and reporting quality

After searching the 3 databases, a total of 512 relevant articles were retrieved. According to the titles and abstracts of publications, 492 records were excluded because of repeats, irrelevance or not being RCTs. The remaining 20 full-text articles were uploaded and assessed for eligibility, and 19 of 20 met our criteria. Thus, 19 RCTs were included for systematic review and meta-analysis. Table 1 shows their characteristics, and Fig. 1 summarizes the inclusion process. Comparators included placebo, dapoxetine, tramadol, sertraline, PDE5Is, fluoxetine, behaviour therapy, local lidocaine gel, duloxetine, escitalopram, and combined therapy. The majority of the included RCTs were 4–12 weeks in duration. Only Wang's and Moudi's trials lasted for 6 months [15, 16]. All of the articles reported similar outcomes involving IELT. Other diffused distribution outcomes included sexual satisfaction score, side effects, premature ejaculation diagnostic tool (PEDT), International Index of Erectile Function (IIEF), premature ejaculation profile (PEP), Arabic Index of Premature Ejaculation (AIPE), libido and frequency of intercourse, which rendered pooled meta-analysis difficult. The only method that we could use was to depict these outcomes. If study data were missing, we attempted to contact the corresponding authors.

Cochrane's risk of bias tool was used to assess the quality of the articles on the basis of random sequence generation, allocation concealment, blinding of participants and personnel, blinding of outcomes assessment, incomplete outcome data, selective report and other biases. Then, a risk of bias summary graph was successfully generated, as Fig. 2 shows. We can see that a large number of RCTs were considered to have an unclear risk of bias because of a lack of adequate information from the articles. Gameel's and Abu's trails were considered at high risk of performance bias due to single blinding. One RCT was considered at high risk of attrition due to incomplete outcome data: there were 1.67, 18.33 and 36.67% of patients in the sildenafil, paroxetine and squeeze therapy groups, respectively, who withdrew from the trial due to little efficacy or side effects [15].

Efficacy

Paroxetine vs. placebo: A total of 7 RCTs met the condition [17–23]. Two RCTs lacked relevant standard deviations [21, 23]. The quality of these articles were described,but they were not included in the meta-analysis. Thus,based on 5 pooled RCTs [17–20, 22], the men treated with paroxetine 20 mg for 4–12 weeks had significantly increased IELT compared with placebo ($p = 0.01$). The MD in IELT was 2.96, in favour of paroxetine [(random effect) 95% confidence interval [Cl], 0.63 to 5.29; $p = 0.01$] (Fig. 3). Meta-analysis of these studies showed a high level of heterogeneity, which might have arisen from the difference in types of PE and treatment periods (Fig. 3). Seven RCTs favoured of paroxetine. One RCT [17] showed PEP changes from the baseline significantly greater than placebo, and two RCTs [18, 20] showed that the change in satisfaction score from baseline was more significant. One RCT reported that paroxetine had a significantly stronger ejaculation-delaying effect than placebo ($p < 0.05$), and it decreased PEDT significantly more than placebo without any side effects [21]. Safarinejad et al. [22] reported that paroxetine had better ability to delay ejaculation than placebo at the end of 12 weeks of treatment. Not only was IELT increased from 31 and 34 to 370 and 55, respectively, with paroxetine ($p < 0.05$) and placebo ($p > 0.05$), but the mean number of coitus episodes and IIEF value improved significantly in the paroxetine group ($p < 0.05$). A similar finding was reported by Abu et al. [23]. The IELT significantly improved from 38.66 to 173.86 in the paroxetine group, while the placebo group showed almost no change. The mean satisfaction score and PEDT in the paroxetine group improved more significant than with placebo. Therefore, paroxetine could have a significantly stronger ejaculation-delaying effect than placebo.

Where reported, side effects related to paroxetine included: headache, fatigue, nausea, dizziness, sleep disturbances, yawning, dry mouth, sweating, and constipation. The pooled relative risk of 3 RCTs [17, 22, 24] was 1.23 [RR (random effect) 95% Cl, 0.38 to 4.04; $p = 0.73$], which indicated no difference between the paroxetine and placebo groups in terms of adverse events (Fig. 4). Our pooled estimate showed significant heterogeneity ($I^2 = 65\%$), which might have arisen from the treatment period, dosage and inclusion criteria. Four RCTs [18–21] that followed up for 3–10 weeks showed no serious treatment-related side effects detected for paroxetine or placebo.

Paroxetine vs. tramadol: Three RCTs [17, 20, 25] provided evidence that suggested that the difference in IELT was not significant between the two groups [MD, 0.81; 95% [Cl], − 2.40 to 4.03; $p = 0.62$] (Fig. 3). One of 3 [17] reported that on-demand tramadol more significantly improved PEP than paroxetine at 4 weeks. Another RCT reported that there was no difference in terms of sexual satisfaction score after one month of on-demand treatment [20]. In addition, Alghobary et al. [25] compared the efficacy of daily paroxetine and on-demand tramadol, paroxetine and tramadol increased IELT after 6 weeks by 11- and 7-fold, respectively. After 12 weeks, the tramadol group decreased IELT to fivefold, while the paroxetine group increased IELT to 22-fold. The tendency of the Arabic Index of PE (AIPE) was consistent with IELT in the two groups. Paroxetine increased libido significantly more than tramadol at 12 weeks. Therefore, a longer treatment time should be used to explore the efficacy and safety of tramadol and paroxetine.

Side effects related to tramadol were sleep disturbance, dry mouth, vomiting and nausea, dizziness, fatigue, sweating, constipation and headache, which were similar with paroxetine ($p = 0.96$) [RR, 1.04; 95%

Table 1 Characteristics of included stuides

RCT, year, dose, duration	Treatment (numbers)	Outcomes	Adverse events	IELT (SD)	PE definition
Gammel et al. [20] 2013 20 mg 4 weeks Sunay et al. [21] 2011 20 mg 4 weeks Safarinejad et al. [22] 2006 20 mg 12 weeks	on-demand tramadol 50 mg/d (29), sildenafil 50 mg/d (30), paroxetine 20 mg/d (28), local lidocaine gel (30), placebo (27) daily paroxetine 20 mg/d (30), acupuncture (30), placebo (30), daily dapoxetine 60 mg/d (104), paroxetine 20 mg/d (105), placebo (100), daily dapoxetine 60 mg/d (104), paroxetine 20 mg/d (105), placebo (100)	IELT, sexual satisfaction scores IELT, PEDT IELT, IIEF, weekly intercourse episodes IELT, IIEF, weekly intercourse episodes	all adverse events were tolerable no side effects were observed well tolerated	5.85 (1.98), 3.8 (1.15), 3.1 (1.08), 2.97 (1.85), 1.35 (0.54) 1.17, 1.17, 0.42 2.98, 6.17, 0.92	IELT < 2 min in > 70% of sexual intercourse episodes IELTs of < 2 min in > 70% of coital attempts IELT < 2 min that occurred in > 90% of episodes of sexual inter course
Gong et al. [18] 2011 20 mg 4 weeks Ozcan et al. [33] 2015 20 mg 1 month	daily paroxetine 20 mg/d (40), placebo (40) daily duloxetine 40 mg/d(40), daily paroxetine 20 mg/d (40)	IELT, sexual satisfaction scores IELT, IIEF, PEP	well tolerated well tolerated	5.75 (1.24), 1.06 (0.28) 2.09 (0.12), 2.14 (0.15)	DSM-IV-TR lifelong PE
Abdel-Hamid et al. [24] 2001 20 mg 4 weeks	on-demand clomipramine 25 mg, on-demand sertraline 50 mg, on-demand paroxetine 20 mg, on-demand sildenafil 50 mg and the pause-squeeze technique	IELT, sexual satisfaction scores	mild to moderate	4, 3, 4, 15, 3	IELT ≤2 min
Abu et al. [23] 2018 30 mg 6 weeks	on-demand sildenafil 50 mg/d combined with dapoxetine 50 mg/d (30), sildenafil 50 mg/d (30), paroxetine 30 mg/d (30), dapoxetine 30 mg/d (30), placebo (30)	IELT, PEDT, sexual satisfaction	well tolerated	4.43, 2.93, 2.90, 2.86, 0.69	IELT ≤1 min
Otunctemur et al. [27] 2014 20 mg 4 weeks	daily fluoxetine 20 mg/d (20), sertraline 50 mg/d (20), paroxetine 20 mg/d (20), healthy control (40)	IELT	not mentioned	2.5 (0.69), 3.09 (1.15), 3.70 (0.86)	IELT < 1 min
Klrecci et al. [29] 2014 20 mg 4 weeks a	daily sertraline 50 mg/d (8), paroxetine 20 mg/d (8), healthy control (11)	IELT, IIEF	not mentioned	1.89 (0.51), 1.92 (0.49)	IELT < 1 min, primary PE
Kirecci et al. [28] 2014 20 mg 4 weeks b	daily sertraline 50 mg/d (20), paroxetine 20 mg/d (20), fluoxetine 20 mg/d (20)	IELT, IIEF	tolerated	1.71 (0.98), 1.78 (0.62), 1.55 (0.64)	lifelong PE (IELT of < 1 min)
Wang et al. [15] 2007 20 mg 6 months	on-demand sildenafil 50 mg/d (59), paroxetine 20 mg/d (649), squeeze technique (38)	IELT, PE grade, intercourse satisfaction score, frequency of intercourse	well tolerated	6.21 (1.86), 4.93 (1.36), 2.62 (0.69)	IELT < 2 min, primary PE
Alghobary et al. [25] 2010 20 mg 6 weeks	on-demand tramadol 50 mg/d (17), daily paroxetine 20 mg/d (18)	IELT, AIPE, libido, erection	well tolerated	3.00,3.84	DSM-IV-TR, lifelong PE
Polat et al. [26] 2015 20 mg 1 month	daily paroxetine 20 mg/d (50), on-demand tadalafil 20 mg (50), on-demand paroxetine 20 mg combined tadalafil 20 mg (50)	IELT, IIEF	well tolerated	1.96 (1.12), 1.84 (0.62), 2.92 (1.00)	lifelong PE
Waldinger et al. [19] 1998 20 mg 6 weeks	placebo (9), fluvoxamine 100 mg/d (10), fluoxetine 20 mg/d (10), paroxetine 20 mg/d (11), sertraline 50 mg/d (11),	IELT	well tolerated	0.48 (0.41), 55 (70), 3.5 (4.18), 7.9 (19.1), 1.95 (1.45)	lifelong PE (IELT of < 1 min)
Shao et al. [32] 2008 20 mg 8 weeks	paroxetine 20 mg/d (40), behaviour therapy (40), paroxetine 10 mg/d combined behaviour therapy (40)	IELT, CIPE-5	well tolerated	4.4 (0.5), 4.2 (0.4), 4.8 (0.5)	not mentioned

Table 1 Characteristics of included stuides *(Continued)*

RCT, year, dose, duration	Treatment (numbers)	Outcomes	Adverse events	IELT (SD)	PE definition
Moudi et al. [16] 2016 10 mg 6 months Zhang et al. [30] 2012 20 mg 12 weeks Hamidi-Madani et al. [17] 2018 20 mg 12 weeks Arafa et al. [31] 2007 20 mg 4 weeks	paroxetine 10 mg/d (50), paroxetine 10 mg/d combined tadalafil 10 mg/d (50) behaviour therapy (22), paroxetine 20 mg/d (32), paroxetine 30 mg/d (32), daily sertraline 50 mg/d (28), daily sertraline 100 mg/d (30) on-demand tramadol 50 mg/d (48), paroxetine 20 mg/d (46), placebo (32) daily fluoxetine 20 mg/d (33), escitalopram 10 mg/d (37), paroxetine 20 mg/d (30)	IELT, IIEF IELT, sexual satisfaction IELT, PEP AIPE, IELT	well tolerated well tolerated well tolerated, well tolerated,	4.8 (1), 5.3 (2)—— 2.29 (1.29), 1.52 (1.23), 1.30 (0.92) 2.4 (0.4), 2.5 (0.3), 2.7 (0.2)	lifelong PE (IELT of < 1.5 min) not mentioned lifelong PE (IELT of < 1 min) IELT ≤2 min

RCT randomized, controlled trial, *IELT* intravaginal ejaculatory latency time, *PEP* premature ejaculation profile, *IIEF* international index of erectile function, *AIPE* Arabic index of premature ejaculation, *CIPE-5* Chinese index of premature ejaculation, *PEDT* premature ejaculation diagnostic tool, *PE* premature ejaculation, *SD* standard deviation, *DSM-IV* Diagnostic and Statistical Manual of Mental Disorders, fourth edition

[Cl] 0.18 to 5.89] (Fig. 4). All of the articles showed that paroxetine and tramadol have well-tolerated side effects [17, 20, 25].

Paroxetine vs. PDE5Is: Five RCTs compared the safety and efficacy of paroxetine with those of tramadol [15, 20, 23, 24, 26]. Because 2 RCTs lacked relevant standard deviations [23, 24],3 other pooled RCTs [15, 20, 26] showed that paroxetine had similar effects to PDE5Is,with between-group difference in IELT of – 0.59 [95% [Cl], – 1.45 to 0.26;$p = 0.17$]. While there was a high level of heterogeneity ($I^2 = 88\%$) (Fig. 3), which may come from the difference type of PE and treatment period. One RCT [20] showed that the on-demand sildenafil group has better sexual satisfaction scores than the daily paroxetine group. Wang et al. [15] reported that 1.7 and 18.3% of patients withdrew from the study in the sildenafil and paroxetine groups, respectively, after 6 months. One

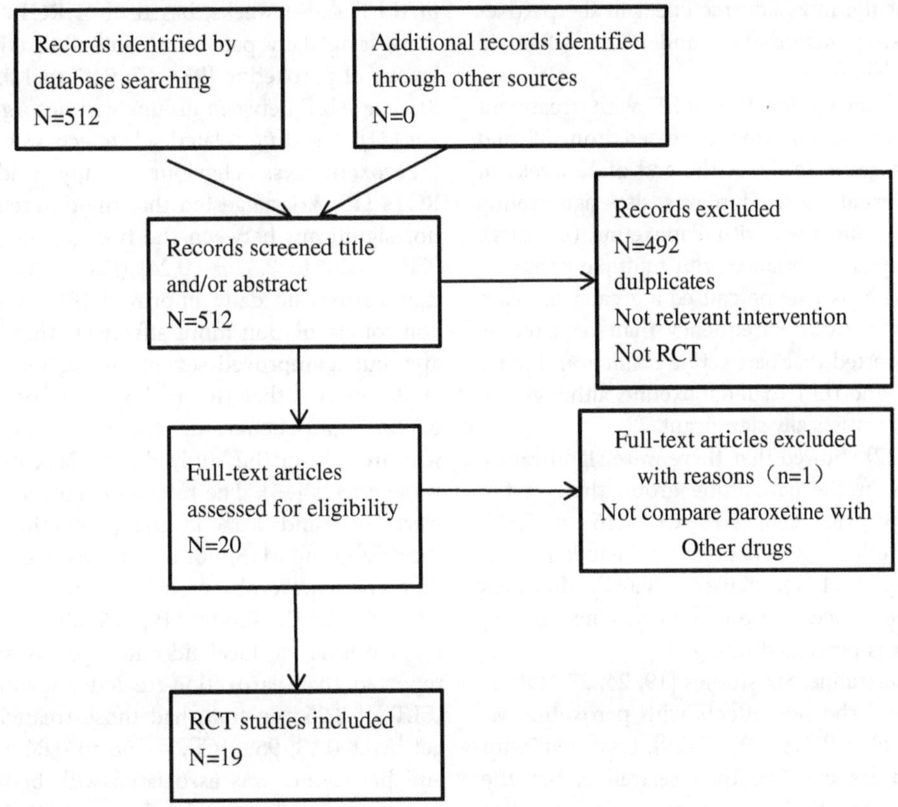

Fig. 1 Flow diagram of the study selection process. RCT = randomized controlled trail

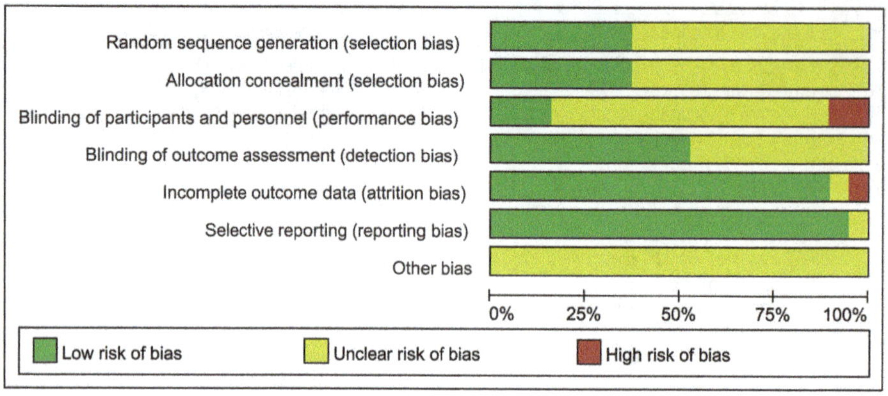

Fig. 2 Overall quality assessment for the selected articles

RCT [23] reported that there was no significant difference in PEDT or satisfaction score after 6 weeks of treatment between the two groups.

The relative risk of side effects between two groups pooled from 3 RCTs [24, 26] was 1.14 [RR (random effect) 95% Cl, 0.76 to 1.73; $p = 0.52$], as shown in Fig. 4. According to 5 RCTs, all side effects were well tolerated. One RCT showed that sleep disturbances, dry mouth, nausea, dizziness, fatigue, vomiting, sweating, headache, flushing, hypotension and nasal congestion were reported with paroxetine and sildenafil [20]. One RCT [23] reported that the most adverse effect in the paroxetine group was sleep disturbance, and in the sildenafil group, it was headache.

Paroxetine vs. dapoxetine: The IELT with treatment using paroxetine and dapoxetine increased from 38 and 31 to 37 and 179, respectively, at the end of 12 weeks in one RCT [22]. Sexual satisfaction was also significantly higher with paroxetine than with dapoxetine ($p = 0.04$). According to analysis of variance with multiple comparisons, treatment with paroxetine caused a greater increase in mean weekly intercourse frequency than dapoxetine. Abu et al. [23] reported that paroxetine resulted in higher satisfaction scores and IELT than dapoxetine, although the difference was not statistically significant.

A single RCT [22] showed that there were significantly more side effects in the paroxetine group than in the dapoxetine group [RR, 2.50; 95% Cl, 1.16 to 5.38]. Drug-related side effects with dapoxetine included headache (6.6%), fatigue (10%), nausea (26.6%), dizziness (10%), sleep disturbances (13.3%) and yawing (16.7%) [23]. A forest plot is presented in Fig. 4.

Paroxetine vs. sertraline: Six studies [19, 24, 27–30] investigated IELT and the side effects with paroxetine vs. sertraline. In 4 pooled RCTs [19, 27–29], treatment with paroxetine was more effective than sertraline, but the difference was not statistically significant [MD, 0.19; 95% Cl, − 0.14 to 0.52; $p = 0.26$] (Fig. 3). There was no evidence of statistical heterogeneity between the groups as assessed by the χ^2 test ($\chi^2 = 3.39$; $I^2 = 12\%$; $p = 0.34$) (Fig. 3). One RCT reported that paroxetine had greater efficacy than sertraline [24], while Zhang et al. [30] showed that there was no difference between the two groups in terms of IELT and sexual satisfaction score. The relative risk of side effects between the two groups pooled from 2 RCTs [24, 30] was 1.01 [RR (random effect)95% Cl, 0.44 to 2.33; $p = 0.98$], as shown in Fig. 4. All side effects were tolerable.

Paroxetine vs. fluoxetine: The between-group difference in IELT at 4–6 weeks, based on 4 RCTs [19, 27, 28, 31] comparing daily paroxetine with fluoxetine, was 0.54 in favour of paroxetine [95% Cl, 0.07 to 1.02; $p = 0.02$] (Fig. 3). The AIEF between groups was not significantly different [31]. The drug-related side effects were tolerable.

Paroxetine vs. behaviour therapy: Evidence from two RCTs [15, 32] suggested that the difference in IELT was not significant between the two groups [MD, 1.25; 95% [Cl], − 0.82 to 3.31; $p = 0.24$] (Fig. 3). One of 2 reported that paroxetine daily improved IELT and the ability to control ejaculation more effectively than behaviour therapy, but it improved sexual satisfaction less [32]. Wang et al. reported that 18.3 and 36.7% of patients in the paroxetine and behaviour therapy groups, respectively, withdrew from the study due to lack of efficacy or adverse effects [15]. The rates of occurrence of side effects were 24.4 and 1.6% in the paroxetine and behaviour therapy groups [15, 30, 32], respectively. No significant differences were observed between the two groups [RR, 8.66; 95% Cl, 0.83 to 90.11; $p = 0.07$] [15, 30, 32] (Fig. 4).

Paroxetine vs. local lidocaine gel: A single RCT [20] reported that paroxetine-treated patients had a longer IELT, of 3.25 min than had those treated with lidocaine gel [MD, 0.13; 95% [Cl], − 0.58 to 0.84, $p = 0.72$] (Fig. 3), and paroxetine was associated with better sexual satisfaction scores than the local anaesthetic of 3.25 and 2.97 points, respectively. The most common side effects were

Study or Subgroup	Paroxetine Mean	SD	Total	comparator Mean	SD	Total	Weight	Mean Difference IV, Random, 95% CI
1.1.1 paroxetine vs placebo-end of study values								
Gameel 2013 20mg 4weeks	3.1	1.08	28	1.35	0.54	27	5.1%	1.75 [1.30, 2.20]
Gong 2011 20mg 4weeks	5.75	1.24	40	1.06	0.28	40	5.2%	4.69 [4.30, 5.08]
Hamidi-Madani 2018 20mg 12week	1.52	1.23	46	1.3	0.92	32	5.0%	0.22 [-0.26, 0.70]
Safarinejad 2006 20mg 12weeks	6.17	11.2	105	0.92	11.2	100	1.2%	5.25 [2.18, 8.32]
Waldinger 1998 20mg 6weeks	7.9	19.1	11	0.48	0.41	9	0.1%	7.42 [-3.87, 18.71]
Subtotal (95% CI)			**230**			**208**	**16.6%**	**2.96 [0.63, 5.29]**
Heterogeneity: Tau² = 5.35; Chi² = 220.74, df = 4 (P < 0.00001); I² = 98%								
Test for overall effect: Z = 2.49 (P = 0.01)								
1.1.2 paroxetine vs. tramadol-end of study values								
Alghobary 2010 20mg 6weeks	6.31	4.9	35	1.62	1.31	35	2.6%	4.69 [3.01, 6.37]
Gameel 2013 20mg 4weeks	3.1	1.08	28	5.85	1.98	29	4.3%	-2.75 [-3.57, -1.93]
Hamidi-Madani 2018 20mg 12week	2.28	1.29	46	1.52	1.23	48	5.0%	0.76 [0.25, 1.27]
Subtotal (95% CI)			**109**			**112**	**11.9%**	**0.81 [-2.40, 4.03]**
Heterogeneity: Tau² = 7.73; Chi² = 81.03, df = 2 (P < 0.00001); I² = 98%								
Test for overall effect: Z = 0.50 (P = 0.62)								
1.1.3 paroxetine vs sertraline-end of study values								
Kirecci 2014 20mg 4weeks b	1.78	0.62	20	1.71	0.98	20	5.0%	0.07 [-0.44, 0.58]
Kirecci 2014 20mg 4weeks a	1.92	0.49	8	1.89	0.51	11	5.1%	0.03 [-0.42, 0.48]
Otunctemur 2014 20mg 4weeks	3.7	0.86	20	3.09	1.15	20	4.7%	0.61 [-0.02, 1.24]
Waldinger 1998 20mg 6weeks	7.9	19.1	11	1.95	1.45	11	0.1%	5.95 [-5.37, 17.27]
Subtotal (95% CI)			**59**			**62**	**14.9%**	**0.19 [-0.14, 0.52]**
Heterogeneity: Tau² = 0.01; Chi² = 3.39, df = 3 (P = 0.34); I² = 12%								
Test for overall effect: Z = 1.12 (P = 0.26)								
1.1.4 paroxetine vs. PDE5 inhibitors-end of study values								
Gameel 2013 20mg 4weeks	3.1	1.08	28	3.8	1.15	30	4.9%	-0.70 [-1.27, -0.13]
Polat 2015 20mg 1month	1.96	1.12	50	1.84	0.62	50	5.2%	0.12 [-0.23, 0.47]
Wang 2007 20mg 6months	4.93	1.36	49	6.21	1.86	59	4.8%	-1.28 [-1.89, -0.67]
Subtotal (95% CI)			**127**			**139**	**14.9%**	**-0.59 [-1.45, 0.26]**
Heterogeneity: Tau² = 0.50; Chi² = 17.13, df = 2 (P = 0.0002); I² = 88%								
Test for overall effect: Z = 1.36 (P = 0.17)								
1.1.5 paroxetine vs. fluoxetine-end of study values								
Arafa 2007 20mg 4weeks	2.7	0.2	30	2.4	0.4	33	5.4%	0.30 [0.15, 0.45]
Kirecci 2014 20mg 4weeks b	1.78	0.62	20	1.55	0.64	20	5.2%	0.23 [-0.16, 0.62]
Otunctemur 2014 20mg 4weeks	3.7	0.86	20	2.5	0.69	20	5.0%	1.20 [0.72, 1.68]
Waldinger 1998 20mg 6weeks	7.9	19.1	11	3.5	4.18	10	0.1%	4.40 [-7.18, 15.98]
Subtotal (95% CI)			**81**			**83**	**15.7%**	**0.54 [0.07, 1.02]**
Heterogeneity: Tau² = 0.14; Chi² = 13.08, df = 3 (P = 0.004); I² = 77%								
Test for overall effect: Z = 2.24 (P = 0.02)								
1.1.6 paroxetine vs. behaviour therapy-end of study values								
Shao 2008 20mg 8weeks	4.4	0.5	40	4.2	0.4	40	5.4%	0.20 [0.00, 0.40]
Wang 2007 20mg 6months	4.93	1.36	49	2.62	0.69	38	5.1%	2.31 [1.87, 2.75]
Subtotal (95% CI)			**89**			**78**	**10.5%**	**1.25 [-0.82, 3.31]**
Heterogeneity: Tau² = 2.20; Chi² = 73.56, df = 1 (P < 0.00001); I² = 99%								
Test for overall effect: Z = 1.18 (P = 0.24)								
1.1.7 paroxetine vs.local lidocaine-end of study values								
Gameel 2013 20mg 4weeks	3.1	1.08	35	2.97	1.85	35	4.6%	0.13 [-0.58, 0.84]
Subtotal (95% CI)			**35**			**35**	**4.6%**	**0.13 [-0.58, 0.84]**
Heterogeneity: Not applicable								
Test for overall effect: Z = 0.36 (P = 0.72)								
1.1.8 paroxetine vs. duloxetine-end of study values								
Ozcan 2015 20mg 1month	2.14	0.15	40	2.09	0.12	40	5.5%	0.05 [-0.01, 0.11]
Subtotal (95% CI)			**40**			**40**	**5.5%**	**0.05 [-0.01, 0.11]**
Heterogeneity: Not applicable								
Test for overall effect: Z = 1.65 (P = 0.10)								
1.1.9 paroxetine vs. escitalopram -end of study values								
Arafa 2007 20mg 4weeks	2.7	0.2	30	2.5	0.3	37	5.4%	0.20 [0.08, 0.32]
Subtotal (95% CI)			**30**			**37**	**5.4%**	**0.20 [0.08, 0.32]**
Heterogeneity: Not applicable								
Test for overall effect: Z = 3.26 (P = 0.001)								
Total (95% CI)			**800**			**794**	**100.0%**	**0.65 [0.27, 1.02]**
Heterogeneity: Tau² = 0.67; Chi² = 805.12, df = 23 (P < 0.00001); I² = 97%								
Test for overall effect: Z = 3.37 (P = 0.0008)								
Test for subgroup differences: Chi² = 18.48, df = 8 (P = 0.02), I² = 56.7%								

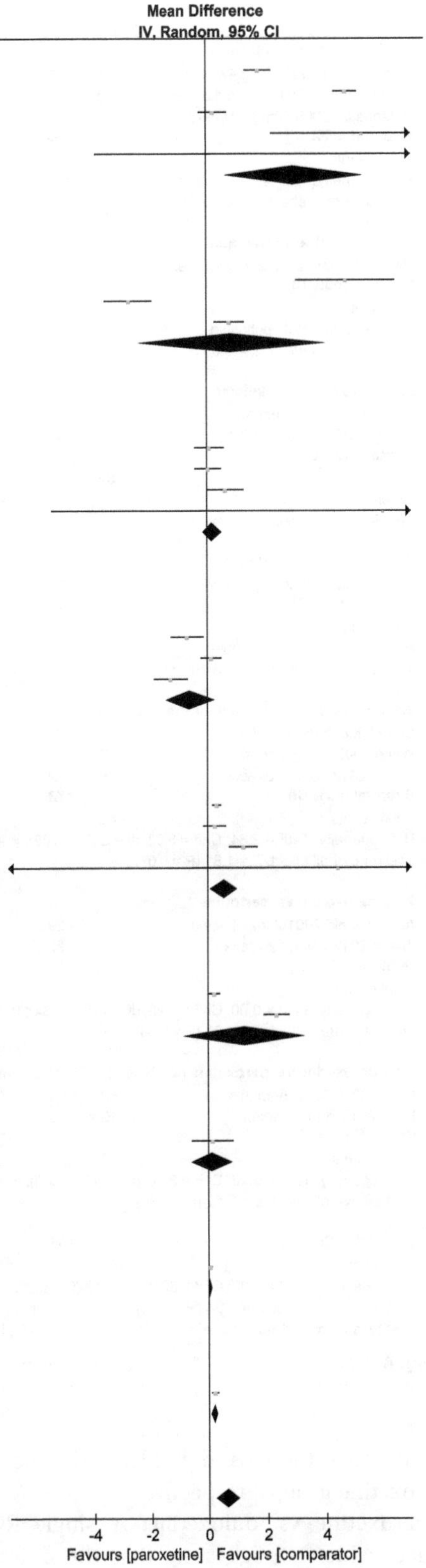

Fig. 3 Forest plot of IELT between paroxetine and other drugs. CI,confidence interval;IELT, intra-vaginal ejaculatory latency time; PDE-5, phosphodiesterase-5 inhibitor; SD, standard deviation

Study or Subgroup	paroxetine Events	paroxetine Total	comparators Events	comparators Total	Weight	Risk Ratio M-H, Random, 95% CI
2.1.1 paroxetine vs placebo						
Abdel-Hamid 2001 20mg 4weeks	3	29	7	28	6.3%	0.41 [0.12, 1.44]
Hamidi-Madani 2018 20mg 12week	3	46	2	48	4.1%	1.57 [0.27, 8.94]
Safarinejad 2006 20mg 12weeks	21	105	8	100	9.7%	2.50 [1.16, 5.38]
Subtotal (95% CI)		**180**		**176**	**20.1%**	**1.23 [0.38, 4.04]**
Total events	27		17			
Heterogeneity: Tau² = 0.71; Chi² = 5.79, df = 2 (P = 0.06); I² = 65%						
Test for overall effect: Z = 0.35 (P = 0.73)						
2.1.2 paroxetine vs tramadol						
Hamidi-Madani 2018 20mg 12week	3	46	2	32	4.1%	1.04 [0.18, 5.89]
Subtotal (95% CI)		**46**		**32**	**4.1%**	**1.04 [0.18, 5.89]**
Total events	3		2			
Heterogeneity: Not applicable						
Test for overall effect: Z = 0.05 (P = 0.96)						
2.1.3 paroxetine vs. tadalafil						
Polat 2015 20mg 1month	15	50	12	50	10.7%	1.25 [0.65, 2.39]
Wang 2007 20mg 6months	17	49	19	59	11.6%	1.08 [0.63, 1.84]
Subtotal (95% CI)		**99**		**109**	**22.3%**	**1.14 [0.76, 1.73]**
Total events	32		31			
Heterogeneity: Tau² = 0.00; Chi² = 0.12, df = 1 (P = 0.73); I² = 0%						
Test for overall effect: Z = 0.64 (P = 0.52)						
2.1.4 paroxetine vs. dapoxetine						
Safarinejad 2006 20mg 12weeks	21	105	8	100	9.7%	2.50 [1.16, 5.38]
Subtotal (95% CI)		**105**		**100**	**9.7%**	**2.50 [1.16, 5.38]**
Total events	21		8			
Heterogeneity: Not applicable						
Test for overall effect: Z = 2.34 (P = 0.02)						
2.1.5 paroxetine vs. behaviour therapy						
Shao 2008 20mg 8weeks	20	80	0	40	2.0%	20.75 [1.29, 334.57]
Wang 2007 20mg 6months	17	60	0	60	1.9%	35.00 [2.15, 569.06]
Zhang 2012 20mg 12weeks	5	32	2	22	4.8%	1.72 [0.37, 8.08]
Subtotal (95% CI)		**172**		**122**	**8.7%**	**8.66 [0.83, 90.11]**
Total events	42		2			
Heterogeneity: Tau² = 2.84; Chi² = 6.02, df = 2 (P = 0.05); I² = 67%						
Test for overall effect: Z = 1.81 (P = 0.07)						
2.1.6 paroxetine vs. sertraline						
Abdel-Hamid 2001 20mg 4weeks	5	29	3	29	5.8%	1.67 [0.44, 6.34]
Zhang 2012 20mg 12weeks	5	32	6	28	7.4%	0.73 [0.25, 2.13]
Subtotal (95% CI)		**61**		**57**	**13.2%**	**1.01 [0.44, 2.33]**
Total events	10		9			
Heterogeneity: Tau² = 0.00; Chi² = 0.90, df = 1 (P = 0.34); I² = 0%						
Test for overall effect: Z = 0.02 (P = 0.98)						
2.1.7 paroxetine vs. paroxetine combined PDE5 inhibitors						
Moudi 2016 10mg 6months	12	50	23	50	11.3%	0.52 [0.29, 0.93]
Polat 2015 20mg 1month	15	50	12	50	10.7%	1.25 [0.65, 2.39]
Subtotal (95% CI)		**100**		**100**	**21.9%**	**0.80 [0.34, 1.88]**
Total events	27		35			
Heterogeneity: Tau² = 0.28; Chi² = 3.88, df = 1 (P = 0.05); I² = 74%						
Test for overall effect: Z = 0.52 (P = 0.60)						
Total (95% CI)		**763**		**696**	**100.0%**	**1.33 [0.88, 2.02]**
Total events	162		104			
Heterogeneity: Tau² = 0.32; Chi² = 32.23, df = 13 (P = 0.002); I² = 60%						
Test for overall effect: Z = 1.34 (P = 0.18)						
Test for subgroup differences: Chi² = 7.30, df = 6 (P = 0.29), I² = 17.8%						

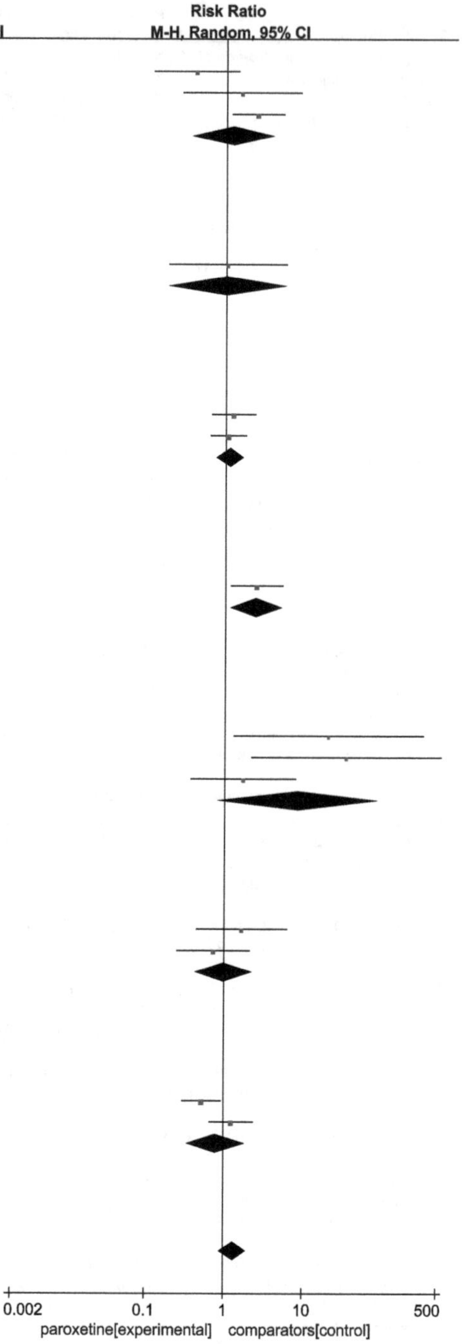

Fig. 4 Pooled estimate of side effects of paroxetine vs. other medical therapy

penile anaesthesia and headache in the lidocaine and paroxetine groups, respectively.

Paroxetine vs. duloxetine: A single RCT [33] provided evidence suggesting that the difference in IELT was not significant between the two groups at 1 month of treatment [MD, 0.05; 95% [CI], −0.01 to 0.11;$p = 0.1$] (Fig. 3). Drug-related side effects included yawning and somnolence (25%), nausea (25%) and asthenia (10%) in the paroxetine group and nausea (25%), headache (12.5%), dry mouth (2.5%), constipation (5%) and dizziness (7.5%) in the duloxetine group.

Paroxetine vs. escitalopram: Only one RCT [31] compared IELT and adverse events between paroxetine and escitalopram groups. Treatment with paroxetine was found to be significantly more effective based on IELT than escitalopram [MD, 0.2; 95% [Cl], 0.08 to 0.32;p = 0.001] (Fig. 3). Both drugs were generally well tolerated.

Paroxetine combined with tadalafil vs. paroxetine: The between-group difference in IELT, based on 2 RCTs [16, 26] comparing daily paroxetine alone with paroxetine combined with tadalafil, was – 0.79 in favour of the latter [95% Cl, – 1.23 to – 0.35;$p = 0.0004$] (Fig. 5), while there was no significant difference in side effects [RR, 0.80; 95% [Cl], 0.34 to 1.88; $p = 0.6$] [16, 26] (Fig. 4).

Paroxetine combined with behaviour therapy vs. paroxetine: A single RCT [32] reported that patients treated with paroxetine combined with behaviour therapy had a significantly longer IELT than had those treated with paroxetine alone [MD, – 0.40; 95% [Cl], – 0.62 to – 0.18;$p = 0.0003$] (Fig. 5). The rates of occurrence of side effects were 10.0 and 40% in the paroxetine and combined groups, respectively, but all side effects, including dizziness, dry mouth, sleep disturbances and fatigue, were tolerable.

Discussion

This meta-analysis, including 19 RCTs comparing the efficacy and safety of paroxetine with other drugs for PE, showed that, compared with placebo, fluoxetine and escitalopram, paroxetine could improve IELT significantly with tolerable side effects. However, when comparing paroxetine with tramadol, sertraline, PDE5Is, local lidocaine gel, behaviour therapy or dapoxetine, we found that the increase in IELT was not statistically significant. Furthermore, paroxetine combined with tadalafil or behaviour therapy was more efficacious than paroxetine alone (all $p < 0.05$). According to published articles from 1998 to 2018, the definition of PE has changed greatly, and the main outcomes only include IELT. Other diffused distribution outcomes included sexual satisfaction score, side effects, PEDT, IIEF, PEP, AIPE, libido and frequency of intercourse, causing difficulty in pooling for meta-analysis. Based on the new ISSM guidelines [11], PE is more than only a short time to ejaculation, and the ability to control ejaculation and personal emotions have been identified as important factors. Therefore, it is not convincing to us to compare IELT only between different drugs in the treatment of PE. Analysing the diffused distribution outcomes, some RCTs reported that paroxetine was associated with better sexual satisfaction than placebo, dapoxetine and lidocaine gel [18, 20, 22, 23], better PEP than placebo and tramadol [17], a better ejaculation-delay effect than placebo and behaviour therapy [21, 22, 32], better mean numbers of coitus episodes than placebo and dapoxetine [22], a better PEDT and IIEF values than placebo and better libido and AIEF than tramadol [21, 23, 25]. Conversely, evidence from other RCTs showed that there was no significant difference in sexual satisfaction between paroxetine and tramadol or dapoxetine [20, 23], no difference in PEDT between paroxetine and PDE5Is [23], and no difference in AIEF between paroxetine and fluoxetine [31]. The possible reasons for these results include the different types of PE and treatment periods.

The ejaculation reflex mainly includes two pathways: peripheral and central. First, during intercourse, the glans of the penis is stimulated, triggering the pudendal sensory nerves; the signal is then transferred to the spinal cord. After the spinal cord receives the signal, the sensory information is converted into secretory and motor signal output, which induces contraction of the epididymis, vas deferens, seminal vesicles, prostate and bladder neck, in turn rhythmically leading to ejaculation through the distal urethra [34]. The ejaculation reflex is also associated with serotonin and dopamine in the central nervous system. The most researched neurotransmitter is 5-HT. Some subtypes (5-HT1a) reduce ejaculatory latency, and other subtypes (5-HT1b, 5-HT2c) prolong ejaculatory latency [35–37]. Paroxetine is one of the SSRIs that increases the amounts of 5-HT in postsynaptic membrane receptors and thus delays

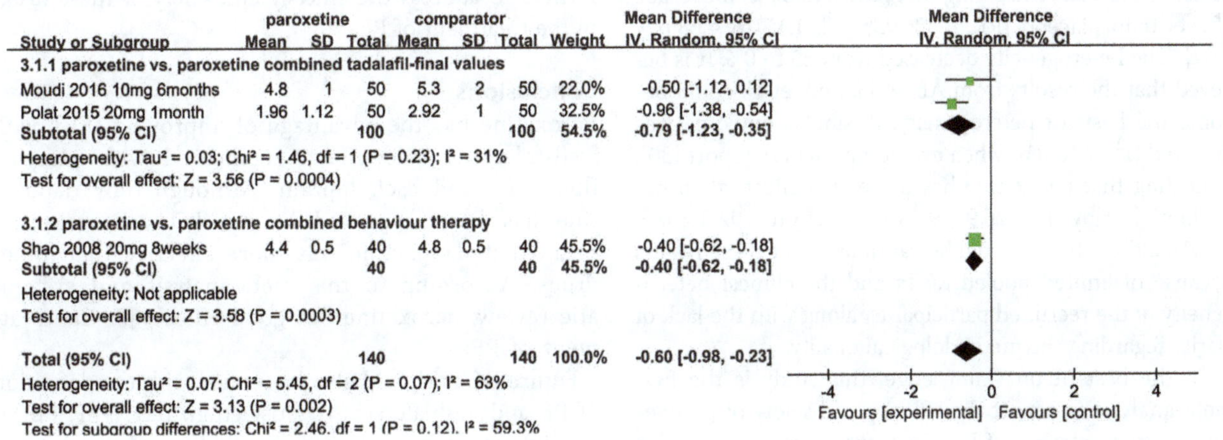

Fig. 5 Pooled estimate of IELT of paroxetine vs. combined therapy

ejaculation. Although not approved by the FDA, compared with the dapoxetine, it has the advantage of lower dropouts and cost with almost identical effects [12, 13]. According to a single RCT [22], paroxetine increased IELT significantly more than dapoxetine ($p = 0.01$). Furthermore, weekly intercourse frequency and satisfaction score were also improved, and the side effects were well tolerated [22, 23]. The difference in IELT between paroxetine and dapoxetine requires more RCTs to confirm.

We evaluated the heterogeneity of each comparison regarding the pooled results by excluding single studies sequentially. The results showed that the heterogeneity remained at a high level in the paroxetine vs. placebo group and the paroxetine vs. tramadol group, validating the rationality of our outcomes. The reasons for this finding might have arisen from the different types of PE, treatment periods and sample sizes. However, in the paroxetine vs. PDE5Is and paroxetine vs. fluoxetine groups, when excluded Polat's and Otunctemur's articles, the results showed that the heterogeneity decreased from 88 and 77% to 46 and 0%, respectively. Analysing the data from Polat's study, a similar IELT value following treatment with paroxetine or PDE5Is might be the cause of this situation. However, Based on data from Otunctemur's study, the heterogeneity might have been due to several design differences among the studies,including patient selection and limited sample sizes. With this point in mind, we excluded their research, and the results of the sensitivity analysis showed that the between-group difference in IELT, based on 2 RCTs [15, 20] comparing daily paroxetine with PDE5Is, was − 0.98 in favour of PDE5Is [95% Cl, − 1.55 to − 0.41; $p = 0.0007$]. Further, based on 3 pooled RCTs [19, 28, 31], the patients treated with paroxetine 20 mg had significantly increased IELT, compared with fluoxetine ($p < 0.0001$). The MD in IELT was 0.29 in favour of paroxetine [(random effect) 95% [Cl], 0.15 to 0.43; $p <$ 0.0001]. The between-group difference in side effects, after excluding 1 RCT [24] comparing daily paroxetine with placebo, was 2.32, indicating that paroxetine has more side effects than placebo [RR, 2.32; 95% Cl, 1.15 to 4.68;$p =$ 0.02]. The heterogeneity decreased from 65 to 0%. It is believed that the results from Abdel-Hamidi et al. could become the basis of heterogeneity. A similar outcome was detected (I^2 67 to 0%) when excluding Zhang's report [30], indicating that paroxetine has more side effects than behaviour therapy [RR, 26.93; 95% [Cl], 3.76 to 192.88; $p =$ 0.001], although we should be cautious about these results because of limited pooled RCTs and the clinical heterogeneity of the recruited participants, along with the lack of clarify regarding the methodological quality.

To the best of our knowledge, this study is the first meta-analysis to report the efficacy and safety of paroxetine in the treatment of PE. Therefore, it is necessary for urologists to update these articles because paroxetine is still not approved by the FDA. Furthermore, the incidence of drug-related side effects, such as dizziness, dry mouth, sleep disturbances and fatigue, could be pooled and evaluated between different drugs.

There were some limitations to this meta-analysis. First, the definition of PE is controversial. The new characteristics of PE are described above [11]. While more than 8 types of definition could be seen in 19 RCTs, mainly IELT, some RCTs defined PE as IELT< 2 min, < 1 min, and < 1.5 min, and some articles used the DSM-IV guideline, which might have influenced the results in the end. For example, if patient A improved primarily in IELT from 25 s to 59 s (PE defined as IELT < 1 min), and patient B improved in IELT from 119 s to 125 s (PE defined as IELT < 2 min) after treatment, it indicated that patient A had better efficacy in light of the change from baseline. However, an increase in IELT from 25 to 59 s (still < 1 min) was likely not clinically relevant based on the definition of PE, and we could only compare the end values, such as 59 and 125, regarding IELT. Therefore, the difference between the two groups could have caused false positives. It is recommended that subgroup analysis be performed according to the same definition of PE in the future. Second, the majority of the included RCTs were 4–12 weeks in duration. Only Wang's and Moudi's trials lasted 6 months [15, 16]. A longer-term follow-up should be performed to explore the efficacy and safety of paroxetine. Third, we searched PubMed, Embase and Cochrane Central Register but excluded quasi-randomized trials, non-randomized trials, observational studies, case reports, abstract and letters, which resulted in a sample that was not large. Fourth, funnel plots could not be used to assess publication bias because of insufficient RCT comparisons. Finally, only one RCT compared local lidocaine, duloxetine and escitalopram with paroxetine in meta-analysis, which could have increased the likelihood of false negatives and false positives. In all, more high-quality RCTs should be performed to address the efficacy and safety of these drugs in the treatment of PE.

Conclusions

Paroxetine has the advantage of improving IELT with well-tolerated side effects, compared with placebo, fluoxetine and escitalopram. Although only dapoxetine has been approved by the FDA, it does not mean that dapoxetine was more effective than other drugs. According to this meta-analysis and systematic review, paroxetine has good efficacy in the treatment of PE.

Future RCTs should also be unified with the definition of PE and evaluate sexual satisfaction, IIEF, PEP, PEDT, etc. A longer-term follow-up should be performed to explore the efficacy and safety of paroxetine.

Abbreviations

SSRIs: Selective serotonin reuptake inhibitors; PE: Premature ejaculation; IELT: Intra-vaginal ejaculatory latency time; RCTs: Randomized controlled trials; PDE5Is: Phosphodiesterase 5 inhibitors; ISSM: International Society for Sexual Medicine; FDA: Food and Drug Administration; 5-HT: 5-hydroxytryptamine; MD: Mean difference; RR: Relative risk; PEDT: Premature ejaculation diagnostic tool; IIEF: International Index of Erectile Function; PEP: Premature ejaculation profile; AIPE: Arabic index of Premature Ejaculation; CIPE-5: Chinese index of premature ejaculation; PEDT: Premature ejaculation diagnostic tool; PE: Premature ejaculation; SD: Standard deviation; DSM-IV: Diagnostic and statistical manual of mental disorders, fourth edition; CI: Confidence interval

Acknowledgements

Not applicable.

Authors' contributions

All authors participated in the conception of the paper.DZ and ZJY made substantial contributions to design, acquire the data. DZ drafted the manuscript. KRW and YC analysed and interpreted the data. ZJY,QM and JHJ commented on revisions to the manuscript. All authors read and approved the final manuscript.

References

1. Porst H, Montorsi F, Rosen R C, Gaynor L,Grupe S, Alexander J. The premature ejaculation prevalence and attitudes (PEPA) survey: prevalence, comorbidities, and professional help-seeking [J] Eur Urol, 2007,51(3):816–823, 824. DOI:https://doi.org/10.1016/j.eururo.2006.07.004. PMID:16934919
2. Kempeneers P, Andrianne R, Cuddy M, Blairy S. Sexual cognitions, trait anxiety, sexual anxiety, and distress in men with different subtypes of premature ejaculation and in their partners [J]. J Sex Marital Ther, 2018,44(4):319–332. DOI: https://doi.org/10.1080/0092623X.2017.1405299 .PMID:29161211.
3. Saitz T R, Serefoglu E C. Advances in understanding and treating premature ejaculation [J]. Nat Rev Urol, 2015,12(11):629–640. DOI:https://doi.org/10.1038/nrurol.2015.252 .PMID:26502991.
4. Safarinejad MR. Retraction statement: analysis of association between the 5-HTTLPR and STin2 polymorphisms in the serotonin-transporter gene and clinical response to a selective serotonin reuptake inhibitor (sertraline) in patients with premature ejaculation [J]. BJU Int. 2015;115(3):E9. 25830184. https://doi.org/10.1111/bju.13062.
5. Jern P, Eriksson E, Westberg L. A reassessment of the possible effects of the serotonin transporter gene linked polymorphism 5-HTTLPR on premature ejaculation [J]. Arch Sex Behav. 2013;42(1):45–9. 22810993. https://doi.org/10.1007/s10508-012-9991-x.
6. Mourikis I, Antoniou M, Matsouka E, Vousoura E, Tzavara C, Ekizoglou C, et al. Anxiety and depression among Greek men with primary erectile dysfunction and premature ejaculation [J]. Ann General Psychiatry. 2015;14:34. 26516337. https://doi.org/10.1186/s12991-015-0074-y.
7. Brody S, Weiss P. Erectile dysfunction and premature ejaculation: interrelationships and psychosexual factors [J]. J Sex Med. 2015;12(2):398–404. 25382712. https://doi.org/10.1111/jsm.12738.
8. Salama N, Eid A, Swedan A, Hatem A. Increased prevalence of premature ejaculation in men with metabolic syndrome [J]. Aging Male. 2017;20(2):89–95. 28367661. https://doi.org/10.1080/13685538.2016.1277515.
9. Lee JH, Lee SW. Relationship between premature ejaculation and chronic prostatitis/chronic pelvic pain syndrome [J]. J Sex Med. 2015;12(3):697–704. 25475760. https://doi.org/10.1111/jsm.12796.
10. Sansone A, Romanelli F, Jannini EA, Lenzi A. Hormonal correlations of premature ejaculation [J]. Endocrine. 2015;49(2):333–8. 25552341. https://doi.org/10.1007/s12020-014-0520-7.
11. Serefoglu EC, McMahon CG, Waldinger MD, Althof SE, Shindel A, Adaikan G, et al. An evidence-based unified definition of lifelong and acquired premature ejaculation: report of the second international society for sexual medicine ad hoc committee for the definition of premature ejaculation [J]. Sex Med. 2014;2(2):41–59. https://doi.org/10.1002/sm2.27.PMID:25356301.
12. Jern P, Johansson A, Piha J, Westberg L, Santtila P. Antidepressant treatment of premature ejaculation: discontinuation rates and prevalence of side effects for dapoxetine and paroxetine in a naturalistic setting [J]. Int J Impot Res. 2015;27(2):75–80. 25410962. https://doi.org/10.1038/ijir.2014.37.
13. Simsek A, Kirecci SL, Kucuktopcu O, Ozgor F, Akbulut MF, Sarilar O, et al. Comparison of paroxetine and dapoxetine, a novel selective serotonin reuptake inhibitor in the treatment of premature ejaculation [J]. Asian J Androl. 2014;16(5):725–7. 24830690. https://doi.org/10.4103/1008-682X.128467.
14. Higgins JP, Altman DG, Gotzsche PC, Jüni P, Moher D, Oxman AD, et al. The Cochrane Collaboration's tool for assessing risk of bias in randomised trials [J]. BMJ. 2011;343:d5928. 22008217. https://doi.org/10.1136/bmj.d5928.
15. Wang WF, Wang Y, Minhas S, Ralph DJ. Can sildenafil treat primary premature ejaculation? A prospective clinical study [J]. Int J Urol. 2007;14(4):331–5. 17470165. https://doi.org/10.1111/j.1442-2042.2007.01606.x.
16. Moudi E, Kasaeeyan AA. Comparison between Tadalafil plus paroxetine and paroxetine alone in the treatment of premature ejaculation [J]. Nephrourol Mon. 2016;8(1):e32286. 26981497. https://doi.org/10.5812/numonthly.32286.
17. Hamidi-Madani A, Motiee R, Mokhtari G, Nasseh H, Esmaeili S, Kazemnezhad E. The efficacy and safety of on-demand tramadol and paroxetine use in treatment of life long premature ejaculation: a randomized double-blind placebo-controlled clinical trial [J]. J Reprod Infertil. 2018;19(1):10–5. 29850442.
18. Gong ZY, Tang TL, Cui S, Wang JZ, Deng XZ. [Oral paroxetine for premature ejaculation: a randomized controlled study][J]. Zhonghua Nan Ke Xue. 2011;17(10):923–5. 22049798.
19. Waldinger MD, Hengeveld MW, Zwinderman AH, Olivier B. Effect of SSRI antidepressants on ejaculation: a double-blind, randomized, placebo-controlled study with fluoxetine, fluvoxamine, paroxetine, and sertraline [J]. J Clin Psychopharmacol. 1998;18(4):274–81. 9690692.
20. Gameel TA, Tawfik AM, Abou-Farha MO, Bastawisy MG, El-Bendary MA, Ael-N E-G. on-demand use of tramadol, sildenafil, paroxetine and local anaesthetics for the management of premature ejaculation: a randomised placebo-controlled clinical trial [J]. Arab J Urol. 2013;11(4):392–7. 26558110. https://doi.org/10.1016/j.aju.2013.05.003.
21. Sunay D, Sunay M, Aydogmus Y, Bağbancı S, Arslan H, Karabulut A, et al. Acupuncture versus paroxetine for the treatment of premature ejaculation: a randomized, placebo-controlled clinical trial [J]. Eur Urol. 2011;59(5):765–71. 21256670. https://doi.org/10.1016/j.eururo.2011.01.019.
22. Safarinejad MR. Comparison of dapoxetine versus paroxetine in patients with premature ejaculation: a double-blind, placebo-controlled, fixed-dose, randomized study [J]. Clin Neuropharmacol. 2006;29(5):243–52. 16960468. https://doi.org/10.1097/01.WNF.0000228210.12194.46.
23. Abu E M, Abdelhamed A. Comparison of the clinical efficacy and safety of the on-demand use of paroxetine, dapoxetine, sildenafil and combined dapoxetine with sildenafil in treatment of patients with premature ejaculation: A randomised placebo-controlled clinical trial [J]. Andrologia, 2018,50(1). DOI:https://doi.org/10.1111/and.12829. PMID:28497478
24. Abdel-Hamid IA, El NE, El GA. Assessment of as needed use of pharmacotherapy and the pause-squeeze technique in premature ejaculation [J]. Int J Impot Res. 2001;13(1):41–5. 11494085. https://doi.org/10.1038/sj.ijir.3900705.
25. Alghobary M, El-Bayoumy Y, Mostafa Y, Mahmoud el-HM,Amr M. Evaluation of tramadol on demand vs. daily paroxetine as a long-term treatment of lifelong premature ejaculation [J]. J Sex Med, 2010,7(8):2860–2867. DOI: https://doi.org/10.1111/j.1743-6109.2010.01789.x. PMID:20367773
26. Polat EC, Ozbek E, Otunctemur A, Ozcan L, Simsek A. Combination therapy with selective serotonin reuptake inhibitors and phosphodiesterase-5 inhibitors in the treatment of premature ejaculation [J]. Andrologia. 2015;47(5):487–92. 24811578. https://doi.org/10.1111/and.12289.
27. Otunctemur A, Ozbek E, Kirecci SL, Ozcan L, Dursun M, Cekmen M, et al. Relevance of serum nitric oxide levels and the efficacy of selective serotonin reuptake inhibitors treatment on premature ejaculation: decreased nitric oxide is associated with premature ejaculation [J]. Andrologia. 2014;46(9):951–5. 24118023. https://doi.org/10.1111/and.12179.
28. Kirecci SL, Simsek A, Gurbuz ZG, Mimaroglu S, Yuksel A, Vural P, et al. Relationship between plasma melatonin levels and the efficacy of selective serotonin reuptake inhibitors treatment on premature ejaculation [J]. Int J Urol. 2014;46(10):1169–75. 24712716. https://doi.org/10.1111/iju.12461.
29. Kirecci SL, Simsek A, Gurbuz ZG, Gurdal H, Gurbuz ZG, Usanmaz S. "relevance of seminal plasma nitric oxide levels and the efficacy of SSRI treatment on lifelong premature ejaculation." [J]. Andrologia. 2014;21(9):921–2. 24354496. https://doi.org/10.1111/and.12210.
30. Zhang WX, Qin JC, Wang R, Lei W, Jie Z. Effect evaluation of paroxetine and sertraline in the treatment of premature ejaculation [J]. Chinese journal of andrology. 2012;26(2):41–43,47. https://doi.org/10.3969/j.issn.1008-0848.2012.02.011

31. Arafa M, Shamloul R. A randomized study examining the effect of 3 SSRI on premature ejaculation using a validated questionnaire [J]. Ther Clin Risk Manag. 2007;3(4):527–31. 18472973.
32. Shao XY, Li JB. Clinical study on treatment of premature ejaculation with paroxetine and behavior-therapy [J]. Chinese journal of andrology. 2008; 22(1):18–20.
33. Ozcan L, Polat EC, Otunctemur A, Ozbek E. Duloxetine, dual serotonin and norepinephrine reuptake inhibitor, versus paroxetine, selective serotonin reuptake inhibitor, in the treatment for premature ejaculation [J]. Int Urol Nephrol. 2015; 47(2):283–7. 25557853. https://doi.org/10.1007/s11255-014-0905-9.
34. Puppo V, Puppo G. Comprehensive review of the anatomy and physiology of male ejaculation: premature ejaculation is not a disease [J]. Clin Anat. 2016;29(1):111–9. 26457680. https://doi.org/10.1002/ca.22655.
35. Giuliano F, Clément P. Serotonin and premature ejaculation: from physiology to patient management. [J]. Eur Urol. 2006;50:454–66. 16844284. https://doi.org/10.1016/j.eururo.2006.05.055.
36. Jannuni EA, Carosa E, Pepe M, Lombardo F, Lenzi A. Update on pathophysiology of premature ejaculation: the bases for new pharmacological treatments. [J]. EAU-EBU Update Series. 2006;4:141–9. https://doi.org/10.1016/j.eeus.2006.05.002.
37. Janssen PK, van Schaik R, Zwinderman AH, Olivier B, Waldinger MD. The 5-HT(1) a receptor Caucasian men with lifelong premature ejaculation [J]. Pharmacol Biochem Behav. 2014;121:184–8. 24440118. https://doi.org/10.1016/j.pbb.2014.01.004.

22

Urethral cavernous hemangioma: A highly misdiagnosed disease

Fang Yong[1†], Lin Juan[2†], Wei Jinhuan[1], Yao Haohua[1], Chen Wei[1], Mo Jiacong[1], Luo Junhang[1] and Wang Wenwei[1*]

Abstract

Background: Diagnosis of urethral cavernous hemangioma (UCH) is very rare. It can be easy to misdiagnose and mistreat due to its atypical clinical manifestations and a lack of relevant knowledge. The study is to explore the diagnosis, differential diagnosis, and treatment of UCH.

Case presentation: The first patient was a 15-year-old male, who was admitted to the hospital for more than 1 year with repeated hematuria. UCH was diagnosed by cystoscope biopsy, and cured with local injection of pingyangmycin. The second patient was a 49-year-old male, who was admitted for repeated painless gross hematuria and intermittent urethral bleeding after penile erection for more than 20 years. The case had been misdiagnosed as seminal vesiculitis, urethritis, or prostatitis, for over 20 years, until it was diagnosed as UCH by MR examination of the penis. It was treated by injection of pingyangmycin into the hemangioma's lumen and base. A small incision in the ventral penile area was separated from the location of the hemangioma, which was injected with pingyangmycin again. A biopsy of resected tissue further confirmed the diagnosis of UCH.

Conclusions: UCH is an easily misdiagnosed disease. Intermittent painless hematuria is important characteristic of UCH. Local injection of pingyangmycin is a good option for treatment of UCH.

Keywords: Urethra cavernous hemangioma, Urethremorrhage, Pingyangmycin

Background

Urethral cavernous hemangioma (UCH) is an unusual disease and a few cases have been reported [1–7]. It can be easy to misdiagnose and mistreat UCH due to its atypical clinical manifestations and a lack of relevant knowledge. Two patients were admitted in our hospital in November 2002 and April 2013 respectively that were misdiagnosed during the preliminary diagnoses. The diagnoses were corrected by cystourethroscopy or imaging. The clinical characteristics and treatment methods of these cases are summarized here.

* Correspondence: wang_wenwei1@sina.com
†Fang Yong and Lin Juan contributed equally to this work.
[1]Department of Urology, First Affiliated Hospital of Sun Yat-sen university, Guangzhou 510080, China
Full list of author information is available at the end of the article

Case presentation

The first patient was a 15-year-old male. After 1 year of repeated gross hematuria, he was admitted to the Department of Nephrology in our hospital on November, 2002. Urinary system ultrasound, intravenous pyelography, contrast enhancement and plain CT scans of the kidney, and renal biopsy were performed. However a cause of the patient's hematuria could not be identified. Later, the patient was transferred to pediatric surgery and cystourethroscopy was performed. The results showed urethral mucosa edema, mass and miliary bulging, and bleeding of the membranous urethra. The urethral mucosa biopsy was also performed, and the pathological report displayed submucosal vascular dilatation of the urethra which is consistent with UCH (Fig. 1). Two weeks after the cystourethroscopy, pingyangmycin was injected under the cystoscope in the outpatient department of urology. In the operation, 4 mg of pingyangmycin was injected into the bulge on the urethral

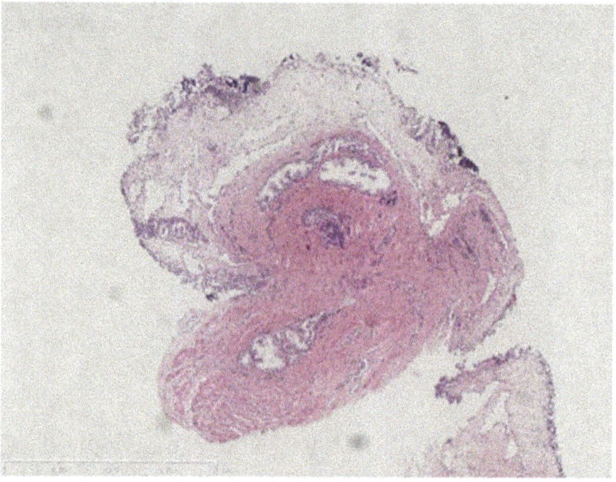

Fig. 1 The pathological tissue originates from the urethral mucosa, displaying submucosal vascular dilatation of the urethra, which is consistent with urethra cavernous hemangioma (UCH)

membrane. The urethral catheter was retained and removed after 3 days. At the follow-ups 1 year, 12 years, and 15 years after treatment, gross hematuria did not recur, and micturition and erectile function were normal.

The second patient was a 49-year-old male with repeated painless gross hematuria and discontinuous urethral bleeding after penile erection for more than 20 years, which had been aggravated for 4 months. He was admitted to the Department of Urology of our hospital on April 29, 2013. The patient had also been misdiagnosed in a local hospital over the course of 20 years with seminal vesitis, urethritis, or prostatitis. No obvious improvement was observed with treatment. Cystoscopy performed in local hospitals, revealed no obvious abnormalities. After artificial erection by tightening the root of the penis and injecting saline into the corpus cavernosum, a small amount of bloody liquid could be detected in the urethra. The penis MR showed an abnormal signal on the right side of the urethra cavernous body at the front of the penis. The range was about 1.1 × 2.4 cm. The distal portion closed to the urethral meatus. The proximal portion was at a distance of 2.4 cm from urethral meatus and invaded the right side of the glans (Fig. 2, 3 and 4). After artificial erection of the penis, urethroscopy examination showed that there was a 0.3 cm fissure located in the 11 o'clock urethral mucosa 2 cm away from the urethral meatus. The fissure bled and the bleeding was aggravated when the penis was squeezed (Additional file 1: Video S1). Pingyangmycin was injected into the lumen and basal side of the tumor under the urethroscope. We took a biopsy from the small incision on the ventral side of the penis that separated the hemangioma and continued to inject pingyangmycin. The total dose of pingyangmycin was 8 mg. The

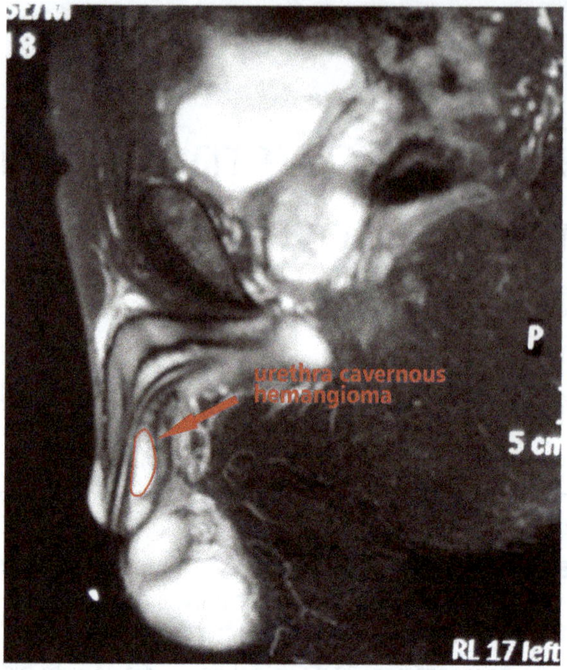

Fig. 2 Preoperative penis sagittal MRI shows a high signal on the urethra cavernous body at the front of the penis. The range was about 1.1 × 2.4 cm

catheter inserted after injection was removed 3 days after the operation. The postoperative pathological report reported a diagnosis of UCH. At 1 year and 5 years of follow-ups, no bleeding occurred during or after penile erection, no gross hematuria recurred, and penile erection and voiding were normal.

Discussion and conclusions

As the tissue of the urethral cavernous body is half-wrapped around the glans and the cavernous body of the penis, along with in the relative depth of the penis, the growth of the hemangioma is limited. Therefore, UCH often has no obvious signs. However, if it breaks through to the urethra it becomes noticeable, making gross hematuria the most important clinical feature of the diseases.

UCH can occur at any age in males, and is more likely to occur in young people. Local trauma and urinary tract inflammation are often the main factors of tumor rupture and bleeding. Penile erection in adult males leads to vascular dilatation and venous flow obstruction, which can also cause rupture and bleeding of UCH. Blockage of the urethra can cause dysuria, in which a larger UCH can form or bleeding can result in a blood clot [1]. In sum, intermittent painless gross hematuria and gross hematuria are the most important features of this disease.

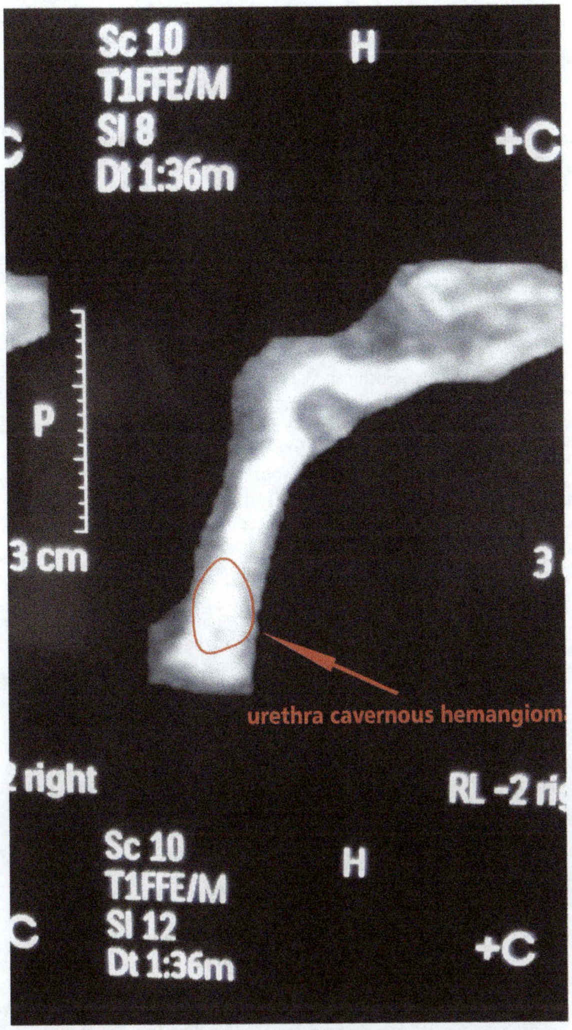

Fig. 3 Preoperative penis MRI reconstruction shows a high signal at the front of the penis

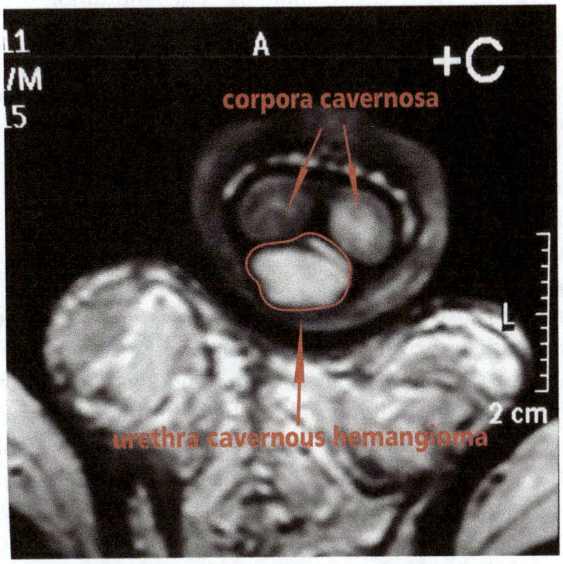

Fig. 4 Preoperative penis coronal MRI shows a high signal on the ventral side of the penis, and underneath the urethra cavernous bodies of the penis

However, the atypical features of UCH lead the disease being easily misdiagnosed and mistreated for a long time. In this report, the first patient was misdiagnosed as nephritis, which was removed from the diagnosis until the invasive renal biopsy was performed. The second patient was misdiagnosed and mistreated for more than 20 years. Therefore, for the painless hematuria that has been excluded from the urinary system related diseases such as inflammation, malignant tumor and stone, especially for young people, cystoscopy is an important means of examination.

Another important feature is that hematuria is often aggravated after penile erection, especially for the sexually active adult male, even visible blood dripping from the urethral meatus. This is very similar to the characteristics of seminal vesicle inflammation and is also one of the reasons for misdiagnosis. In the second patient, as a 49-year-old adult male patient, the most frequent misdiagnosis was seminal vesicle inflammation. The reason why we could correct the misdiagnosis is we noted that the urethral bleeding after the patient's sexual activity was not discharged with the semen. Therefore, for incurable hemospermia of patients' complaining, we should pay more attention to the way that the blood is discharged from the urethra and the relationship with the excretion of sperm so as to distinguish between the semen with blood (the so-called true hemospermia) or the urethral bleeding caused by sexual activity.

At present, the common treatment of hemangioma includes drugs, physical therapy, and surgery. Drug treatments include oral propranolol, oral or injection of glucocorticoid, local injection of pingyangmycin, etc. [8, 9]. Physical therapies include direct current copper needle, laser, radiation, microwave, etc. [10–13]. Surgery treatment includes local excision, the purse-string closure method, etc. [14]. In particular, minimally invasive urological surgery like transurethral Holmium laser therapy is also suitable for the treatment of hemangioma of the urinary system, which has been successfully applied to urethral hemangioma [15]. The surgical excision of UCH is a complex operation with significant trauma because of the deep location of the mass and proximity to the urethra. Urethral stricture may be caused by scarring after the operation or the surgical injury leads to acquired hypospadias. Radiation therapy also causes radiation orchitis, which may affect reproductive function [16].Therefore, both patients were treated with the interventional technology pingyangmycin injection, and satisfactory results were achieved.

Pingyangmycin is a commonly used antitumor drug. This drug mainly inhibits the synthesis of deoxynucleic acid and ribonucleic acid, decomposes deoxyribonucleic acid, breaks the DNA chain and produces oxygen free radicals, prevents DNA replication, and interferes with cell division and proliferation [17]. Hemangioma is caused by abnormal proliferation of vascular endothelial cells. Injection of pingyangmycin in the tumor, can quickly inhibit the proliferation of immature vascular endothelial cells. At the same time, its chemical stimulation can cause aseptic inflammation of vascular endothelium and destroy the endothelium of the blood sinus, resulting in damage of the vascular endothelium and extensive formation of microthrombus, causing local tissue degeneration. Necrosis and coagulation eventually leads to tissue fibrosis, bringing about the gradual disappearance of hemangioma [18]. Further mechanistic studies have shown that pingyangmycin can induce apoptosis and reduce cell invasiveness by inhibiting the PI3K/Akt pathway [19] and by up-regulating P53 inducing P53-dependent apoptosis [20].

Our study is limited because it included only two patients from China. And no female patients included. Our application of pingyangmycin injection for treatment of UCH may be optimal only to patients with small tumor size.

In conclusion, UCH is a hemangioma deep in the penis. The most common presentation of UCH is intermittent hematuria which is typically painless. This disease is easily misdiagnosed. For patients complaining with long lasting hematuria or bloody sperm, we should inquire about the characteristics of urinating blood and its relationship with the discharge of sperm. For suspected patients, we should take a cystoscopy and MR of the penis. It is advisable to apply pingyangmycin injection for treatment, and the prognosis is generally good.

Additional file

Additional file 1: Video S1. Urethroscopy examination video. After artificial erection of the penis, urethroscopy showed that the 0.3 cm fissure located in the 11 o'clock urethral mucosa 2 cm away from the urethral meatus. The fissure bled and the bleeding was aggravated when the penis was squeezed. (AVI 2906 kb)

Abbreviations

MR: Magnetic resonance; UCH: Urethra cavernous hemangioma

Acknowledgements

We gratefully acknowledge the kind cooperation of Dr. Guo Yan in the preparation of imaging data.

Authors' contributions

WW designed the study. FY, LJ, WJ, and YH participated in acquisition of data. CW, MJC, LJ, and WW participated in analysis and interpretation of data. All authors read and approved the final manuscript to be published. All authors agreed to be accountable for all aspects of the work.

References

1. Saito S. Posterior urethral hemangioma: one of the unknown causes of hematuria and/or hematospermia. Urology. 2008;71(1):168.e11–4.
2. Efthimiou I, Kavouras D, Vasilakis P, Katsanis S. Hemangioma of penile urethra-treatment with simple transurethral excision: a case report. Cases J. 2009;2:6199.
3. Hamada A, Hattahara K, Oyama R, Hirayama K, Masui K, Shichiri Y. Urethral hemangioma with repeated urinary retention by posterection hematuria. Hinyokika Kiyo. 2017;63(12):533–5.
4. Ongun S, Celik S, Aslan G, Yorukoglu K, Esen A. Cavernous hemangioma of the female urethra: a rare case report. Urol J. 2014;11(2):1521–3.
5. Rohan VS, Hanji AM, Patel JJ, Tankshali RA. Female urethral hemangioma. Saudi J Kidney Dis Transpl. 2008;19(4):647–8.
6. Rao AR, Motiwala H. Urethral hemangioma. Urology. 2005;65(5):1000.
7. Tabibian L, Ginsberg DA. Thrombosed urethral hemangioma. J Urol. 2003; 170(5):1942.
8. Keller RG, Stevens S, Hochman M. Modern Management of Nasal Hemangiomas. JAMA Facial Plast Surg. 2017;19(4):327–32.
9. Wu X, Mao W, He P, Wei C. Curative effect of chemotherapy, KTP lasers, and CO2 lasers combined with chemotherapy in the treatment of adult laryngeal hemangioma. Acta Otolaryngol. 2018;138(6):567–73.
10. Zhang D, Zhang H, Sun P, Li P, Xue A, Jin X. A creative therapy in treating cavernous hemangioma of penis with copper wire. J Sex Med. 2014;11(10): 2605–10.
11. Darrow DH. Management of Infantile Hemangiomas of the Airway. Otolaryngol Clin N Am. 2018;51(1):133–46.
12. Park S, Yoon SM, Lee S, Park JH, Song SY, Lee SW, et al. Role of fractionated radiotherapy in patients with hemangioma of the cavernous sinus. Radiat Oncol J. 2017;35(3):268–73.
13. Ziemlewicz TJ, Wells SA, Lubner MA, Musat AI, Hinshaw JL, Cohn AR, et al. Microwave ablation of giant hepatic cavernous hemangiomas. Cardiovasc Intervent Radiol. 2014;37(5):1299–305.
14. Grzesik P, Wu JK. Current perspectives on the optimal management of infantile hemangioma. Pediatric Health Med Ther. 2017;8:107–16.
15. Soleimani MJ, Shadpour P, Mehravaran K, Kashi AH. Laser treatment for urethral hemangiomas: report of three cases. Urol J. 2017;14(3):3094–9.
16. Khan S, Adhikari JS, Rizvi MA, Chaudhury NK. Radioprotective potential of melatonin against (6)(0)Co gamma-ray-induced testicular injury in male C57BL/6 mice. J Biomed Sci. 2015;22:61.
17. Wang C, Liu J, Pan W, Wang X, Gao Q, Hou S. Pingyangmycin loaded bovine serum albumin microspheres for chemoembolization therapy--in vitro and in vivo studies. Int J Pharm. 2008;351(1–2):219–26.
18. Huang Y, Li P, Xia S, Zhuo Y, Wu L. Proapoptotic effect and the mechanism of action of pingyangmycin on cavernous hemangiomas. Exp Ther Med. 2014;7(2):473–7.
19. Peng LX, Zhao P, Zhao HS, Pan E, Yang BB, Li Q. Phosphoinositide 3-kinase/ Akt pathway is involved in pingyangmycininduced growth inhibition, apoptosis and reduction of invasive potential in EOMA mouse hemangioendothelioma cells. Mol Med Rep. 2015;12(6):8275–81.
20. Tu JB, Li QY, Jiang F, Hu XY, Ma RZ, Dong Q, et al. Pingyangmycin stimulates apoptosis in human hemangioma-derived endothelial cells through activation of the p53 pathway. Mol Med Rep. 2014;10(1):301–5.

23

Penile metastasis from recurrent sarcoma in a teenager

Chi-Fang Chen[1], Tzu-Ying Tang[2,3], Marcelo Chen[1,3] and Li-Chen Chen[1*]

Abstract

Background: Metastatic tumors of the penis are uncommon, and fewer than 500 cases have been reported since 1870. Most penile secondary tumors originate in organs of the genitourinary tract, followed by the gastrointestinal tract. Primary tumors of sarcoma origin are extremely rare. Herein, we present a teenager who had recurrent sarcoma of the right femur with penile metastasis.

Case presentation: The 20-year-old male patient was diagnosed with sarcoma of the right femur when he was 16 days old. He was stable following combination chemotherapy with the VAC regimen (vincristine, adriamycin, and cyclophosphamide) and debulking surgery. In January 2018, five months ago, he presented with right leg pain and swelling, and a recurrent tumor was found. Following excision of the tumor showed recurrent sarcoma. However, 2 months after the operation, right thigh swelling with tenderness occurred. A firm nodule on the glans of the penis was also noted. Penile metastasis was suspected and a biopsy was performed. The final pathology report disclosed pleomorphic sarcoma with penile metastasis. Symptoms including priapism and inguinal lymph node enlargement progressed rapidly within 2 weeks. He also complained of voiding difficulty with urine retention. The patient died 35 days after admission due to pneumonia with septic shock.

Conclusion: Penile metasitasis largely occurs from organs in the pelvis. To the best of our knowledge, this is the first case of a teenager with a secondary penile tumor, metastasizing from sarcoma of the bone. It presented as a palpable mass, and then progressed into priapism. The patient had a dismal prognosis and the symptoms progressed faster than his physicians anticipated.

Keywords: Secondary penile tumor, Metastasis, Malignant priapism, Sarcoma

Background

Secondary penile tumors are a rare clinical entity, despite the rich vascularization and circulation between neighbouring organs. Fewer than 500 cases have been reported reviews since 1870 [1–3]. The vast majority of primary tumors occur in the genitourinary organs, followed by the recto-sigmoid region [4]. To date, penile tumors secondary from sarcoma origins are extremely rare [5]. Herein, we report a teenager with recurrent sarcoma with penile nodular lesions which were proven to be sarcoma metastases. We discusses the possible metastatic routes and clinical factors associations.

* Correspondence: cetaceachen@gmail.com
[1]Department of Urology, MacKay Memorial Hospital, No.92, Sec. 2, Zhongshan N. Rd., Zhongshan Dist, Taipei City 10449, Taiwan
Full list of author information is available at the end of the article

Case presentation

The 20-year-old male patient was diagnosed with spindle cell sarcoma of the right femur in Aug. 1998, when he was 16 days old, at Mackay Memorial hospital (consent was obtained from his mother for the publication). Due to right thigh enlargement with a palpable mass, excisional biopsy were performed, and pathology disclosed a spindle cell sarcoma with hypercellularity (Fig. 1a). The patient was administered five courses of combination chemotherapy with vincristine, adriamycin, and cyclophosphamide. Debulking excision of the tumor was performed when he was 11 months old. He was regularly followed up at the orthopedics department over the next 20 years and he recieved reconstruction surgery, after which he was able to walk and run. Until 5 months ago, January 2018, he complained of progressive right thigh pain with radiation to the right lower leg, which continued for 5 months. The patient also complained of right

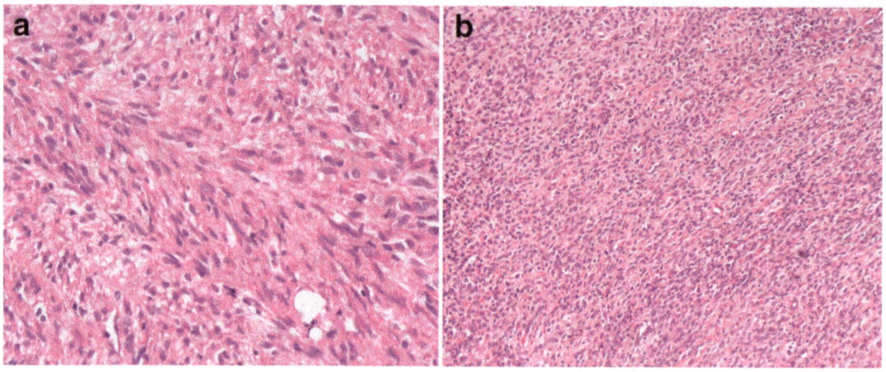

Fig. 1 Pathology of locally recurrence tumor. **a** 400x H&E of the original low-grade neoplasm from 1999 composed of monotonous atypical spindle cells arranged in long sweeping bundles. **b** 200x H&E of a recurrent lesion in 2018 with the presence of a round cell component

leg numbness and weakness. Follow-up magnetic resonance imaging (MRI) revealed an infiltrative tumor mass measuring 3.6 × 3.3 × 10.4 cm in the medial proximal right thigh. The patient underwent tumor excision in May 2018. A tumor was removed from beneath the sciatic nerve and the pathology report showed recurrent sarcoma with a round cell pattern (Fig. 1b).

Two months after the surgery, the patient complained of progressive right thigh swelling with tenderness and swelling of the glans penis with painful nodules. Leg computed tomography (CT) revealed a huge intraoseous cystic lesion in the right femoral shaft. Penile swelling was thought to be an balanitis at first. Urologists were then consulted for the penis lesion and 2 firm nodules about 1 to 2 cm in size were identified on the glans of the penis. No discharge, ulceration or necrosis was noted on the the overlying skin of the glans (Fig. 2a). Morning erection were unaffected; however, 3 days later the nodules had not shrunk and became a mild purple in color (Fig. 2b). Furthermore, progressive penile pain and swelling from the glans to the shaft was noted (Fig. 2c). Priapism with venous thrombosis was suspected; He compained of voiding difficulty and urine retention, but only a 14 Fr Foley tube could be inserted due to compression. In Aug. 2018, one week after admission, biopsies of the right leg and penis were performed. During the operation, a 16 Fr cystoscope could only reach the distal urethra and a 6 Fr ureteroscope revealed mucosal swelling throughout the urethra. Gross hematuria with blood clot retention in the urinary bladder and right inguinal lymph node enlargement was noted. Two weeks after admission, a suprapubic cystostomy was performed for blood clot evacuation, as it was difficult to insert a cystoscope into the urethra. An open biopsy of the right inguinal lymph node was also performed. The penile biopsy showed a hypercellular lesion with an infiltrating border, spindle fascicles with collagen deposition, and cellular pleomorphism. Histopathological examination of the recurrent tumor on the right thigh, penile lesion and inguinal lymph node showed presence of the same type of enlarged bizarre tumor cells with prominent cellular atypia. Immunohistochemistry staining of the recurrent tumor and metastasis lesion showed Gata3 (−) CD45 (−) ALK-P (−) melanA(−), S100 (−) and INI-1 with an intact expression. A FISH (Fluorescence in situ hybridization) study showed the absence of the ETV6-NTRK3 gene (a characteristic gene fusion identified in infantile fibrosarcoma). Thereby ruling out urothelial carcinoma, lymphoma, inflammatory myofibroblastic tumor, melanoma, infantile sarcoma and epithelioid tumor.

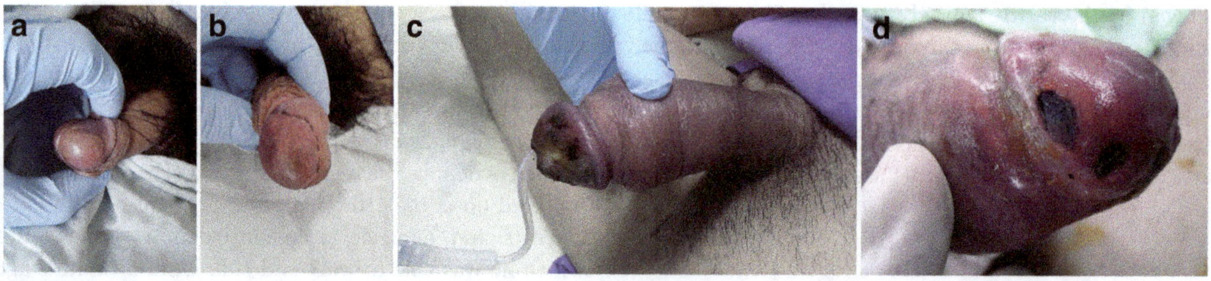

Fig. 2 Gross pictures. **a** Painless firm nodules over the glans of the penis on admission **b** Mild swelling with purple congestion change. **c** Priapism with urine retention and an s/p nephrostomy tube and penis biopsy **d** Gangrene change over the glans of the penis

The final pathology was penile metastasis and inguinal lymph node metastasis of high-grade pleomorphic/epithelioid sarcoma (Fig. 3a,b,c). Compared to previous tumor morphology (Fig. 1), the tumor recurred became of spindle cell with round cell pattern. And then, it transformed with biphasic bizarre anaplastic epithelidoid cell (Fig. 3) in 2 months.

Four weeks after admission, the patient still had persistent priapism with gross hematuria, and poor appetite with progressive cachexia. The biopsy wound over the glans developed gangrene (Fig. 2d). Fever with pneumonia occurred during the hospitalization. The patient died due to septic shock with respiratory failure 35 days after the penile swelling first ocurred.

Discussion and conslusion

The majority of secondary metastatic penile tumors origniate from adjacent organ systems in the pelvis, including the genitourinary organs or the rectum. Previous reviews reported that the most common metastatic organs were the prostate and bladder, followed by the colorectal system. Fewer than 10% of cases are from other organs, such as the lung, liver and bone [2].

Nearly 500 cases of penile metastasis tumors have been reported, but only 3 previous cases have reported a primary tumor site with sarcoma origin. The first reported case was a 37-year-old male patient with penile metastasis from the primary site of chondrosarcoma in the jaw [6]. The second case was a 35-year-old male who had primary extraosseous penis osteosarcoma [7] and the third case was a 42-year-old male with a history of ischial tuberosity osteosarcoma with pulmonary metastasis and a painful penile metastatic lesion [5].

To the best of our knoweldge, the present study is the first case of sarcoma with multiple recurrences, where the first metastatic site was the penis. In addition, the present case is the first reported in a teenager. In a previous case series, the patients with penile metastasis were aged between 60 and 80 years [8] and most patient had disseminated disease condition. The metastasic route and mechanism have yet to be elucidated. The most accepted mechanisms of metastasis are as follows: 1) A retrograde venous route, 2) a retrograde lymphatic route, 3) arterial spread, 4) direct extension, and 5) implantation secondary to instrumentation [1] The retrograde venous route is the most likely mechanism of metastasis because there is communication between the dorsal penile venous system and the pelvic organs, and therfore bladder and prostate tumors are able to reach the penile circulation. In our case, the retrograde lymphatic route could not be ruled out, because he also presented with right leg swelling and lymph node enlargement.

It is difficult to identify penile lesions except by an open biopsy. There is no classic presentation or symptom complex in penile metastasis. Our patient had unusual symptoms of priapism, urine retention and gross hematuria. Previous cases series, mostly presented with painless nodule lesions over the penis, followed by priapism and pain [1, 2, 9]. However, the metastatic manifestation of priapism is uncommon. The mechanism could be either occlusion of the draining vein or secondary tumor thrombus occlusion of carvernosal spaces. Unlike a previous case report, urine retention and gross hematuria developed after priapism in our case. Malignant priapism was also noted in the case with disseminated metastasis; however, only locally advanced recurrence in the right thigh with primary metastasis to the penis was noted in our case. Unfortunately, the disease progressed rapidly before the biopsy report revealed the final diagnosis. Due to the rapidly-changing morphology of recurrent tumor cells, and shorter recurrent intervals, tumor progression with penile metastasis was likely.

Penile metastasis is an indicator of a poor prognosis. The median survival time after the diagnosis of penile metastasis is 10 months (range 6–18 months) and the patient presenting with priapism and those with metastasis from

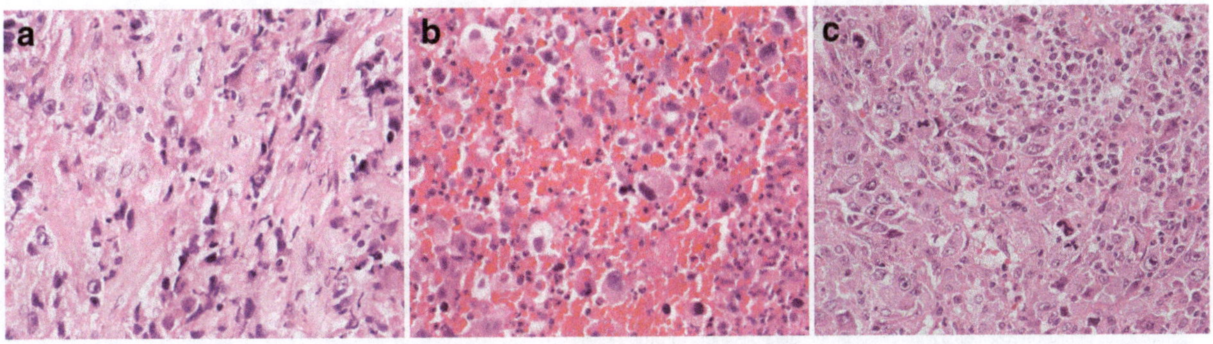

Fig. 3 Pathology of metastatis tumors. The presence of high grade anaplastic epithelioid cells arranged in a nodular pattern. Frequent mitosis and abundant lymphoplasmacytic infiltrates can be found in these metastatic lesions. **a** Right thigh open biopsy. **b** Penile biopsy **c** Inguinal lymph node biopsy

non-urologic tumors have a significantly worse prognosis [9]. Our 20-year-oldeee male patient died 35 days after penile metastasis due to cachexia status and septic shock. We believe that the poor disease outcome and dramatic progression were related to the tumor cell transformation. The recurrent sarcoma underwent anaplastic transformation into high grade pleomophic sarcoma, which then progressed with both local recurrence and penile and right inguinal lymph node metastasis in 2 months.

Secondary malignancy of the penis rarely occurs in young patients, and it mostly originates from the genitourinary organs. A literature review showed that the current case is the first case of metastatic penile tumor originateing from sarcoma of the femur in a teenager. He presented with a palpable mass and subsequently developed priapism and gross hematuria. Because the overall outcome is poor, most patients will need early palliative or supportive care.

Abbreviations

CT: Computed tomography; FISH: Fluorescence in situ hybridization); MRI: Magnetic resonance imaging; VAC: Vincristine, adriamycin, and cyclophosphamide

Acknowledgements

Not applicable.

Authors' contributions

CFC made contributions to the acquisition of history, image and wrote the manuscript. TYT carried out the pathology part interpretation and description. LCC performed the treatment, and reviewed the manuscript to give clinical opinions. MC made supervision and helped reviewing the manuscript. The All the authors read and approved the final manuscript.

Author details

[1]Department of Urology, MacKay Memorial Hospital, No.92, Sec. 2, Zhongshan N. Rd., Zhongshan Dist, Taipei City 10449, Taiwan. [2]Department of Pathology, Tamsui branch, MacKay Memorial Hospital, No.45, Minsheng Rd., Tamsui Dist, New Taipei City 25160, Taiwan. [3]School of Medicine, MacKay Medical College, No.46, Sec. 3, Zhongzheng Rd., Sanzhi Dist, New Taipei City 252, Taiwan.

References

1. Cherian J, Rajan S, Thwaini A, Elmasry Y, Shah T, Puri R. Secondary penile tumours revisited. Int Semin Surg Oncol. 2006;3:33.
2. Chaux A, Amin M, Cubilla AL, Young RH. Metastatic tumors to the penis: a report of 17 cases and review of the literature. Int J Surg Pathol. 2011;19:597–606.
3. Efared B, Ebang GA, Tahirou S, Tahiri L, Sidibe IS, Erregad F, Sow A, Hammas N, Farih MH, Chbani L, et al. Penile metastasis from rectal adenocarcinoma: a case report. BMC Res Notes. 2017;10:564.
4. Perez LM, Shumway RA, Carson CC 3rd, Fisher SR, Hudson WR. Penile metastasis secondary to supraglottic squamous cell carcinoma: review of the literature. J Urol. 1992;147:157–60.
5. Liu N, Man LB, Huang GL. Penile metastasis of osteosarcoma: a rare case report. Asian J Androl. 2013;15:841–2.
6. Cardoso Guimaraes G, Rodrigues De Souza R, Paiva Gadelha Guimaraes A, Filho WD, Valeschka De Matos Granja N, Karan Kalil R, Augusto Soares F, Lopes A. Penile metastasis of chondrosarcoma of the jaw. Urology. 2003;61:837.
7. Shringarpure SS, Kumar A, Shankar S, Menon M. A case of primary extraosseous penile osteosarcoma and review of the literature. Indian J Urol. 2012;28:102–4.
8. Osther PJ, Lontoft E. Metastasis to the penis. Case reports and review of the literature. Int Urol Nephrol. 1991;23:161–7.
9. Cocci A, Hakenberg OW, Cai T, Nesi G, Livi L, Detti B, Minervini A, Morelli G, Carini M, Serni S, et al. Prognosis of men with penile metastasis and malignant priapism: a systematic review. Oncotarget. 2018;9:2923–30.

Vasitis: A rare diagnosis mimicking inguinal hernia

Chih-Wei Chen[1], Chin-Ho Lee[1], Tsung-Yi Huang[2] and Yi-Ming Wang[1*]

Abstract

Background: Vasitis or inflammation of the vas deferens is a rare condition, and few case reports with computed tomography images have been published since 1980.

Case presentation: A 50-year-old man presented with severe right inguinal and lower abdominal pain. Initial diagnosis at the emergency department was incarcerated or strangulated inguinal hernia. The computed tomography scan revealed diffuse edematous changes of right spermatic cord and vas deferens with peripheral fat stranding. Correlating with his clinical symptoms, signs, and imaging findings, the diagnosis of vasitis was made. We report a case of acute vasitis about the cause, symptom, pathogen, differential diagnoses, image findings, and treatment.

Conclusion: Although very rare, vasitis should be listed as one of the differential diagnosis for inguinal mass lesions. Cross-sectional imaging may be necessary to confirm the diagnosis and exclude differentials such as an inguinal hernia. Recognition of the characteristic image findings can help to make the correct diagnosis and avoid unnecessary surgery.

Keywords: Hernia, Vasitis, Vas deferens, Inguinal hernia

Background

Acute vasitis or inflammation of the vas deferens is an extremely rare disease, with only about twenty adult case reports published since 1980. Few of these contain computed tomography (CT) images [1–10]. Clinically, it presents with nonspecific symptoms of inguinal swelling and local pain that can mimic orchitis, epididymitis, testicular torsion, and inguinal hernia. Familiarity with symptoms, image findings, and differential diagnoses is essential to prevent unnecessary surgery, especially when symptoms mimic an inguinal hernia.

Case presentation

A middle-aged male presented to our emergency department with severe right inguinal and lower abdominal pain, exaggerated by walking and Valsalva's maneuver. He did not have a fever or chillness. The patient has no other prior medical history, no trauma history, no recent travel history, and no habitual alcohol and cigarette consumption. The patient is of Han Chinese origin and is currently working as an office clerk. He denied any family history of similar symptoms, no recent heavy lifting activities, and no high-risk sexual behaviors. The physical examination revealed tenderness and swelling in the right inguinal area. The laboratory tests revealed leukocytosis (11.39 × 103 /uL), elevated C reactive protein (35.4 mg/L) and leukocyturia, but a negative result of the urine culture. Due to the progression of localized right inguinal pain, the emergency doctor arranged computed tomography scan to rule out incarcerated inguinal hernia. The scan revealed diffuse edematous changes of right spermatic cord and vas deferens with peripheral fat stranding and no herniated bowel loop [Figs. 1, 2]. Correlating the patient's clinical symptoms, signs, and, imaging findings, the emergency doctor was able to overturn the initial diagnosis of an inguinal hernia and confirm vasitis. Empirical antibiotic treatment (Levofloxacin) was prescribed with good response.

* Correspondence: ohyala@gmail.com
[1]Department of Radiology, Kaohsiung Medical University Hospital, Kaohsiung Medical University, No. 100, Ziyou 1st Rd., Sanmin District, Kaohsiung City 80756, Taiwan, Republic of China
Full list of author information is available at the end of the article

Timeline

Dates	Patient Relevant Past Medical History and Interventions		
No previously medical or surgical history. No family medical history.			
Dates	Summaries from Initial Emergency and Follow-up Visits	Diagnostic Testing	Interventions
2017-Feb	Came to the emergency department due to severe right inguinal and lower abdominal pain.	Physical examination: Right inguinal mass with pain, exaggerated when walking and Valsalva's maneuver. laboratory data: leukocytosis, elevated C reactive protein and leukocyturia, CT: Revealed unilateral edematous spermatic cord without evidence of herniated bowel loop.	Prescribed oral antibiotic use: 500 mg of Levofloxacin (Cravit) daily for two weeks.
7 Days later	Out-patient department follow-up.	Symptoms improved.	
14 Days later	Out-patient department follow-up.	Symptoms improved.	

Discussion and Conclusions

Inflammation of the vas deferens or vasitis is a rare condition categorized by Chan and Schlegel as acutely painful infective vasitis or asymptomatic vasitis nodosa [8]. Vasitis nodosa was first described in 1943 by Benjamin [9] as asymptomatic, chronic inflammatory reactions associated with blockage of the vas deferens, which causes high intra-luminal pressure with spermatozoa leakage and inflammatory process. Clinical presentation is with asymptomatic nodular lesions in the vas deferens, and most cases have a history of vasectomy. No specific treatment is required [4].

Acute infective vasitis is thought to be due to the retrograded spread of common urinary pathogens including *Haemophilus influenza* and *Escherichia coli*. However, urinary culture is usually negative. Other rare pathogens reported include Chlamydia trachomatis and *Mycobacterium tuberculosis* [4, 6].

Most cases of the previously reported vasitis patients have histories of surgeries in close proximity to the affected vas deferens. Due to the low prevalence nature of acute vasitis, other risk factors have not been credited to this condition. A retrospective review was conducted by Clavijo et al. in 2010 where the clinical characteristics of eleven patients were thoroughly evaluated [10]. Of the eleven subjects, eight had previous surgeries in the neighboring regions, such as herniorrhaphy, prostatectomy, and perianal fistulectomy. The review also proposed other risk factors such as trauma history, concurrent human immunodeficiency virus/herpes simplex virus infections, and smoking habits [10]. Interestingly, our patient had none of the aforementioned risks factors.

Clinical symptoms include localized pain or palpable mass in the scrotal or inguinal region, some of them with leukocytosis or fever. Acute vasitis could be classification as three groups depending on involved site: scrotal, suprascrotal, and prepubic. It can be easily confused when there is isolated site involvement [11].

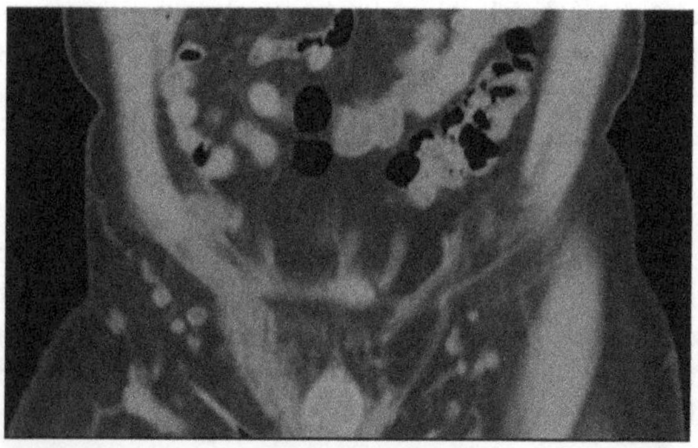

Fig. 1 Non-enhanced coronal CT image revealed diffuse edematous change of right spermatic cord (white arrow)

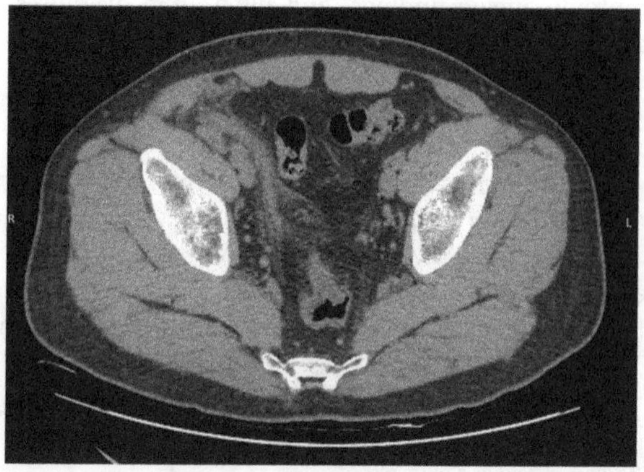

Fig. 2 Non-enhanced axial CT image revealed dilated right vas deferens with peripheral fat stranding (white arrows)

The common differential diagnoses include orchitis, epididymitis, testicular torsion, and inguinal hernia. Correct diagnosis is essential because the treatment of vasitis is via antibiotics, and operation is not required [6].

The diagnosis of vasitis could be a challenge by its rarity and unclear image findings. We review past reports that suggest appropriate tools include ultrasound, computed tomography and magnetic resonance imaging (MRI). Ultrasound can be used to exclude orchitis, epididymitis, and testicular torsion by color Doppler. Acute vasitis often reveals heterogeneous, hypoechoic spermatic cord and echogenic fat surrounding the lesions. However, ultrasound is relatively challenging to differentiate from incarcerated inguinal hernia to vasitis [12]. CT and MRI are more recommended to confirm the diagnosis. Spiral CT has high resolution and short scanning time. Acute vasitis typically reveals unilateral edematous spermatic cord without evidence of herniated bowel loop. MRI can provide more soft tissue detail, abnormal signal intensities of inflamed or ischemic structures, with the additional benefits of no radiation exposure [3, 6, 7, 12].

Based on the available literature, the majority of the reported vasitis can be resolved with the use of anti-inflammatories and antibiotics alone [3, 8]. Some authors prescribed oral antibiotics while others started with intravenous antibiotics in combination with oral antibiotics [6]. A reported pediatric vasitis case suggested only partial regression of the inguinal swelling symptoms with 7 days of oral antibiotic use, and the patient was later admitted and treated successfully with intravenous antibiotics [13]. Surgical exploration and drainage may be necessary in more severe cases that are not responsive to antibiotic treatment [10]. En bloc excision of the vas deferens is uncommon and is usually performed for the exceptionally rare cases of Tuberculous vasitis [14]. For our patient, we prescribed empirical antibiotic treatment with 500 mg of Levofloxacin once daily for two weeks. The patient's symptoms improved drastically upon the scheduled weekly follow-ups.

In summary, we present a rare case mimicking incarcerated inguinal hernia, and although vasitis is very rare, physicians should keep in mind that patients might present with similar symptoms, especially when the patient has risk factors such as previous vasectomy and concurrent leukocyturia. CT or MRI scan can play an important role to prevent unnecessary surgery.

Abbreviations

CT: Computed tomography; MRI: Magnetic resonance imaging

Acknowledgements

Not applicable.

Authors' contributions

CC and YW were responsible for the concept and drafted the manuscript. CL and TH gave intellectual content and critically reviewed the manuscript. YW was responsible for the official radiology report. All authors have given final approval of the version to be published. All authors have participated sufficiently in the work to take public responsibility for appropriate portions of the content; and agreed to be accountable for all aspects of the work in ensuring that questions related to the accuracy or integrity of any part of the work are appropriately investigated and resolved.

Author details

[1]Department of Radiology, Kaohsiung Medical University Hospital, Kaohsiung Medical University, No. 100, Ziyou 1st Rd., Sanmin District, Kaohsiung City 80756, Taiwan, Republic of China. [2]Department of Urology, Kaohsiung Medical University Hospital, Kaohsiung Medical University, Kaohsiung City, Taiwan.

References

1. Wilson SR, Katz DS. Computed tomography demonstration of epididymitis with extension to vas deferens. Urology. 2006;68:1339–40.
2. Yang DM, Kim HC, Lee HL, et al. Sonographic findings of acute vasitis. J Ultrasound Med. 2010;29:1711–5.
3. Eddy K, Connell D, Goodacre B, et al. Imaging findings prevent unnecessary surgery in vasitis: an under-reported condition mimicking inguinal hernia. Clin Radiol. 2011;66:475–7.
4. Dylewksi J, Sygal V. Infectious vasitis caused by chlamydia trachomatis. Infec Dis Clin Pract. 2014;22:e16–7.
5. You SH, Sung DJ, Han NY, et al. Emphysematous vasitis misdiagnosed as strangulated inguinal hernia. J Emerg Med. 2014;47:e15–7.
6. Patel K, Lamb B, Pathak S, Peters J. Vasitis: the need for imaging and clinical acumen. BMJ Case Rep. 2014;2014. https://doi.org/10.1136/bcr-2014-206994.
7. Kerkeni W, Saadi A, Ben Miled A, et al. Vasitis: an uncommon diagnosis mimicking incarcerated inguinal hernia. Urology. 2016;93:e1.
8. Chan PTK, Schlegel PN. Inflammatory conditions of the male Excurrent ductal system. Part II. J Androl. 2002;23:461–9.
9. Benjamin JA, Robertson TD, Cheetham JG. Vasitis nodosa: a new clinical entity simulating tuberculosis of the vas deferens. J Urol. 1943;49:575–82.
10. Clavijo RI, Rose-Nussbaumer J, Turek PJ. Clinically symptomatic vasitis: clinical correlations in a rare condition. Syst Biol Reprod Med. 2010;56(6):445–9.
11. Middleton WD, Dahiya N, Naughton CK, et al. High-resolution sonography of the normal extrapelvic vas deferens. J Ultrasound Med. 2009;28:839–46.
12. Eddy K, Piercy GB, Eddy R. Vasitis: clinical and ultrasound confusion with inguinal hernia clarified by computed tomography. Can Urol Assoc J. 2011;5:E74–6.
13. Schurr E, Cytter-Kuint R, Ehrlichman M, Weiser G. Pediatric vasitis: a rare complication of epididymitis. Can Urol Assoc J. 2014;8(5–6):E436–8.
14. Yang DM, Kim HC, Kim SW, Lee HL, Min GE, Lim SJ. Sonographic findings of tuberculous vasitis. J Ultrasound Med. 2014;33(5):913–6.

25

The distribution of Preputial vessels in different severity of rat congenital hypospadias model: Imaging study using micro-computerized tomography

Defu Lin[1,2], Pei Liu[1,2], Guannan Wang[1,2], Weiping Zhang[1,2] and Ning Sun[1,2*]

Abstract

Background: Micro-computerized tomography (micro-CT) is considered as an innovative non-invasive and high-resolution imaging technology. The current research aims to reconstruct the distribution of preputial vessels in different severity of rat congenital hypospadias model by micro-CT, and to provide an anatomic basis for the selection of preputial vessel pedicle flaps in surgery.

Methods: Pregnant rats were exposed to finasteride from gestational day 12 to 17. Depending on the position of the urethral meatus, the pups were divided into normal, mild hypospadias and severe hypospadias groups. Six months after birth, the preputial blood vessels were observed in vascular perfusion with Microfil (a silicone-based polymer) and scanned by micro-CT. CTvox and NRecon were utilized to reconstruct 3-dimentional (3D) images. A pathological analysis of the specimen was taken in order to determine the position of Microfil.

Results: The normal group and the mild hypospadias group had similar preputial image characteristics. At the junction of the inner and outer prepuce, the deep layer vessels of the superficial fascia were transversely distributed and formed a vascular ring-like structure. Among the severe hypospadias group, five had sufficient blood circulation while six had insufficient blood circulation. In sufficient blood circulation type, the ring-like vessels were found at the junction of the inner and outer prepuce similar to that of the normal and mild hypospadias group. However, only a small amount of capillary supply to this area in the insufficient type.

Conclusion: The junction of the inner and outer prepuce with abundant blood circulation was suitable to be a vascular pedicle flap. The tubularized preputial island flaps were consistent with the ring-like vessels area, and the original blood supply was retained to the greatest extent.

Keywords: Prepuce, Blood vessel, Micro-CT, Hypospadias, Rat model

Background

The incidence of hypospadias is approximately 1:200~1:300 male births, which have doubled over the past three decades. The preputial skin is the principal grafting material to the urethroplasty [1, 2]. However, postoperative complications are about 5–25% [3], including urethral fistula, stricture and diverticula. The occurrences of urethral fistula and stricture are correlated to the blood supply of molding material for urethral reconstruction [4]. To create a more reasonable preputial vessel pedicle flap design to minimize the disruption of blood circulation, anatomical study is required to have a better understanding on the distribution of preputial vasculature.

The anatomic characteristic of the blood supply is difficult to detect, because the capillaries of prepuce are the terminal branch and measured in micron [5]. Micro-CT scanners reach spatial resolution in submicron level [6–9]. So far little research has been carried out in the study of preputial vascular distribution of patients with hypospadias. Previous literature has reviewed the anatomy of hypospadias preputial

* Correspondence: doctorsn@163.com
[1]National Center for Children's Health, Beijing, China
[2]Department of Urology, Beijing Children's Hospital affiliated to Capital Medical University, No.56 Nanlishilu Rd, West District, Beijing, China

vessels using methods such as trans-illumination, microscopic observation and 3D computer reconstruction [10–12]. Although these approaches have studied the vascular anatomy, the preputial vascular networks are still difficult to measure in 3D.

Exposure to finasteride, estrogen and other anti-androgens in pregnant rat can induce congenital hypospadias model [13–16]. This is the first study identifying the distribution of the preputial vessels in rat hypospadias mode. The micro-CT, which was used extensively to detect the anatomy of the animal, was used to scan the rat hypospadias penile specimens to produce the 3D images of the preputial vessels [17].

It is hypothesized that the deep layer vessels of the superficial fascia were transversely distributed at the junction of the inner and outer prepuce. According to this distribution, a transvers preputial island flap was selected to preserve the blood supply to the greatest extent. The current research aims to reconstruct the distribution of preputial vessels in different severity of rat congenital hypospadias model by micro-CT, and to provide a theoretical basis for the selection of preputial vessel pedicle flaps in surgery.

Methods

Hypospadias rat model

The animal ethics committee's approval was achieved by the Institutional Animal Care and Use Committee of Beijing Children's Hospital, Capital Medical University prior to the experiment. Total 6 pregnant Wista rats (250-270 g) obtained from Animal Experimental Center (Capital Medical University, China) were housed in a temperature-controlled room in plastic cage (1 animal per cage) with free access to food and water at 22–25 °C on a 12 h light/dark cycle. The pregnant rats were divided into an experimental group ($n = 4$) and control group ($n = 2$). The experimental group received daily finasteride (Yuan Sen pharmaceutical Co. Ltd., Hebei, China) injection of 40 mg/kg to the subcutaneous of the abdominal wall, from 12 to 17 gestational days (GDs). The control group was injected with same volume of normal saline solution only. After delivery (GD22–24), mothers and the newborn rats were fed in one cage. On the 28th day after delivery, hypospadias rat models were selected from the neonatal rats. For testing purpose, rat models with the following features were used in the experiment: deficient foreskin ventrally with dorsal hood; abnormally located urethral meatus; vary degrees of ventral penile curvature.

Silicone rubber compound infusion

Microfil infusion on rat models was started at the age of 6 months. Urethane was given to the rat models through intraperitoneal injection of 6 mL/kg to induce general anesthesia. The abdominal wall was opened using a midline incision. The abdominal aorta and the inferior vena cava were isolated and ligated. 24G indwelling needle was inserted to the abdominal aorta at the distal of the ligation point as an input channel. A 2 mm hole was cut at the inferior vena cava wall as an output channel. The micro-pump was connected (Product model: SDS-MP09, Shan De Shi medical company, Beijing, China), and 50 ml 40 °C heparin saline (50 U/ml) at 5 ml/min was input to dilate blood vessels and anticoagulation. Microfil (MV^{-122} compound 4 ml, diluent solution10ml, curing agent 0.7 ml, Circulation Tech Company, America) 2 mL/min was added to replace heparin when the viscera turned pale. The perfusion was finished until the viscera became yellow. The specimens were stored at 25 °C to clot the Microfil, then the penile specimen was cut and stored in 4 °C environments. The specimens were saved in 10% formalin. After experiment, animals were deeply anesthetized by intraperitoneal injection of urethane to minimize the pain.

Micro-CT scan

The Bruker SkyScan 1172 micro-CT system (Bruker, Kontich, Belgium) was utilized. Technical protocol of the Scanning was specified as follows: voltage of 59 kV and current of 167 μA with a 0.5-mm aluminum attenuation filter. A 6.88-μm resolution was obtained. Acquisition time for each specimen was 120 min. Raw projection image files were reconstructed using the Fledkamp cone-beam algorithm in NRecon Reconstruction and CTvox (Bruker) software [18].

Pathological section

After image acquisition, the samples were embedded in paraffin and horizontally sectioned (7 mm of thickness). Samples were stained with hematoxylin-eosin (HE), rinsed in distilled water and mounted. Sections were assessed and the Microfil particles were detected using light microscopy.

Results

Establishment of hypospadias model

The control group rats gave birth to 24 fetuses, including 10 females and 14 males. All male offspring had normal penis without hypospadias. The experimental group gave birth to 41 fetuses, including 17 females and 24males. Totally, 16 hypospadias offspring were included. According to the location of the meatus, 16 hypospadias pups were further divided into mild group ($n = 3$) and severe group ($n = 13$).

The morphology of the hypospadias model

In the control group (Fig. 1a), the urethral meatus are normally located. Prepuce covered the penis completely, and no ventral penile curvature was found. The urethral

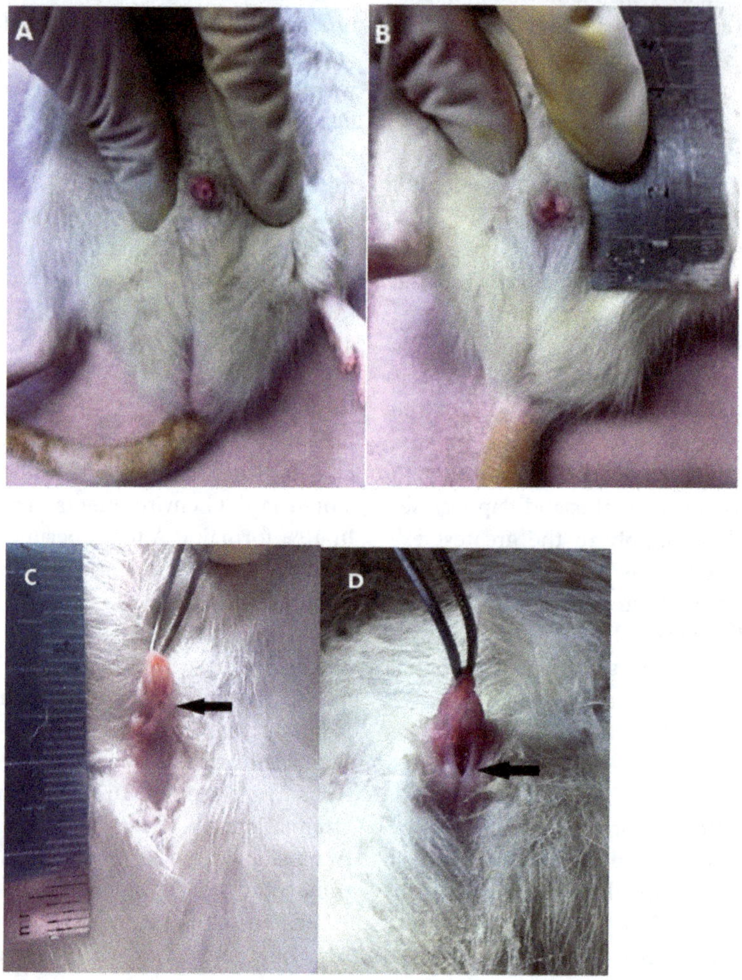

Fig. 1 **a** The normal penis appearance. **b** The "V" shape prepuce of the hypospadias model. **c** Mild hypospadias model. **d** The severe hypospadias model. Arrows show the ectopic urethral meatus

meatus was situated in the ventral of the ventral shaft in the mild hypospadias model (Fig. 1c). In the mild hypospadias group, there was ventral prepuce defect and a "V" shape dorsal prepuce (Fig. 1b). The glans was observed and the ventral penile curvature was not obvious in the normal position. The severe hypospadias model has urethral meatus located at the perineum. While the appearance of the prepuce and glans was similar between the severe and the mild hypospadias model, meatus fibrosis, which may induce penile ventral curvature, was observed on both sides of the ectopic urethral meatus in the severe hypospadias model (Fig. 1d).

Penis images

Tissues of different density were observed easily by adjusting the CT threshold value. The anatomy of penile and preputial dartos vessels, penile dorsal vessels, corpora cavernosa, corpus spongiosum, baculum was visualized clearly. (Fig. 2).

Normal rat preputial blood vessels

The deep layer vessels of the superficial fascia, which was from the external pudendal artery, were axially distributed bilaterally. At the junction of the inner and outer prepuce, bilateral deep layer vessels showed a transverse distribution and form a vascular ring-like structure. The ring-like structure continued to send parallel terminal vessels to the inner preputial skin (Fig. 3b). These terminal vessels formed numerous reticular lateral branches. The superficial layer vessels of the superficial fascia supplied blood to the penile skin. The deep and superficial layers vessels can be observed clearly by adjusting the viewing angle in 3D. There was no noticeable relationship between the superficial and deep vessels of prepuce. The diameter of the superficial vessel was thinner than the deep one, but the superficial one had a greater number of blood vessels and branches (Fig. 3).

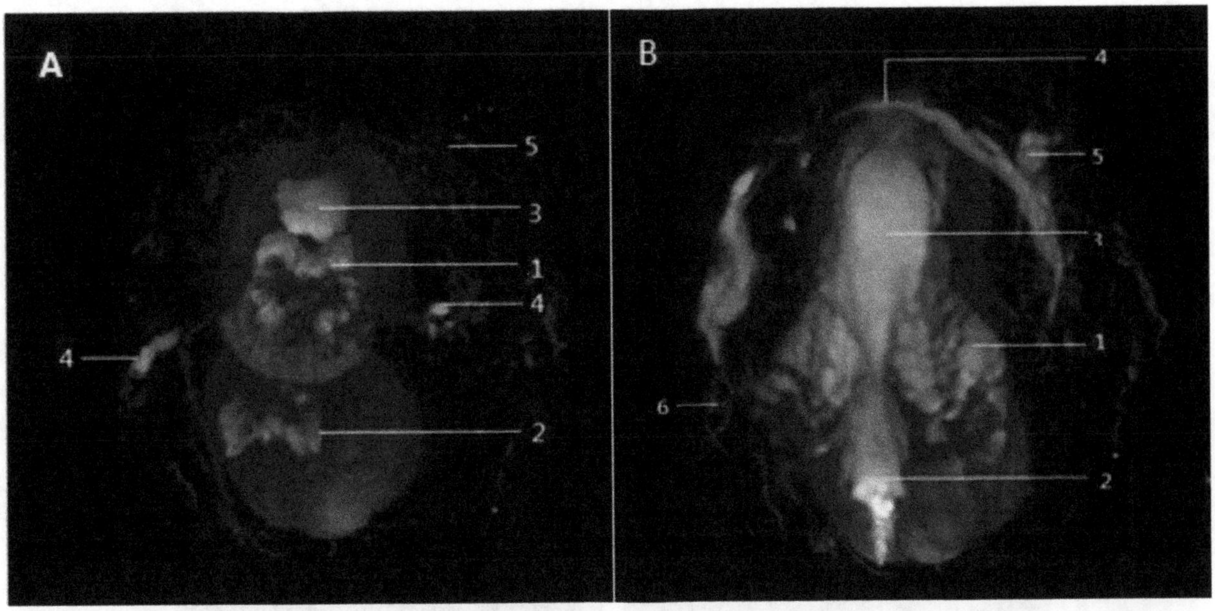

Fig. 2 a Transverse section image at the level penile shaft showing (1) the bilateral corpora cavernosa connected with each other at the midline, (2) the corpus spongiosum was located on the ventral side and relatively smaller than the corpora cavernosa, (3) the dorsal penile vessels, (4) the two deep layer vessels of the superficial fascia were axially distributed at the lateral of the penile shaft in the area between 9- to 8-o'clock and 3- to 4-o'clock positions. (5) Innumerable superficial layer vessels of the superficial fascia were distributed at the surrounding of the penis to supply blood to the skin. **b** Transverse section image at the level of the glans showing (1) the corpora cavernosa separated by the (2) baculum, (3) showing the dorsal penile vessels. (4) The deep layer vessels showed a transverse distribution and formed a 'ring-like structure' at the junction of the inner and outer prepuce. The 'ring-like structure' was oriented from bilateral (5) the deep layer vessel of the superficial fascia

Hypospadias model preputial blood vessels

The distribution and morphology of the deep and the superficial layer vessels were similar between mild hypospadias model and normal penis. The bilateral deep layer vessels were converged to form an intact vascular ring at the junction of the inner and outer prepuce (Fig. 4a).

The severe hypospadias group was divided into two subgroups based on their blood circulation of the deep layer vessels at the junction of inner and outer prepuce. In the good blood circulation group as showing in Fig. 4b, the deep layer vessels converged to form a half ring structure at the dorsal of the prepuce regardless of the fact that there was an absent of ventral prepuce. However, the vascular ring was replaced by a network distribution in the poor circulation group (Fig. 4c).

Pathology

Microfil particles can be found in the arteries, capillary networks and veins. The diameter of Microfil was less than capillaries, so Microfil can fill the entire vascular system. No Microfil leakage was observed outside the blood vessel wall to the surrounding tissue, hence Microfil was an ideal angiography reagent.

Discussion

Hypospadias is among the most common congenital defects in pediatric urology. Due to anterior urethral maldevelopment, the ectopic urethral meatus may be located anywhere from the tip of glans to perineum. Urethroplasty is the only method to treat hypospadias. There are more than 300 surgical techniques to treat this disease, but every technique has some corresponding surgical complications, which are most likely in urethral fistula. So far, there are no common standard surgical techniques have been approved by all pediatric urologists [19–21]. To figure out this problem, we analyzed the preputial vessels in different severity of the rat hypospadias model by micro-CT. It is generally believed that blood vessels in the prepuce have two layers which can be easily separated [10]. The junction of the inner and outer prepuce has the most abundant blood supply from the deep layer vessels and can serve as a preputial vessel flap. Innumerable superficial layer vessels are distributed at the surrounding of the penis to supply blood to the skin. This type of vascular distribution is the anatomic basis of tubularized preputial island flaps procedure, as it not only ensures blood supply to the flap, but also prevents penis skin necrosis, which has been demonstrated once again in this study.

The vascular ring structure was originated from the deep layer vessels of the superficial fascia. Four main types of the deep layer vessels had been described in human: single branch predominant type (41%), two branches

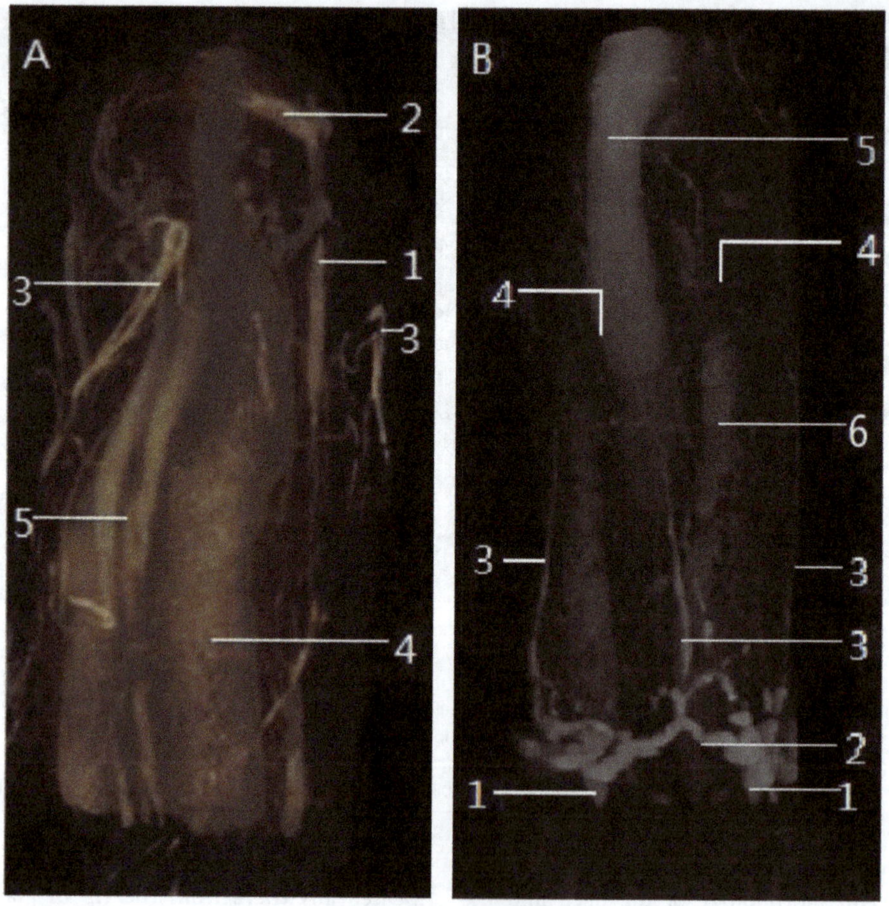

Fig. 3 a The penis and preputial appearance in the nature position. (1) The deep layer of the penile dartos vessels go along with penile shaft at the dorsolateral position. At the junction of the inner and outer prepuce, the vessel transversely oriented terminal bifurcations anastomose with similar vessels of contralateral side and form a (2) vascular ring-like structure. (3) The superficial layer of the dartos vessels. (4) The corpora cavernosa, (5) the corpus spongiosum. **b** Reflecting the prepuce to the level of penopubic junction. (1) The bilateral deep layer of the penile dartos vessels converged and formed (2) the vascular ring, and then send (3) some parallel terminal blood vessels to the inner preputial dartos, these terminal blood vessels (4) anastomosis with each other. (5) The dorsal penile vessels. (6) The corpora cavernosa

predominant type (25%), arching H-type (12.5%), or net-like type (21%). The qualities of the vascular pedicle and the urethral-plate were the two important surgical variables [22].

Tubularized preputial island flaps are the ideal single-stage repairs for the proximal hypospadias. For patients with severe hypospadias and ventral curvature, two-stage operation is still meaningful [23]. Clinical data indicates that penile curvature corrected in the first phase. Urethroplasty is done in the second phase to reduce the incidence of complications. Two-stage surgery reduces the difficulty of the operation somewhat, on the other hand it increases surgical operation time and prolonged treatment time [24]. This experiment verified that in the normal group and the mild hypospadias group, the blood vessels at the junction of the inner and outer prepuce had a wider caliber and formed a vascular ring. While in the group with severe hypospadias, the blood vessels at the junction of the inner and outer prepuce had a relatively smaller caliber displayed a net-like distribution and could not constitute a clear and complete vascular ring. These results may explain patients with severe hypospadias are most likely to suffer from postoperative complications than the ones with mild hypospadias.

We divided the severe hypospadias group into two types based on their vascular morphology: The first type has a sufficient blood supply. Although the blood vessels at the junction of the inner and outer prepuce could not form a vascular ring completely due to the ventral prepuce defect, there was a semi-circular vessel structure, which diverges small branches into the inner preputial skin to ensure an efficient supply of blood; For the second type, there was no semi-vascular ring to support the efficient blood circulation. The vessels were netlike distributed and contained mainly capillaries so there was no sufficient supply of blood to the preputial vessel pedicle flap. This result may

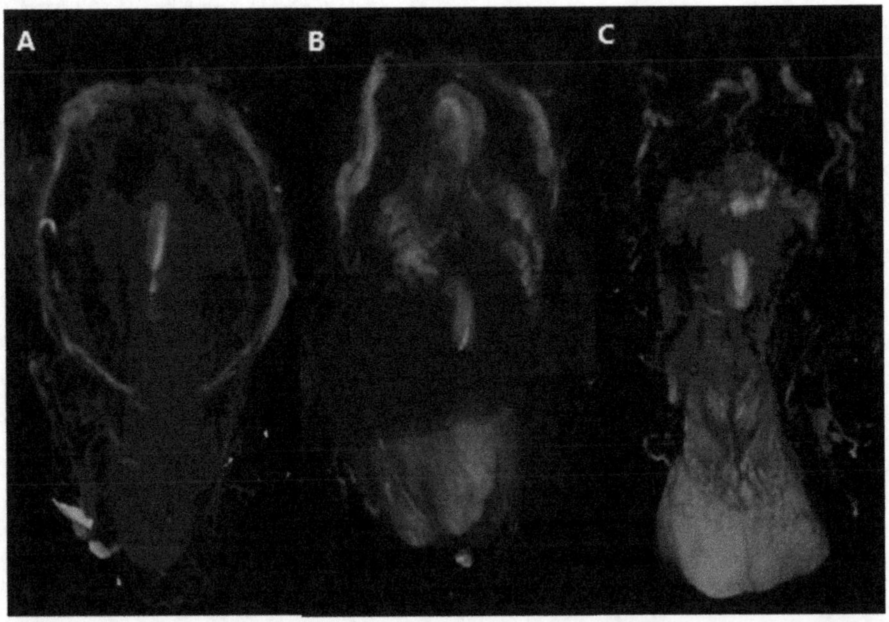

Fig. 4 The 3D images reconstructed by the micro-CT.(A) Mild hypospadias. (B) Severe hypospadias with good blood circulation. (C) Severe hypospadias with poor blood circulation. **a** The terminal branches originated from the deep layer of the penile dartos vessels formed an intact vascular ring and covered the glans. **b** Because of the ventral part prepuce defected, the deep layer vessels converge to form a half ring structure at the dorsal of the glans. **c** The severe hypospadias with insufficient blood circulation, which was absent of dominant vessels, the vascular ring was replaced by a network structure

explain the fact that patients with severe hypospadias achieved satisfactory results without postoperative complications after one stage surgery because their blood vessels at the junction of inner and outer prepuce provided a sufficient amount of blood for a better survival of the flap. At the same time, we concluded that patients with severe hypospadias with poor vessels structures were highly recommended to undergo two-stage surgery to reduce postoperative complications.

The prepuce vessels are the terminal branch, and the capillaries are extremely narrow, hence knowledge about the vessels is limited. Considerable work has been done to study prepuce vessels, such as transillumination with endoscopic cold light source, microscopic observation of gelation and India ink perfusion, 3D reconstruction of histological sections [10–12]. In this study, an advanced technology, micro-CT scanning, was used to analyze the distribution of preputial vessels. Micro-CT is an innovative non-invasive and high-resolution imaging technology. O'Neill et al. found the results of virtual sectioning at micro-CT and conventional histologic sectioning are highly correlated [18]. The CTvox (Bruker) software can be utilized to observe the samples by transverse, sagittal, and coronal section image, and established 2- or 3-dimensional reconstruction on interesting parts. The highest resolution can reach 0.5 μm, while the mean diameter of capillary vessels is 6 to 9 μm, so micro-CT can be used to micro vessels scanning [25].

The limitation of this study is that human penile anatomy is different from penile anatomy of rats. This study may not represent such anatomy of the humans. The next step, the clinical experiment will be carried out to detect the exact relationship between the postoperative complication and the anatomy of the preputial vessels.

Conclusion

The application of Microfil and contrasted micro-CT scanning improve our understanding on the anatomy of the hypospadias, especially the preputial vascular structure in 3D. The junction of the inner and outer prepuce with abundant blood circulation would be a suitable vessel pedicle flap. The tubularized preputial island flaps were consistent with the ring-like vessels area, and the original blood supply was retained to the greatest extent.

Abbreviations

3D: 3-dimentional; GDs: Gestational days; HE: Hematoxylin-eosin; Micro-CT: Micro-computerized tomography

Acknowledgements

Not applicable.

Authors' contributions

DFL and PL conceived of the study and performed the experiments and wrote the manuscript. GNW was done the acquisition of data, or analysis and interpretation of date. WPZ participated in the design of the study and provided technical advice. NS was involved in the design of the study, in discussions and reviewed the manuscript. All authors read and agreed to the final manuscript.

References

1. Mesrobian HG, Canning DA. Surgical technique for antegrade dissection of the preputial vascular pedicle during hypospadias repair. J Pediatr Urol. 2012;8(3):282–4. https://doi.org/10.1016/j.jpurol.2011.03.020.
2. Singal AK, Dubey M, Jain V. Transverse preputial onlay island flap urethroplasty for single-stage correction of proximal hypospadias. World J Urol. 2016;34(7):1019–24. https://doi.org/10.1007/s00345-015-1686-1.
3. Long CJ, Canning DA. Hypospadias: are we as good as we think when we correct proximal hypospadias? J Pediatr Urol. 2016;12(4):196.e1-5. https://doi.org/10.1016/j.jpurol.2016.05.002.
4. Westenfelder M. Treatment of hypospadias. Urologe A. 1992;31(333–341): 1992 (In German).
5. Cagri SM, Kapucuoglu N, Gursoy K, Baspinar S. The microvessel density of the hypospadiac prepuce in children. J Pediatr Urol. 2011;2(7):162–5. https://doi.org/10.1016/j.jpurol.2010.04.017.
6. Schambach SJ, Bag S, Schilling L, Groden C, Brockmann MA. Application of micro-CT in small animal imaging. Methods. 2010;50(1):2–13. https://doi.org/10.1016/j.ymeth.2009.08.007.
7. Razavi H, Dusch MN, Zarafshar SY, Taylor CA, Feinstein JA. A method for quantitative characterization of growth in the 3-D structure of rat pulmonary arteries. Microvasc Res. 2012;83(2):146–53. https://doi.org/10.1016/j.mvr.2011.12.003.
8. Weber SM, Peterson KA, Durkee B, Qi C, Longino M, Warner T, Lee FT, Weichert JP. Imaging of murine liver tumor using micro CT with a hepatocyte-selective contrast agent: accuracy is dependent on adequate contrast enhancement. J Surg Res. 2004;119(1):41–5. https://doi.org/10.1016/S0022-4804(03)00357-3.
9. Chugh BP, Lerch JP, Yu LX, Pienkowski M, Harrison RV, Henkelman RM, Sled JG. Measurement of cerebral blood volume in mouse brain regions using micro-computed tomography. Neuroimage. 2009;47(4):1312–8. https://doi.org/10.1016/j.neuroimage.2009.03.083.
10. Zhao Z, Sun N, Mao X. Vascularization of vessel pedicle in hypospadias and its relationship to near-period complications. Exp Ther Med. 2018;16(3): 2408–12. https://doi.org/10.3892/etm.2018.6475.
11. Perovic SV, Radojicic ZI. Vascularization of the hypospadiac prepuce and its impact on hypospadias repair. J Urol. 2003;169(3):1098–100 discussion 1101.
12. Ceyhan L, Cagri SM, Baspinar S, Duman L, Büyükyavuz BI. The correlation between preputial blood flow and microvessel density in distal hypospadias: a prospective clinical study. J Pediatr Urol. 2014;10(1):103–6. https://doi.org/10.1016/j.jpurol.2013.07.003.
13. An N, Peng J, He G, Fan X, Li F, Chen H. Involvement of activation of mitogen-activated protein kinase (MAPK)/extracellular signal-regulated kinase (ERK) signaling pathway in proliferation of urethral plate fibroblasts in Finasteride-induced rat hypospadias. Med Sci Monit. 2018;24:8984–92. https://doi.org/10.12659/MSM.911271.
14. Martinez AG, Pardo B, Gamez R, Mas R, Noa M, Marrero G, Valle M, Garcia H, Curveco D, Mendoza N, Goicochea E. Effects of in utero exposure to D-004, a lipid extract from Roystonea regia fruits, in the male rat: a comparison with finasteride. J Med Food. 2011;14(12):1663–9. https://doi.org/10.1089/jmf.2010.0279.
15. Kim KS, Torres CR Jr, Yucel S, Raimondo K, Cunha GR, Baskin LS. Induction of hypospadias in a murine model by maternal exposure to synthetic estrogens. Environ Res. 2004;94(3):267–75. https://doi.org/10.1016/S0013-9351(03)00085-9.
16. Yucel S, Desouza A, Baskin LS. In utero prednisone exposure affects genital development. J Urol. 2004;172(4 Pt 2):1725–30.
17. Durkee BY, Weichert JP, Halberg RB. Weichert and R.B. Halberg, small animal micro-CT colonography. Methods. 2010;50(1):36–41. https://doi.org/10.1016/j.ymeth.2009.07.008.
18. O'Neill M, Huang GO, Lamb DJ. Novel application of micro-computerized tomography for morphologic characterization of the murine penis. J Sex Med. 2017;14(12):1533–9. https://doi.org/10.1016/j.jsxm.2017.10.065.
19. Hueber PA, Antczak C, Abdo A, Franc-Guimond J, Barrieras D, Houle AM. Long-term functional outcomes of distal hypospadias repair: a single center retrospective comparative study of TIPs, Mathieu and MAGPI. J Pediatr Urol. 2015;11(2):68e1–7. https://doi.org/10.1016/j.jpurol.2014.09.011.
20. Al-Adl AM, El-Karamany TM, Bassiouny AS. Distal extension of the midline urethral-plate incision in the Snodgrass hypospadias repair: An objective assessment of the functional and cosmetic outcomes. Arab J Urol. 2014; 12(2):116–26. https://doi.org/10.1016/j.aju.2014.02.002.
21. Chalmers DJ, Siparsky GL, Wiedel CA, Wilcox DT. Distal hypospadias repair in infants without a postoperative stent. Pediatr Surg Int. 2015;31(3):287–90. https://doi.org/10.1007/s00383-014-3647-y.
22. Yucel S, Guntekin E, Kukul E, Karaguzel G, Ciftcioglu A, Melikoglu M, Baykara M. Comparison of hypospadiac and normal preputial vascular anatomy. J Urol. 2004;172:1973–6.
23. McNamara ER, Schaeffer AJ, Logvinenko T, Seager C, Rosoklija I, Nelson CP, Retik AB, Diamond DA, Cendron M. Management of Proximal Hypospadias with 2-stage repair: 20 year experience. J Urol. 2015;194(4):1080–5. https://doi.org/10.1016/j.juro.2015.04.105.
24. Fan ZQ, Sun JT, Huangfu XH, Chen GX, Hao JW, Liu ZH. Prefabricated partial distal urethral in 2-staged repair of proximal hypospadias with severe chordee. Int J Clin Exp Med. 2015;8(2):2453–8.
25. Bastos AN, Oliveira LR, Ferrarez CE, de Figueiredo AA, Favorito LA, Bastos Netto JM. Structural study of prepuce in hypospadias--does topical treatment with testosterone produce alterations in prepuce vascularization? J Urol. 2011;185(6 Suppl):2474–8. https://doi.org/10.1016/j.juro.2011.01.035.

26

Sexual pain and IC/BPS in women

Su Jin Kim[1,5], Jayoung Kim[2,3*] and Hana Yoon[4*]

Abstract

Interstitial cystitis/bladder pain syndrome (IC/BPS) and female sexual dysfunction (FSD) are common conditions that substantially reduce women's health. In particular, women with IC/BPS show vulvodynia, a kind of FDS that originates from consistent pain around the vulvar area. There have been many studies attempting to find the underlying mechanisms that induce the chronic pain associated with IC/BPS and vulvodynia and explain why these two conditions often coexist. Proposed theories suggest that pain hypersensitivity is being mediated by peripheral and central sensitization. However, there are still many unknown factors, such as etiologies, that can evoke pain hypersensitivity and may be linking the casual relationship between IC/BPS and vulvodynia. At present, knowledge regarding IC/BPS and vulvodynia are insufficient when considering their clinical importance. Therefore, efforts are necessary to elucidate the issues surrounding IC/BPS and vulvodynia.

Keywords: Cystitis, interstitial, Sexual dysfunction, Chronic pain, Vulvodynia, Lower urinary tract symptoms, Quality of life

Background

Female sexual dysfunction (FSD) and interstitial cystitis/ bladder pain syndrome (IC/BPS) are two conditions affecting women's health. A study on the association between sexual and general well-being found that women reported better quality of life (QoL) with higher sexual satisfaction, regardless of age and/or menopausal status [1]. Both FSD and IC/BPS significantly impairs a woman's abilities to pursue and enjoy sexual relations. Approximately 40–50% of women experience FSD and 0.5–12% experience IC/BPS. Considering these incidence rates, both FSD and IC/BPS present serious challenges for patients and clinicians [2–6].

Chronic pain deteriorates not only personal health and wellness, but also QoL. Chronic pain can induce sexual dysfunction, such as arousal disorder, and relationship problems [7]. Furthermore, studies have shown that significantly more women with chronic pelvic pain (CPP) show FSD compared to those without CPP. Women with CPP and FSD reported various types of sexual dysfunctions, including hypoactive sexual desire disorder, sexual arousal disorder, orgasmic disorder, and sexual pain disorder [8].

* Correspondence: Jayoung.Kim@csmc.edu; wowhana@ewha.ac.kr
[2]Departments of Surgery and Biomedical Sciences, Cedars-Sinai Medical Center, Los Angeles, CA 90048, USA
[4]Department of Urology, Medical Research Center, Ewha Womans University School of Medicine, Seoul, Republic of Korea
Full list of author information is available at the end of the article

The symptoms of IC/BPS, such as urinary frequency, urgency, and pelvic pain, can have a negative impact on sexual activity and QoL [9]. Women with overactive bladder (OAB) frequently have a risk for sexual dysfunction [10]. In the postmenopausal group, women with scores indicating severe OAB reported worse sexual function, particularly in the arousal, lubrication, orgasm, pain, and total domains [11]. Despite the known association between FSD and bladder diseases, contributing risk factors have yet to be explored. Evaluating the impact of duration, severity, pain localization, sexual trauma history, anxiety, and depression associated with sexual dysfunction may help elucidate risk factors. Increasing our knowledge about sexual dysfunction as it relates to bladder diseases may aid in clinical diagnoses, treatment strategies, and overall symptom improvement. This review will provide an overview of studies that address FSD in women with IC/BPS.

Pain in FSD

According to consensus from the 4th Internaional Consultation on Sexual Medicine (ICSM), FSD is classified as hypoactive sexual desire dysfunction, female sexual arousal dysfunction, female orgasmic dysfunction, female-genital-pelvic pain dysfunction, persistent genital arousal disorder, postcoital syndrome, hypohedonic orgasm, or painful orgasm [2, 12]. Guidelines from the 4th ICSM also define pain-associated FSD as female-genital-pelvic pain dysfunction and include all conditions that inhibit sexual intercourse or induce negative effects on sexual functions. Female-genital-pelvic pain dysfunction is different from the previous classification characterized as pain associated with FSD, which includes sexual pain disorder including dyspareunia and vaginismus [13]. According to the ICSM, female-genital-pelvic pain dysfunction includes persistent or recurrent difficulties with at least one of the following: (1) vaginal penetration during intercourse, (2) marked vulvovaginal or pelvic pain during genital contact, (3) marked fear or anxiety about vulvovaginal or pelvic pain in anticipation of, during, or as a result of genital contact, or (4) marked hypertonicity or overactivity of pelvic floor muscles with or without genital contact [14]. Painful orgasm also falls under this category and is defined as genital and/or pelvic pain during or shortly after orgasm [2]. These recent new definitions reflect the evolving concept behind pain-associated FSD as it also now includes pain in the vulvovaginal and pelvic area and pelvic floor hypertonicity. The new categorization of female-genital-pelvic pain dysfunction has broadened the view on pain-associated FSD and has differentiated it from its previous classification, which confined symptoms to each organ or single disease. This recent change in classification by the ICSM considers pain-associated FDS as a complex condition influenced by psychological and physical factors and supports the general thought that FSD is multifactorial.

Previously, vulvodynia had been generalized under chronic vulvar pain with no precise discrimination for it. However, recent consensus has redefined chronic vulvar pain as vulvar pain associated with specific diseases, such as inflammation, neoplasm, and/or injury. This was conducted at a conference with the International Society for the Study of Vulvovaginal Disease, the International Society for the Study of Women's Sexual Health, and the International Pelvic Pain Society [15]. Vulvodynia can have diverse pain characteristics; therefore, pain-based classification helps in identification, diagnosis, and treatment. Vulvodynia can be characterized as either general (entire vulva) or localized (parts of the vulva). Additionally, based on the situation of the pain, vulvodynia can be classified as either provoked (triggered by physical contact) or unprovoked (spontaneous occurrence without specific triggers) [16]. Women of all ages can experience vulvodynia, and provoked vulvodynia is the most commonly diagnosed [17, 18]. Provoked vulvodynia is thought to be more widely diagnosed than unprovoked because its symptoms can be better recognized by doctors. Therefore, there is an great need to better identify unprovoked vulvodynia patients.

Sexual pain and IC/bps

IC/BPS is a disorder that induces chronic pain or discomfort in the bladder and surrounding pelvic organs [19, 20]. At present, IC/BPS is not a disease confined to just the bladder and pelvic area; it is a complex disease that includes the outside of the genitourinary tract. Tripp et al. [21] investigated the pain characteristics of IC/BPS using whole-body diagram pain locators. They found that women with IC/BPS reported significantly more pain all over their body, compared to healthy women without. Only 52 of the 193 IC/BPS diagnosed women (27%) presented pain restricted to the bladder and pelvic area. Moreover, IC/BPS patients had various co-morbidities. Diseases, such as irritable bowel syndrome, fibromyalgia, vulvodynia, chronic pelvic pain, endometriosis, OAB, allergies and chronic fatigue syndrome, were found to coexist in IC/BPS patients [22–28].

In addition, there are several reports that IC/BPS can increase the risk for or worsen other diseases, including FSD. A population-based study found higher prevalence of FSD in women with IC/BPS [29]. FSD incidence also increased depending on the severity of IC/BPS symptoms, suggesting that FSD is a factor may be worsening IC/BPS. In regards to the pain associated with FSD, vulvodynia may be contributing to flare-ups of IC/BPS symptoms and could be the reason why IC/BPS patients avoid sexual activity [9, 30].

Can FSD and IC/bps be generalized as one disease?

Diseases characterized with lower urinary tract symptoms (LUTS) in females, such as incontinence and OAB, are known to have a negative impact on all domains in female sexual function. Symptoms of IC/BPS can also deteriorate patient's sexual activities and QoL. A significant number of IC/BPS patients avoid sexual activity because of pain. In addition, FSD and IC/BPS share similar clinical characteristics and comorbidities, making it difficult to discriminate between the two [31–33]. As mentioned previously, there are many clinical reports presenting an association between IC/BPS and vulvodynia, mainly due to shared FSD conditions.

Although the mechanisms of the association between IC/BPS and vulvodynia are unclear, visceral nerve cross-talking and the anatomic relationship between genital organs and the bladder offer a simple proximity explanation. Another possible mechanism behind the relationship is abnormal pain hypersensitivity induced by peripheral and central sensitization. The abnormal pain response frequently observed in vulvodynia patients is caused by central or peripheral maladaptive pain processing from local insult, injury, or trauma (Fig. 1).

Role of peripheral sensitization in the pain hypersensitivity of vulvodynia and IC/BPS

Exposure of nociceptors to repetitive pain stimulation reduces the pain threshold and amplifies the responsiveness of nociceptors. Therefore, this can abnormally increase peripheral transduction of sensitivity and lead to the

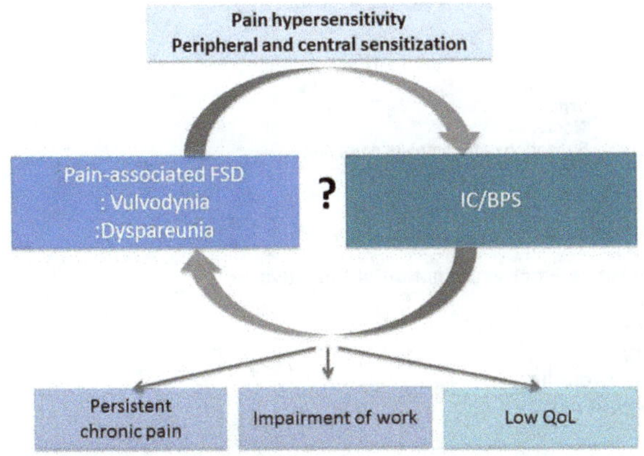

Fig. 1 FSD and IC/BPS: FSD; Female sexual dysfunction, *IC/BPS* Interstitial cystitis/bladder pain syndrome, *QoL* Quality of life

development of peripheral pain hypersensitivity [34–36]. The potential underlying mechanism of peripheral pain hypersensitivity noted in both vulvodynia and IC/BPS could be due to sensory nerve upregulation. Previous studies have shown that sensory nerve density is significantly increased in the vulva vestibule and bladder. Compared to the normal controls, patients with vulvodynia were found to have increased nociceptors in their vulvar vestibule [37–40]. Consequentially, this increased density of peripheral nociceptors results in increased sensitivity. It was also found that transient receptor potential V1 (TRPV1) exists in these nociceptive nerve endings and enhances pain signaling [37, 41, 42]. Pukall CF et al. [43] and Giesecke J et al. [44] reported increased peripheral tactile, pressure, and pain sensitivity in the patients with vulvodynia and confirmed histologic and molecular changes of peripheral nociceptors is associated with clinical manifestations. Similarly with vulvodynia, it has been reported that IC/BPS patient bladders have upregulated sensory innervation and TRPV1 expression [45–47].

Role of central sensitization in the pain hypersensitivity of vulvodynia and IC/BPS

Central sensitization is an important mechanism underlying various conditions associated with chronic pain and induces pain hypersensitivity through pathologically enhanced pathways that are not normally associated with nociception. For example, the low-threshold Aδ fiber, that is mostly used for temperature and pressure signaling, can be sensitized to pain. Chronic pain induced by central sensitization is persistent even after initiation of the signal and disappearance of the peripheral cause [48]. Studies have shown that the pain characteristics of central sensitization can be found in vulvodynia patients. Foster DC et al. [49] observed that vulvar vestibulitis syndrome patients experienced hyperalgesia and allodynia more often than normal controls after intradermal foot and forearm capsaicin injections. In addition, pelvic organ crosstalk has an important role in central sensitization because pelvic organs, such as the bladder, colon and vulva, are controlled by the same neural pathway [50]. Thus, afferent signals from other pelvic organs can provoke pain through neural crosstalk even though the initiation and peripheral causes of vulvodynia and IC/BPS have gone. Therefore, central sensitization plays an important role in the chronic pain observed in vulvodynia and IC/BPS. Clinically, similar manifestations of vulvodynia and IC/BPS have also existed. Moreover, recently, there has been an attempt to categorize various pain-associated conditions due to central sensitization as central sensitivity syndrome (CSS). Vulvodynia and IC/BPS are considered subgroups of CSS [51]. Previous studies on clinical findings support the notion that the same mechanisms associated with central sensitization are involved in the pain behind vulvodynia and IC/BPS [52–54].

Recently, evidence supporting central sensitization using functional and structural brain imaging were reported in vulvodynia and IC/BPS. Previously, Pukall et al. [55] showed that increased perception and activation of pain-related brain regions were observed in women with vulvar vestivulitis syndrome, compared to normal women, after tacticle stimulation of the vulvar vestibule. Other studies have reported that vulvodynia patients show increased grey matter density in pain-modulating and stress-related regions of the brain as well as alterations in the intrinsic connectivity of regions comprising the sensorimotor, salience, and default mode resting state networks [56, 57]. Similarly, women with IC/BPS showed alterations of oscillation frequency and functional connectivity of brain regions previously reported in other chronic pain conditions [58] and various white matter (right anterior thalamic radiation, left forceps major, and right longitudinal fasciculus, right superior and bilateral inferior longitudinal fasciculi) abnormalities that correlated with severity of pain, urinary symptoms, and impaired QoL [59]. Fig. 2 shows common therapeutic approaches and points of divergence among IC/BPS, IC/BPS + vulvodynia, and vulvodynia patient groups.

Approach and management of vulvodynia and IC/bps patients

Clinically, vulvodynia and IC/BPS often coexists and differentiation between the two is not easy, especially when the patient reports LUTS combined with pain. A majority of patients also seek medical care after relatively longer periods of initially feeling pain, leading to central sensitization that has been firmly established. Furthermore, clinical manifestations of chronic pain found in various other comorbidities can mask vulvodynia and IC/BPS, making it confusing and difficult to officially diagnose.

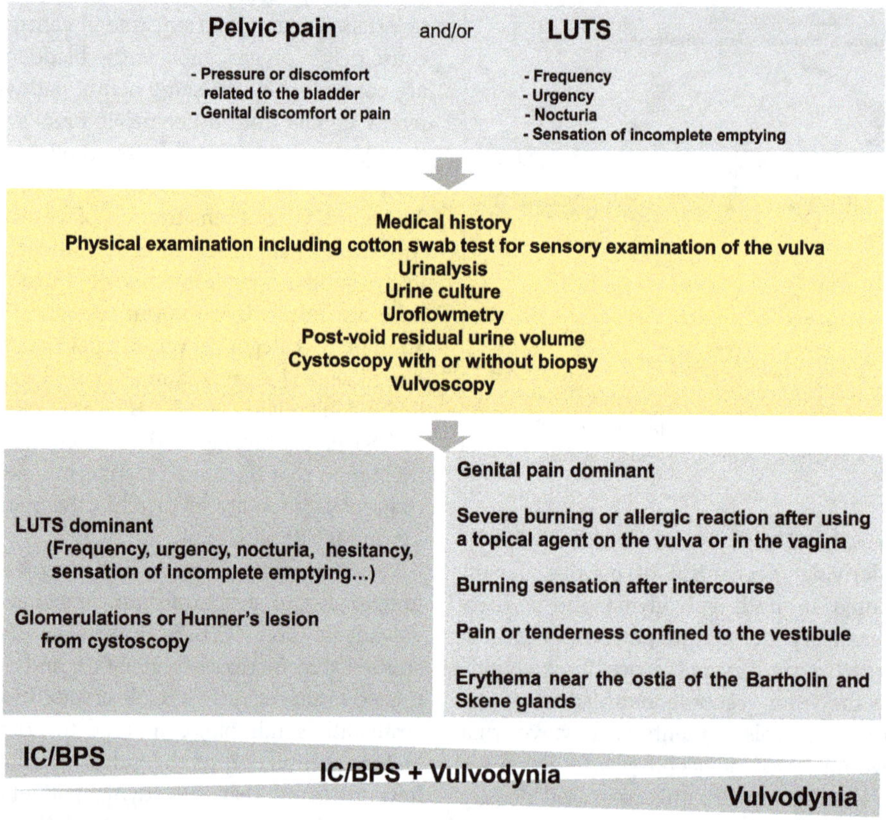

Fig. 2 Approach for differential diagnosis of IC/BPS, vulvodynia, and IC/BPS + vulvodynia (*LUTS* lower urinary tract symptoms, *IC/BPS* interstitial cystitis/bladder pain syndrome)

Table 1 Characteristics of FSD observed in women with IC/BPS

	Age	Types of FSD	Prevalence (%)	Other associated conditions
Verit et al. [8][a]	34.73 ± 8.07 years	NA	67.8 (78 of 112)	NA
Gardella et al. [28]	38.7 ± 12 years	Vulvodynia Dyspareunia	Vulvodynis: 85.1 (40 of 47) Vaginal burning: 65.9 (31 of 47) Dyspareunia: 31.9 (15 of 47)	LUTS (frequency, urgency)
Carrico et al. [24]	52 years (range, 19–90)	Vulvodynia	Vulvar pain: 48.1 (91/189) Pain with intercourse: 66.9 (117/175)	Sexually transmitted infections (genital warts, positive HPV, gonorrhea, chlamydia)
Yoon et al. [9]	51.0 ± 14.7 years	Vulvodynia Dyspareunia	NA	LUTS (frequency, urgency)
Bogart et al. [27]	43.6 ± 16.7 years	NA	Women experienced with sexual dysfunction symptoms: 88 (866/985)	NA
Gardella et al. [23]	38.2 ± 11.3 years	Vulvodynia Dyspareunia	Spontaneous vulvodynia: 23.4 (11 of 47) Provoked vulvodynia: 74.5 (35/47) Localized vulvodynia: 80.9 (38/47) Generalized vulvodynia: 17 (8/47) Dyspareunia: 87.2 (41/47)	NA

[a]This study was done in the women diagnosed of chronic pelvic pain. *FSD* female sexual dysfunction, *IC/BPS* interstitial cystitis/bladder pain syndrome, *LUTS* lower urinary tract symptom, *NA* Not applicable

Many previous studies have revealed a close correlation between LUTS and impaired sexual function; IC/BPS is not an exception. Besides, it is not uncommon to have trouble differentiating sexual pain and IC/BPS-related genital pain in women. Unfortunately, despite the growing population of affected individuals, there is a lack of comprehensive studies regarding sexual dysfunction and IC/BPS (Table 1). Clinicians should take more concern regarding sexual dysfunction and pain in IC/BPS patients, and more randomized controlled studies should be conducted to better understand correlations and diagnostic differentiations.

Conclusions

Both vulvodynia and IC/BPS are common and irritable conditions that disrupt normal life and reduce QoL in women. Vulvodynia also manifests itself along with IC/BPS and there are several reports supporting an association between the two diseases. Unfortunately, knowledge concerning vulvodynia and IC/BPS is inadequate when considering the clinical impact and importance of these two conditions. Therefore, there is an essential need for further studies that delve into discovering the features of vulvodynia and IC/BPS.

Abbreviations

CPP: Chronic pelvic pain; CSS: Central sensitivity syndrome; FSD: Female sexual dysfunction; IC/BPS: Interstitial cystitis/bladder pain syndrome; ICSM: International consultation on sexual medicine; LUTS: Lower urinary tract symptoms; OAB: Overactive bladder; QoL: Quality of life; TRPV1: Transient receptor potential V1

Acknowledgements

The authors would like to thank Mr. Taeeun Daniel Park and Mr. Austin Yeon for careful review and editing the manuscript.

Authors' contributions

HY and JK made substantial contributions to conception and design and involved in critically for important intellectual content. SK was involved in acquisition of data, interpretation of data, and drafting the manuscript. All authors gave final approval of the version to be published.

Author details

Department of Urology, Seoul St. Mary's Hospital, The Catholic University of Korea College of Medicine, Seoul, Republic of Korea. [2]Departments of Surgery and Biomedical Sciences, Cedars-Sinai Medical Center, Los Angeles, CA 90048, USA. [3]Department of Medicine, University of California Los Angeles, Los Angeles, CA 90095, USA. [4]Department of Urology, Medical Research Center, Ewha Womans University School of Medicine, Seoul, Republic of Korea. [5]Current address: Department of Urology, Yonsei University Wonju College of Medicine, Wonju, Republic of Korea.

References

1. Davison SL, Bell RJ, LaChina M, Holden SL, Davis SR. The relationship between self-reported sexual satisfaction and general well-being in women. J Sex Med. 2009;6:2690–7.
2. McCabe MP, Sharlip ID, Lewis R, Atalla E, Balon R, Fisher AD, Laumann E, Lee SW, Segraves RT. Incidence and prevalence of sexual dysfunction in women and men: a consensus statement from the fourth international consultation on sexual medicine 2015. J Sex Med. 2016;13:144–52.
3. Leppilahti M, Tammela TL, Huhtala H, Auvinen A. Prevalence of symptoms related to interstitial cystitis in women: a population based study in Finland. J Urol. 2002;168:139–43.
4. Clemens JQ, Meenan RT, O'Keeffe Rosetti MC, Brown SO, Gao SY, Calhoun EA. Prevalence of interstitial cystitis s Urology 2009 Mar;73(3):494–498. https://doi.org/10.1016/j.urology.2008.01.053. Epub 2009 Jan.
5. Lifford KL, Curhan GC. Prevalence of painful bladder syndrome in older women. Urology. 2009;73:494–8.
6. Clemens JQ, Link CL, Eggers PW, Kusek JW, Nyberg LM Jr, McKinlay JB; BACH Survey Investigators. Prevalence of painful bladder symptoms and effect on quality of life in black, Hispanic and white men and women. J Urol 2007;177:1390–1394.
7. Ambler N, Williams AC, Hill P, Gunary R, Cratchley G. Sexual difficulties of chronic pain patients. Clin J Pain. 2001;17:138–45.
8. Verit FF, Verit A, Yeni E. The prevalence of sexual dysfunction and associated risk factors in women with chronic pelvic pain: a cross-sectional study. Arch Gynecol Obstet. 2006;274:297–302.
9. Yoon HS, Yoon H. Correlations of interstitial cystitis/painful bladder syndrome with female sexual activity. Korean J Urol. 2010;51:45–9.
10. Juliato CRT, Melotti IGR, Junior LCS, Britto LGO, Riccetto CLZ. Does the severity of overactive bladder symptoms correlate with risk for female sexual dysfunction? J Sex Med. 2017;14:904–9.
11. Cohen BL, Barboglio P, Gousse A. The impact of lower urinary tract symptoms and urinary incontinence on female sexual dysfunction using a validated instrument. J Sex Med. 2008;5:1418–23.
12. Jayasena CN, Alkaabi FM, Liebers CS, Handley T, Franks S, Dhillo WS. A systematic review of randomized controlled trials investigating the efficacy and safetyof testosterone therapy for female sexual dysfunction in postmenopausal women. Clin Endocrinol. 2019;90:391–414.
13. Leiblum SR. Classification and diagnosis of female sexual disorders. In: Goldstein I, Meston CM, Davis S, Traish AM, editors. Women's sexual function and dysfunction: study, diagnosis and treatment. London: Taylor and Francis; 2005. p. 323–31.
14. McCabe MP, Sharlip ID, Atalla E, Balon R, Fisher AD, Laumann E, Lee SW, Lewis R, Segraves RT. Definitions of sexual dysfunctions in women and men: a consensus statement from the fourth international consultation on sexual medicine 2015. J Sex Med. 2016;13:135e143.
15. 2015 Consensus terminology and classification of persistent vulvar pain. http://www.isswsh.org/images/PDF/Consensus_Terminology_of_Vulvar_Pain.pdf
16. Haefner HK. Report of the International Society for the Study of vulvovaginal disease terminology and classification of vulvodynia. J Low Genit Tract Dis. 2007;11:48–9.
17. Clare CA, Yeh J. Vulvodynia in adolescence: childhood vulvar pain syndromes. J Pediatr Adolesc Gynecol. 2011;24:110–5.
18. Reed BD, Harlow SD, Sen A, Legocki LJ, Edwards RM, Arato N, Haefner HK. Prevalence and demographic characteristics of vulvodynia in a population-based sample. Am J Obstet Gynecol. 2012;206:170.e1–9.
19. Barr S. Diagnosis and management of interstitial cystitis. Obstet Gynecol Clin N Am. 2014;41:397–407.
20. Hanno P, Nordling J, van Ophoven A. What is new in bladder pain syndrome/interstitial cystitis? Curr Opin Urol. 2008;18:353–8.
21. Tripp DA, Nickel JC, Wong J, Pontari M, Moldwin R, Mayer R, Carr LK, Doggweiler R, Yang CC, Mishra N, Nordling J. Mapping of pain phenotypes in female patients with bladder pain syndrome/interstitial cystitis and controls. Eur Urol. 2012;62:1188–94.
22. Nickel JC, Tripp DA, Pontari M, Moldwin R, Mayer R, Carr LK, Doggweiler R, Yang CC, Mishra N, Nordling J. Interstitial cystitis/painful bladder syndrome and associated medical conditions with an emphasis on irritable bowel syndrome, fibromyalgia and chronic fatigue syndrome. J Urol. 2010;184: 1358–63.
23. Chelimsky G, Heller E, Buffington CA, Rackley R, Zhang D, Chelimsky T. Co-morbidities of interstitial cystitis. Front Neurosci. 2012;6:114.
24. Alagiri M, Chottiner S, Ratner V, Slade D, Hanno PM. Interstitial cystitis: unexplained associations with other chronic disease and pain syndromes. Urology. 1997;49:52–7.
25. Gardella B, Porru D, Nappi RE, Dacco MD, Chiesa A, Spinillo A. Interstitial cystitis is associated with vulvodynia and sexual dysfunction—a case-control study. J Sex Med. 2011;8:1726–34.
26. Carrico DJ, Sherer KL, Peters KM. The relationship of interstitial cystitis/painful bladder syndrome to vulvodynia. Urol Nurs. 2009;29:233–8.
27. Pontari MA. Chronic prostatitis/chronic pelvic pain syndrome and interstitial cystitis: are they related? Curr Urol Rep. 2006;7:329–34.
28. Elliott CS, Payne CK. Interstitial cystitis and the overlap with overactive bladder. Curr Urol Rep. 2012;13:319–26.

29. Bogart LM, Suttorp MJ, Elliott MN, Clemens JQ, Berry SH. Prevalence and correlates of sexual dysfunction among women with bladder pain syndrome/interstitial cystitis. Urology. 2011;77:576–80.
30. Gardella B, Porru D, Ferdeghini F, Martinotti Gabellotti E, Nappi RE, Rovereto B, Spinillo A. Insight into urogynecologic features of women with interstitial cystitis/painful bladder syndrome. Eur Urol. 2008;54:1145–51.
31. Groysman V. Vulvodynia: new concepts and review of the literature. Dermatol Clin. 2010;28:681–96.
32. Shah M, Hoffstetter S. Vulvodynia. Obstet Gynecol Clin N Am. 2014;41:453–64.
33. Dasgupta J, Tincello DG. Interstitial cystitis/bladder pain syndrome: an update. Maturitas. 2009;64:212–7.
34. Hucho T, Levine JD. Signaling pathways in sensitization: toward a nociceptor cell biology. Neuron. 2007;55:365–76.
35. Chen X, Tanner K, Levine JD. Mechanical sensitization of cutaneous C-fiber nociceptors by prostaglandin E2 in the rat. Neurosci Lett. 1999;267:105–8.
36. Petho G, Derow A, Reeh PW. Bradykinin-induced nociceptor sensitization to heat is mediated by cyclooxygenase products in isolated rat skin. Eur J Neurosci. 2001;14:210–8.
37. Bohm-Starke N, Hilliges M, Falconer C, Rylander E. Increased intraepithelial innervation in women with vulvar vestibulitis syndrome. Gynecol Obstet Investig. 1998;46:256–60.
38. Bohm-Starke N, Hilliges M, Falconer C, Rylander E. Neurochemical characterization of the vestibular nerves in women with vulvar vestibulitis syndrome. Gynecol Obstet Investig. 1999;48:270–5.
39. Tympanidis P, Terenghi G, Dowd P. Increased innervation of the vulval vestibule in patients with vulvodynia. Br J Dermatol. 2003;148:1021–7.
40. Goetsch MF, Morgan TK, Korcheva VB, Li H, Peters D, Leclair CM. Histologic and receptor analysis of primary and secondary vestibulodynia and controls: a prospective study. Am J Obstet Gynecol. 2010;202:614.e1–8.
41. Halperin R, Zehavi S, Vaknin Z, Ben-Ami I, Pansky M, Schneider D. The major histopathologic characteristics in the vulvar vestibulitis syndrome. Gynecol Obstet Investig. 2005;59:75–9.
42. Tympanidis P, Casula MA, Yiangou Y, Terenghi G, Dowd P, Anand P. Increased vanilloid receptor VR1 innervation in vulvodynia. Eur J Pain 2004; 8129–33.
43. Pukall CF, Binik YM, Khalifé S, Amsel R, Abbott FV. Vestibular tactile and pain thresholds in women with vulvar vestibulitis syndrome. Pain. 2002;96:163–75.
44. Giesecke J, Reed BD, Haefner HK, Giesecke T, Clauw DJ, Gracely RH. Quantitative sensory testing in vulvodynia patients and increased peripheral pressure pain sensitivity. Obstet Gynecol. 2004;104:126–33.
45. Hanno P, Andersson KE, Birder L, Elneil S, Kanai A, Pontari M. Chronic pelvic pain syndrome/bladder pain syndrome:taking stock, looking ahead: ICI-RS 2011. Neurourol Urodyn. 2012;31:375–83.
46. Amaya F, Oh-hashi K, Naruse Y, Iijima N, Ueda M, Shimosato G, Tominaga M, Tanaka Y, Tanaka M. Local inflammation increases vanilloid receptor 1 expression within distinct subgroups of DRG neurons. Brain Res. 2003;963:190–6.
47. Liu BL, Yang F, Zhan HL, Feng ZY, Zhang ZG, Li WB, Zhou XF. Increased severity of inflammation correlates with elevated expression of TRPV1 nerve fibers and nerve growth factor on interstitial cystitis/bladder pain syndrome. Urol Int. 2014;92:202–8.
48. Latremoliere A, Woolf CJ. Central sensitization: a generator of pain hypersensitivity by central neural plasticity. J Pain. 2009;10:895–926.
49. Foster DC, Dworkin RH, Wood RW. Effects of intradermal foot and forearm capsaicin injections in normal and vulvodynia-afflicted women. Pain. 2005; 117:128–36.
50. Klumpp DJ, Rudick CN. Summation model of pelvic pain in interstitial cystitis. Nat Clin Pract Urol. 2008;5:494–500.
51. Yunus MB. Editorial review: an update on central sensitivity syndromes and the issues of nosology and psychobiology. Curr Rheumatol Rev. 2015;11:70–85.
52. Kayhan F, Küçük A, Satan Y, İlgün E, Arslan Ş, İlik F. Sexual dysfunction, mood, anxiety, and personality disorders in female patients with fibromyalgia. Neuropsychiatr Dis Treat. 2016;12:349–55.
53. Bel LG, Vollebregt AM. Van der Meulen-de Jong AE, Fidder HH, ten Hove WR, Vliet-Vlieland CW, Ter Kuile MM, de Groot HE, both S. sexual dysfunctions in men and women with inflammatory bowel disease: the influence of IBD-related clinical factors and depression on sexual function. J Sex Med. 2015;12:1557–67.
54. Clemens JQ, Elliott MN, Suttorp M, Berry SH. Temporal ordering of interstitial cystitis/bladder pain syndrome and non-bladder conditions. Urology. 2012; 80:1227–31.
55. Pukall CF, Strigo IA, Binik YM, Amsel R, Khalifé S, Bushnell MC. Neural correlates of painful genital touch in women with vulvar vestibulitis syndrome. Pain. 2005;115:118–27.
56. Schweinhardt P, Kuchinad A, Pukall CF, Bushnell MC. Increased gray matter density in young women with chronic vulvar pain. Pain. 2008;140:411–9.
57. Gupta A, Rapkin AJ, Gill Z, Kilpatrick L, Fling C, Stains J, Masghati S, Tillisch K, Mayer EA, Labus JS. Disease-related differences in resting-state networks: a comparison between localized provoked vulvodynia, irritable bowel syndrome, and healthy control subjects. Pain. 2015;156:809–19.
58. Kilpatrick LA, Kutch JJ, Tillisch K, Naliboff BD, Labus JS, Jiang Z, Farmer MA, Apkarian AV, Mackey S, Martucci KT, Clauw DJ, Harris RE, Deutsch G, Ness TJ, Yang CC, Maravilla K, Mullins C, Mayer EA. Alterations in resting state oscillations and connectivity in sensory and motor networks in women with interstitial cystitis/painful bladder syndrome. J Urol. 2014;192:947–55.
59. Farmer MA, Huang L, Martucci K, Yang CC, Maravilla KR, Harris RE, Clauw DJ, Mackey S, Ellingson BM, Mayer EA, Schaeffer AJ, Apkarian AV, Research Network MAPP. Brain white matter abnormalities in female interstitial cystitis/bladder pain syndrome: a MAPP Network neuroimaging study. J Urol. 2015;194:118–26.

The impact of Mirabegron on sexual function in women with idiopathic overactive bladder

Marilena Gubbiotti[1,2*], Antonella Giannantoni[3], Simona Cantaluppi[4], Anna Chiara Coluccia[4], Fabio Ghezzi[4] and Maurizio Serati[4]

Abstract

Background: Overactive bladder (OAB) can frequently exert a negative effect on female sexual function. Mirabegron, a β3 receptor agonist, improves OAB symptoms, but there are very few information about its role on female sexual dysfunction (FSD). Aim of the study was to assess the impact of Mirabegron on FSD in women affected by OAB.

Methods: Fifty sexually active women suffering from idiopathic OAB were included in the study. Patients were assessed by means of a urogynecologic physical examination and were asked to complete the 3-day voiding diary, the International Consultation on Incontinence Questionnaire- Short Form (ICIQ-SF), the Female Sexual Function Index (FSFI) questionnaire and VAS, before and 12 weeks after treatment with Mirabegron. In addition, at the same time points, patients underwent uroflowmetry with the measurement of post- void residual volume (PVR).

Results: At baseline all patients were affected by OAB symptoms, with 49/50 patients (98%) presenting with FSD. At 12- weeks follow- up, OAB symptoms improved significantly in all patients, with 59.5% of subjects achieving a complete urinary continence. FSFI Total Score significantly improved in 42/50 patients (84%) from 18.9 ± 4.3 to 21.8 ± 4.5 ($p < 0.0001$). Sixteen cases (32%) presented with no FSD. Also mean ± SD scores of ICIQ-SF and VAS significantly improved (from 17.1 ± 5 to 7.9 ± 4.8 and from 3.9 ± 1.2 to 6.9 ± 1.2 respectively, $p < 0.000$).

Conclusions: Mirabegron not only is able to control urinary symptoms in women with OAB, but also induces a significant improvement in their sexual life.

Keywords: Mirabegron, Overactive bladder, Sexual dysfunction, Women

Brief summary

Women with OAB may suffer from sexual dysfunction. This study shows that Mirabegron is also able to improve female sexual function.

Background

According to the International Continence Society, Overactive Bladder (OAB) is a symptom syndrome suggestive of lower urinary tract dysfunction and includes urgency, increased day- time and night- time urinary frequency and Urge Urinary Incontinence (UUI) [1]. Prevalence of OAB has been reported to be 12.2% in women, becoming higher in patients aged > 40 years [2]. To date very few studies have investigated the impact of OAB symptoms on female sexual function [3, 4]. One of previous studies demonstrated a great deterioration in sexual Quality of Life (QoL) in women with OAB than in those with only urinary incontinence. In addition, it has been demonstrated that the improvement in OAB symptoms, as induced by a pharmacological treatment, can determine an amelioration also in female sexual life [5]. Mirabegron is a β3- agonist recently introduced in the treatment of OAB, with proven efficacy in reducing urgency and UUI, and with a good safety and tolerability profiles [6–8]. Moreover, Mirabegron has also been shown to exert a beneficial impact on health related QoL in treated patients [9]. Actually, there are no data

* Correspondence: marilena.gubbiotti@gmail.com
[1]Department of Surgical and Biomedical Sciences, Uro- Oncology Section, University of Perugia, S. Maria della Misericordia Hospital, 06132 Perugia, Italy
[2]Istituto Serafico di Assisi, Centro di Ricerca "InVita", 06081 Assisi, Perugia, Italy
Full list of author information is available at the end of the article

on the impact of Mirabegron on sexual function in women affected by OAB. Aim of the study was to determine whether Mirabegron, used as a treatment for OAB symptoms, can have a positive effects also on Female Sexual Dysfunction (FSD) and to identify possible relationships between the improvement in urinary symptoms and changes in female sexual life.

Methods

This was an observational, analytical, prospective study performed in two Italian centers. The procedures were performed in accordance with the Declaration of Helsinki and approved by the local Ethics Committee (CEAS No. 12394/18). Patients gave their informed written consent to the study. Fifty sexually active women, with a confirmed diagnosis of idiopathic OAB, attending the Urogynecology outpatient clinic were consecutively enrolled. OAB was defined using the International Continence Society definition [10]: patients having urinary symptoms of urgency with or without UUI, with frequency and nocturia. All patients reported day- time urinary frequency of 8 or more times per day, urgency that may or may not accompanies UUI, urinary symptom's duration of 3 months or longer. Subjects were excluded from participation if they had documented recurrent urinary tract infections (UTIs ≥3 episodes/year), urinary retention or clinically relevant Post- Void Residual volume (PRV), clinically significant voiding dysfunction (symptoms of hesitancy, slow streaming, intermittency, straining to void, feeling of incomplete bladder emptying), previous anti- incontinence or prolapse surgery, presence of a neurological cause of OAB, Pelvic Organ Prolapse Quantification (POPQ ≥ stage II), any medical condition contraindicating the use of β3- agonist medications and previous pharmacological treatment or intradetrusor injections of botulinum toxin for OAB during the previous 3 months. Not sexually active women were also excluded from the study.

Screening visit

At the screening visit, patients underwent medical history, including a detailed sexual history, urogynecologic assessment (performed with the patient in the lithotomy position, and POP classified during a maximal Valsalva manoeuvre according to the POPQ system), blood pressure measurement, urinalysis and cultures, uroflowmetry with PVR, and VAS to score the impact of urinary symptoms on QoL (0 = worse; 10 = best). A 3- day voiding diary was used to record daily urgency and UUI episodes and day- time and night- time urinary frequencies. Patients underwent a validated Italian version of "International Consultation on Incontinence Questionnaire-Short Form" (ICIQ-SF) questionnaire. ICIQ-SF is a specific and brief questionnaire: it has four questions that rapidly assess the impact of UI and qualify the urinary losses of analysed patients in terms of frequency and severity, and eight self- diagnostic items related to causes or situations of UI experienced by patients. The questionnaire has a 0–10 numerical scale for assessment of the UI impact. Zero indicates little interference of UI in the interviewer's daily life, and 10 represents a lot of interference. The total score is obtained by summing the questions related to frequency, quantity and impact on daily life, and can vary from 0 to 21 [11].

The assessment of sexual function and sexual QoL were performed by patient- reported questionnaires [12]. All patients were asked to complete the Female Sexual Function Index (FSFI) questionnaire, by using its validated Italian version [13]. FSFI is one of the most frequently adopted questionnaires in assessing female sexual function and dysfunction, and it has been strongly recommended from the latest report of International Consultation on Sexual Medicine. [14, 15] FSFI allows to study and classify the following domains: (a) desire (b) arousal (c) lubrication (d) orgasm (e) satisfaction and (f) pain. A total FSFI score of 26.5 is the cut-off to discriminate women with and without sexual dysfunction [16].

Treatment

All patients received a 12- week oral Mirabegron (50 mg once a day). We considered patients to be compliant only if they adhered to the therapy every day for 12 weeks.

Follow- up

At the 12- week follow- up examination, patients underwent blood pressure measurement, the 3- day voiding diary, uroflowmetry with PVR and ICIQ-SF and FSFI questionnaires and VAS.

Objective efficacy outcomes

Were: changes from baseline in the mean number of day-time and night- time urinary frequency, urgency and UUI; maximum flow rate at uroflowmetry with PVR.

Subjective efficacy outcomes

Were: changes from baseline in ICIQ-SF and FSFI scores and in VAS scores.

Side effect

Presence of side effects possibly related to the use of Mirabegron, such as hypertension, nasopharyngitis, and urinary tract infection was investigated. A daily blood pressure recording was performed during the first week of treatment and at the end of the study.

Data were prospectively collected into a specifically designed digital database.

Statistical analysis

Statistical analysis was performed with IBM-SPSS v.17 for Windows (IBM Corp, Armonk, NY, USA). Student's t test and the Mann–Whitney U test were performed to compare continuous parametric and nonparametric variables, as appropriate. Continuous variables were reported as median and Interquartile Range (IQR) or mean ± SD. Relationships between differences in FSFI and ICIQ-SF, urgency episodes, UUI, and frequency, were evaluated by Pearson coefficient analysis. A P value less than or equal to .05 was considered significant. Power calculation were done and we estimated that with 50 participants, the study would have 80% or greater power to detect a mean difference between the pre- and the post treatment FSFI total score of at least 3 points (considered clinically relevant), assuming a standard deviation of 2 and a two-sided type I error rate of 0.05.

Results

All the 50 patients completed the study. Mean ± SD age was 49.3 ± 11.3 years. All patients completed the questionnaires at the start of the study and at 12- week follow- up. Baseline characteristics of the study population are summarized in Table 1.

Clinical results

At initial evaluation (Table 2), all patients had increased day- time urinary frequencies and all complained of urgency. Forty- seven (94%) patients presented with UUI. At the 12- week follow- up, mean ± SD day- time and night- time urinary frequencies, daily urgency and UUI episodes decreased significantly ($p < 0.0001$). Twenty-eight/fifty (56%) patients achieved a complete urinary continence. On uroflowmetry, we did not observe any significant difference in the Maximum Flow rate (Q_{max}) and in PVR between the pre- treatment and post- treatment values. Mean ± SD ICIQ-SF score significantly increased, from 17.1 ± 5 (pathologic value) to 7.9 ± 4.8 (normal value; $p < 0.0001$). Mean ± SD VAS score significantly increased, from 3.9 ± 1.2 to 6.9 ± 1.2 ($p < 0.0001$).

Table 1 Baseline characteristics of 50 women affected by idiopathic OAB with sexual dysfunction, treated with oral Mirabegron, 50 mg/day for 12 weeks

	$N = 50$
Age (years)	50 (36–60)
BMI (kg/m^2)	23.3 (23–28)
Obese (BMI ≥ 30	5 (10%)
Menopausal	19 (38%)
Previous vaginal deliveries	1 (1–2)
Macrosome (≥4000 g)	10 (20%)
Operative delivery (vacuum/forceps)	5 (10%)

Data are expressed as absolute number (%) or median (IQR)

Table 2 Urinary symptoms and uroflowmetry results in 50 women affected by idiopathic OAB and sexual dysfunction before and 12- weeks after treatment with oral Mirabegron, 50 mg/day

Urinary symptoms and uroflowmetry results	Baselin (mean ± SD)	12 weeks f-up (mean ± SD)	*p* value
Day-time urinary frequency/day	10.1 ± 2.2	6 ± 1.1	< 0.0001
Night-time urinary frequency/day	1.6 ± 1.2	0.7 ± 0.8	0.0001
Daily urgency episodes	5.2 ± 2.3	2.3 ± 1.8	< 0.0001
Urge urinary incontinence frequency/day	2.1 ± 1.3	0.7 ± 0.9	< 0.0001
Q_{max}(ml/sec)	25.1 ± 8.3	25.2 ± 7.9	0.83
Post-void residual volume(ml)	5.8 ± 9.5	3 ± 5.8	0.32

Sexual function and sexual QoL

At initial evaluation, 49/50 patients (98%) presented with FSD (FSFI Total Score < 26.55). At 12- weeks follow- up, 42/50 patients (84%) reported improvements in the FSFI Total Score and 16 patients (32%) had no FSD (Table 3). Mean ± SD FSFI Total Score significantly increased from 18.9 ± 4.3 to 21.9 ± 4.5 ($p < 0.0001$). The domains most relevantly impaired were arousal and lubrication, orgasm and pain. After treatment with Mirabegron, an improvement was noted in all the domains but pain remained unchanged (Table 3). At the 12- weeks follow- up, when comparing changes in sexual function between the 28 continent patients and the remaining incontinent ones, FSFI domains significantly improved in those patients who obtained a complete urinary continence. (Table 4).

We found a significant relationship between improvements in ICIQ-SF and FSFI scores after treatment ($r = 0.5$; $p = 0.007$). Moreover, we could detect a significant relationship between the reduction in daily urgency episodes and the improvement in FSFI score ($r = 0.45$; $p = 0.03$). On the contrary, the relationship between daily UUI episodes, urinary frequency and FSFI total score was not statistically significant ($r = -0.1$; $p = 0.35$).

Table 3 FSFI scores in 50 patients affected by idiopathic OAB symptoms and sexuadysfunction, before and 12 weeks after treatment with oral Mirabegron, 50 mg/day

FSFI domains	Baseline (mean ± SD)	12-weeks f-up (mean ± SD)	*p* value
Desire	3.03 ± 0.65	3.51 ± 0.88	0.04
Arousal	2.87 ± 0.61	3.35 ± 0.94	< 0.0001
Lubrication	3.31 ± 0.72	3.93 ± 1.06	0.0008
Orgasm	3.36 ± 0.74	3.80 ± 0.96	0.0001
Satisfaction	3.33 ± 0.91	4.04 ± 1.05	0.0008
Pain	3.24 ± 0.88	3.52 ± 0.93	0.58
Total FSFI score	18.9 ± 4.3	21.9 ± 4.5	< 0.0001

Table 4 FSFI scores in 50 women affected by idiopathic OAB symptoms and sexual dysfunction, before and 12 weeks after treatment with oral Mirabegron, 50 mg/day

Patients (No.)	FSFI Total Score baseline (mean ± SD)	FSFI Total Score 12-weeks f-up (mean ± SD)
Continent (28)	22 ± 3.7	27.5 ± 3.5
Incontinent (22)	14.1 ± 3.1	21 ± 3.2

Comparison between continent and incontinent patients before and after treatment with Mirabegron

Side effects

None of the patients reported any increase in systolic and/or diastolic pressure along the whole follow- up. At the 12- week follow- up, 2 patients presented with UTIs.

Discussion

This study seems to show that the treatment of OAB with Mirabegron 50 mg per day for 12 weeks is able to improve sexual function in female patients with OAB.

In the last years, an enormous interest has emerged in sexual life of patients affected by OAB. Nevertheless, there is still limited knowledge about the impact of OAB therapies on sexual function.

This study was addressed to evaluate whether treatment with the β3- agonist Mirabegron and a corresponding improvement in OAB symptoms could be associated with an amelioration on FSD. Herein we demonstrate for the first time that Mirabegron, given to control OAB in women, was able not only to improve urinary symptoms but also many aspects of sexual life of these patients in the short- term follow- up.

Specifically, we found that all OAB symptoms and ICIQ-SF total score significantly improved at the 12-week follow- up. At the same time point, a significant amelioration was found also in sexual dysfunction, as assessed by the FSFI questionnaire. In addition, the impact of urinary symptoms on QoL, as assessed by VAS, also showed a significant reduction. Worth of noting, ameliorations in urinary urgency and in ICIQ-SF scores were significantly related to the improvement in FSFI scores, with desire, arousal, satisfaction, lubrication and orgasm being the most improved domains.

Indeed, at baseline, our patients presented with FSFI scores (mean ± SD: 18.9 ± 4.3) lower than that reported in the accepted definition of FSD (FSFI ≤26.5), with arousal, lubrication, orgasm- related problems and pain most relevantly impaired. Twelve weeks after treatment with Mirabegron, FSFI total score significantly improved, particularly in those patients who achieved a complete urinary continence, although patients still presented with low FSFI values (mean ± SD: 21.9 ± 4.5), which did not reach the suggested cut- off. In the literature, the cut- off point in the FSFI score to define clinical improvement is unclear and FSFI is adopted as an assessment tool to determine any change post- treatment.

Few data exist in the literature regarding the effect of OAB treatments on female sexual function. Sand et al. demonstrated that women treated with transdermal oxybutynin reported improvements in sexual function at 6 months [17]. In the study of Hajebrahimi et al., 30 sexually active OAB women underwent treatment with tolterodine immediate release in order to control their OAB symptoms. In these patients, significant improvements have been reported not only in urinary symptoms but also in the mean ASEX score at all the considered follow- up time points [18]. In a randomized, placebo-controlled study, Rogers and co-workers observed a significant amelioration in urinary symptoms and sexual dysfunction in female patients treated with tolterodine extended- release, as compared to those treated with placebo, at 3 months follow up [19]. Finally, significant improvements in total FSFI score and in OAB symptoms have been observed also in patients undergoing sacral neuromodulation or onabotulinumtoxin A intradetrusor injections [5, 20]. Although Mirabegron has been demonstrated to be effective and safe in the treatment of OAB in naïve patients or in those refractory to anticholinergics [21], to date data related to an eventual effect on sexual dysfunction are completely lacking. The results in our study may be in favour of a causal relationship between urinary symptoms and sexual dysfunction in women [22]. Since Mirabegron induced improvements in all OAB symptoms and a complete urinary continence in a large proportion of patients, we retain that the positive effect on sexual dysfunction could be attributed to an indirect effect by the urologic clinical and QoL amelioration. Overall, Mirabegron was well tolerated without any systemic side effects along the whole follow- up and it did not affect the bladder emptying, as already demonstrated in the literature.

Possible limitations of the present study are the short-term follow- up and the lack of a control or a placebo group. Indeed, no patient was lost to follow- up, and the limited improvement in sexual function observed in patients not reaching a complete urinary continence can strengthen these results.

Conclusion

This study could advance the understanding of FSD in women with OAB and the possibility of intervening with new pharmacologic oral agents in the treatment of OAB. In our study the improvement in sexual dysfunction observed in patients treated with Mirabegron can be explained by the amelioration in OAB symptoms and in urinary incontinence. However, future trials with a larger patient population should confirm these preliminary findings. In conclusion, according to our research, treatment of OAB with Mirabegron 50 mg per day for 12 weeks is able to improve sexual function in women affected by OAB. This finding can improve our counseling when we prescribe this pharmacological therapy of OAB.

Abbreviations
BMI: Body Mass Index; FSD: Female Sexual Dysfunction; FSFI: Female Sexual Function Index; ICIQ-SF: International Consultation on Incontinence Questionnaire-Short Form; IQR: Interquartile Range; OAB: Overactive Bladder; POP(Q): Pelvic Organ Prolapse (Quantification); PVR: Post- Void Residual volume; Q_{max}: Maximum Flow rate; QoL: Quality of Life; SD: Standard Deviation; UTIs: Urinary Tract Infections; UUI: Urge Urinary Incontinence

Acknowledgements
None.

Authors' contributions
MG, AG and MS contributed to conception and design, collected data, contributed to the analysis and interpretation of data, drafted the manuscript and revised it critically for important intellectual content. SC, ACC analyzed and interpreted the patient data. FG contributed to conception, design of data. All authors read and approved the final manuscript.

Author details
[1]Department of Surgical and Biomedical Sciences, Uro- Oncology Section, University of Perugia, S. Maria della Misericordia Hospital, 06132 Perugia, Italy. [2]Istituto Serafico di Assisi, Centro di Ricerca "InVita", 06081 Assisi, Perugia, Italy. [3]Department of Medical and Surgical Sciences and Neuroscience, Urology Section, University of Siena, Siena 53100, Italy. [4]Department of Obstetrics and Gynecology, University of Insubria, Varese 21100, Italy.

References
1. International Continence Society. First report on the standardization of terminology of lower urinary tract function. Br J Urol. 1976;48:39.
2. Irwin DE, Milsom I, Hunskaar S, et al. Population- based survey of urinary incontinence, overactive bladder, and other lower urinary tract symptoms in five countries: results of the EPIC study. Eur Urol. 2006;50:1306.
3. Patel AS, O'Leary ML, et al. The relationship between overactive bladder and sexual activity in women. Int Braz J Urol. 2006;32:77.
4. Rogers R, Bachmann G, Jumadilova Z, et al. Efficacy of tolterodine on overactive bladder symptoms and sexual and emotional quality of life in sexually active women. Int Urogynecol J Pelvic Floor Dysfunct. 2008;19:1551.
5. Giannantoni A, Proietti S, Giusti G, et al. OnabotulinumtoxinA intradetrusorial injections improve sexual function in female patients affected by multiple sclerosis: preliminary results. World J Urol. 2015;33:2095.
6. Chapple CR, Kaplan SA, Mitcheson D, et al. Randomized double-blind, active-controlled phase 3 study to assess 12-month safety and efficacy of mirabegron, a beta(3)-adrenoceptor agonist, in overactive bladder. Eur Urol. 2013;63:296.
7. Khullar V, Amarenco G, Angulo JC, et al. Efficacy and tolerability of mirabegron, a beta(3)-adrenoceptor agonist, in patients with overactive bladder: results from a randomised European-Australian phase 3 trial. Eur Urol. 2013;63:283.
8. Tubaro A, Batista JE, Nitti VW, et al. Efficacy and safety of daily mirabegron 50 mg in male patients with overactive bladder: a critical analysis of five phase III studies. Ther Adv Urol. 2017;9:137.
9. Freeman R, Foley S, Rosa Arias J, et al. Mirabegron improves quality-of-life, treatment satisfaction, and persistence in patients with overactive bladder: a multi-center, non-interventional, real-world, 12-month study. Curr Med Res Opin. 2017;18:1.
10. Abrams P, Cardozo L, Fall M, et al. The standardisation of terminology in lower urinary tract function: report from the standardisation sub-committee of the international continence society. Urology. 2003;61:37.
11. Tubaro A, Zattoni F, Prezioso D, et al. Flow study group. Italian validation of the international consultation on incontinence questionnaires. BJU Int. 2006; 97:101.
12. Hatzichristou D, Rosen RC, Broderick G, et al. Clinical evaluation and management strategy for sexual dysfunction in men and women. J Sex Med. 2004;1:49.
13. Filocamo MT, Serati M, Li Marzi V, et al. The female sexual function index (FSFI): linguistic validation of the Italian version. J Sex Med. 2014;11:447.
14. Hatzichristou D, Kirana PS, Banner L, et al. Diagnosing sexual dysfunction in men and women: sexual history taking and the role of symptom scales and questionnaires. J Sex Med. 2016;13:1166.
15. Zachriou A, Filiponi M. The effect of extended release tolterodine used for overactive bladder treatment on female sexual function. Int Braz J Urol. 2017;43:713.
16. Wiegel M, Meston C, Rosen R. The female sexual function index (FSFI): cross-validation and development of clinical cutoff scores. J Sex Marital Ther. 2005;31:1.
17. Sand PK, Goldberg RP, Dmochowski RR, et al. The impact of the overactive bladder syndrome on sexual function: a preliminary report from the multicenter assessment of transdermal therapy in overactive bladder with oxybutynin trial. Am J Obstet Gynecol. 2006;195:1730.
18. Hajebrahimi S, Azaripour A, Sadeghi- Bazargani H. Tolterodine immediate release improves sexual function in women with overactive bladder. J Sex Med. 2008;5:2880.
19. Rogers RG, Bachmann G, Scarpero H, et al. Effects of tolterodine ER on patient-reported outcomes in sexually active women with overactive bladder and urgency urinary incontinence. Curr Med Res Opin. 2009;25: 2159.
20. Signorello D, Seitz CC, Berner L, et al. Impact of sacral neuromodulation on female sexual function and his correlation with clinical outcome and quality of life indexes: a monocentric experience. J Sex Med. 2011; 8:1147.
21. Serati M, Leone Roberti Maggiore U, Sorice P, et al. Publication Committee of the Italian Society of Urodynamics. Is mirabegron equally as effective when used as first- or second-line therapy in women with overactive bladder? Int Urogynecol J. 2017;28:1033.
22. Juliato CRT, Melotti IGR, Junior LCS, et al. Does the severity of overactive bladder symptoms correlate with risk for female sexual dysfunction? J Sex Med. 2017;14:904.

28

Ureteroenteric strictures: A single center experience comparing Bricker versus Wallace ureteroileal anastomosis in patients after urinary diversion for bladder cancer

Frank Christoph[1*], Franziska Herrmann[2], Peter Werthemann[2], Thomas Janik[2], Martin Schostak[1], Christian Klopf[2] and Steffen Weikert[2]

Abstract

Background: To evaluate the outcome and complication rate in a single institution experience using the two most commonly used techniques of ureteroenteric anastomosis, the Bricker and Wallace anastomosis.

Methods: A total of 137 patients underwent ileal conduit for bladder cancer. Ureters were anastomosed by two experienced surgeons, one performing a Bricker and the other, a Wallace anastomosis. Stricture was identified during clinical follow-up.

Results: Seventy-five patients underwent a Bricker anastomotic, and 65 received a Wallace anastomosis. The average age was 70 in both groups, males were predominant (66% Bricker, 70% Wallace). Follow up period was 36.5 months in Bricker group and 17 months in Wallace group. In both groups, the body mass index (BMI) was similar (26.1 kg/m^2 Bricker and 26.4 kg/m^2 Wallace). We observed that the stricture rate after performing the Bricker anastomosis technique was 25.3% (19/75) as compared to 7.7% (5/65) after Wallace anastomosis technique, which was statistically significant ($p = 0.001$). In the Bricker group, patients with strictures had higher BMI (28.3 vs. 25.7 kg/m^2, $p = 0.05$). On average it took 8.5 months in the Bricker group and three months in the Wallace group ($p = 0.6$) to develop stricture.

Conclusions: The stricture rate was significantly higher when Bricker technique was applied. Although the BMI was not different in both groups, patients with a higher BMI were more likely to develop stricture. We believe that the approach of the separate and refluxing technique of Bricker anastomosis especially in obese patients poses a higher risk for anastomotic stricture formation.

Keywords: Bricker, Wallace, Ureteroenteric anastomosis, Stricture, Hydronephrosis

Background

Bladder cancer is the second most common malignancy of urological cancers. In 2017 about 20.000 men and women were diagnosed with bladder cancer in Germany [1]. Approximately only one third of these patients will have muscle invasive disease and subsequent radical cystectomy with urinary diversion [2]. The commonly used types of urinary diversion involve a segment of bowel, typically the ileum, which is then anastomosed to the ureter [3]. However, this ureteroenteric anastomosis is at risk for developing strictures. The postoperative stricture rates range from 3 to 10%; the etiology of which is attributed to local ischemia caused by poor neovascularization after excessive dissection for inflammation, or urinary leakage leading to further scarring of the affected ureter [4]. Thus, a uni- or bilateral obstruction of the ureter may subsequently lead to renal hydronephrosis impairing renal function [5].

The most commonly used forms of ureteroenteric anastomosis techniques are the Bricker (separate) and

* Correspondence: praxis@urologie-christoph.de
[1]University of Urology, Otto-von-Guericke-Universität, Magdeburg, Leipziger Str. 44, 39120 Magdeburg, Germany
Full list of author information is available at the end of the article

the Wallace (conjoined) anastomosis. The Bricker anastomosis was first described by Eugene M. Bricker in 1956 whereas David Wallace described his technique in the British Journal of Urology in 1966 [6, 7]. But until today, there have only been four publications and one meta-analysis that evaluate the benefits and harms of each implantation strategy of the ureter [8–12].

The aim of our study was to retrospectively evaluate the outcomes of these two different techniques that were performed on 140 patients without preoperative hydronephrosis between 2009 and 2014. The mean follow up was two years. We sought to identify potential risk factors for developing ureteral stricture and to analyze the incidence and pathologic variables that are associated with ureteroenteric strictures after urinary diversion.

Methods

Written informed consent to participate in the study was obtained from all participants. The local database was reviewed for patients who underwent radical cystectomy and had either Bricker or Wallace ureterenteric anastomosis performed on them. Only patients without preoperative hydronephrosis or radiotherapy were included.

Each procedure was performed by an experienced surgeon. All cystectomy cases were conducted utilizing open surgical approach. The decision whether to perform Bricker or Wallace anastomosis was dependent upon surgeons' preference, one using Bricker (T.J.) other using Wallace (S.W.) anastomosis.

All patients underwent heterotopic urinary diversion (ileal conduit). Routinely, patients were discharged from hospital after seven to ten days when leakage from anastomosis could be excluded through radiography. Further follow-up consisted of ultrasound every three months until one to two years after procedure, every six months for another two years, and annual ultrasounds thereafter.

Evidence of hydronephrosis was identified by ultrasound, loopogram, and intravenous pyelogram (IVP); in selected cases by renal scintigraphy depending on patient renal function. A computed tomography was done to exclude extrinsic obstruction. in some cases. If extrinsic obstruction was evidenced, patients were excluded. Only patients with proven narrowing of the ureteroanastomotic region were included in the study. Time until diagnosis and type of treatment was recorded and was defined as time to stricture presentation from the date of surgery e.g. cystectomy.

Statistical analysis was performed using SPSS statistics (IBM SPSS Statistics 25). For comparison of categorical variables Fisher's exact test and chi-square tests were used. Kaplan-Meier analysis and Log-rank test were used to compare potential treatment success or failure by risk factors on univariate analysis. Univariate Cox proportional hazard regression models were performed for association of significant variables to identify independent predictors of stricture formation.

Results

Our study examined 140 patients, of which 75 patients underwent Bricker anastomosis and 65 patients underwent Wallace anastomosis, following radical cystectomies and urinary diversion for urothelial malignancies (urothelial carcinoma. Patients who received either radiation therapy or neoadjuvant chemotherapy were excluded.

The demographics of the two cohorts are depicted in Table 1. The median age for both the Bricker and the Wallace group was 71 (mean age in Bricker group 70 and 69.8 in Wallace). The percentage of males in the Bricker group was 66 and 70% in the Wallace group.

The mean follow-up period was 36.5 months for the Bricker group and 17.0 months for the Wallace group. The body mass index (BMI) was 26.1 kg/m^2 in patients treated with Bricker and 26.4 kg/m^2 in patients treated with Wallace anastomosis (p-value > 0.05). In the Bricker group, patients who developed stricture had a mean BMI of 28.3 kg/m^2 and those who did not develop stricture had a mean BMI of 25.7 kg/m^2

Table 1 Comparison of patients undergoing Bricker or Wallace anastomosis

	Bricker *n* = 75	Wallace *n* = 65
Surgeon	J.H.	S.W.
Male	50 (67%)	46 (70%)
Female	25 (33%)	19 (30%)
Median Age	71	71
Smoking history	24 (32%)	21 (32.3%)
Hypertension	47 (62.6%)	41 (63.1%)
Diabetes type 2	5 (6.6%)	4 (6.1%)
BMI kg/m^2	26.2	26.4
Pathologic stage		
No tumor	5 (6.6%)	4 (6.2%)
Tumor		
≤ T2	46 (65.7%)	40 (65.6%)
≥ T3	24 (34.3%)	21 (34.4%)
Any T N+	9 (12.8%)	7 (11.5%)
Mean preop creatinine mg/dl	1.02	1.01
Mean postop creatinine mg/dl	1.14	1.12
Median est. blood loss/ ml	166	175
Median operating room time/ min	299	285
Median hospital stay/ days	11.3	10.5
Median Follow up months	36.5	17.0

which was statistically significant (p-value = 0.05). In the Wallace group, the mean BMI was 26.1 kg/m^2 in both (stricture and no stricture) groups (Table 2).

The strictures were diagnosed as hydronephrosis in regular postsurgical ultrasound examination after initial Bricker or Wallace implantation. Subsequent radiographic imaging confirmed the presence of an anastomotic stricture.

In the Bricker group 19 out of 75 (25.3%) were diagnosed with hydronephrosis and evidenced to have an ureteroenteric anastomotic stricture (Table 2). In the Wallace group five out of 65 (7.7%) were diagnosed with hydronephrosis and stricture. This was statistically significant (chi-quadrat test, $p = 0.001$) and still seen when Cox Regression after age adjustment was applied ($p = 0.024$). There was no predominant laterality in any of the groups, Bricker or Wallace (Table 2). The median time to develop hydronephrosis was 8.5 months in the Bricker group and three months in the Wallace group ($p = 0.6$).

Of the 19 patients that experienced anastomotic stricture in the Bricker group, 12 received double J stent placement and seven nephrostomy tubes. In the Wallace group one patient had a double J stent and four were treated with nephrostomy tube.

Reporting renal function, as monitored by measuring the serum creatinine level shortly before and two weeks after surgery, the mean creatinine level was 1.02 mg/dl before and 1.14 mg/dl after surgery in the Bricker group. In the Wallace group serum creatinine level was 1.01 mg/dl before and 1.12 mg/dl after surgery. This was not statistically significant (Table 1).

Discussion

Although Bricker and Wallace anastomotic techniques belong to the most common surgical procedures used in urinary diversion, few studies have addressed their postsurgical outcome [8, 11–14]. Every surgical technique has its advantages and disadvantages, which explains why several techniques have been used to connect the conduit to the distal ureter. However, as only few studies provide sufficient evidence for the superiority of one technique, the decision as to which technique to utilize depends on the surgeons' own preference.

In our study we have observed that stricture rates were significantly higher in patients receiving Bricker (separate and refluxing) as compared to Wallace (conjoined and refluxing) anastomosis. Kouba et al. have reported on stricture rates that were 2% after Bricker and did not appear after Wallace anastomosis technique in a large series of 186 patients [12]. Follow-up was 34 months and did not differ amongst the two groups. However, in their study, among the group with a higher stricture rate, the BMI was significantly higher (29 vs. 25 kg/m^2). Obesity and a greater BMI have been proposed as a potential risk factor, because extensive manipulation and mobilization is required, the blood supply is compromised thus unfortunately provoking fibrosis and stricture development. In our study, the mean BMI was almost identical in both groups (26.2 vs. 26.4 kg/m^2) but a significant difference in the stricture rate was still evident. Further analysis in the Bricker group revealed a higher BMI in the group that developed stricture. In our study, the BMI in the stricture-developing group was 28.3 kg/m^2 and is thus in accordance with the findings from Kouba et al. Obesity seems to be a risk factor for stricture risk when the Bricker technique is applied.

Other studies, dating back to the 1970s, have not shown one technique being superior to the other. In 1974, Wiederhorn et al. have published a series, comparing 51 Bricker to 15 Wallace type anastomosis [14]. As strictures were not found in the small Wallace group no reliable conclusions could be drawn. In contrast, Esho at al. published their results from 33 Bricker and 33 Wallace anastomosis types also in 1974: After a follow-up of two years, no difference was detected [15]. However, this was a pediatric study and obviously different from the group we are discussing in this study.

A more recent study, published by Evangelidis et al. in 2006, was conducted in a cohort of 237, including post-radiation patients, failed to prove any difference in risk for strictures after Bricker anastomosis. The stricture rate was remarkably low (2.9%) and, although not significant, higher in the Wallace group (4.5%) as compared to the Bricker group (1.8%). Information about mean patient BMI was not provided in this study [8]. In contrast to other studies, no laterality was observed. Several studies have shown that postoperatively, left sided hydronephrosis is predominant and the extensive mobilization of the left ureter required for rectosigmoidal tunneling has been suggested as the etiology [9, 16]. Ischemia at the distal ureter following

Table 2 Comparison of patients with or without stricture undergoing Bricker or Wallace anastomosis

	Bricker ($n = 75$)		Wallace ($n = 65$)		
	stricture	no stricture	stricture	no stricture	p-value
Patients (%)	19 (25.3)†	56 (74.7)	5 (7.7)†	60 (92.3)	0.001†
mean age	69	70	71	72	n.s.
BMI*	28.3*	25.7*	26.1	26.1	0.05*
right side	4	–	1	–	n.s.
left side	6	–	2	–	n.s.
both sides	9	–	2	–	n.s.

The Symbol Renates Tod Thema Bricker Group, means significance was only obtained in the Group with the † or *

extensive dissection can lead to fibrosis, scarring and stricture. However, we have not observed this in our study but in the Bricker group 6 had left sided and 4 had a right sided hydronephrosis.

In the view of the rising use of robotic surgery, a study from 2014 published by Desai et al. has addressed various issues when orthotopic neobladder was reconstructed completely intracorporally. Besides being a feasibility study, they reported an overall stricture rate of 3.8% performing Wallace type anastomosis in 65% and Bricker type anastomosis in 35%. It is noteworthy, that even though the follow-up largely differed between 1 month and 9.8 years and operation time was between 6 to 8 h, the resulting stricture rate was similar to the rate observed by using an open approach [13]. A comment in European Urology by Giannarini et al. stated, that this type of surgery should be offered to a well selected group of patients, however a higher risk of stricture formation rate when robotic intracorporal anastomotic technique is applied could be excluded [17].

Of the eligible, published studies, one meta-analysis by Davis et al. has summarized the most relevant issues when Bricker and Wallace techniques are compared [10]. In this analysis, they included a prospective trial conducted by Liu et al., that did not find one technique to be superior to the other [11]. Stricture rate was 3.8% (Bricker) as compared to 2.2% (Wallace) which was not statistically significant in a study group of 99 patients. Interestingly, they also reported a higher stricture rate in patients with elevated BMI ($25.2\,kg/m^2$) when compared to the group without stricture formation ($23.3\,kg/m^2$) ($p = 0.008$). In their meta-analysis, Davis et al. concluded that despite complication rates in earlier studies of up to 14%, the Bricker ureteroenteric anastomosis was not associated with a higher rate of ureteroenteric stricture. The authors also stress that follow-up data are only available at short term. However, as ureteroenteric strictures are most likely to develop within the first 12 months following urinary diversion and all publications included in the analysis reported follow up data of between from two to four years. Furthermore, oncologic outcomes did not differ with regard to each of the anastomotic techniques employed, which is consistent with previous published studies. Davis and colleagues concluded that, based upon current available data, the final selection of the diversion method should be based on the surgeons' experience and preference.

Thus, even today not much can be said about superiority or inferiority of either technique in demonstrating a higher or lower risk for stricture formation. This might relate to the retrospective character of all these studies or heterogeneous patient groups. However, in line with the data published by Liu et al. and Kouba et al., we suggest higher risk for stricture building in patients with elevated BMI [11, 12].

Addressing the question of time to first appearance of hydronephrosis, no conclusion can be drawn due to the small number of patients in our study that became symptomatic in the Wallace group ($n = 5$). One could hypothesize, that the wide spatulation of the ureters will build up more scare tissue and thus has an impact on building of fibrotic tissue which takes longer than the direct attachment of the ureter ends to the bowel segment. If narrowing becomes apparent in the Wallace group, it might be related to early building of scar tissue in the anastomotic region.

Interestingly, neither anastomotic technique affected the patients' overall renal function. Postoperative creatinine levels four weeks after surgery and removal of the stents remained stable and did not differ significantly from the levels prior surgery.

There are some notable limitations to the study: firstly, the study was conducted in a retrospective manner and the mean follow up of the groups differed. However, as noted above, strictures at the ureteroenteric anastomosis typically present within 12 months after surgery. In this study, the median follow-up of the shorter follow-up group (Wallace) was 17 months. In their study of 124 patients undergoing open ureteroenteric anastomotic revision, Packiam et al. have shown a median time to stricture of 9 months [18]. Secondly, as there were two different surgeons each performing only one type of technique, it is impossible to separate the outcomes from the influence of the surgeon. In the absence of a prospective, randomized trial with a single surgeon, many studies have compared the outcomes of a specific surgical technique (Bricker vs. Wallace) among multiple surgeons. Sha et al., reported retrospectively on 100 patients operated by eight different surgeons and Evangelidis et al. published their study with five surgeons. In both studies, the decision whether to perform Wallace or Bricker technique was dependent upon surgeons' choice [4, 8].

Conclusion

This is one of the few studies that have dealt with the incidence rate of anastomotic strictures by comparing two widely used techniques. We conclude, that there is a significantly higher stricture rate when Bricker anastomosis is performed which seems to be even more likely in obese patients. The findings of this study have led to a change: Whereas Bricker technique has been used before, nowadays the less harmful Wallace technique is employed at our institution.

Abbreviations
BMI: Body mass index; IVP: Intravenous pyelogram

Acknowledgements
Not applicable.

Authors' contributions
Each author has participated sufficiently in the work and takes public responsibility for appropriate portions of the content. The authors have agreed to be accountable for all aspects of the work and ensure that questions related to the accuracy or integrity of any part of the work are appropriately investigated and resolved. FC created the design and concept of the study together with FH and SW. Supported by PW and TJ they acquired the scientific data and implemented the clinical trial. Literature research was conducted by FC, MS and CK. The manuscript was prepared by FC and FH. Statistical analysis was carried out by FH and PW. All authors reviewed and edited the manuscript.

Author details
[1]University of Urology, Otto-von-Guericke-Universität, Magdeburg, Leipziger Str. 44, 39120 Magdeburg, Germany. [2]Department of Urology, Vivantes Humboldt Klinikum Berlin, Am Nordgraben 2, 13509 Berlin, Germany.

References
1. Verbreitung von Krebserkrankungen in Deutschland, Entwicklungen der Prävalenzen in Deutschland zwischen 1990 und 2010, Robert-Koch Institut, www.krebsdaten.de.
2. Stenzl A, Cowan N, De Santis M, et al. Treatment of muscle invasive and metastatic bladder cancer: update of EAU guidelines. Eur Urol. 2011;59: 1009–18.
3. Hautmann R, Abol-Enein H, Lee T, et al. Urinary diversion: how experts divert. Urology. 2015;85:233–8.
4. Shah S, Movassaghi K, Sinner D, et al. Ureteroenteric strictures after open radical cystectomy and urinary diversion: the University of Southern California experience. Urology. 2015;86:87–91.
5. Skinner EC, Fairey AS, Groshen S, et al. Randomized trial of Studer pouch versuch T-pouch orthotopic ileal neobladder in patients with bladder cancer. J Urol. 2015;194:433–9.
6. Bricker EM. Bladder substitution after pelvic evisceration. Surg Clin North Am. 1950;30:1511–21.
7. Wallace DM. Ureteric diversion using a conduit: a simplified technique. Br J Urol. 1966;38:522–7.
8. Evangelidis A, Lee E, Karellas M, et al. Evaluation of ueretrointestinal anastomosis: Wallace vs Bricker. J Urol. 2006;175:1755–8.
9. Richards K, Cohn J, Large M, et al. The effect of length of ureteral resection on benign ureterointestinal stricture rate in ileal conduit or ileal neobladder urinary diversion following radical cystectomy. Urol Oncol. 2015;33:65 e 1–8.
10. Davis N, Burke J, McDermott T, et al. Bricker versus Wallace anastomosis: a meta-analysis of ureteroenteric stricture rates after ileal conduit urinary diversion. Can Urol Assoc J. 2015;9:E284–90.
11. Liu L, Chen M, Li Y, et al. Technique selection of bricker or Wallace ureteroileal anastomosis in ileal conduit urinary diversion: a strategy based on patient characteristics. Ann Surg Oncol. 2014;8:2808–12.
12. Kouba E, Sands M, Lentz A, et al. A comparison of the Bricker versus Wallace ureteroileal anastomosis in patients undergoing urinary diversion for bladder cancer. J Urol. 2007;178:945–9.
13. Desai M, Gill I, de Castro AA, et al. Robotic intracorporeal orthotopic neobladder during radical cystectomy in 132 patients. J Urol. 2014;192: 1734–40.
14. Wiederhorn A, Roberts M. Comparison of Wallace and Bricker techniques. Urology. 1974;3:168–70.
15. Esho J, Vitko R, Ireland G, Cass A. Comparison of Bricker and Wallace methods of ureteroileal anastomosis in urinary diversions. J Urol. 1974;111: 600–2.
16. Westermann M, Parker W, Viers B, et al. Malignant ureteroenteric anastomotic stricture following radical cystectomy with urinary diversion: Patterns, risk factors and outcomes. Urol Oncol. 2016;34:485 e 1–6.
17. Giannarini G, Palumbo V, Ficarra V. Re: robotic intracorporeal orthotopic neobladder during radical cystectomy in 132 patients. Eur Urol. 2015;67: 1191–2.
18. Packiam V, Agrawal V, Cohen A, et al. Lessons from 151 ureteral reimplantations for postcystectomy ureteroenteric strictures: A single center experience over a decade. Urol Oncol. 2017;35:112 e 19–15.

29

Multidisciplinary management of a large pheochromocytoma presenting with cardiogenic shock

Umberto Maestroni[1], Francesco Ziglioli[1], Marco Baciarello[2*], Valentina Bellini[2], Raffaele Dalla Valle[3], Simona Cataldo[4], Giada Maspero[2] and Elena Bignami[2]

Abstract

Background: Pheochromocytoma is well-known for sudden initial presentations, particularly in younger patients. Hemodynamic instability may cause serious complications and delay a patient's ability to undergo surgical resection. Larger tumors present a further challenge because of the risk of catecholamine release during manipulations. In the case we present, increases in systemic vascular resistance caused cardiogenic shock, and the size of the lesion prompted surgeons to veer off from their usual approach.

Case presentation: A 38-year-old female patient was admitted to our intensive care unit with hypertension and later cardiogenic shock. Profound systolic dysfunction (left ventricular ejection fraction of 0.12) was noted together with severely increased systemic vascular resistance, and gradually responded to vasodilator infusion. A left-sided 11-cm adrenal mass was found with computed tomography and confirmed a pheochromocytoma with a meta-iodo-benzyl-guanidine scintigraphy. Surgical treatment was carefully planned by the endocrinologist, anesthesiologist and surgeon, and was ultimately successful. After prolonged hemodynamic stabilization, open adrenalectomy and nephrectomy were deemed safer because of lesion size and the apparent invasion of the kidney. Surgery was successful and the patient was discharged home 5 days after surgery. She is free from disease at almost 2 years from the initial event.

Conclusions: Large, invasive pheochromocytoma can be safely and effectively managed with open resection in experienced hands, provided all efforts are made to achieve hemodynamic stabilization and to minimize. Catecholamine release before and during surgery.

Keywords: Pheochromocytoma, Adrenalectomy, Cardiogenic shock, Case report

Background

The classical triad of headache, sweating and hypertension in patients with cathecolamine-secreting adrenal tumors is hardly ever seen lately. In an era of aggressive pharmacological management of primary hypertension, only half pheochromocytoma patients are diagnosed during workup of blood pressure anomalies [1] Occasionally, however, patients present with extremely elevated blood pressure and heart rate, causing single or multiple organ failure in what has been termed "pheochromocytoma crisis" [2].

While surgical resection of large, symptomatic adrenal masses is standard practice, the choice of a laparoscopic vs open surgical approach is still controversial [3, 4].

We present the case of a patient whose first symptoms were catastrophic hypertension and tachycardia leading to cardiogenic shock. We will discuss our decision to proceed with open resection and the importance of a MDT in this context. This manuscript is written in accordance to the 2018 SCARE statement [5].

Case presentation

A 38-year-old woman of Eastern European descent was admitted to the emergency department of a peripheral hospital for headache, dizziness, nausea and vomiting. She had a history of migraine and she had taken NSAIDs

* Correspondence: marco.baciarello@unipr.it
[2]Department of Medicine and Surgery, Anesthesia, Critical Care and Pain Medicine, University of Parma, Parma, Italy
Full list of author information is available at the end of the article

in the previous days to mitigate the headache. She was a secundipara with two vaginal deliveries, and had no further medical history.

On presentation she was hypertensive (170 over 130 mmHg) and tachycardic (130 bpm); peripheral blood oxygen saturation was low for her age at 90% in room air, and her tympanic temperature was 36.7 °C. She was rapidly approaching respiratory fatigue, with generalized cyanosis, accessory muscle recruitment and orthopnea. Peripheral pulses were noted to be barely palpable bilaterally. On echocardiography, global systolic function was depressed, with an ejection fraction of 0.25. Electrocardiogram showed mild ST-segment elevation in V5 and V6. The patient was initially hypervigilant and anxious, but her mental status deteriorated to the point that she was tracheally intubated to secure airway patency; there were no focal neurological deficits.

She was transferred to the ICU of the tertiary medical center, the University Hospital of Parma.

The main finding during secondary examination was a severely impaired systolic function (ejection fraction 0.12, calculated using a modified Simpson's rule). As systolic BP reached values above 220 mmHg, sodium nitroprusside and labetalol were started in continuous infusion to lower BP and HR, respectively, and a pulmonary artery catheter was inserted. Thermodilution confirmed the diagnosis of cardiogenic shock due to severely increased peripheral vascular resistance.

Because of the patient's unremarkable medical history and abruptness of the crisis, a total body CT scan was requested in search of a diagnosis. The brain scan was negative; lungs were remarkable for diffuse ground glass infiltrates; finally, a 11.4-cm adrenal mass occupying the superior cap of the left kidney was found. It had cystic and solid components (Fig. 1). There were also areas of increased bone density in the the inferior endplates of the D12, L1 and L3 vertebrae.

Urine analysis confirmed the hypothesis that norepinephrine levels were particularly elevated with respect to epinephrine. The patient then underwent a [123I]-MIBG to formalize the diagnosis of left-sided adrenal pheochromocytoma (Fig. 2) extending to the ipsilateral kidney.

The patient was extubated on the 4th day of admission, but she required noninvasive CPAP ventilation to maintain adequate oxygenation and avert respiratory muscle fatigue, despite her left ventricular ejection fraction having increased to 0.42. Her ICU stay was complicated by right lower lobe VAP which prolonged weaning from ventilation and delayed surgery, in order to complete a full course of vancomycin and piperacillin/tazobactam. Intravenous vasoactive drugs were weaned over 2 weeks and substituted with doxazosin 4 mg *tid*, bisoprolol 5 mg and amlodipine 10 mg daily. Blood pressure was stabilized but persistently elevated, around 150/95 mmHg, with HR closer to the lower normal range.

Since [123I]-MIBG scans have inferior sensitivity for pheochromocytoma metastases [6] and the disease was high-grade, a confirmatory [18F]-DOPA PET scan was also performed as soon as the patient was extubated. Both studies showed no uptake by the vertebral lesions, whereas the primary tumor had consistently increased signal.

Once pneumonia resolved and hemodynamics were confirmed stable, some 20 days after admission, the patient was transferred to an internal medicine ward and a MDT was assembled to take charge of the patient. A radiologist, a urologist, an endocrinologist and an anesthesiologist convened to offer open resection of the malignancy, to include nephrectomy because of the apparent invasion, under general anesthesia with epidural analgesia. It was convened that the combined results of the functional and morphological imaging studies did not warrant a vertebral biopsy, particularly in such a high-risk patient, and active monitoring was proposed. Our patient then consented to surgery with planned postoperative surgical ICU admission.

In the preoperative holding area, an epidural catheter was sited at the T10–T11 interspace and loaded with 10 µg of sufentanil, a potent short-acting opioid; the anesthesiologist opted to reserve LA administration until hypertensive crises developed. Monitoring included radial and pulmonary artery catheters, the latter to better assess systemic vascular resistances and systemic oxygen delivery vs consumption in case of hypotension after tumor resection.

As expected, a hypertensive crisis developed during tumor isolation, and it was managed with continuous infusions of sodium nitroprusside and esmolol, as well as generous lidocaine boluses (up to 80 mg every 10–15 min) via the epidural catheter, to induce pharmacological sympathectomy with vasodilation in the lower half of the body. During such management, cardiac systolic function remained at the lower end of the normal range, as did mixed venous saturation, which was never below 70%.

A left subcostal incision was chosen, which provided the surgeons with optimal exposure, confirming its usefulness in the excision of larger adrenal masses. Left kidney invasion was confirmed upon direct inspection. The renal vein was ligated first in order to block incretion of catecholamines, followed by the artery. The tumor's size and the inflammatory reaction around it complicated cleavage, which took more time than expected; resection *en bloc* with the kidney was nevertheless completed in 100 min, with an estimated blood loss of 550 ml.

Hydrocortisone (200 mg daily in continuous infusion after an intraoperative 100-mg loading dose) was

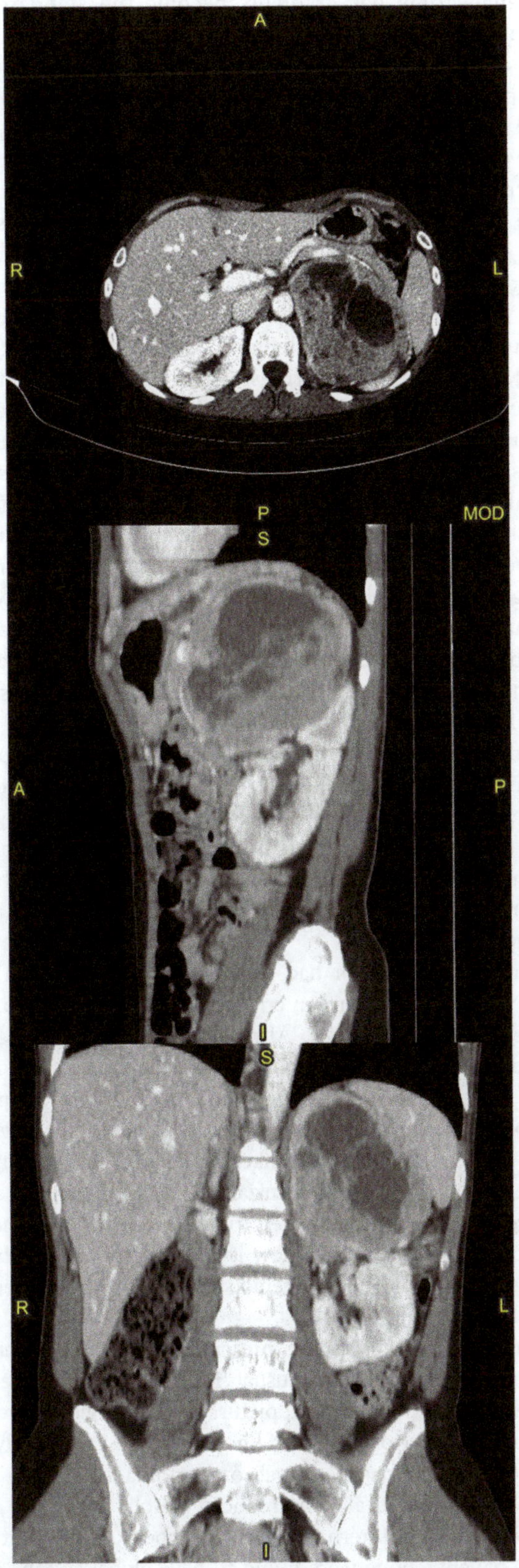

Fig. 1 Multiplanar reconstruction of a contrast-enhanced abdominal computed tomography scan. The left adrenal mass has a maximum diameter of 11.2 cm, and is seen displacing the gastric fundus antero-superiorly and the spleen laterally; cleavage from the kidney is unclear around the pelvis in the coronal image, suggesting cancerous infiltration

selected to transition the patient during the expected transient acute adrenal insufficiency, in the first 48 h. Hypotension developed as soon as the renal vein was ligated, and required norepinephrine infusion in addition to discontinuation of the previous short-acting vasoactive drugs. One additional 100-mg hydrocortisone bolus was also given during surgery.

The patient was transferred to the surgical ICU for monitoring. She was weaned from ventilation and extubated shortly after admission. Norepinephrine was also gradually discontinued within the first 18 h. Doxazosin and amlodipine were withheld the same day, whereas bisoprolol was tapered off over 3 days. Hydrocortisone was tapered to 100 mg/day and replaced with same-dose oral cortisone; total cortisol and ACTH levels were monitored to guide therapy and maintained within normal ranges. On postoperative day 1, slightly elevated serum troponin I and urine dopamine concentrations were detected; in light of the overall satisfactory clinical condition, this was attributed to the mineralocorticoid activity of the exogenous steroids. On postoperative day 2 the patient was transferred to the Urology floor. Her stay there was unremarkable, and she was discharged home in good conditions 4 days later. One month later, urinary metanephrine and particularly normetanephrine levels were half the preoperative values, yet still elevated (~ 900 µg/24 h), but there were no associated signs or symptoms; cortical hormones were within the normal range throughout the whole postoperative period.

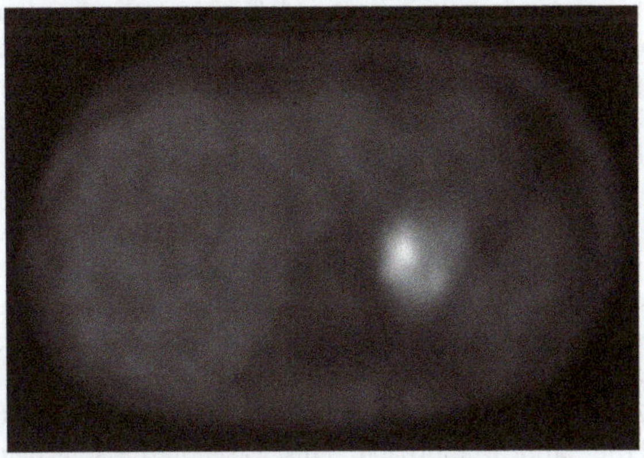

Fig. 2 [123I]-MIBG gamma ray emission scan showing intense emission from a left-sided adrenal pheochromocytoma extending into the ipsilateral kidney

Histopathology findings were adrenal pheochromocytoma and chronic pyelonephritis, which had resembled malignant invasion in imaging studies and during surgery. Immunohystochemistry analyses were positive for chromogranin A, synaptophysin and neuron-specific enolase. Final PASS [7] was 10. The score is compatible with high risk of malignant behavior. In the absence of obvious metastases and of recurrent signs or symptoms, the MDT opted to offer close follow-up and to withhold further treatment.

Two years after diagnosis and surgery, the patient has discontinued all drugs and enjoys a disease-free life. Metabolic tests were normalized since the first follow-up, 6 months after surgery. She was tested for genetic variants of lactate dehydrogenase, succinate dehydrogenase and for mutations associated with multiple endocrine neoplasia, type 2; results were negative. She is being followed up with urine cathecolamine tests twice a year, and surveillance magnetic resonance imaging every other year.

Discussion and conclusions

Pheochromocytoma is a rare neuroendocrine tumor, which may occur sporadically [8] but is more typically associated with inheritable syndromes. A significant proportion of pheochromocytomas may be clinically silent, with up to 58% classifying as adrenal "incidentalomas" [9]. While hypertension is a typical feature of symptomatic pheochromocytoma, its unexpected onset in certain patients may be mistaken for more typical conditions for that population; migraine was the first diagnosis in our patient, and in the absence of a trigger event, physicians could not immediately associate her hypertensive crisis and subsequent shock to the presence of cathecolamine-producing tumor. Abdominal surgery is likely the most common trigger, but there are reports associating crises with glucocorticoid administration [10], anesthesia induction [11] and even low back massage [12]. Our patient presented with life-threatening signs and symptoms, and the successful management was first and foremost the result of coordination between specialties. One of the peculiar aspects of this case is how the patient stayed in the ICU well after the initial crisis resolved. This was initially a deliberate choice which allowed stable hemodynamics control and optimization of the patient's respiratory function; development of VAP caused an unexpected delay in discharge and surgery, but its management in the ICU (where advanced monitoring and treatment are possible) averted any trigger events it might have caused.

Another crucial point in management was the choice of the surgical approach. This was not the sole decision of a surgeon, but instead it was the result of contributions from all members of the MDT. Since the original descriptions by Garner and coll [13]. VL adrenalectomy has gradually become the standard of care for resections of large adrenal masses [14–16]. Advantages of laparoscopy include shorter length of hospital stay, lower morbidity and postoperative pain, and better cosmetic results. In the case of clinically active pheochromocytoma, however, greater caution is warranted, as it is a hormone-secreting tumor in which size can make a significant difference when choosing the surgical approach [17]. It is generally agreed that a maximum pheochromocytoma diameter > 6 cm identifies a "large" tumor, and that VL resection is feasible, though technically challenging [18–20]. Conzo et al. [21], as well as de Fourmestraux and coll [18], retrospectively compared results of VL resection in large vs normal (*ie*, < 6 cm) pheochromocytomas; they reported no significant differences in terms of blood loss or surgical time, which is also, in this context, a (poor) surrogate measure of the extent of tumor manipulation. Other more recent studies demonstrate significantly longer surgery duration and more blood loss with laparoscopy [3, 4]. Perhaps counterintuitively, laparoscopic resection does not invariably result in greater hemodynamic stability [22, 23]. This may be surprising for intraoperative hypertension/tachycardia (often the product of tumor manipulations), as one would expect laparoscopic surgery to be "gentler" on the mass. However, hypotension should be expected to be as likely in VL as in open surgery, since it is initially associated with renal vein ligature and interruption of catecholamine incretion, followed by relative adrenal insufficiency later on.

Our patient's tumor had a maximum diameter of 11.4 cm, very large by common criteria, and it appeared to infiltrate the kidney diffusely. Although the surgeon, UM, has good experience with laparoscopic adrenalectomy [15, 16], the open approach allowed us to minimize tumor mobilization until the renal vein was ligated, to a degree that we believe would be unlikely in laparoscopic resection of such a large mass. Minimization of catecholamine discharge during surgery was felt to be the top safety concern for this patient, seeing as how it had caused vasoconstriction to the point of cardiogenic shock even in the absence of a trigger event.

Finally, the catastrophic presentation of our patient's pheochromocytoma is unusual in that her cardiogenic shock did not fit the typical picture of adrenergic or stress-related cardiomyopathy (also known as TS). In an analysis of 80 case reports of pheochromocytoma-associated TS, 20% demonstrated globally reduced systolic function [24]; however, in the International Takotsubo Registry, out of 1750 patients, none were found to have global systolic depression, as opposed to focal ballooning [25].

We hypothesize that in a sizable proportion of pheochromocytoma crisis patients, acute heart failure results from severely increased systemic vascular resistance, as was the case with our patient. Takotsubo in pheochromocytoma is typically focal and may be a result of myocardial inflammation due to high levels of circulating catecholamines [26]. By contrast, our patient responded well to vasodilators and she did not require the use of inotropic agents. Her left ventricular contractility recovered rapidly as BP was stabilized, whereas many patients with pheochromocytoma-related TS suffer from recurrences (17.7% in Y-Hassan's review) [24]. A combination of alpha-adrenergic blockade as well as non-antiadrenergic vasodilators are recommended in addition beta-blockers to minimize the risk of further hemodynamic deterioration [27]; to this end, an older drug such as labetalol is still a good choice.

Our choice of monitoring the vertebral lesions is highly debatable; since the primary tumor had an elevated PASS score, a biopsy might have been the most prudent option. However, the lesions showed no uptake of markers which were avidly absorbed by the primary lesion, and there weren't any osteolytic regions within the sclerotic areas [28]. Bone sclerosis is a relatively common sign found in the general population, especially in the presence of degenerative disc disease, whether or not they suffer from low back pain [29]. Had the vertebral lesions turned out to be metastases, there is anecdotal evidence of symptom improvement at 6–12 months, but no clear survival benefit [30]. In our case, complete resection would have entailed a three-level corpectomy, which we doubt would have been feasible, or at least compatible with acceptable quality of life.

In conclusion, we report a case of pheochromocytoma initially presenting with headache and hypertension, rapidly evolving into cardiogenic shock secondary to increased afterload. Blood pressure control with alpha- and beta-adrenergic antagonists led to stabilization of myocardial function but the patient's course was complicated by VAP. A MDT selected what they felt was the safest approach to surgery given the large mass and its secretory potential; open adrenalectomy and nephrectomy were performed with alpha- and beta-blockers, epidural analgesia and general anesthesia with advanced cardiovascular monitoring.

Aside from the specific case presentation, the concurrent involvement of different specialists was instrumental for successful management. Preoperative stabilization was obtained by intensivists and endocrinologists; the anesthesia team treated intraoperative hemodynamic imbalances which might have resulted in serious complications; the surgical team's judgment and experience helped make the choice of the technique, which resulted in minimal impact on the patient. Our case shows that multidisciplinary management is critical for minimizing the risk of complications in decompensated pheochromocytoma.

Abbreviations

ACTH: adrenocorticotropic hormone; BP: blood pressure; CPAP: continuous positive airway pressure; DOPA: 3,4-dihydroxyphenylalanine; HR: heart rate; ICU: intensive care unit; LA: local anesthetic; MDT: multidisciplinary team; MIBG: meta-iodo-benzyl-guanidine; OR: operating room; PASS: Pheochromocytoma of the Adrenal gland Scaled Score; PET: positron-emission tomography; TS: takotsubo syndrome; VAP: Ventilator-associated pneumonia; VL: video laparoscopy

Acknowledgments

None.

Authors' contributions

UM and RDV were the lead surgeons on the case; GM was the anesthesiologist and helped collect the clinical data; SC was the lead endocrinologist; EB collected relevant bibliography and helped compare the current case with the literature; VB collected most of the clinical data, including images; MB and FZ wrote the manuscript. All authors read and approved the final manuscript.

Author details

[1]Department. of General and Specialty Surgery, Urology Unit, University Hospital of Parma, Parma, Italy. [2]Department of Medicine and Surgery, Anesthesia, Critical Care and Pain Medicine, University of Parma, Parma, Italy. [3]Department of Medicine and Surgery, Hepatobiliary Surgery Unit, University of Parma, Parma, Italy. [4]Department of Medicine, Endocrinology and Metabolic Diseases Unit, University Hospital of Parma, Parma, Italy.

References

1. Baguet JP, Hammer L, Mazzuco TL, Chabre O, Mallion JM, Sturm N, et al. Circumstances of discovery of phaeochromocytoma: a retrospective study of 41 consecutive patients. Eur J Endocrinol. 2004;150(5):681.
2. Kakoki K, Miyata Y, Shida Y, Hakariya T, Takehara K, Izumida S, et al. Pheochromocytoma multisystem crisis treated with emergency surgery: a case report and literature review. BMC Res Notes. 2015;8:758.
3. Carter YM, Mazeh H, Sippel RS, Chen H. Safety and feasibility of laparoscopic resection for large (≥ 6 CM) pheochromocytomas without suspected malignancy. Endocr Pract. 2012;18(5):720–6.
4. Natkaniec M, Pędziwiatr M, Wierdak M, Białas M, Major P, Matłok M, et al. Laparoscopic adrenalectomy for pheochromocytoma is more difficult compared to other adrenal tumors. Wideochir Inne Tech Maloinwazyjne. 2015;10(3):466–71.
5. Agha RA, Borrelli MR, Farwana R, Koshy K, Fowler AJ, Orgill DP, et al. The SCARE 2018 statement: updating consensus surgical CAse REport (SCARE) guidelines. Int J Surg. 2018;60:132–6.
6. Ilias I, Divgi C, Pacak K. Current role of metaiodobenzylguanidine in the diagnosis of pheochromocytoma and medullary thyroid cancer. Semin Nucl Med. 2011;41(5):364–8.
7. Thompson LD. Pheochromocytoma of the adrenal gland scaled score (PASS) to separate benign from malignant neoplasms: a clinicopathologic and immunophenotypic study of 100 cases. Am J Surg Pathol. 2002;26(5): 551–66.
8. Neumann HP, Bausch B, McWhinney SR, Bender BU, Gimm O, Franke G, et al. Germ-line mutations in nonsyndromic pheochromocytoma. N Engl J Med. 2002;346(19):1459–66.
9. Motta-Ramirez GA, Remer EM, Herts BR, Gill IS, Hamrahian AH. Comparison of CT findings in symptomatic and incidentally discovered pheochromocytomas. Am J Roentgenol. 2005;185(3):684.
10. Rosas AL, AA K-Z, Papierska L, Bass BL, Pacak K, Eisenhofer G. Pheochromocytoma crisis induced by glucocorticoids: a report of four cases and review of the literature. Eur J Endocrinol. 2008;158(3):423–9.
11. Holldack HJ. Induction of anesthesia triggers hypertensive crisis in a patient with undiagnosed pheochromocytoma: could rocuronium be to blame? J Cardiothorac Vasc Anesth. 2007;21(6):858–62.
12. Pereira-da-Silva T, Abreu J, Ramos R, Galrinho A, Fortuna P, Tavares NJ, et al. Unexpected triggers for pheochromocytoma-induced recurrent heart failure. Int Arch Med. 2014;7:30.
13. Gagner M, Lacroix A, Bolté E. Laparoscopic adrenalectomy in Cushing's syndrome and pheochromocytoma. N Engl J Med. 1992;327(14):1033.

14. Castillo OA, Vitagliano G, Secin FP, Kerkebe M, Arellano L, et al. Laparoscopic adrenalectomy for adrenal masses: does size matter? Urology. 2008;71(6): 1138–41.
15. Feo CV, Portinari M, Maestroni U, Del Rio P, Severi S, Viani L, et al. Applicability of laparoscopic approach to the resection of large adrenal tumours: a retrospective cohort study on 200 patients. Surg Endosc. 2016; 30(8):3532–40.
16. Maestroni U, Vicente D, Del Rio P, Ziglioli F, Dinale F, Campobasso D, et al. Laparoscopic adrenalectomy for large adrenal masses: a challenge or a routine? Minerva Chir. 2014;69(2):59–64.
17. Lenders JW, Duh QY, Eisenhofer G. Gimenez-Roqueplo AP, grebe SK, Murad MH, et al. Pheochromocytoma and paraganglioma: an endocrine society clinical practice guideline. J Clin Endocrinol Metab. 2014;99(6): 1915–42.
18. de Fourmestraux A, Salomon L, Abbou CC, Grise P. Ten year experience of retroperitoneal laparoscopic resection for pheochromocytomas: a dual-Centre study of 72 cases. World J Urol. 2015;33(8):1103–7.
19. Naya Y, Suzuki H, Komiya A, Nagata M, Tobe T, Ueda T, et al. Laparoscopic adrenalectomy in patients with large adrenal tumors. Int J Urol. 2005;12(2): 134–9.
20. Shen WT, Sturgeon C, Clark OH, Duh QY, Kebebew E. Should pheochromocytoma size influence surgical approach? A comparison of 90 malignant and 60 benign pheochromocytomas. Surgery. 2004;136(6): 1129–37.
21. Conzo G, Musella M, Corcione F, De Palma M, Avenia N, Milone M, et al. Laparoscopic treatment of pheochromocytomas smaller or larger than 6 cm. A clinical retrospective study on 44 patients. Laparoscopic adrenalectomy for pheochromocytoma. Ann Ital Chir. 2013;84(4):417–22.
22. Kasahara T, Nishiyama T, Takahashi K. Laparoscopic adrenalectomy for pheochromocytoma: evaluation of experience and strategy at a single institute. BJU Int. 2009;103(2):218–22.
23. Kercher KW, Park A, Matthews BD, Rolband G, Sing RF. Heniford BT. Laparoscopic adrenalectomy for pheochromocytoma urg Endosc. 2002; 16(1):100–2.
24. Y-Hassan S. Clinical features and outcome of Pheochromocytoma-induced Takotsubo syndrome: analysis of 80 published cases. Am J Cardiol 2016; 117(11):1836–1844.
25. Templin C, Ghadri JR, Diekmann J, Napp LC, Bataiosu DR, Jaguszewski M, et al. Clinical features and outcomes of Takotsubo (stress) cardiomyopathy. N Engl J Med. 2015;373(10):929–38.
26. Gil-Barrionuevo E, Balibrea JM, Caubet E, Gonzalez O, Vilallonga R, Fort JM, et al. Adrenergic cardiomyopathy and cardiogenic shock as initial presentation of pheochromocytoma. A case report and review of the literature. Int J Surg Case Rep. 2018;49:145–148.
27. Sibal L, Jovanovic A, Agarwal SC, Peaston RT, James RA, Lennard TW, et al. Phaeochromocytomas presenting as acute crises after beta blockade therapy. Clin Endocrinol. 2006;65(2):186–90.
28. Leung K, Stamm M, Raja A, Low G. Pheochromocytoma: the range of appearances on ultrasound, CT, MRI, and functional imaging. Am J Roentgenol. 2013;200(2):370–8.
29. Raastad J, Reiman M, Coeytaux R, Ledbetter L, Goode AP. The association between lumbar spine radiographic features and low back pain: a systematic review and meta-analysis. Semin Arthritis Rheum. 2015;44(5):571–85.
30. Liu S, Song A, Zhou X, Kong X, Li WA, Wang Y, Liu Y. Malignant pheochromocytoma with multiple vertebral metastases causing acute incomplete paralysis during pregnancy: literature review with one case report. Medicine (Baltimore). 2017;96(44):e8535.

30

Giant urethral calculus in anterior urethral diverticulum

Maokun Sun[1], Wanting Xu[2], Shuai Guo[1], Wenyi Ma[1], Haiyue Xu[3] and Ruili Sun[1*]

Abstract

Background: In this case report, giant calculus in the urethral diverticulum was found through ureteroscopy investigation, the pneumatic lithotripsy combined with ultrasound lithotripsy (PLCUL) was successfully performed to break down this rare and giant urethral calculus in the diverticulum without open surgery.

Case presentation: A 82-year-old male presented to the urology department, complaining of frequent urination and dysuria. One giant, dark brown stone (6.5 × 6 × 5.5 cm) was revealed in the diverticulum of the anterior urethra using combination of local ultrasound, pelvic Computer Tomography (CT) and Magnetic Resonance Imaging (MRI). The stone was then successfully broken down via the PLCUL, and the emptied anterior urethral diverticulum was left untreated. In the 18 months' follow-up, no new calculus was found in urethral tract, anterior diverticula became gradually smaller, eventually disappeared.

Conclusion: In the treatment of giant calculus in the urethral diverticulum, this case report provides an effective method of lithotripsy in the clinical trials.

Keywords: Urethral calculus, Lithotripsy, Diverticulum

Background

Urethral calculus in male often cause dysuria with urinary tract irritation and acute urinary retention, which is considered as a urological emergency. Usually, small stones can be discharged naturally. Those small ones located at the anterior or more deep positions in urinary tract can be squeezed out followed by application of lubricants with low pressure injection. If the procedure fails, open surgical interventions may be adopted. For the huge anterior urethral diverticulum with urethral calculus, open surgery (i.e. diverticulum resection and urethrostomy) is conventional approach. Krystian [1] performed one open surgery to remove the urethral calculus and the following urethroplasty in a previous reported case of urethral giant stones complicated with multiple urethral stricture due to multiple pelvic fracture. Clinical results showed the postoperative recovery was very good. Nonetheless, for the open surgery procedure, patients always undergo major open wounds and slow recovery, associated with the risk of urinary tract infections, stenosis and urinary fistula complications. In this case, a rare giant urethral calculus was found in the urethral diverticulum of a male patient, PLCUL technique was performed to break down the giant urethral calculus in the diverticulum without open surgery, this case study provides a feasible and effective method in the treatment of giant calculus in the urethral diverticulum.

Case presentation

A 82-year-old male presented to the urological department, complaining of swelling and pain in perineal region, along with a frequent, painful, and difficult urination, when initially started 6 years ago. The patient was diagnosed with prostatitis and treated with quinolone antibiotics in several local hospitals. However, the symptoms did not ease and the patient showed up in our hospital where he was referred to our urology department. After multiple urinalysis, it was confirmed the patient had urinary tract infection. Blood parameters, biochemical, coagulation mechanisms, virus screening and other indicators were in normal level. In the physical examination, swelling and tenderness were observed in bilateral scrotum and perineum. A hard mass with a size of 7 × 7 × 6 cm was detected below the scrotal skin

* Correspondence: sunrl6004@sina.com
[1]Department of Urology, Liaocheng People's Hospital, Liaocheng, Shandong, China
Full list of author information is available at the end of the article

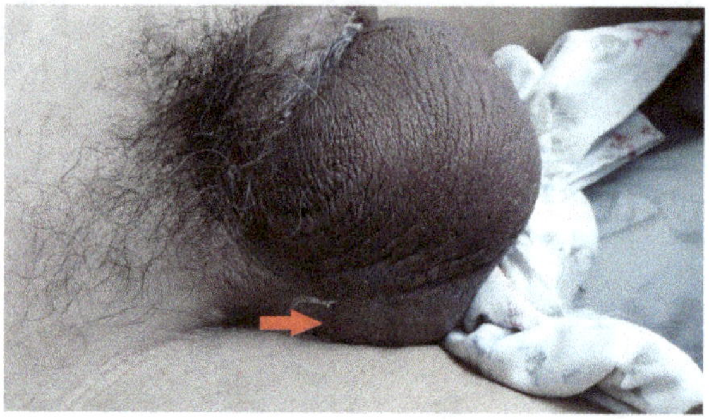

Fig. 1 Physical examination showed swelling and tenderness located below the scrotal skin near the root of penis, the arrow indicates the position of calculus was underneath the skin

near the root of penis. The surrounding tissue boundaries of the mass was not clear. The patient experienced pain during the physical examination of the mass (Fig. 1). In the enhanced urinary CT scan, a compact shadow of round shape with a size of 6.5 × 6 × 5.5 cm was observed below the pubic symphysis. Without a significant enhancement, the shadow has a clear border and uniform density in the scan. Enlargement of the scrotal volume was also observed. A disorder structure of internal scrotum with multiple low-density liquid regions was detected (Fig. 2). In the MRI scan of prostate gland, irregular clumps of T1 and T2 signals was observed in the subcutaneous posterior scrotum. SPAIR signals was high and without a clear border. There were no obvious high signals in DWI. The prostate gland showed a normal morphology, without significant abnormal signals in the scan (Fig. 3). On the urethroscopy investigation, a giant, dark brown stone was revealed to be ventrally attached to the urethral wall, which is located at the rear of the urethral bulb (Fig. 4).

The patient was treated with pneumatic lithotripsy combined with ultrasound lithotripsy (PLCUL) via LithoClast® Master (EMS, Nyon, Switzerland), the procedure lasted a total of 60 min and the amount of bleeding was about 15 ml. The stone was successfully broken down and removed (Figs. 5 and 6). Urethral diverticulum was left untreated. At the end of procedure, a catheter was left to support the urethra for 1 week. After the discharge, patient followed the doctors' advice to squeeze urethral diverticulum to extrude residual urine to prevent the formation of new stones at the end of each urination. The patient was examined, for the presence of new stones formation or diverticulum changes, via

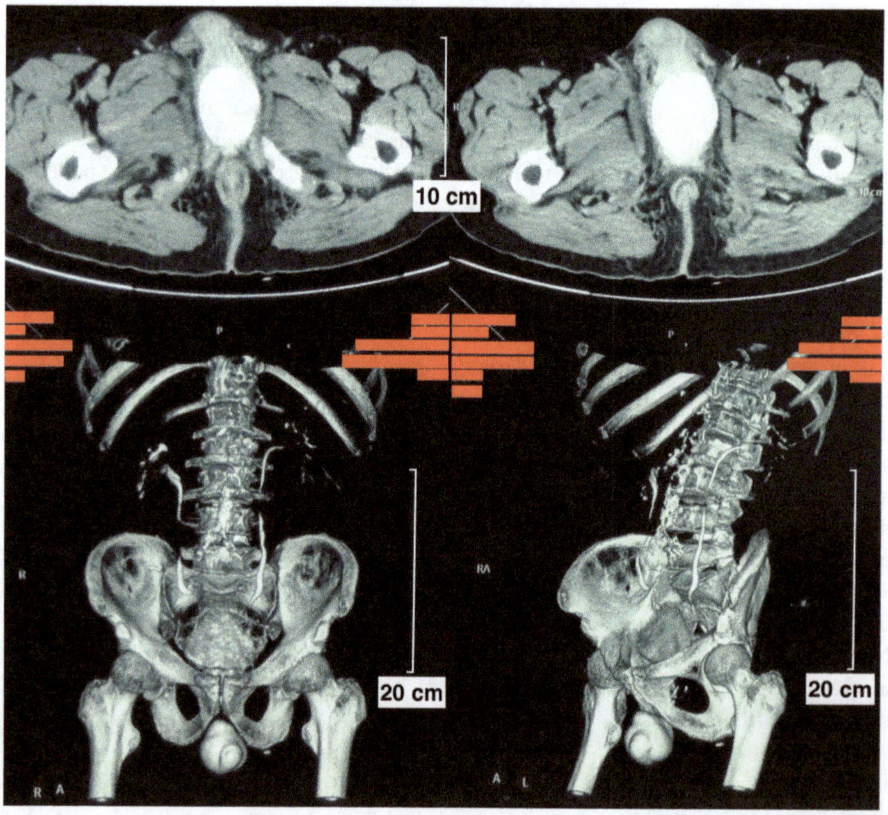

Fig. 2 A giant urethral calculus with a size of 6.5 × 6 × 5.5 cm was observed below the pubic symphysis in the enhanced urinary CT

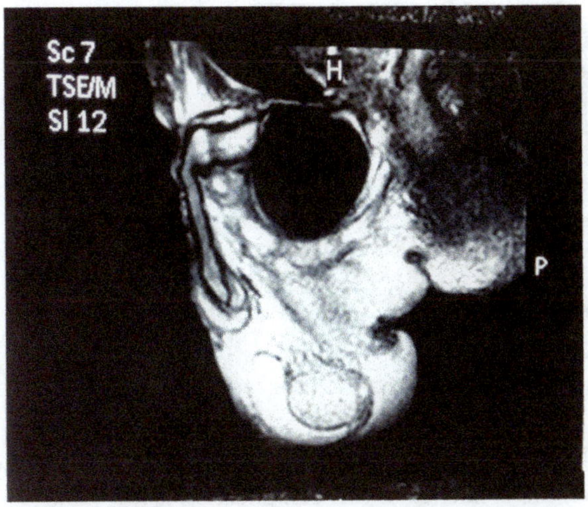

Fig. 3 Irregular clumps was observed in the subcutaneous posterior scrotum in the prostate MR scan before lithotripsy

ultrasound and urethraloscopy every 6 months in the outpatient clinic. Results showed that there was no formation of new stones in the urethral diverticulum and diverticula returned to the normal size (result not shown). The patient had normal functional urination until this paper is reported.

Discussion and conclusions

Urethral calculus is always found on the site of prostatic urethra, bulbar and fossa navicularis. Koga [2], paulk [3] and Sharfi [4] reported most urethral stones occurred in the posterior urethra, whereas Amin [5] and Englisch [6] reported high occurrence in the anterior urethra. The majority of urethral calculus is actually kidney and bladder stones which accumulated or embedded in the urethra. However, there are a few occurrences of urethral calculus reported due to the urethral stricture, foreign body inside or primary urethral calculus in the urethra diverticulum. Urethral diverticulum is a protrusion of the urethra through the periurethral fascia [7]. In this case, the urethral diverticulum was considered to be caused by stones in the urinary tract, long-term stay of the urethral calculus led to local necrosis fibrosis, further to the formation of diverticula, along with repeated inflammations.

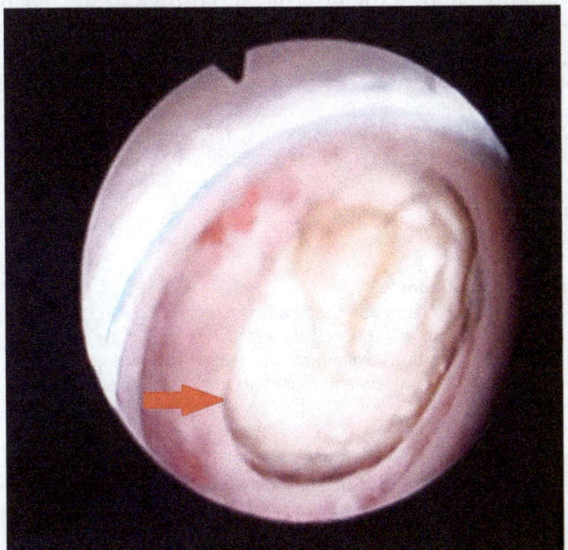

Fig. 4 A giant, dark brown stone was revealed to located in the urethral diverticulum through ureteroscopy investigation, the arrow indicates the calculus in the urethral diverticulum

X-ray, urethrography, CT, MRI and urethral physical examination are usually used to confirm the presence of urethral calculus. In this case, urethral calculus and urethral diverticulum were basically diagnosed by physical examination (Fig. 1), CT (Fig. 2) and MRI (Fig. 3). In a further diagnosis, stones were clearly seen using cystoscopy (Fig. 4). This direct observation also helped to differentiate the tumor from the calculus in the urethra.

In the treatment of giant calculus in the urethral diverticulum, open surgery is commonly used in the clinical trials as described before. However, with advancement in technology and new equipment, endovascular treatment techniques are becoming more popular. Some authors reported the use of low energy extracorporeal shock wave lithotripsy (ESWL) and endoscopic ultrasonography in the treatment of urethral calculus. However, because the low energy ESWL equipped with the shock waves and X-ray radiation can cause damage to the surrounding tissue, it is not preferred in clinical trials. The heat generated by high-frequency vibration in endoscopic ultrasonography can also damage the surrounding tissue, the procedure also needs a lot of circulating water to cool sonophoretic probe, which is susceptible to damage during clinical use [8]. Various types of lasers were also used in clinical trials, but they were less efficient in treating large stones in urinary tract [9].

Pneumatic lithotripsy overcome the above shortcomings and suitable for almost all urinary tract stones. Pneumatic lithotripsy is the new lithotripsy technology invented in the 1990s [10]. It has a reliable lithotripsy function, minor tissue injury, no thermal effects, low cost of treatment and other advantages. The fourth generation of Electronic Systems Management (ESM) pneumatic system is equipped with ultrasound lithotripsy system to break down the stones, and the active negative pressure to clean the debris. PLCUL technique has high efficiency in the clinic trials. Olbert [11] reported that PLCUL significantly increased the clearance of renal stones. Also, Juan [12] used PLCUL in the treatment of the bladder stones. PLCUL has the advantages of less operating time, less tissue injury, less bleeding and

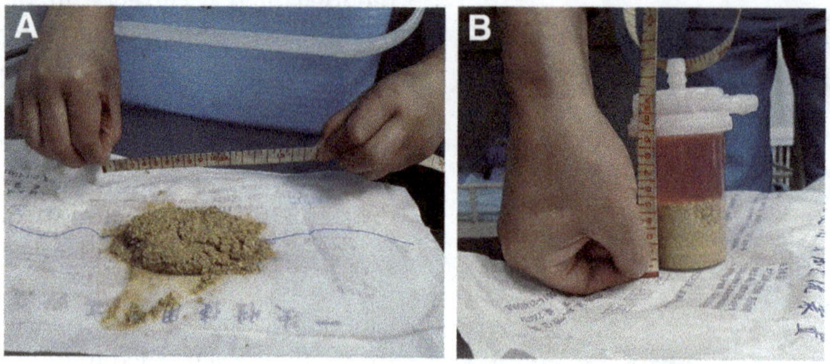

Fig. 5 Urethral calculus was removed after the lithotripsy, the metric rulers within unit of centimeter (e.g. number 8 means 8 cm in length) indicate **a**) the estimate size of stone after break-down, and **b**) the estimated volume of shredded calculus was calculated as 100 mL

higher lithotripsy efficiency than holmium laser treatment. Also, in our case report, PLCUL was successfully performed to treat the giant urethral calculus in the diverticulum (Figs. 5 and 6).

Urethral lithotripsy has been successfully performed with any type of efficient energy source: ballistic [13], ultrasonic [14], electrohydraulic [15], laser [16, 17], etc. The success rate for the endoscopic approach of urethral lithiasis is almost 100%, regardless if they are fragmented in situ, in the prostatic cavity, or in the urinary bladder [15]. For the complications associated with endoscopic surgery, injuries may vary from simple abrasions to false passages. It is necessary to carefully perform the extraction of larger stones or fragments of stones, as to ensure the compliance of the lumen in order to avoid tearing or avulsion of the urethral wall [18]. Bleeding may also be a consequence of parietal injury during lithotripsy, although it is usually clinically insignificant. The bleeding management requires insertion of a larger caliber urethra-vesical catheter [18]. In addition, the endoscopic treatment may also generate a urethral stricture, However, the incidence of this complication is low [18].

For the treatment of emptied urethral diverticulum after lithotripsy, if the open surgery is performed to remove the stone, the diverticulum resection and urethral modeling are usually performed. For endovascular calculus removal without open surgery, several conservative treatments on the emptied urethral diverticulum has been reported, such as urethral massage and prophylactic use of antibiotics, tamponade of cellulose or injection of teflon, but the effect was not as expected [19]. In our case report, the urethral diverticulum was located in the bulbous urethra and was easily touched by hand. After the removal of calculus, urethral diverticulum was left without treatment, the patient followed the doctors' advice to massage the urethral diverticulum site after each urination by squeezing out the residual urine in the diverticular cavity. Eventually there was no new formation of urethral stones, the diverticula returned to the normal size.

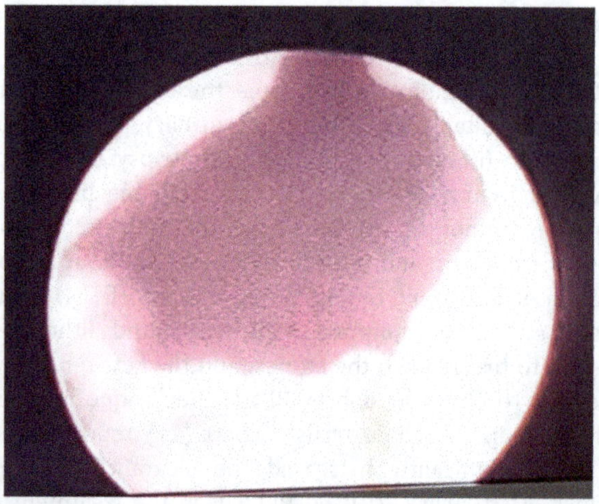

Fig. 6 No residue of urethral calculus left in the urethral diverticulum after calculus removal through ureteroscopy investigation

Abbreviations

CT: Computer Tomography; ESM: Electronic Systems Management; ESWL: Extracorporeal Shock Wave Lithotripsy; MRI: Magnetic Resonance Imaging; PLCUL: Pneumatic lithotripsy combined with ultrasound lithotripsy

Acknowledgements

Not applicable.

Authors' contributions

MS, SG, WM, and RS has made contributions to conception and design, or acquisition of data, or analysis and interpretation of data in the clinical trials;WX and HX has been drafting the manuscript and revising it critically for important intellectual content. All authors read and approved the final manuscript.

Author details

[1]Department of Urology, Liaocheng People's Hospital, Liaocheng, Shandong, China. [2]Liaocheng Food and Drug Administration, Liaocheng, Shandong, China. [3]Division of Molecular Pharmaceutics and Drug Delivery, The University of Texas at Austin, College of Pharmacy, Austin, TX, USA.

References

1. Kaczmarek K, Gołąb A, Soczawa M, Słojewski M. Urethral stone of unexpected size: case report and short literature review. Open Medicine. 2016;11(1):7 10.

2. Koga S, Arakaki Y, Matsuoka M, Ohyama C. Urethral calculi. BJU Int. 1990; 65(3):288–9.
3. Paulk SC, Khan AU, Malek R, Greene LF. Urethral calculi. J Urol. 1976;116(4): 436–9.
4. Sharfi A. Presentation and management of urethral calculi. BJU Int. 1991; 68(3):271–2.
5. AMIN HA. Urethral calculi. BJU Int. 1973;45(2):192–9.
6. Englisch J. Uber eigelagere and einges achle stein der Hanrohre. Arch Klin Chir. 1904;72:487–93.
7. El-Nashar SA, Bacon MM, Kim-Fine S, Weaver AL, Gebhart JB, Klingele CJ. Incidence of female urethral diverticulum: a population-based analysis and literature review. Int Urogynecol J. 2014;25(1):73–9.
8. Artifon EL, Couto DS Jr, Goñi S. Endoscopic ultrasonography-guided common bile duct stone removal. World J Gastrointest Endosc. 2010;2(6):210.
9. Naqvi S, Khaliq M, Zafar M, Rizvi S. Treatment of ureteric stones. Comparison of laser and pneumatic lithotripsy. BJU Int. 1994;74(6):694–8.
10. Kostakopoulos A, Stavropoulos N, Picramenos D, Kyriazis P, Deliveliotis C. The Swiss lithoclast: an ideal intracorporeal lithotripter. Urol Int. 1995;55(1): 19–20.
11. Olbert P, Weber J, Hegele A, Varga Z, Heidenreich A, Hofmann R. Combining Lithoclast and ultrasound power in one device for percutaneous nephrolithotomy: in vitro results of a novel and highly effective technology. Urology. 2003;61(1):55–9.
12. Gong J, Ge J, Zhou S, Wei Z, Xu S, Wei W. Clinical comparison of three treatment methods of vesical Calculus. J Clin Urol. 2010;1:3.
13. Wadhwa S, Hemal A, Sharma R. Intracorporeal lithotripsy with the Swiss lithoclast. Br J Urol. 1994;74(6):699–702.
14. Durazi M, Samiei M. Ultrasonic fragmentation in the treatment of male urethral calculi. Br J Urol. 1988;62(5):443–4.
15. Selli C, Barbagli G, Carini M, Lenzi R, Masini G. Treatment of male urethral calculi. J Urol. 1984;132(1):37–9.
16. Walker BR, Hamilton BD. Urethral calculi managed with transurethral holmium laser ablation. J Pediatr Surg. 2001;36(9):16–7.
17. Maheshwari PN, Shah HN. In-situ holmium laser lithotripsy for impacted urethral calculi. J Endourol. 2005;19(8):1009–11.
18. Geavlete P, Mulţescu R, Georgescu D, Geavlete B. Chapter 6 - Treatment of Urethral Lithiasis and Foreign Bodies. In: Geavlete PA, editor. Endoscopic Diagnosis and Treatment in Urethral Pathology. San Diego: Academic Press; 2016. p. 105-27.
19. Alexander AR, Morrisseau PM, Leadbetter G Jr. Urethral-hymenal adhesions and recurrent post-coital cystitis: treatment by hymenoplasty. J Urol. 1972; 107(4):597.

31

The relationship between prevalence and severity of lower urinary tract symptoms (LUTS) and body mass index and mid-abdominal circumference in men in a resource-poor community in Southeast Nigeria

Ikenna I. Nnabugwu[1,2*], Fredrick O. Ugwumba[1], Emeka I. Udeh[1], Solomon K. Anyimba[3] and Louis T. Okolie[3]

Abstract

Background: There is paucity of information on the community-based prevalence and severity of lower urinary tract symptoms (LUTS) in men who are 40 years and older in the southeast region of Nigeria. This study seeks to determine the community-based prevalence of LUTS and the relationship between LUTS, and body mass index (BMI) and mid-abdominal circumference (MAC) in men.

Methods: An interviewer-administered, questionnaire-based survey. Three of nine settlement clusters were randomly selected while systematic random sampling of 1 in 3 eligible subjects was used to select participants. Analysis was done using SPSS® version 20.

Results: One thousand three hundred and nineteen duly completed questionnaires were analyzed. The respondents are within ages 40-92 years with mean age 54.2 ± 10.2 years, mean BMI 25.97 ± 4.18Kg/m^2 and mean MAC 89.80 ± 12.43 cm. Overall prevalence of LUTS is 20.2%. Nocturia at a prevalence of 19.2% is the most prevalent lower urinary tract symptom and also the earliest to manifest. LUTS prevalence and severity increases with increasing age. About 9.6% report moderate LUTS while 2.3% report severe LUTS. Storage LUTS are reported more frequently than voiding LUTS. LUTS did not vary significantly with BMI, MAC or Wealth-Index.

Conclusion: LUTS prevalence and severity vary with age, but not with BMI, MAC or Wealth-Index.

Keywords: Men, LUTS, BMI, Mid-abdominal circumference

Background

Generally, the prevalence of lower urinary tract symptoms (LUTS) increases with increasing age in men. This may partly be as a result of increasing bladder outlet resistance consequent upon an enlarging prostate and partly due to other dysfunctional states of the lower urinary tract [1, 2].

* Correspondence: ikenna.nnabugwu@unn.edu.ng
[1]Department of Surgery, College of Medicine, University of Nigeria Ituku-Ozalla, KM 20 Enugu-PortHarcourt Highway, Enugu PMB 01129, Nigeria
[2]Department of Health Administration and Management, University of Nigeria Enugu Campus, Enugu, Nigeria
Full list of author information is available at the end of the article

Though the prevalence of LUTS among men may vary from community to community [3, 4], the onset of these symptoms is usually insidious and the course usually progressive.

Notably, the severity of these lower urinary tract symptoms tend to worsen over time from mild less bothersome symptoms to severe quite bothersome symptoms [5], though there may be intermittent remissions in symptoms of varying durations within this natural history of symptom progression. At any point in the course of LUTS, the International Prostate Symptom Score (IPSS) is recognized globally as a tool for assessing

LUTS severity especially LUTS due to benign prostate enlargement [6].

Hospital-based estimates of the prevalence of LUTS in southeast Nigeria, a higher low-income country, has been documented [7], but community-based prevalence of LUTS in the region is essentially lacking. And figures from other resource-poor settings suggest that there could be wide variations between hospital-based prevalence and community-based prevalence of LUTS within a community [8]. There are indications as well that storage LUTS may be more prevalent than voiding LUTS and post-void LUTS [4].

Similarly, studies have suggested some association between LUTS in men and recognized indices of obesity such as body mass index (BMI) [9], abdominal circumference, and serum lipid parameters [4]. Arguably, higher BMI may be associated with higher income societies [10], and within a community, higher BMI may be prevalent among men with higher wealth-index [11]. However, there are no indications that a similar relationship is obtainable between LUTS and higher income or wealth-index.

As increasing proportions of the global population age due to improving living conditions and healthcare services, and with estimates indicating that Africa will be one of the continents with greatest increase in LUTS in the coming years [12], a firsthand knowledge of the prevalence of LUTS and its relationship with body mass index (BMI) among men in communities in Africa is relevant for planning.

Therefore, this study aims to provide the community-based prevalence of LUTS in an aging population of men in a resource-poor community in southeast Nigeria, and to identify the nature of the relationship between LUTS, and BMI and mid-abdominal circumference (MAC) among these men.

Methods

An interviewer-administered quantitative questionnaire-based survey was conducted from March 5th to May 25th, 2018 in Enugu, the regional capital of southeast Nigeria with an estimated population of 983,000 persons, 22.0% of which are men who are 40 years and above, and are mostly civil servants and regional businessmen [13].

The first section of the survey questionnaire captured the age, weight, height and mid-abdominal circumference of the respondent, the second section was the validated International Prostate Symptom Score (IPSS) chart [14], and the thirdsection, adapted from Nigeria-General Household Survey, Panel 2015–2016, Wave 3 [15], assessed household living conditions and durable assets from which wealth indices were computed for individual respondents.

Face and construct validity of the study questionnaire were confirmed by experts in the field while reliability test yielded Cronbach's $\alpha = 0.735$ for the third section of the questionnaire. The questionnaires were administered by pre-tutored trainee surgeons and intern doctors.

A sample size of 372 was worked out using the formula $n = \frac{Z^2 P(1-P)}{d^2}$ where P is 0.591 [16]; Z is 1.96 and d is 0.05. An additional 10% of calculated sample size was included to cater for possible errors in data collection bringing the estimated minimum number of participants to 410.

Three of nine settlement clusters were randomly selected in Enugu urban for the study. Within the clusters, the study participants were selected through a systematic random sampling technique of 1 in every 3 eligible men. A minimum number of 410 participants was expected from each of the 3 selected clusters. Men dwelling in the communities who were 40 years and older were recruited. Written informed consent was obtained from each eligible participant before questionnaire was administered. Men who are known Diabetics, those who have spinal injury, urethral injury/stricture or cerebrovascular accident, and those on known diuretic drugs were excluded.

Simple frequency was used to determine prevalence of LUTS. Independent t test was used for comparison of means of BMI and MAC of men reporting LUTS against those of men reporting no LUTS. Principal Component Analysis (PCA) was used to create wealth indices using household durable assets and living conditions. Binary Logistic Regression Analysis was used to evaluate associations between the predictor variables (age, BMI, MAC, wealth index) and the dependent variable (presence of LUTS). Significance was set at $p < 0.05$. All analyses were done with SPSS® version 20. The University of Nigeria Teaching Hospital Bioethics Committee approved of the study.

Results

Of the 1337 questionnaires administered and retrieved during the study, 1319 (98.6%) questionnaires were adequately completed and therefore could be analyzed. The socio-demographic characteristics of respondents are shown in Table 1.

Two hundred and sixty-seven respondents reported at least one lower urinary tract symptom giving a crude LUTS prevalence rate of 20.2% from this survey. Among these 267 respondents, 111 (41.6%) reported mild LUTS (IPSS 1–7), 126 (47.2%) reported moderate LUTS while 30 (11.2%) reported severe LUTS.

Sorting the respondents according to age reveals that the prevalence of LUTS from 40 years of age increases with increasing age as shown in Fig. 1. Similarly, the

Table 1 Shows the socio-demographic characteristics of respondents ($N = 1319$)

Variables	Frequency (%)
Age of Respondents (years)	
40–49	500 (37.9%)
50–59	420 (31.8%)
60–69	277 (21.0%)
70–79	110 (8.3%)
80–89	10 (0.8%)
90–99	2 (0.2%)
Body Mass Index (BMI) Kg/m^2	
15.00–19.99	79 (6.0%)
20.00–24.99	522 (39.6%)
25.00–29.99	522 (39.6%)
30.00–34.99	158 (12.0%)
35.00–39.99	26 (2%)
40.00–44.99	11 (0.8%)
45.00–50.99	1 (0.1%)
Mid-Abd Circumference (cm)	
50.00–69.00	52 (3.9%)
70.00–89.00	617 (46.8%)
90.00–109.00	564 (42.8%)
110.00–129.00	85 (6.4%)
130.00–149.00	1 (0.1%)
Formal Education	
≤6 years	466 (35.3%)
>6 years	853 (64.7%)

Table 1 reveals that 90.7% of the respondents are below the age of 70 years, 39.6% are overweight while 14.9% are obese. Majority of the respondents (89.6%) have MAC between 70 cm and 109 cm about 64.7% had formal education beyond the primary level. The mean age of respondents is 54.2 ± 10.2 years, the mean BMI is 26.0 ± 4.18 kg/m^2, the mean MAC is 89.80 ± 12.43 cm and the mean duration of formal education is 10.5 ± 5.3 years

prevalence of moderate to severe LUTS increases with age (r 0.368; $p < 0.001$; Fig. 2) and there exists a positive correlation between LUTS severity and LUTS quality of life index (r 0.586; $p < 0.001$).

The bar chart in Fig. 2 displays the severity of LUTS according to age: the prevalence of moderate to severe LUTS increases with age while that of mild LUTS decreases with age (χ^2 28.421; df 10; p 0.002).

The body mass index (BMI) and the mid abdominal circumference (MAC) of respondents experiencing LUTS are compared against those of respondents who do not experience any LUTS using independent t test. There is no evidence (p 0.35) of difference in mean BMI of respondents experiencing LUTS (26.18 ± 3.99Kg/m^2) and of those not experiencing LUTS (25.91 ± 4.23Kg/m^2). There is also weak evidence, if any, (p 0.04) of a difference in mean MAC of respondents experiencing LUTS (90.20 ± 13.31 cm) and of those who are not experiencing LUTS (89.45 ± 12.18 cm). In addition, cross-tab analysis showed no evidence of any association between men reporting LUTS and wealth-index (χ^2 6.22; p 0.18). Essentially therefore, there is no difference in the body sizes and the wealth-index of the 2 groups. Further analysis shows no evidence as well of correlation between LUTS severity and BMI (r 0.01; p 0.86), or between LUTS severity and MAC (r − 0.09; p 0.13). However, there is strong evidence of significant association between LUTS and age of respondents (χ^2 96.32; $p < 0.001$).

Table 2 shows that from the age of 40 years among men in this community, the odds that an older man will experience LUTS compared to a younger man is estimated to be 1.065 (95%CI 1.051–1.080).

Discussion

Majority of the participants in this study are between the ages of 40 and 70 years, had more than 6 years of formal education and are still actively involved in some form of economic activity (Table 1). The overall prevalence of LUTS from this study is 20.2% while the prevalence of moderate to severe LUTS is 11.9% (Table 3). These values are lower than the prevalence rates from the studies by Ojewola et al. [16], Olapade-Olaopa et al. [17] in southwest Nigeria and Chokkalingam et al. [18] in Accra, Ghana. The difference in prevalence rates may be partly explained by the observation that the study population in this study is younger than those in the other studies. At these observed prevalence rates, LUTS deserve some attention as a non-communicable disorder of importance in public health discussions in Nigeria. This is especially so in view of the existing misconceptions about LUTS in men, the significant delay in seeking medical care, and the attendant consequences thereof [19]. Commonly highlighted non-communicable chronic diseases such as systemic hypertension, Diabetes Mellitus, osteoarthritis, have similar prevalence rates, outcomes of management and consequences of neglect [20] compared to LUTS in men, and yet LUTS in men appear to receive less attention. Akin to many other studies [16], this study observes that storage LUTS are more prevalent than voiding LUTS, and nocturia is the most prevalent lower urinary tract symptom.

The survey also shows succinctly that the prevalence rates of LUTS increases with advancing age (Fig. 1) similar to reports from other studies [21, 22] In addition, the severity of LUTS significantly worsens with advancing age (χ^2 28.421; df 10; p 0.002; Fig. 2). These findings are in keeping with the recognized progressive nature of the chronic symptom complex [23]., Though remissions in symptoms of various durations can, and do, occur during the natural course of these lower urinary tract symptoms [24], the aggregate outlook is usually that the

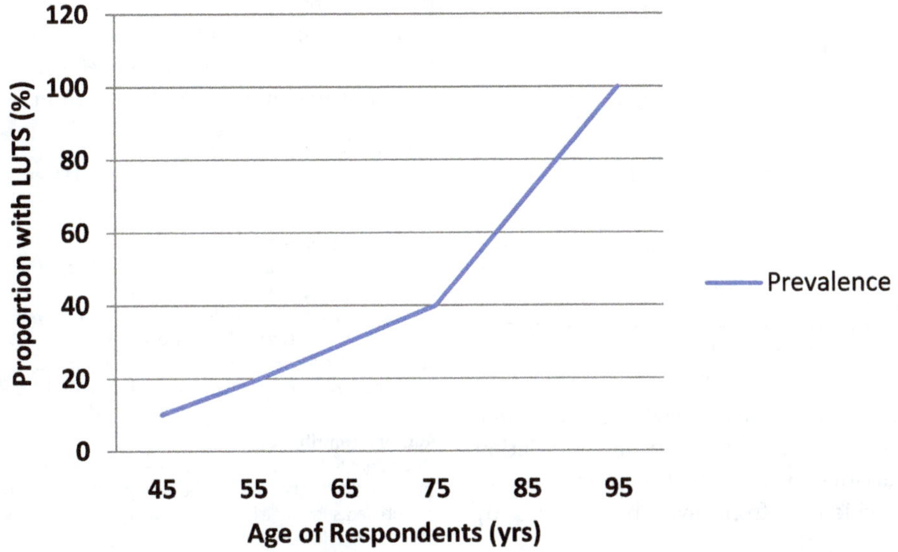

Fig. 1 A line chart showing the relationship between respondents' age and the proportion of respondents experiencing at least one lower urinary tract symptom ($N = 1319$). This figure shows that there is a gradual increase in the prevalence of LUTS from 40 years of age. The increase is at the rate of 7% per decade from 40 to 70 years. Beyond 70 years of age the rate of increase is nearly tripled

symptoms gradually worsen, or at the best, persist as age progresses. The odds that an older man from the age of 40 years in the community will report LUTS, controlling for BMI, MAC and higher wealth index, is 1.065 ($p < 0.001$) (Table 2).

Though there is very weak evidence of any significant difference in MAC of men reporting LUTS and those reporting no LUTS (t – 2.057; df 1317; p 0.04), there exists no evidence of any significant difference in BMI of the 2 groups (t 0.938; df 1317; p 0.35). Similar studies in southwest Nigeria [25], in Korea Republic [26], in Italy [27] and in USA [5] report, as well, the absence of any significant difference in LUTS among men of various anthropometric dimensions. The explanation for this may be that while LUTS occurrence and progression are related to aging, BMI and MAC are not consistent in their relationship with aging. On the contrary, some other studies have reported significant positive correlation [28] or negative correlation [29] between LUTS and BMI as well as other components of metabolic syndrome. These conflicting observations suggest that there may be no direct causal relationship between

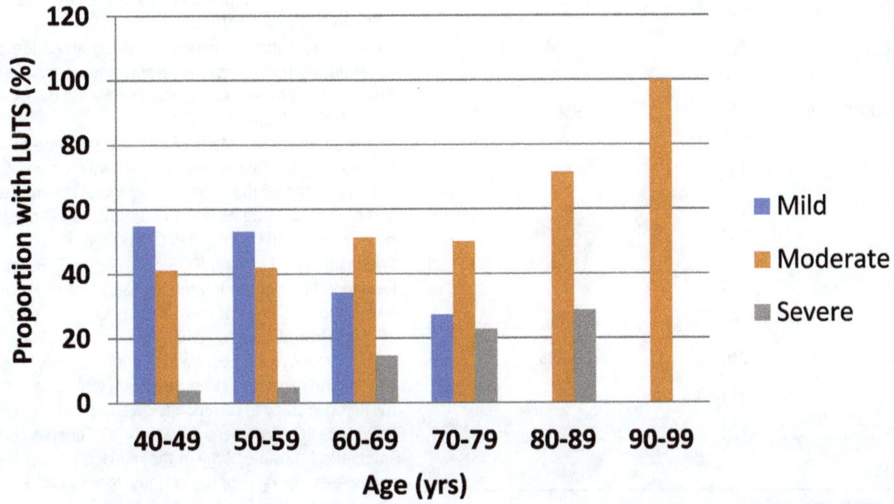

Fig. 2 A cluster bar chart showing severity of lower urinary tract symptoms within the various age categories of respondents with LUTS ($N = 267$) Before the age of 60 years, mild LUTS is more prevalent, while beyond the age of 70 years, moderate to severe LUTS become more prevalent. This pattern is significant statistically

Table 2 The outcome of Binary Logistic Regression analysis of factors relating with presence or not of LUTS

Variable	OR	95% CI		
		Lower Limit	Upper Limit	*p* value
Age of Respondent	1.065	1.051	1.080	< 0.001
BMI	1.007	0.969	1.046	0.732
MAC	1.010	0.997	1.022	0.139
Wealth Index	0.909	0.821	1.006	0.066

[*OR* Odds Ratio, *CI* Confidence Interval, *BMI* Body Mass Index, *MAC* Mid-Abdominal Circumference]
There is no evidence from this table, that the obesity indices BMI and MAC and the wealth index significantly influence LUTS in men, controlling for age

LUTS, BMI, MAC and other metabolic syndrome components. Such absence of a significant correlation between these variables is the conclusion from a recent review of evidences from available studies by Sebastianelli & Gacci [30].

Conclusions

This survey reveals that the overall prevalence rate of LUTS among men 40 years and older in this community is 20.2% with 58.4% of them experiencing moderate to severe LUTS. LUTS prevalence and severity increases with increasing age, but not with increasing obesity indices, BMI and MAC, or with increasing wealth-index. These observations suggest that attention should be given to the disorder during public health discuss. In addition, the observations contribute knowledge to the nature of the relationship between LUTS, aging, obesity and affluence in black African men in Nigeria,

Table 3 Shows the frequency distribution of the various lower urinary tract symptoms among all respondents ($N = 1319$)

Variables	Frequency (n)	Proportion (%)
Frequency of urination	180	13.6%
Urgency	175	13.3%
Nocturia ≥ 1 per night	253	19.2%
Nocturia ≥ 2 per night	229	17.4%
At Least 1 Storage Symptom with Nocturia ≥ 1	263	19.9%
At Least 1 Storage Symptom with Nocturia ≥ 2	262	19.9%
Weak Stream	131	9.9%
Intermittency	104	7.9%
Straining	109	8.3%
Incomplete Emptying	125	9.4%
At Least 1 Voiding Symptom	181	13.7%
Any Lower Urinary Tract Symptom	**267**	**20.2%**
Mild LUTS (IPSS 1–7)	111	8.4%
Moderate LUTS (IPSS 8–19)	126	9.6%
Severe LUTS (IPSS 20–35)	30	2.3%

[*LUTS* lower urinary tract symptoms]
The table indicates that nocturia defined as any void during night sleep or as greater than 1 void during night sleep is the most prevalent lower urinary tract symptom; storage LUTS are generally more prevalent than voiding LUTS and 11.9% reported moderate to severe LUTS

Abbreviations

BMI: Body Mass Index; IPSS: International Prostate Symptom Score; LUTS: Lower Urinary Tract Symptoms; MAC: Mid-abdominal Circumference

Acknowledgements

Dr. Jude Edeh, Dr. Ekeoma Nwosu, Dr. Uko Uko, Dr. Casmir Nnadi, Dr. Nonso Iwenofu, Dr. Pascal Maduabuchi, Dr. Wilson Onoh, Dr. Kingsley Onyia, Dr. Njideka Oragunye, Dr. Maxwell Isiwu, Dr. Chimuanya Mogbo, Dr. Hyginus Odoh, Dr. Pamela Okafor, Dr. Princewill Osueke, Dr. Arinze Onyia, Dr. Kingsley Bassey and Dr. Nwoku Amy, Dr. Chimuanya Mogbo, Dr. Bassey K Bassey, and Dr. Chinenye Eneh are acknowledged for their roles during data collection.

Authors' contributions

IIN contributed substantially in conception, design, acquisition, analysis and interpretation of data, and in the drafting of the manuscript. FOU contributed substantially in design, analysis and interpretation of acquired data and revision of manuscript. EIU contributed substantially in design, analysis and interpretation of acquired data, and drafting of manuscript. SKA contributed substantially in design of study, acquisition of data, analysis and interpretation of acquired data, and drafting the manuscript. LTO contributed substantially in design of study, acquisition of data, analysis and interpretation of acquired data, and drafting the manuscript. All Authors read and approved of the final version being submitted and agreed to be accountable for all parts of the research work.

Author details

[1]Department of Surgery, College of Medicine, University of Nigeria Ituku-Ozalla, KM 20 Enugu-PortHarcourt Highway, Enugu PMB 01129, Nigeria. [2]Department of Health Administration and Management, University of Nigeria Enugu Campus, Enugu, Nigeria. [3]Department of Surgery, University of Nigeria Teaching Hospital Ituku-Ozalla, Enugu, Nigeria.

References

1. Drake MJ, Morris N, Apostolidis A, Rahnama'I MS, Marchesi JR. The urinary microbiome and its contribution to lower urinary tract symptoms; ICI-RS 2015. Neurourol Urodyn. 2017;36(4):850–3. https://doi.org/10.1002/nau.23006.
2. Irwin DE, Milsom I, Hunskaar S, Reilly K, Kopp Z, Herschorn S, Coyne K, Kelleher C, Hampel C, Artibani W, Abrams P. Population-based survey of urinary incontinence, overactive bladder, and other lower urinary tract symptoms in five countries: results of the EPIC study. Eur Urol. 2006;50(6): 1306–14 discussion 1314-5.
3. Bajunirwe F, Stothers L, Berkowitz J, Macnab AJ. Prevalence estimates of lower urinary tract symptom severity among men in Uganda and sub-Saharan Africa based on regional prevalence data. Can Urol Assoc J. 2018. https://doi.org/10.5489/cuaj.5105.
4. Martin SA, Haren MT, Marshall VR, Lange K, Wittert GA. Members of the Florey Adelaide male ageing study. Prevalence and factors associated with uncomplicated storage and voiding lower urinary tract symptoms in community-dwelling Australian men. World J Urol. 2011;29(2):179–84. https://doi.org/10.1007/s00345-010-0605-8.
5. Parsons JK, Wilt TJ, Wang PY, Barrett-Connor E, Bauer DC, Marshall LM, Osteoporotic Fractures in Men Research Group. Progression of lower urinary tract symptoms in older men: a community based study. J Urol. 2010;183(5): 1915–20. https://doi.org/10.1016/j.juro.2010.01.026.
6. Kok ET, Groeneveld FP, Gouweloos J, Jonkheijm R, Bosch JL, Thomas S, Bohnen AM. Determinants of seeking of primary care for lower urinary tract symptoms: the Krimpen study in community-dwelling men. Eur Urol. 2006;50(4):811–7.
7. Ugwumba FO, Ozoemena OF, Okoh AD, Echetabu KN, Mbadiwe OM. Transvesical prostatectomy in the management of benign prostatic hyperplasia in a developing country. Niger J Clin Pract. 2014;17(6):797–801. https://doi.org/10.4103/1119-3077.144402.
8. Stothers L, Macnab AJ, Bajunirwe F, Mutabazi S, Berkowitz J. Associations between the severity of obstructive lower urinary tract symptoms and care-seeking behavior in rural Africa: a cross-sectional survey from Uganda. PLoS One. 2017;12(3):e0173631. https://doi.org/10.1371/journal.pone.0173631.

9. Burgio KL, Johnson TM 2nd, Goode PS, Markland AD, Richter HE, Roth DL, Sawyer P, Allman RM. Prevalence and correlates of nocturia in community-dwelling older adults. J Am Geriatr Soc. 2010;58(5):861–6. https://doi.org/10.1111/j.1532-5415.2010.02822.x.
10. Wang YC, McPherson K, Marsh T, Gortmaker SL, Brown M. Health and economic burden of the projected obesity trends in the USA and the UK. Lancet. 2011;378(9793):815–25. https://doi.org/10.1016/SD140-6736(11)60814-3.
11. Asiki G, Mohamed SF, Wambui D, Wainana C, Muthuri S, Ramsay M, Kyobutungi C, as members of AWI-Gen the H3Africa Consortium. Sociodemographic and behavioural factors associated with body mass index among men and women in Nairobi slums: AWI-gen project. Glob Health Action. 2018;11(sup2):1470738. https://doi.org/10.1080/16549716.2018.1470738.
12. Irwin DE, Kopp ZS, Agatep B, Milsom I, Abrams P. Worldwide prevalence estimates of lower urinary tract symptoms, overactive bladder, urinary incontinence and bladder outlet obstruction. BJU Int. 2011;108(7):1132–8. https://doi.org/10.1111/j.1464-410X.2010.09993.x.
13. Aliyu AA, Amadu L. Urbanization, cities, and health: the challenges to Nigeria –a review. Ann Afr Med. 2017;16(4):149–58. https://doi.org/10.4103/aam.aam_1_17.
14. IPSS Form. Accessed from (www.urospec.com/uro/Forms/ipss.pdf) on Dec 4th 2017.
15. Nigeria, UNDP. Human Development Report, Nigeria, 2008–2009. Abuja, Nigeria: United Nation Development Programme, 2009. Accessed from (www.nigerianstat.gov.ng) on Feb 20th 2018.
16. Ojewola RW, Oridota ES, Balogun OS, Ogundare EO, Alabi TO. Lower urinary ract symptoms: prevalence, perceptions, and healthcare-seeking behavior amongst Nigerian men. World J Mens Health. 2016;34(3):200–8. https://doi.org/10.5534/wjmh.2016.34.3.200.
17. Olapade-Olaopa EO, Owoaje ET, Ladipo MM, Fadimu OA, Muoka O, Adedeji TG. Frequency and pattern of lower urinary tract symptoms in a screened population of men above 40 years in Ibadan, southwestern Nigeria. J West Afr Coll Surg. 2015;5(4):60–78.
18. Chokkalingam AP, Yeboah ED, Demarzo A, Netto G, Yu K, Biritwum RB, Tettey Y, Adjei A, Jadallah S, Li Y, Chu LW, Chia D, Niwa S, Partin A, Thompson IM, Roehrborn C, Hoover RN, Hsing AW. Prevalence of BPH and lower urinary tract symptoms in west Africans. Prostate Cancer Prostatic Dis. 2012;15(2):170–6. https://doi.org/10.1038/pcan.2011.43.
19. Suen LKP, Cheng HL, Yeung SKW, Au-Yeung CH, Lee JCY, Ho KKY, Lau NMY, Ng CKF, Chan IWS. Qualitative insights into the experiences of living with moderate-to-severe lower urinary tract symptoms among community-dwelling ageing males. PLoS One. 2017;12(10):e0187085. https://doi.org/10.1371/journal.pone.0187085.
20. Janssens W, Goedecke J, de Bree GJ, Aderibigbe SA, Akande TM, Mesnard A. The financial burden of non-communicable chronic diseases in rural Nigeria: wealth and gender heterogeneity in health care utilization and health expenditures. PLoS One. 2016;11(11):e0166121. https://doi.org/10.1371/journal.pone.0166121.
21. Egan KB. The epidemiology of benign prostatic hyperplasia associated with lower urinary tract symptoms. Prevalence and incident rates Urol Clin North Am. 2016;43(3):289–97. https://doi.org/10.1016/j.ucl.2016.04.001.
22. Rohrmann S, Katzke V, Kaaks R. Prevalence and progression of lower urinary tract symptoms in an aging population. Urology. 2016;95:158–63. https://doi.org/10.1016/j.urology.2016.06.021.
23. De Ridder D, Roumeguère T, Kaufman L. Urgency and other lower urinary tract symptoms in men aged ≥ 40 years: a Belgian epidemiological survey using the ICIQ-MLUTS questionnaire. Int J Clin Pract. 2015;69(3):358–65. https://doi.org/10.1111/ijcp.12541.
24. Pöyhönen A, Häkkinen JT, Kosskimäki J, Tammela TL, Auvinen A. Natural course of lower urinary tract symptoms in men not requiring treatment: a 5-year longitudinal population-based study. Urology. 2014;83(2):411–5. https://doi.org/10.1016/j.urology.2013.10.003.
25. Badmus TA, Asaleye CM, Badmus SA, Takure AO, Ibrahim MH, Arowolo OA. Benign prostate hyperplasia: average volume in southwestern Nigerians and correlation with anthropometrics. Niger Postgrad Med J. 2013;20(1):52–6.
26. Lee SH, Lee SK, Choo MS, Ko KT, Shin TY, Lee WK, Batsaikhan T, Quan S, Jeong JY, Kim DH. Relationship between metabolic syndrome and lower urinary tract symptoms: Hallym aging study. Biomed Res Int. 2015;130917. https://doi.org/10.1155/2015/130917.
27. Yang HJ, Doo SW, Yang WJ, Song YS. Which obesity index best correlates with prostate volume, prostate-specific antigen, and lower urinary tract symptoms? Urology. 2012;80(1):187–90. https://doi.org/10.1016/j.urology.2012.04.003.
28. He Q, Babcook MA, Shukla S, Shankar E, Wang Z, Liu G, Erokwu BO, Flask CA, Lu L, Daneshgari F, MacLennan GT, Gupta S. Obesity-initiated metabolic syndrome promotes urinary voiding dysfunction in a mouse model. Prostate. 2016;76(11):964–76. https://doi.org/10.1002/pros.23185.
29. Yelsel K, Alma E, Eken A, Gülüm M, Erçil H, Ayyıldız A. Effect of obesity on international prostate symptom score and prostate volume. Urol Ann. 2015;7(3):371–4. https://doi.org/10.4103/0974-7796.152056.
30. Sebastianelli A, Gacci M. Current status of the relationship between metabolic syndrome and lower urinary tract symptoms. Eur Urol Focus. 2018;4(1):25–7. https://doi.org/10.1016/j.euf.2018.03.007.

32

The etiology and prevalence of urinary tract infection and asymptomatic bacteriuria in pregnant women in Iran

Milad Azami[1,2], Zahra Jaafari[3], Mansour Masoumi[4], Masoumeh Shohani[5], Gholamreza Badfar[6], Leily Mahmudi[7] and Shamsi Abbasalizadeh[2*]

Abstract

Background: Urinary tract infection (UTI) is a common clinical problem in pregnant women. Bacteriuria in pregnancy without antibiotic treatment could result in complications. This study aims to investigate the etiology and prevalence of UTI and asymptomatic bacteriuria (ASB) in pregnant women in Iran.

Method: This meta-analysis follows the Preferred Reporting Items for Systematic Reviews and Meta-Analyses (PRISMA) guidelines. To avoid bias, all steps of the study were carried out independently by two researchers. We conducted a comprehensive search on all the related literature in national databases, including IranDoc, SID, Barakat Knowledge Network System, RICST, Magiran, Iranian National Library and international databases, including Scopus, Embase, Science Direct, PubMed/ Medline, Cochrane Library, Web of Sciences, EBSCO, as well as Google Scholar search engine until June 2018. After considering the inclusion/exclusion criteria and qualitative evaluation, studies were analyzed based on random effects model using Comprehensive Meta-Analysis Software Version 2.

Results: In 31 studies with a sample size of 20,309, the prevalence of ASB in pregnant Iranian women was estimated to be 8.7% (95%CI: 7.2–10.4). The lowest and highest prevalence of ASB were observed in the third trimester (6.1% [95%CI: 2.1–16.4]) and first trimester (11.7% [95%CI: 7.9–16.9]), respectively. Subgroup analysis of the prevalence of ASB based on geographical region ($P = 0.002$) and province ($P < 0.001$) was significant but for the quality of studies ($P = 0.51$) was not significant. In 17 studies including 48,731 pregnant women, the prevalence of UTI was estimated to be 9.8% (95%CI: 7.6–12.5). The test for subgroup differences of prevalence of UTI for province ($P < 0.001$) was significant but for geographical region ($P = 061$) and quality of studies ($P = 0.11$) was not significant. Meta-regression model for the prevalence of UTI and ASB in pregnant women in Iran based on year of the studies was significant ($P < 0.001$). The most common microorganism involved in the etiology of UTI (61.6% [95%CI: 51.6–70.7]) and ASB (63.22% [95%CI: 51.2–73.8]) was *E. coli*.

Conclusion: UTI and ASB are prevalent in pregnant women in Iran. Therefore, UTI screening is essential in pregnant women. The most common microorganism involved in the etiology of UTI and ASB in pregnant women in Iran is *E.coli*.

Keywords: Etiology, Urinary tract infection, Asymptomatic bacteriuria, Pregnant women, Iran

* Correspondence: shamciabbasalizadeh@gmail.com
[2]Department of Obstetrics & Gynecology, Women's Reproductive Health Research Center, School of Medicine, Tabriz University of Medical Sciences, Tabriz, Iran
Full list of author information is available at the end of the article

Background

Urinary tract infection (UTI) is a common clinical problem that constitutes about 1–6% of medical referrals and includes urinary tract, bladder and kidney infections [1]. UTI may be symptomatic or asymptomatic, while asymptomatic bacteriuria (ASB) is of particular importance due to lack of any symptom [2, 3]. UTI and its related complications cause about 150 million deaths per year around the world [4].

In pregnant women, physiological and anatomical changes in the urinary tract, as well as immune system changes during pregnancy increase the prevalence of ASB and in some cases lead to the symptomatic infection, resulting in serious risks for both mother and fetus. Increasing age, parity, diabetes, sickle cell anemia, history of UTI, urinary tract disorders and immune deficiency may increase the risk of UTI in pregnant women [5–7].

Bacteriuria in pregnancy without antibiotic treatment could result in complications such as preterm labor, pre-eclampsia, hypertension, pyelonephritis, anemia, amnionitis, low birth weight, neonatal deaths (stillbirths), bacteremia and toxic septicemia [8–10]. Treatment of bacteriuria in pregnancy reduces the risk of complications. Therefore, screening for early diagnosis and treatment of bacteriuria in women during pregnancy is necessary to prevent its complications [11].

The overall prevalence of bacteriuria in pregnant Iranian women was reported to be 2–41% [11–54]. Therefore, there is inconsistency in the results of studies. Thus, determining the prevalence of ABS, UTI and the most common pathogenic microorganisms involved in its creation is a valuable diagnostic capability in different countries.

Because of the inconsistency in different reports, reviewing various studies cannot be sufficient to achieve this goal. In systematic reviews, examining all related documents and combining them through meta-analysis provides a more complete picture of the dimensions of a problem [55–57].

This study aims to assess the prevalence of UTI, ASB and pathogens involved in bacteriuria among pregnant women in Iran.

Methods

Study protocol

This systematic review and meta-analysis follows the Preferred Reporting Items for Systematic Reviews and Meta-Analyses (PRISMA) guidelines [57]. To avoid bias, all steps of study were carried out independently by two researchers and in case of controversies, the problem was resolved by a third researcher.

Inclusion and exclusion criteria

Inclusion criteria according to PICO (Evidence-Based Medicine) [58] were as follows [1]: **P**opulation: The epidemiologic studies that investigated UTI, ASB and etiology among pregnant women [2]; **I**ntervention: Urine culture for confirmed UTI and ASB [3]; **C**omparison: That can show the prevalence of UTI and ASB based on geographical region, province and trimester of pregnancy [4]; **O**utcome: Studies that estimated the UTI, ASB and etiology prevalence in pregnant women.

The exclusion criteria were: 1. Non-random sampling; 2. Non-pregnant Iranian women; 3. Irrelevance with the subject of the research; 4. Incomplete information such as failing to report the prevalence; 5. Qualitative studies; 6. Review articles, case reports and editorials; 7. Duplicates.

Search strategy and study selection

We conducted a comprehensive search on all English and Persian related literature in national databases, including Iranian Research Institute for Information Science and Technology (IranDoc) (https://irandoc.ac.ir), Scientific Information Database (SID) (http://www.sid.ir/), Barakat Knowledge Network System (http://health.barakatkns.com), Regional Information Center for Science and Technology (RICST) (http://en.ricest.ac.ir/), Magiran (http://www.magiran.com/), Iranian National Library (http://www.nlai.ir/) and international databases, including Scopus, PubMed/Medline, Science Direct, Cochrane Library, Embase, Web of Sciences, EBSCO, as well as Google Scholar search engine until June 2018. We searched the articles using English MeSH keywords and Persian equivalents: "Pregnant", "Gestational", "Pregnancy", "Prenatal Care", "Urinary Tract Infection", "Bacteriuria", "Iran" and all possible combinations of keywords using "AND" and "OR" operators for English databases. In addition, the manual search was conducted to find more studies by screening the reference list of all articles included in the meta-analysis. PubMed combination search was as follows: ("Pregnant"[Title/Abstract] OR "Pregnancy"[Title/Abstract]) OR "Gestational"[Title/Abstract] OR "Prenatal Care"[Title/Abstract] AND ("Urinary Tract Infection"[Title/Abstract] OR "Bacteriuria"[Title/Abstract] AND "Iran"[Title/Abstract/Affiliation].

It is worth noting that 'High Sensitive Searching' was used in databases; in addition, the search was conducted by qualified researchers and experts in the field of database searching ("M. Azami" and "Z. Jaafari").

Quality assessment

Authors assessed the quality of studies according to the modified Newcastle Ottawa Scale (NOS) for cross-sectional studies [59], which includes eight sections, and evaluated the selected articles from the selection, comparability, exposure assessment, and outcome. Points of 0–5, 6–7 and 8–10 were considered as low quality, moderate quality and high quality, respectively. A minimum score of 6 was considered as a criterion to include an article.

Data extraction

The checklist was designed based on goals. This checklist included: authors, place, province, region, year of publication, year of study, study design, mean age, sample size, prevalence of UTI, ASB and microorganisms involved in bacteriuria. Sample size and prevalence of UTI and ASB for the first, second and third trimester of pregnancy were independently extracted by two researchers.

Statistical analysis

Binomial distribution formula was used to estimate the standard error for the prevalence of UTI, ASB and pathogens involved in bacteriuria. The heterogeneity of the studies was assessed using Cochran's Q test and I^2 index, and interpreted as follows: 0–24% may not be important, 25–49% indicates moderate heterogeneity, 50–75% indicates substantial heterogeneity and over 75% indicates considerable heterogeneity [60]. To combine data in high heterogeneity, we used the random effects model. To explore the potential sources of heterogeneity, subgroup analysis was preformed based on geographical region, province and trimester of pregnancy [61, 62]. We used the meta-regression model for the prevalence of UTI and ASB according to year of the study. Publication bias was measured by reviewing the funnel plots and through Begg and Egger's tests. Meta-analysis of data was performed using Comprehensive Meta-Analysis Software Version 2 and the significance level was considered less than 0.05.

Results

Search results

In the systematic review, 520 potentially relevant articles were identified, and after screening the titles and abstracts, 260 studies were excluded because of being duplicate, and the full text of 260 possibly related articles was studied. After the evaluation of exclusion/inclusion criteria and the quality of articles, 42 eligible studies, published from 1995 to 2015, were included in meta-analysis (Fig. 1).

Study characteristics

42 eligible articles (17 studies for UTI and 31 studies for ASB) including 67,776 pregnant women were investigated. Mean and standard deviation (SD) for age was 26.47 ± 5.47 years. Other study characteristics are shown in Table 1.

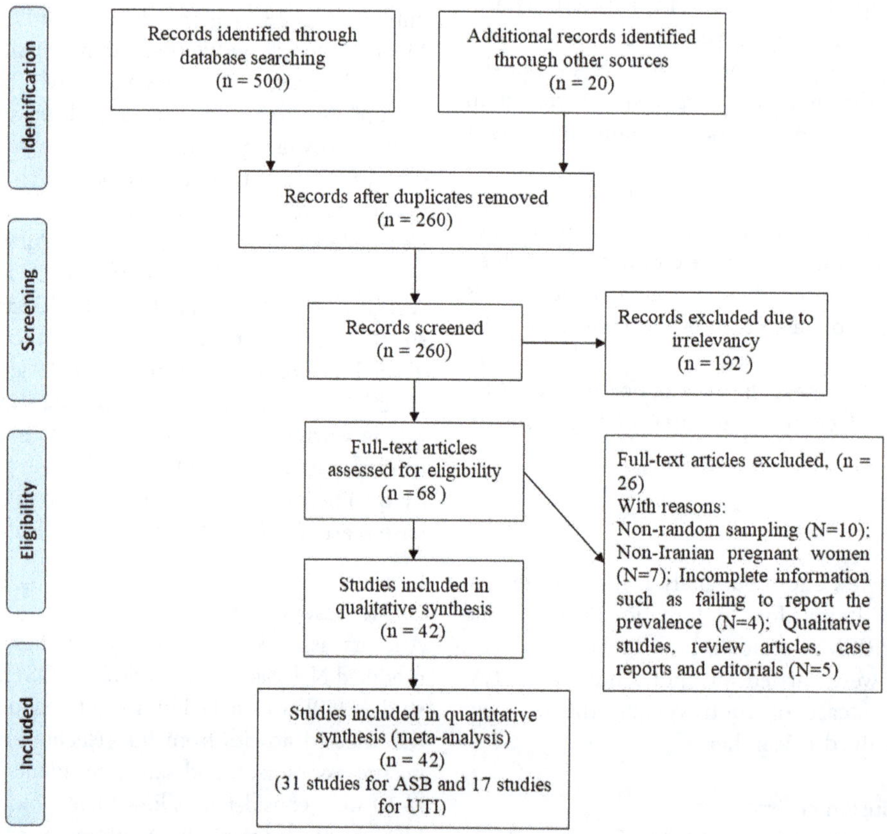

Fig. 1 A flow diagram following the PRISMA template

Table 1 Characteristics of studies on asymptomatic bacteriuria and urinary tract infections among pregnant Iranian women

Ref	First author, published year	Place	Year of study	Sample size	(Mean±SD[a]) age	Prevalence of ASB[b]	Prevalence of UTI[c]	Test	Most common microorganisms
[12]	Vejdani MH, 1998	Tabriz	1995	950		10.5		Culture	E.coli[d]
[13]	Farajzadegan Z, 2008	Isfahan	2008	100	25.1 ± 3.6	2		Culture	
[14]	Shirazi MH, 2007	Hamadan	2007	377		10.1		Culture	E.coli
[15]	Safari M, 2008	Yasuj	2006	715	25 ± 5.3		6	Culture	
[16]	Mobsheri E, 2002	Gorgan	2000	900		3.7		Culture	E.coli
[17]	Kameli M, 2013	Torbat Haidaria	2013	1250		10		Culture	*Staphylococcus epidermidis*
[18]	Soofizadeh N, 2012	Sanandaj	2009	1500	28.4 ± 6.1	7.6		Culture	–
[19]	Azizzadeh Sh, 1999	Tehran	1997	547		12.7		Culture	E.coli
[20]	Aaron H, 2008	Kerman	2007	323		24.1		Culture	–
[21]	Aghaee alamouti M, 2010	Tehran	2009	826		8.7		Culture	–
[22]	Yousofzadeh Sh, 1995	Kashan	1995	400		4.7	7.5	Culture	–
[23]	Necohesh L, 2005	Ghods	2004	100		14		Culture	E.coli
[24]	Namazi A, 2012	Guilan	2008	710	27.48 ± 6.0	21.1		Culture	–
[25]	Shojaee H, 2000	Shahrekord	1999	864		4.3	8.8	Culture	E.coli
[26]	Zarganj Fard A, 2000	Arak	2000	1736		6.3		Culture	E.coli
[27]	Khorshidi A, 1997	Kashan	1996	350	24 ± 5.5	5.4		Culture	E.coli
[28]	Hazhir S, 2007	Tabriz	2007	1100		6.1		Culture	–
[29]	Motaghi M, 2012	Mashhad	2008	150		10.7		Culture	E.coli
[30]	Dadkhah F, 2011	Tehran	2010	1246		9		Culture	–
[31]	Kalantar E, 2008	Sanandaj	2008	1505	28.4 ± 4.6	8.9		Culture	E.coli
[32]	Kasraeian M, 2009	Shiraz	2007	389	26.3 ± 4.2	5.1		Culture	E.coli
[33]	Jazayeri Moghadas A, 2009	Semnan	2007	297		3.3		Culture	E.coli
[34]	Alavi-Naini R, 2003	Zahedan	2002	490		14.9		Culture	E.coli
[34]	Alavi-Naini R, 2003	Zahedan	2002	478		10.5		Culture	E.coli
[34]	Alavi-Naini R, 2003	Zahedan	2002	463		16.2		Culture	E.coli
[35]	Rahmani E, 2012	Kermanshah	2011	500	27.4 ± 5.8		19.8	Culture	–
[36]	Norouzzadeh M, 1997	Karaj	1997	300			22.7	Culture	E.coli
[37]	Mardanian F, 2004	Isfahan	2004	543		10.4		Culture	–
[37]	Mardanian F, 2004	Isfahan	2004	911		9.9		Culture	–
[37]	Mardanian F, 2004	Isfahan	2004	891		2.0		Culture	–
[38]	Fakhimi L, 2002	Zanjan	2002	1012			13	Culture	–
[39]	Azizi A, 2015	Sanqor	2001	3157	26.5 ± 5.5		5.8	Culture	–
[40]	Jalali M, 2014	Karaj	2013	180	26 ± 5.8		19.8	Culture	E.coli
[41]	Zakeri Hamidi M, 2006	Mazandaran	2004	300			8.33	Culture	–
[42]	Shahhosseini Z, 2012	Sari	2009	428	24.5 ± 4.8		2.8	Culture	–
[43]	Rahimkhani M, 2008	Tehran	2012	86	26.8 ± 5.5	29.1		Culture	Staphylococcus epidermidis
[44]	Golestan M, 2011	Yazd	2008	5897			6.98	Culture	–
[45]	Rahmanian M, 2014	Semnan	2012	160	27.8 ± 5.4	5.6		Culture	–
[46]	Shams MR, 2000	Tehran	1996	205		6.8		Culture	–
[47]	Alijahan R, 2014	Ardabil	2011	2496			9.7	Culture	E.coli
[48]	Saffar MJ, 2008	Sari	2002	5600			12.6	Culture	E.coli

Table 1 Characteristics of studies on asymptomatic bacteriuria and urinary tract infections among pregnant Iranian women *(Continued)*

Ref	First author, published year	Place	Year of study	Sample size	(Mean±SD[a]) age	Prevalence of ASB[b]	Prevalence of UTI[c]	Test	Most common microorganisms
[49]	Soleimani Zadeh L, 2004	Bam	2001	850	25.5 ± 6.6		12.3	Culture	–
[50]	Modars Sh, 1998	Tehran	1996	462		10.8		Culture	E.coli
[51]	Sharemi H, 2013	Rasht	2012	330	27.9 ± 5.8		23.6	Culture	–
[52]	Sohrabi D, 2011	Zanjan	2007	3102			5.83	Culture	–
[53]	Amiri M, 2015	Dezful	2012	22,600		10.5	5	Culture	E.coli

[a]Standard deviation; [b] Asymptomatic bacteriuria; [c] Urinary tract infections; [d]*Escherichia coli*

*Some studies estimated the prevalence of UTI or ASB for more than 1 year and also regions. Each data was considered separately because of assessing the slope of prevalence in the years and estimating which region is the highest or lowest

Total prevalence of ASB and sensitivity analysis

The heterogeneity rate for the prevalence of ASB was high ($I^2 = 93.38$, $P < 0.001$). In 31 studies with a sample size of 20,309, the prevalence of ASB in pregnant Iranian women was estimated to be 8.7% (95% CI:7.2–10.4) (Fig. 2). The lowest and highest prevalence of ASB were 2 and 29.1% in the studies of Farajzadegan [13] and Rahimkhani [43], respectively (Fig. 2). Sensitivity analysis for the prevalence of ASB in Fig. 3 shows that after removing a study at a time, the result is still robust.

Subgroup analysis of the prevalence of ASB based on geographical region and province

The lowest prevalence of ASB in pregnant women was estimated to be in the South of Iran (5.1% [95% CI: 3.3–7.8]) and Golestan province (3.7% [95% CI: 2.6–5.2]). The

Study name, published year	Event rate	Lower limit	Upper limit	Z-Value	p-Value	Relative weight
Vedjdani MH, 1998	0.105	0.087	0.126	-20.247	0.000	3.53
Farajzadegan Z, 2008	0.020	0.005	0.076	-5.449	0.000	1.30
Shirazi MH, 2007	0.101	0.074	0.136	-12.791	0.000	3.33
Mobsheri E, 2002	0.037	0.026	0.052	-18.456	0.000	3.31
Kameli M, 2013	0.100	0.085	0.118	-23.305	0.000	3.56
Soofizadeh N, 2012	0.076	0.064	0.091	-25.638	0.000	3.56
Azizzadeh Sh, 1999	0.127	0.102	0.158	-15.012	0.000	3.47
Aaron H, 2008	0.241	0.197	0.291	-8.818	0.000	3.47
Aghaee alamouti M, 2010	0.087	0.070	0.108	-19.041	0.000	3.49
Yousofzadeh Sh, 1995	0.048	0.030	0.073	-12.755	0.000	3.07
Necohesh L, 2005	0.140	0.085	0.223	-6.299	0.000	2.83
Namazi A, 2012	0.211	0.183	0.243	-14.327	0.000	3.57
Shojaee H, 2000	0.043	0.031	0.059	-18.500	0.000	3.34
Zarganj Fard A, 2000	0.063	0.052	0.075	-27.328	0.000	3.55
Khorshidi A, 1997	0.054	0.035	0.083	-12.107	0.000	3.06
Hazhir S, 2007	0.061	0.048	0.077	-21.701	0.000	3.48
Motaghi M, 2012	0.107	0.067	0.167	-8.033	0.000	2.94
Dadkhah F, 2011	0.090	0.075	0.107	-23.372	0.000	3.55
Kalantar E, 2008	0.089	0.076	0.104	-25.693	0.000	3.57
Kasraeian M, 2009	0.051	0.033	0.078	-12.686	0.000	3.09
Jazayeri Moghadas A, 2009	0.033	0.018	0.061	-10.398	0.000	2.67
Alavi-Naini R, 2003	0.149	0.120	0.183	-13.737	0.000	3.48
Alavi-Naini R, 2003	0.105	0.081	0.136	-14.362	0.000	3.40
Alavi-Naini R, 2003	0.162	0.131	0.198	-13.029	0.000	3.48
Mardanian F, 2004	0.104	0.081	0.133	-15.319	0.000	3.43
Mardanian F, 2004	0.099	0.081	0.120	-19.907	0.000	3.52
Mardanian F, 2004	0.020	0.013	0.032	-16.264	0.000	3.05
Rahimkhani M, 2008	0.291	0.205	0.395	-3.751	0.000	3.06
Rahmanian M, 2014	0.056	0.029	0.104	-8.215	0.000	2.58
Shams MR, 2005	0.068	0.041	0.112	-9.436	0.000	2.88
Modars Sh, 1998	0.108	0.083	0.140	-14.086	0.000	3.40
Random effects model	0.087	0.072	0.104	-23.233	0.000	

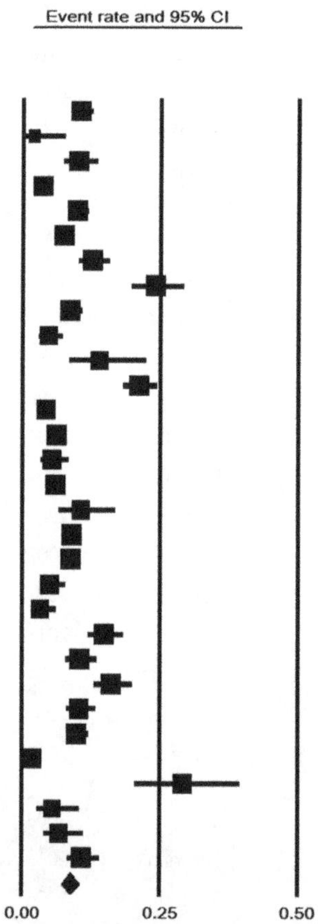

Meta Analysis

Fig. 2 Prevalence of asymptomatic bacteriuria in pregnant women in Iran

Study name, published year	Statistics with study removed				
	Point	Lower limit	Upper limit	Z-Value	p-Value
Vedjdani MH, 1998	0.086	0.071	0.104	-22.291	0.000
Farajzadegan Z, 2008	0.089	0.074	0.106	-22.978	0.000
Shirazi MH, 2007	0.086	0.072	0.104	-22.644	0.000
Mobsheri E, 2002	0.090	0.075	0.107	-23.173	0.000
Kameli M, 2013	0.086	0.071	0.104	-22.114	0.000
Soofizadeh N, 2012	0.087	0.072	0.105	-22.262	0.000
Azizzadeh Sh, 1999	0.086	0.071	0.103	-22.664	0.000
Aaron H, 2008	0.084	0.070	0.100	-24.673	0.000
Aghaee alamouti M, 2010	0.087	0.072	0.105	-22.393	0.000
Yousofzadeh Sh, 1995	0.089	0.074	0.106	-22.794	0.000
Necohesh L, 2005	0.086	0.071	0.103	-22.993	0.000
Namazi A, 2012	0.084	0.071	0.100	-25.241	0.000
Shojaee H, 2000	0.089	0.074	0.107	-23.017	0.000
Zarganj Fard A, 2000	0.088	0.073	0.106	-22.609	0.000
Khorshidi A, 1997	0.088	0.073	0.106	-22.751	0.000
Hazhir S, 2007	0.088	0.073	0.106	-22.666	0.000
Motaghi M, 2012	0.086	0.072	0.104	-22.838	0.000
Dadkhah F, 2011	0.087	0.072	0.105	-22.163	0.000
Kalantar E, 2008	0.087	0.072	0.105	-22.046	0.000
Kasraeian M, 2009	0.088	0.074	0.106	-22.769	0.000
Jazayeri Moghadas A, 2009	0.089	0.074	0.107	-22.867	0.000
Alavi-Naini R, 2003	0.085	0.071	0.102	-22.938	0.000
Alavi-Naini R, 2003	0.086	0.071	0.104	-22.585	0.000
Alavi-Naini R, 2003	0.085	0.071	0.102	-23.141	0.000
Mardanian F, 2004	0.086	0.071	0.104	-22.540	0.000
Mardanian F, 2004	0.086	0.071	0.104	-22.309	0.000
Mardanian F, 2004	0.091	0.076	0.108	-23.504	0.000
Rahimkhani M, 2008	0.084	0.070	0.100	-23.965	0.000
Rahmanian M, 2014	0.088	0.073	0.105	-22.802	0.000
Shams MR, 2005	0.088	0.073	0.105	-22.757	0.000
Modars Sh, 1998	0.086	0.071	0.104	-22.604	0.000
Random effects model	0.087	0.072	0.104	-23.233	0.000

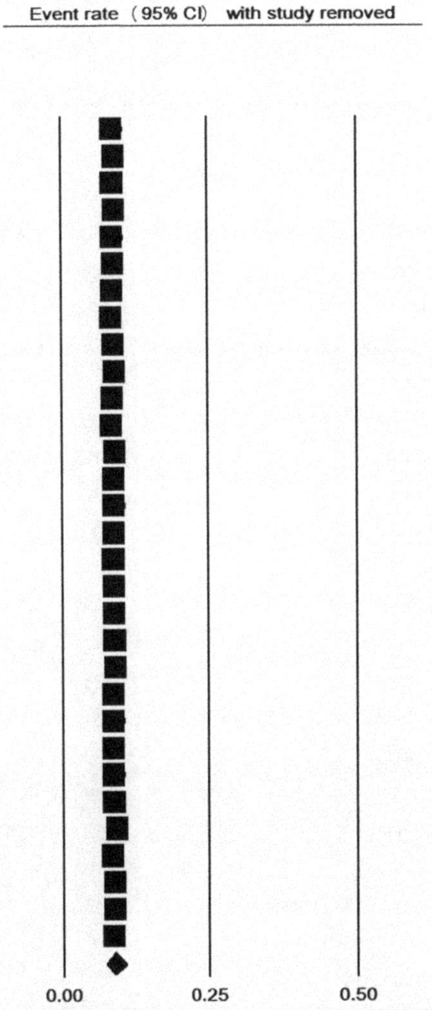

Meta Analysis

Fig. 3 Sensitivity analysis for the prevalence of asymptomatic bacteriuria in pregnant women in Iran

highest prevalence of ASB in pregnant women was estimated to be in the East of Iran (13.9% [95% CI: 10.3–18.6]) and Kerman province (24.1% [95% CI: 19.7–29.1]). The test for subgroup differences for geographical region ($P = 0.002$) and province ($P < 0.001$) was significant (Table 2).

Subgroup analysis of the prevalence of ASB based on quality of studies

The prevalence of ASB among pregnant women in terms of quality of studies based on NOS checklist was estimated to be 9.3% [95% CI: 7.1–12.1]) and 8.3% [95% CI: 6.4–10.6]) in moderate-quality and high-quality studies, respectively. No significant difference was found ($P = 0.51$) (Table 2).

The prevalence of ASB based on trimester of pregnancy

The lowest and highest prevalence of ASB were estimated in the third trimester (6.1% [95% CI: 2.1–16.4]) and first trimester (11.7% [95% CI: 7.9–16.9]), respectively (Fig. 4).

Prevalence of UTI in pregnant women

The heterogeneity rate for the prevalence of UTI was high ($I^2 = 98.12\%$, $P < 0.001$). In 17 studies including 48,731 pregnant Iranian women, the prevalence of UTI was estimated to be 9.8% (95% CI: 7.6–12.5). The lowest prevalence was in the study of Shahhosseini (2.8%) and the highest prevalence was in the study of Sharemi (23.6%) (Fig. 5). Sensitivity analysis by removing a study at a time showed that the result for the prevalence of UTI was robust (Fig. 6).

Subgroup analysis of the prevalence of UTI based on geographical region and province

The prevalence of UTI among pregnant women in the South of Iran (7.2% [95% CI: 3.9–13.1]) and Khuzestan

Table 2 subgroup analysis for the prevalence of asymptomatic bacteriuria and urinary tract infections in pregnant women in Iran

Variable	Asymptomatic bacteriuria						Urinary tract Infection					
	Studies (N^a)	Sample (N)	Heterogeneity		95%CI[b]	Pooled prevalence (%)	Studies (N)	Sample (N)	Heterogeneity		95%CI	Pooled prevalence (%)
			I^2	*P*-Value					I^2	*P*-Value		
Region												
Center	17	9724	90.01	< 0.001	5.8–9.4	7.4	6	11,575	96.42	< 0.001	6.7–13.8	9.7
East	6	3154	90.19	< 0.001	10.3–18.6	13.9	–	–	–	–	–	–
North	3	2560	98.08	< 0.001	3.9–22.1	9.7	6	9334	94.77	< 0.001	8.2–15.6	11.4
South	1	389	–	–	3.3–7.8	5.1	3	24,165	97.55	< 0.001	3.9–13.1	7.2
West	4	4482	68.68	0.023	6.6–9.6	8.0	2	3657	99.04	< 0.001	3.1–32.4	11.0
Test for subgroup differences: Q = 17.07, df(Q) = 4, *P* = 0.002							Test for subgroup differences: Q = 1.77, df(Q) = 3, *P* = 0.61					
Province												
East Azarbaijan	2	2050	92.25	< 0.001	4.7–13.5	8.1	1	400	–	–	5.3–10.5	7.5
Isfahan	6	3195	91.29	< 0.001	3.1–8.8	5.2	–	–	–	–	–	–
Hamedan	1	377	–	–	7.4–13.6	10.1	–	–	–	–	–	–
Golestan	1	900	–	–	2.6–5.2	3.7	–	–	–	–	–	–
Khorasan Razavi	2	1400	0	0.78	8.6–11.8	10.1	–	–	–	–	–	–
Kurdistan	2	3005	40.25	0.19	7.1–9.6	8.3	–	–	–	–	–	–
Tehran	7	3472	85.23	< 0.001	8.8–15.3	11.7	–	–	–	–	–	–
Kerman	1	323	–	–	19.7–29.1	24.1	1	850	–	–	10.3–14.7	12.3
Chaharmahal and Bakhtiari	1	864	–	–	4.7–13.5	8.1	1	864	–	–	7.1–10.9	8.8
Markazi	1	1736	–	–	5.2–7.5	6.3	–	–	–	–	–	–
Fars	1	389	–	–	3.3–7.8	5.1	–	–	–	–	–	–
Semnan	2	457	26.81	0.24	2.5–7.1	4.3	–	–	–	–	–	–
Guilan	1	710	–	–	18.3–24.3	21.1	1	330	–	–	19.3–28.5	23.6
Sistan and Baluchestan	3	1431	71.41	0.03	10.8–17.5	13.8	–	–	–	–	–	–
Kohgiloyeh and Boyerahmad	–	–	–	–	–	–	1	715	–	–	4.5–8.0	6.0
Kermanshah	–	–	–	–	–	–	2	3657	99.04	< 0.001	3.1–32.4	11.0
Alborz	–	–	–	–	–	–	2	480	0	0.45	18.2–25.6	21.6
Zanjan	–	–	–	–	–	–	2	4114	98.11	< 0.001	3.9–18.5	8.8
Mazandaran	–	–	–	–	–	–	3	6328	94.07	< 0.001	3.2–14.6	7.0
Ardebil	–	–	–	–	–	–	1	2496	–	–	8.6–10.9	9.7
Yazd	–	–	–	–	–	–	1	5897	–	–	6.4–7.7	7.0
Khuzestan	–	–	–	–	–	–	1	22,600	–	–	4.7–5.3	5.0
Test for subgroup differences: Q = 289.16, df(Q) = 13, *P* < 0.001							Test for subgroup differences: Q = 491.83, df(Q) = 11, *P* < 0.001					
Quality												
High	19	12,500	94.19	< 0.001	6.4–10.6	8.3	11	45,355	98.42	< 0.001	6.4–11.5	8.6
Moderate	12	7809	92.25	< 0.001	7.1–12.1	9.3	6	3376	93.11	< 0.001	8.7–17.6	12.5
Test for subgroup differences: Q = 0.42, df(Q) = 1, P = 0.51							Test for subgroup differences: Q = 2.45, df(Q) = 1, P = 0.11					

[a]Number; [b] Confidence interval

province (5% [95% CI: 4.7–5.3]) were the lowest and in the North of Iran (11.4% [95% CI: 8.2–15.6]) and Alborz province (21.6% [95% CI: 18.2–25.6]) were the highest. The test for subgroup differences for geographical region (*P* = 061) was not significant but for province (*P* < 0.001) was significant (Table 2).

Subgroup analysis of the prevalence of UTI based on quality of studies

The prevalence of UTI among pregnant women in terms of quality of studies based on NOS checklist was estimated to be 12.5% [95% CI: 8.7–17.6]) and 8.6% [95% CI: 6.4–11.5]) in moderate-quality and high-quality studies,

A

Study name, year published	Event rate	Lower limit	Upper limit	Z-Value	p-Value	Relative weight
Shirazi MH, 2007	0.101	0.074	0.136	-12.791	0.000	12.98
Soofizadeh N, 2012	0.076	0.064	0.091	-25.638	0.000	13.70
Namazi A, 2012	0.211	0.183	0.243	-14.327	0.000	13.75
Khorshidi A, 1997	0.043	0.019	0.092	-7.447	0.000	9.35
Hazhir S, 2007	0.067	0.039	0.112	-9.172	0.000	11.35
Alavi-Naini R, 2003	0.149	0.120	0.183	-13.737	0.000	13.45
Mardanian F, 2004	0.104	0.081	0.133	-15.319	0.000	13.32
Rahimkhani M, 2008	0.291	0.205	0.395	-3.751	0.000	12.10
Random effects model	0.117	0.079	0.169	-9.214	0.000	

Meta Analysis

B

Study name, year published	Event rate	Lower limit	Upper limit	Z-Value	p-Value	Relative weight
Farajzadegan Z, 2008	0.020	0.005	0.076	-5.449	0.000	4.63
Khorshidi A, 1997	0.050	0.023	0.107	-7.000	0.000	10.10
Hazhir S, 2007	0.068	0.049	0.095	-14.333	0.000	20.59
Kasraeian M, 2009	0.051	0.033	0.078	-12.686	0.000	18.01
Alavi-Naini R, 2003	0.105	0.081	0.136	-14.362	0.000	22.39
Mardanian F, 2004	0.099	0.081	0.120	-19.907	0.000	24.29
Random effects model	0.072	0.053	0.097	-15.172	0.000	

Meta Analysis

C

Study name, year published	Event rate	Lower limit	Upper limit	Z-Value	p-Value	Relative weight
Khorshidi A, 1997	0.077	0.037	0.153	-6.317	0.000	23.38
Hazhir S, 2007	0.051	0.034	0.076	-13.368	0.000	25.38
Alavi-Naini R, 2003	0.162	0.131	0.198	-13.029	0.000	26.04
Mardanian F, 2004	0.020	0.013	0.032	-16.264	0.000	25.19
Random effects model	0.061	0.021	0.164	-4.847	0.000	

Meta Analysis

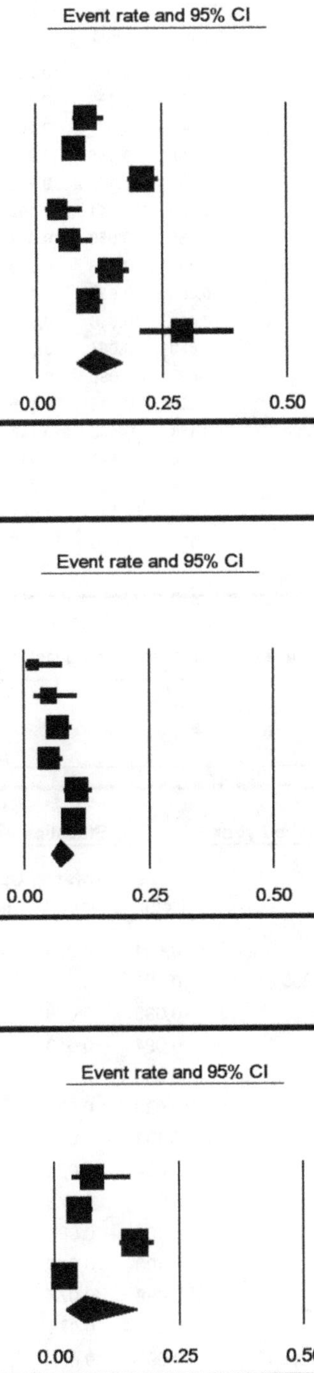

Fig. 4 Prevalence of asymptomatic bacteriuria in the first (**a**), second (**b**) and third (**c**) trimesters in Iran

Study name, published year	Event rate	Lower limit	Upper limit	Z-Value	p-Value	Relative weight
Safari M, 2008	0.060	0.045	0.080	-17.473	0.000	5.77
Yousofzadeh Sh, 1995	0.075	0.053	0.105	-13.234	0.000	5.58
Shojaee H, 2000	0.088	0.071	0.109	-19.471	0.000	5.95
Rahmani E, 2012	0.198	0.165	0.235	-12.464	0.000	5.98
Norouzzadeh M, 1997	0.227	0.183	0.278	-8.890	0.000	5.87
Fakhimi L, 2002	0.130	0.111	0.152	-20.337	0.000	6.06
Azizi A, 2015	0.058	0.050	0.067	-36.610	0.000	6.11
Jalali M, 2014	0.198	0.146	0.263	-7.479	0.000	5.60
Zakeri Hamidi	0.083	0.057	0.120	-11.479	0.000	5.46
Shahhosseini Z, 2012	0.028	0.016	0.049	-12.106	0.000	4.88
Golestan M, 2011	0.070	0.064	0.077	-50.675	0.000	6.17
Alijahan R, 2014	0.097	0.086	0.109	-32.988	0.000	6.13
Saffar MJ, 2008	0.126	0.118	0.135	-48.097	0.000	6.19
Soleimani Zadeh L, 2004	0.123	0.103	0.147	-18.809	0.000	6.01
Sharemi H, 2013	0.236	0.193	0.285	-9.061	0.000	5.91
Sohrabi D, 2011	0.058	0.051	0.067	-36.306	0.000	6.11
Amiri M, 2015	0.050	0.047	0.053	-96.473	0.000	6.21
Random effects model	0.098	0.076	0.125	-15.892	0.000	

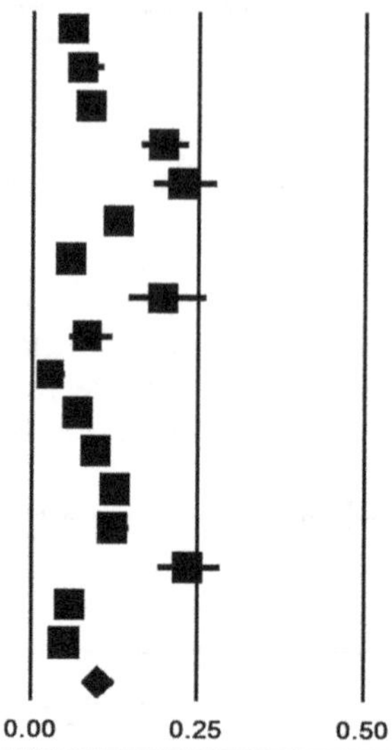

Meta Analysis

Fig. 5 Prevalence of urinary tract infection in pregnant women in Iran

Study name, published year	Point	Lower limit	Upper limit	Z-Value	p-Value
Safari M, 2008	0.101	0.078	0.130	-15.097	0.000
Yousofzadeh Sh, 1995	0.100	0.077	0.128	-15.225	0.000
Shojaee H, 2000	0.099	0.076	0.127	-15.139	0.000
Rahmani E, 2012	0.094	0.073	0.119	-16.353	0.000
Norouzzadeh M, 1997	0.093	0.072	0.118	-16.426	0.000
Fakhimi L, 2002	0.096	0.074	0.124	-15.485	0.000
Azizi A, 2015	0.101	0.078	0.131	-14.781	0.000
Jalali M, 2014	0.094	0.073	0.120	-15.965	0.000
Zakeri Hamidi	0.099	0.076	0.127	-15.298	0.000
Shahhosseini Z, 2012	0.104	0.081	0.133	-15.100	0.000
Golestan M, 2011	0.100	0.076	0.131	-14.144	0.000
Alijahan R, 2014	0.098	0.075	0.127	-14.796	0.000
Saffar MJ, 2008	0.096	0.075	0.124	-15.615	0.000
Soleimani Zadeh L, 2004	0.097	0.075	0.124	-15.411	0.000
Sharemi H, 2013	0.093	0.072	0.118	-16.614	0.000
Sohrabi D, 2011	0.101	0.078	0.131	-14.782	0.000
Amiri M, 2015	0.103	0.082	0.128	-17.111	0.000
Random effects model	0.098	0.076	0.125	-15.892	0.000

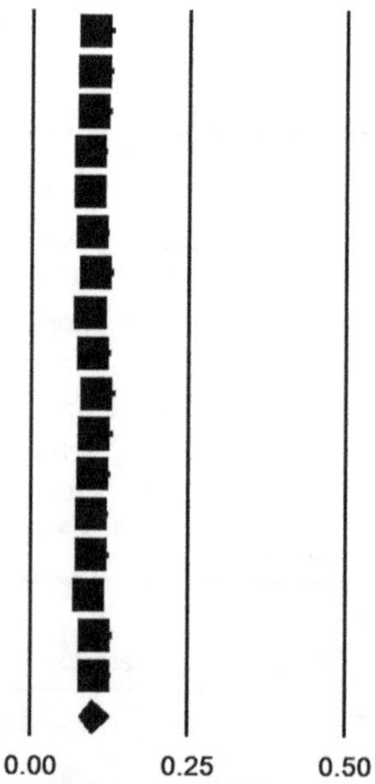

Meta Analysis

Fig. 6 Sensitivity analysis for the prevalence of urinary tract infection in pregnant women in Iran

A

Study name, published year	Event rate	Lower limit	Upper limit	Z-Value	p-Value	Relative weight
Safari M, 2008	0.060	0.045	0.080	-17.473	0.000	7.44
Yousofzadeh Sh, 1995	0.075	0.053	0.105	-13.234	0.000	7.11
Shojaee H, 2000	0.088	0.071	0.109	-19.471	0.000	7.78
Fakhimi L, 2002	0.130	0.111	0.152	-20.337	0.000	7.97
Azizi A, 2015	0.058	0.050	0.067	-36.610	0.000	8.08
Zakeri Hamidi M, 2006	0.083	0.057	0.120	-11.479	0.000	6.91
Shahhosseini Z, 2012	0.028	0.016	0.049	-12.106	0.000	5.95
Golestan M, 2011	0.070	0.064	0.077	-50.675	0.000	8.19
Alijahan R, 2014	0.097	0.086	0.109	-32.988	0.000	8.12
Saffar MJ, 2008	0.126	0.118	0.135	-48.097	0.000	8.23
Soleimani Zadeh L, 2004	0.123	0.103	0.147	-18.809	0.000	7.90
Sohrabi D, 2011	0.058	0.051	0.067	-36.306	0.000	8.07
Amiri M, 2015	0.050	0.047	0.053	-96.473	0.000	8.26
Random effects model	0.076	0.060	0.097	-18.572	0.000	

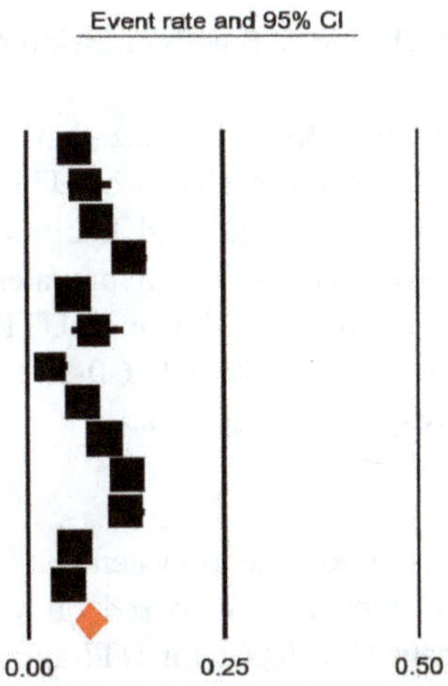

Meta Analysis

B

Study name, published year	Event rate	Lower limit	Upper limit	Z-Value	p-Value	Relative weight
Vedjdani MH, 1998	0.105	0.087	0.126	-20.247	0.000	4.12
Farajzadegan Z, 2008	0.020	0.005	0.076	-5.449	0.000	1.03
Shirazi MH, 2007	0.101	0.074	0.136	-12.791	0.000	3.72
Mobsheri E, 2002	0.037	0.026	0.052	-18.456	0.000	3.68
Kameli M, 2013	0.100	0.085	0.118	-23.305	0.000	4.18
Soofizadeh N, 2012	0.076	0.064	0.091	-25.638	0.000	4.17
Azizzadeh Sh, 1999	0.127	0.102	0.158	-15.012	0.000	4.00
Aghaee alamouti M, 2010	0.087	0.070	0.108	-19.041	0.000	4.03
Yousofzadeh Sh, 1995	0.048	0.030	0.073	-12.755	0.000	3.26
Necohesh L, 2005	0.140	0.085	0.223	-6.299	0.000	2.88
Shojaee H, 2000	0.043	0.031	0.059	-18.500	0.000	3.74
Zarganj Fard A, 2000	0.063	0.052	0.075	-27.328	0.000	4.16
Khorshidi A, 1997	0.054	0.035	0.083	-12.107	0.000	3.25
Hazhir S, 2007	0.061	0.048	0.077	-21.701	0.000	4.01
Motaghi M, 2012	0.107	0.067	0.167	-8.033	0.000	3.05
Dadkhah F, 2011	0.090	0.075	0.107	-23.372	0.000	4.16
Kalantar E, 2008	0.089	0.076	0.104	-25.693	0.000	4.20
Kasraeian M, 2009	0.051	0.033	0.078	-12.686	0.000	3.29
Jazayeri Moghadas A, 2009	0.033	0.018	0.061	-10.398	0.000	2.63
Alavi-Naini R, 2003	0.149	0.120	0.183	-13.737	0.000	4.00
Alavi-Naini R, 2003	0.105	0.081	0.136	-14.362	0.000	3.87
Alavi-Naini R, 2003	0.162	0.131	0.198	-13.029	0.000	4.01
Mardanian F, 2004	0.104	0.081	0.133	-15.319	0.000	3.92
Mardanian F, 2004	0.099	0.081	0.120	-19.907	0.000	4.10
Mardanian F, 2004	0.020	0.013	0.032	-16.264	0.000	3.23
Rahmanian M, 2014	0.056	0.029	0.104	-8.215	0.000	2.51
Shams MR, 2000	0.068	0.041	0.112	-9.436	0.000	2.96
Modars Sh, 1998	0.108	0.083	0.140	-14.086	0.000	3.86
Random effects model	0.078	0.067	0.090	-29.821	0.000	

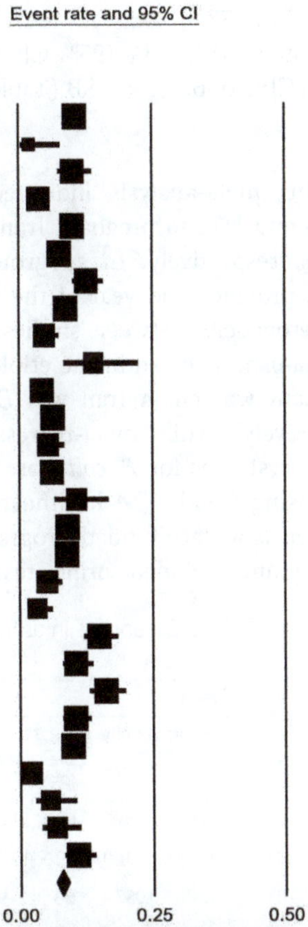

Meta Analysis

Fig. 7 Prevalence of urinary tract infection (**a**) and asymptomatic bacteriuria (**b**) in pregnant women in Iran with deleted high prevalence reports (4 studies for prevalence of UTI: Rahmani, Norouzzadeh, Jalali and Sharemi and 3 studies for ASB: Namazi, Rahimkhani and Aaron) respectively. No significant difference was found ($P = 0.11$) (Table 2).

Total prevalence of UTI and ASB with omission of high prevalence reports

Four studies (Rahmani [35], Norouzzadeh [36], Jalali [40] and Sharemi [51]) for prevalence of UTI and three studies (Namazi [24], Aaron [20] and Rahimkhani [43]) for prevalence of ASB reported high prevalence. After omitting these studies, the prevalence of UTI and ASB was estimated to be 7.6% (95% CI: 6.0-9.7) and 7.8% (95% CI: 6.7–9.0), respectively (Fig. 7).

Meta-regression

Meta-regression model for the prevalence of UTI and ASB in pregnant women in Iran based on year of the studies was significant ($P < 0.001$ for UTI and $P < 0.001$ for ASB) (Fig. 8).

The prevalence of microorganisms

The most common microorganism involved in the etiology of UTI (61.6% [95% CI: 51.6–70.7]) and ASB (63.22% [95% CI: 51.2–73.8]) was *E. coli*. The lowest prevalence was Proteus with 2.6% (95% CI: 1.9–3.4) for UTI and 3.6% (95%CI: 2.0–6.3) for ASB (Table 3).

Discussion

The results of this meta-analysis indicated that the prevalence of ASB and UTI in pregnant Iranian women was 8.7 and 9.8%, respectively. In subgroup analysis, geographic region, province and year of the studies can be a cause of heterogeneity between studies. The most common microorganism involved in the etiology of ASB and UTI in pregnant women in Iran was *E. coli* (63.2 and 61.6%, respectively), while meta-regression model based on year of the studies for *E. coli* (for ASB) had a significantly decreasing trend. The healthcare structure for pregnant women is a state funded program running in Iran. This program included urine testing (urine culture test and urine analysis) in the first prenatal visit [12–15].

Prevalence of bacteriuria in pregnancy is affected by several factors such as multiple pregnancies, age, previous history of UTI, diabetes, urinary tract anatomic abnormalities, lack of personal hygiene and socioeconomic status [63, 64]. In a systematic review conducted in Iran in 2015, ASB prevalence in pregnant women was reported to be 13% (95% CI: 9–7) [65] after combining 20 articles (sample size: 15,108). In the present meta-analysis combining 31 studies with a sample size of 20,309 Iranian pregnant women, the prevalence of ASB was 8.7% (95% CI: 7.2–10.4). The strengths of this study compared to previous published meta-analyses include bigger sample size, the use of cross-sectional studies, excluding studies with a non-randomized sample [66, 67] and removal of the duplicate articles that published the results more than once [14, 16, 68, 69]. Each of the suggested factors can affect the final evaluation and accuracy of the prevalence while this was not considered in the previous meta-analyses [65].

The prevalence of ASB in pregnant Iranian women based on trimester of pregnancy shows that the highest prevalence occurs in the first trimester of pregnancy (11.7% [95% CI: 7.9–16.9]). Given that screening for UTI is done before the pregnancy and at 6–10 weeks of gestation in Iran, lack of care before pregnancy may increase the risk of UTI in pregnant women in the first trimester. However, trimester of pregnancy can be one of the causes of diverse prevalence of ASB in Iranian studies ($P = 0.02$).

There seem to be a geographical variation in the ASB prevalence, and we could not find the causes, but a possible reason might include differences in race (there is much racial diversity in Iran), socioeconomic factors, education, quality health care and women's health services communities [70, 71].

The prevalence of ASB among pregnant women in other countries, including India (7.3%), Nigeria (24.7–

Table 3 The prevalence of Micro-Organisms in asymptomatic bacteriuria and urinary tract infections among Pregnant Iranian women

Micro-Organisms	Asymptomatic bacteriuria							Urinary tract Infection						
	Studies (N[a])	Sample (N)	Heterogeneity		Pooled prevalence (%) [95%CI[b]]	Meta-regression		Studies (N)	Sample (N)	Heterogeneity		Pooled prevalence (%) [95%CI]	Meta-regression	
			I^2	P-Value		Trend	P-Value			I^2	P-Value		Trend	P-Value
Escherichia coli	18	1037	91.03	< 0.001	63.2 [51.2–73.8]	DES[c]	< 0.001	6	2255	93.34	< 0.001	61.6 [51.6–70.7]	ASC[c]	0.088
Staphylococcus	15	902	88.09	< 0.001	19.6 [12.7–29.2]	ASC[d]	< 0.001	5	2187	58.99	0.045	9.9 [7.7–12.6]	DES[d]	< 0.001
Klebsiella	12	783	42.86	0.057	6.3 [4.2–9.4]	DES	0.232	3	1448	90.05	< 0.001	13.9 [7.3–25.0]	DES	0.094
Streptococcus	3	145	50.91	0.130	5.2 [1.6–15.9]	ASC	0.046	–	–	–	–	–	–	–
Enterococcus	5	336	24.33	0.259	3.8 [1.8–7.9]	DES	0.165	–	–	–	–	–	–	–
Enterobacter	8	608	29.33	0.194	6.4 [4.1–9.7]	ASC	0.578	2	776	61.51	0.107	7.6 [4.3–13.1]	–	–
Proteus	6	356	0	0.766	3.6 [2.0–6.3]	ASC	0.383	3	1871	0	0.84	2.6 [1.9–3.4]	ASC	0.820

[a]Number; [b] Confidence interval; [c] descending; [d] ascending

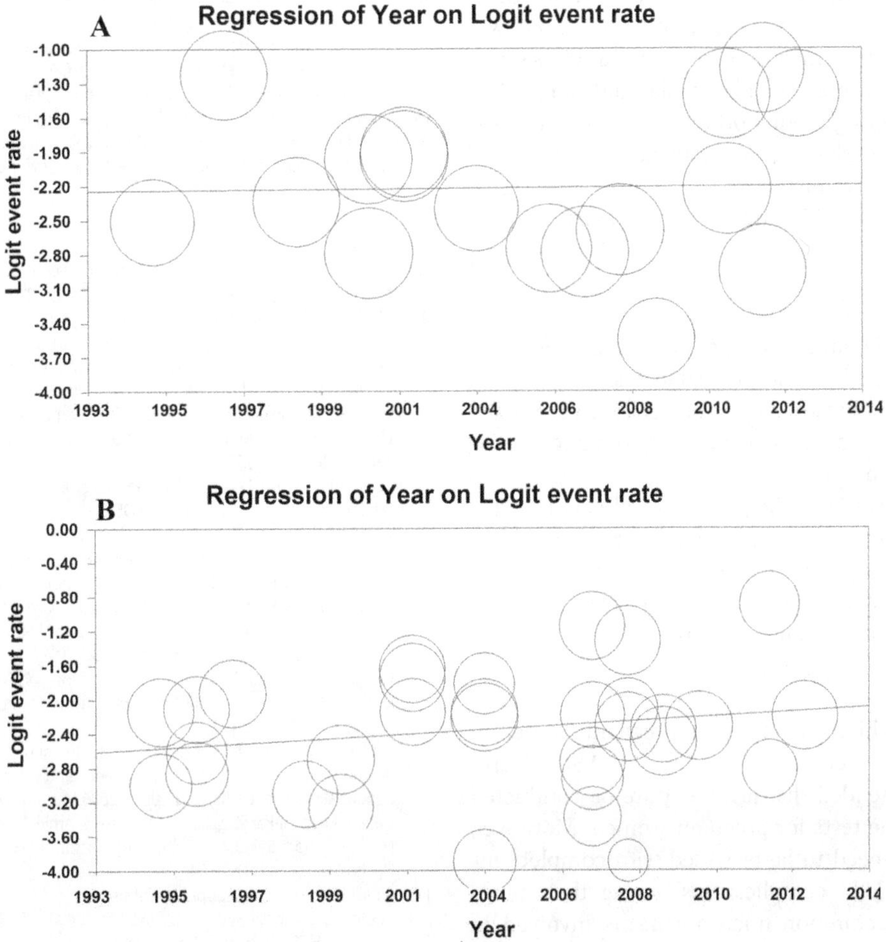

Fig. 8 Meta-regression model for the prevalence of urinary tract infection (**a**) and asymptomatic bacteriuria (**b**) in pregnant women in Iran based on year of the studies

45.3%), Nepal (8.7%) Bangladesh (10.2%) and Ethiopia (21.2%) was reported to be different [71–75].

The prevalence of UTI among young women is about 1–3% [76]. The results of this meta-analysis showed that the prevalence of UTI in pregnant Iranian women is high. Pregnant women prone to UTI are at risk for prematurity, preterm delivery, low birth weight, hypertension/pre-eclampsia, anemia, maternal and perinatal death associated with amnionitis [75, 76].

Studies show that the higher the education level, the lower the frequency of this problem. Hence, the need for education and awareness of pregnant women, especially in those with a lower education level, is necessary [18–20].

A common organism of ASB in pregnant women in Iran was *E.coli* (63.2%). In other studies, the most common organism of ASB in women was *E.coli* [77]. *E.coli* is the underlying cause of ASB in 77% of sexually active young American women [78], 72% of girls of school age [79], and 65–84% of pregnant women [80–83].

E. coli strains isolated from healthy women without symptoms may have a lower frequency of virulence factors, such as adhesions, specific lipopolysaccharide, toxins, mobility factors, and other proteins compared to strains isolated from symptomatic urinary tract infection [84, 85].

The aim of ASB treatment is to maintain sterile urine without causing toxicity in mother or fetus during pregnancy [82]. However, the best way to achieve this is not clear yet. In low-income countries, the situation is worse due to lack of information about the resistance to drugs used for UTI in pregnancy, drug costs and lack of access to information regarding the safety and efficacy of newer antibiotics [86].

In Iran, drug resistance in antibiotics used for UTI is a controversial topic. Different levels of antibiotic resistance and sensitivity has been reported in different studies. For example, in a study by Enaiat et al., high resistance of nalidixic acid, tetracycline and co-trimoxazole and low sensitivity of ampicillin, gentamicin and amikacin to *E. coli* has been reported in regard with bacteriuria in pregnant women [87]. However, in the study of Saffar, *E.coli* was highly sensitive to gentamicin and amikacin and less sensitive to trimethoprim-sulfamethoxazole and ampicillin. Therefore, considering the importance of empiric therapy for physicians, conducting a systematic review and meta-analysis to determine patterns of microbial resistance to drugs against UTI in Iran seems necessary.

Limitations

1. Lack of "AND" and "OR" operators support for a combined search in national databases.
2. Failure to investigate the prevalence of UTI based on trimester of pregnancy due to the limited number of studies.
3. Failure to investigate the prevalence of UTI based on factors such as multiple pregnancies, age, previous history of UTI, diabetes, anatomical abnormalities of urinary tract, lack of personal hygiene and socioeconomic status

Conclusion

UTI and ASB are highly common in pregnant women in Iran and the most common type of UTI is ASB. Therefore, it is recommended that urine culture be conducted as a part of routine tests for pregnant women. Moreover, pregnant women need to be provided with complete information about UTI complications during their pregnancy. The most common microorganisms involved in the etiology of ASB and UTI in pregnant women in Iran are *E.coli* and *Staphylococcus*. Since women and mothers' health is the foundation of the family and the public health, making better management decisions for prevention, screening and treatment of this problem is recommended.

Abbreviations

ASB: Asymptomatic Bacteriuria; IranDoc: Iranian Research Institute for Information Science and Technology; PRISMA: Preferred Reporting Items for Systematic Reviews and Meta-Analyses; RICST: Regional Information Center for Science and Technology; SID: Scientific Information Database; UTI: Urinary tract infection

Acknowledgements

The authors sincerely appreciate the Women's Reproduction Health Research Center of Tabriz University of Medical Sciences who helped us in accomplishing this research.

Authors' contributions

MA, SHA and ZJ performed data extraction. MA and LM performed statistical analysis. MA and SHA wrote the manuscript. ZJ, GHB, MA, MSH and MM performed the literature search and quality evaluation. SHA, GHB, MSH, and MM revised the manuscript. All authors read and approved the final manuscript.

Author details

[1]Faculty of Medicine, Ilam University of Medical Sciences, Ilam, Iran. [2]Department of Obstetrics & Gynecology, Women's Reproductive Health Research Center, School of Medicine, Tabriz University of Medical Sciences, Tabriz, Iran. [3]HIV/STI Surveillance Research Center, and WHO Collaborating Center for HIV Surveillance, Institute for Futures Studies in Health, Kerman University of Medical Sciences, Kerman, Iran. [4]Department of Urology, Faculty of Medicine, Ilam University of Medical Sciences, Ilam, Iran. [5]Department of Nursing, Faculty of Nursing and Midwifery, Ilam University of Medical Sciences, Ilam, Iran. [6]Department of Pediatrics, Behbahan Faculty of Medical Sciences, Behbahan, Iran. [7]Faculty of Medicine, Dezful University of Medical Sciences, Dezful, Iran.

References

1. Gulfareen H, Nishat Z, AftabAfroze M, Ambreen H. Risk factors of urinary tract infection in pregnancy. J Pak Med Assoc. 2010;60(3):213–6.
2. MacLean AB. Urinary tract infection in pregnancy. Int J Antimicrob Agents. 2001;17(4):273–6.
3. Girishbabu RJ, Srikrishna R, Rameshs T. Asymptomatic bacteriuria in pregnancy. Int J Biol Med Res. 2011;2(3):740–2.
4. Totsika M, Moriel DG, Idris A, Rogers BA, Wurpel DJ, Phan MD, et al. Uropathogenic Escherichia coli mediated urinary tract infection. Curr Drug Targets. 2012;13(11):1386–99.
5. Counningham FG, Leveno KJ, Bloom SL, et al. Williams Obstetrics. 22nd ed. New York: McGraw_hill; 2005. p. 1095.
6. Giraldo PC, Araújo ED, Junior JE, Amaral RLGD, Passos MRL, Gonçalves AK. The prevalence of urogenital infections in pregnant women experiencing preterm and full-term labor. Infect Dis Obstetrics Gynecol. 2012;2012:1–4.
7. Raza S, Pandey S, Bhatt CP. Microbiological analysis of isolates in Kathmandu medical college teaching hospital, Kathmandu, Nepal. Kathmandu Univ Med J (KUMJ). 2011;9(36):295–7.
8. Glaser AP, Schaeffer AJ. Urinary Tract Infection and Bacteriuria in Pregnancy. Urol Clin North Am. 2015;42(4):547–60. https://doi.org/10.1016/j.ucl.2015.05.004. Epub 2015 Aug 1.
9. Bánhidy F, Acs N, Puhó EH, Czeizel AE. Maternal urinary tract infection and related drug treatments during pregnancy and risk of congenital abnormalities in the offspring. BJOG. 2006;113:1465–71.
10. Izadi B, Rostami-Far Z, Jalilian N, Khazaei S, Amiri A, Madani SH, Rostami-Far M. Urinary tract infection (UTI) as a risk factor of severe preeclampsia. Glob J Health Sci. 2016;8(11):54364.
11. Smaill F, Vazquez JC. Antibiotics for asymptomatic bacteriuria in pregnancy. Cochrane Database Syst Rev. 2015;8:CD000490.
12. Vejdani MH, Gourabchi H, Nahaie MRSM. Study of asymptomatic bacteriuria in pregnant women and antibiotic-sensitivity of isolated bacteria in Tabriz 1996. J Kerman Uni Med Sci. 1998;5(4):165–70.
13. Farajzadegan Z, Mirmoghtadaee P, Mehrabian F. Screening of asymptomatic bacteriuria:urinalysis or urine culture? Which one is more cost- effective? J Isfahan Med School. 2008;26(89):119–26.
14. Shirazi MH, Ranjbar R, Daneshyar E, Sadeghian S, Sadeghifard N. Urinary tract pathogens in asymptomatic bacteriuria and their antimicrobial resistance in pregnant women in Hamedan. IJIDTM J. 2007;12(36):53–8.
15. Safari M, Yazdanpanah B, Yazdanpanah S. High risk pregnancy and some of related factors in women who Refered to Vasouj health and medical centers. Sci J Hamadan Nurs Midwifery Fac. 2008;16(2):18–28.
16. Mobsheri E, Tabbraei A, Ghaemei E, Mojerloo M, Vakili MA, Dastforooshan M, et al. Distribution of asymptomatic bacteriuria in pregnant women referring to Dezyani Hospital in Gorgan. J Gorgan Uni Med Sci. 2002;4(1):42–6.
17. Kameli M, Badiee M, Rafiee M. Prevalence of asymptomatic bacteriuria and its treatment in pregnant women referred to health centers of Torbat Haydarieh in 2013. J Torbat Heydariyeh Uni Med Sci. 2013;1(3):58–64.
18. Soofizadeh N, Farhadifar F, Kalantar E, Shahsavari S. Evaluating the prevalence of asymptomatic urinary tract infection and Anemia in pregnant women in first trimester. IJOGI. 2012;15(8):11–6.
19. Azizzadeh Sh, Ashtiani M, Baygi D. Evaluate the frequency of asymptomatic bacteriuria in pregnant women and diagnostic value of urine analysis in screening with its during 1999. [dissertation]. Tehran: Tehran Univ Med Sci; 1999.
20. Aaron H, Salari D. The prevalence of asymptomatic bacteriuria in pregnant women referred to Afzalipour haspital in Kerman. [Dissertation]. Kerman: Kerman Univ Med Sci; 2008.
21. Aghaee alamouti M, Moheit M. The prevalence of asymptomatic bacteriuria and social factors that influence the prevalence among women referred to hospitals in Tehran. [Dissertation]. Tehran: Islamic Azad Univ Med Sci; 2010.

22. Yousofzadeh Sh. Determine the prevalence of asymptomatic and symptomatic urinary tract infection in pregnant women referred to prenatal care in Kashan. [Dissertation]. Kashan: Kashan Univ Med Sci; 1995.
23. Necohesh L, Karimi MR. The Survey of bacterial agents of rinary tract infection among pregnant women in Ghods city in 2004–2005. [Dissertation]. Tehran: Islamic Azad Univ Med Sci; 2005.
24. Namazi A, Alizadeh S. The frequency of bacteriuria and its relationship with demographic characters in pregnant women of Gilan, 2009–11. J Kermanshah Univ Med Sci. 2012;16(3):263–8.
25. Shojaee H. Microbiologic evaluation of bacteriuria in pregnant women in Shahrekord 1999. Pejouhandeh Q Res J. 2000;5(19):337–43.
26. Zarganj Fard A. The prevalence of asymptomatic bacteriuria in pregnant women who were referred to health centers of Arak city from November 1998 to March 1999. Arak Univ Med Sci (Rahavard Danesh). 2000;3(10):21–4.
27. Khorshidi A, Khakbazan S, Mousavi SGA, Hoshyaran A. Epidemiologic study of urinary infections without clinical symptoms among pregnant women: Diagnostic values of Nitrate among subjects referred to the Dr.Shabikhani Hospital, 1996. KAUMS Journal (FEYZ). 1997;1(3):53–60.
28. Hazhir S. Asymptomatic bacteriuria in pregnant women. Urol J. 2007;4(1): 24–7.
29. Motaghi M, Sadegh-Al-Hosseini A, Yaghoubi MA. Assessment of the risk factors of asymptomatic bacteriuria among pregnant and non-pregnant married women. Zahedan J Res Med Sci (ZJRMS). 2012;13(suppl 1):4.
30. Dadkhah F, Kashanian M, Noori M. A Comparison between Diagnostic Value of Pyuria and Bacteriuria in Asymptomatic Bacteriuria in Pregnant Women. IJOGI. 2011;14(1):48–53.
31. Kalantar E, Fariba F, Bahram N. Asymptomatic bacteriuria among pregnant women referred to outpatient clinics in Sanandaj, Iran. Int Braz J Urol. 2008; 34(6):699–704.
32. Kasraeian M, Asadi N, Ghaffarpasand F. Prevalence of asymptomatic bacteriuria among pregnant women in shiraz, Iran. Saudi Med J. 2009;30(7): 917–20.
33. Jazayeri Moghadas A, Irajian G. Asymptomatic urinary tract infection in pregnant women. Iran J Pathol. 2009;4(3):105–8.
34. Alavi-Naini R, Sharifi-Mood B, Metanat M. The prevalence and drug resistance of a asymptomatic bacteriuria in pregnant women referring to zahedan ghods hospital. IJOGI. 2003;6(1):58–63.
35. Rahmani E, Karami A, Khalili M, Hasani S. A survey on the urinary tract infection (UTI) prevalence and its consequences in pregnant women referring to health centers in Kermanshah in 2011. J Clin Res Paramed Sci. 2012;1(4):31–8.
36. Norouzzadeh M, Sultandalal MM. Evaluation of Urinary Tract Infection in pregnant women admitted to Kasra hospital in Karaj. . [Dissertation]. Tehran: Islamic Azad Univ Med Sci; 1997.
37. Mardanian F, Atri S, Kian Pour M, Soleimani B, E Arab. Urinary tract infection in pregnancy. J Isfahan Med Sch. 2004;22(74–75):109–14.
38. Fakhimi L, Sohrabi D, Mousavi Nasab N, Fekri SH. Evaluate the frequency and risk factors for PROM in pregnant women referred off to hospital Valiasser in 2002. [Dissertation]. Zanjan: Zanjan Univ Med Sci; 2002.
39. Azizi A. The prevalence of the causes of high-risk pregnancies in pregnant women of Songor city, 2011. IJOGI. 2015;18(153):10–9.
40. Jalali M, Shamsi N, Roozbehani N, Kabir K. Prevalence of urinary tract infection and some factors affected in pregnant women in Iran Karaj City 2013. Middle East J Sci Res. 2014;20(7):781–5.
41. Zakeri Hamidi M. Urinary tract infections in pregnant women with bacterial vaginosis. Physician Lab Mon. 2006;2:47–48.
42. Shahhosseini Z, Esmaeeli Douki Z, Vaezzadeh N, Keshavarz Z. Maternal depression and preterm delivery. World Appl Sci J. 2012;18(1):15–20.
43. Rahimkhani M, Khavari-Daneshvar H, Sharifian R. Asymptomatic bacteriuria and pyuria in pregnancy. Acta Medica Iranica. 2008;46(5):409–12 B.
44. Golestan M, Akhavan Karbasi S, Fallah R. Prevalence and risk factors for low birth weight in Yazd, Iran. Singapore Med J. 2011;52(10):730–3.
45. Rahmanian M, Ghorbani R, Mirza Aghaie MR, Pourazizi M. Association of asymptomatic bacteriuria and preeclampsia in pregnant women. IJOGI. 2014;17(122):1–7.
46. Shams MR, Ghafarnezhad M. Prevalence and risk factors of asymptomatic bacteriuria in pregnancy. Tehran Univ Med J. 2000;58(2):76–9.
47. Alijahan R, Pourfarzi F, Salimi S, Tahmasebi P, Moradi S, Hazrati S. Prevalence of urinary tract infection and associated risk factors in pregnant women. Iran South Med J. 2014;17(4):676–86.
48. Saffar MJ, Enayti AA, Abdolla IA, Razai MS, Saffar H. Antibacterial susceptibility of uropathogens in 3 hospitals, sari, Islamic Republic of Iran, 2002-2003. East Mediterr Health J. 2008;14(3):556–63.
49. Soleimani Zadeh L. Danesh a, basri N, abaszadeh a, arab M. Assessment of high risk pregnancy in bam Mahdieh maternity hospital, 2001. J Shahrekord Univ Med Sci. 2004;6(2):67–73.
50. Modars Sh, Amidi Z. A survey on bacterial agents of asymptomatic bacteriuria in pregnant women in Tehran. Hakim Res J. 1998;2(1):23–6.
51. Sharemi H, Milani F, Zahiri Z, Zendedel M, Salamat F, Rafipour B, Javid Z. Comparison of pre-eclampsia risk factors regarding to its severity in pregnant women referred to Alzahra Hospital of Rasht, Iran, 2012. IJOGI. 2013;16(69):1–8.
52. Sohrabi D, Ghanbari GM. A survey on risk factors and outcomes of women with preterm labor admitted to Valieasr hospital in Zanjan. J Urmia Nurs Midwifery Fac. 2011;9(2):84–9.
53. Amiri M, Lavasani Z, Norouzirad R, Najibpour R, Mohamadpour M, Nikpoor AR, Raeisi M, et al. Prevalence of Urinary Tract Infection Among Pregnant Women and its Complications in Their Newborns During the Birth in the Hospitals of Dezful City, Iran, 2012–2013. Iran Red Crescent Med J. 2015; 17(8):e26946.
54. Azhari S, Mousavi YM, Sojudi MM, EbrahimZadeh S. Accuracy of urine Dipslide to detect asymptomatic bacteriuria in pregnancy. IJOGI. 2011;15(3): 8–14.
55. Sayehmiri K, Tavan H, Sayehmire F, Mohamadi I. Prevalence of Epilepsy in Iran Using Meta-Analysis and Systematic Review. zumsj. 2015;23(97):112–21.
56. Sayehmiri K, Tavan H. Systematic review and Meta- analysis methods prevalence of peptic ulcer in IRAN. J Govaresh. 2015;20(4):250–8.
57. Shamseer L, Moher D, Clarke M, Ghersi D, Liberati A, Petticrew M, et al. PRISMA-P Group. PRISMA-P Group. Preferred reporting items for systematic review and meta-analysis protocols (PRISMA-P) 2015:elaboration and explanation. BMJ. 2015;349:g7647.
58. Richardson WS, Wilson MC, Nishikawa J, Hayward RS. The well-built clinical question:a key to evidence-based decisions. ACP J Club. 1995;123:A12–3.
59. Wells GA, Shea B, O'Connell D, Peterson J, Welch V, Losos M, et al. The Newcastle-Ottawa Scale (NOS) for assessing the quality of nonrandomized studies in meta-analyses. 2011. Available from:http://www.ohri.ca/programs/clinical_epidemiology/oxford.asp. [cited 2012 Nov 25]
60. Guyatt GH, Oxman AD, Kunz R, Brozek J, Alonso-Coello P, Rind D, et al. GRADE guidelines 6. Rating the quality of evidence--imprecision. J Clin Epidemiol. 2011;64:1283–93. 21839614.
61. DerSimonian R, Laird N. Meta-analysis in clinical trials. Control Clin Trials. 1986;7:177–88.
62. Ades AE, Lu G, Higgins JP. The interpretation of random-effects Meta-analysis in decision models. Med Decis Mak. 2005;25(6):646–54.
63. Al-Haddad AM. Urinary tract infection among pregnant women in Al-Mukalla district, Yemen. East Mediterr Health J. 2005;11:505–10.
64. Bandyopadhyay S, Thakur JS, Ray P. Kumar R:high prevalence of bacteriuria in pregnancy and its screening methods in North India. J Indian Med Assoc. 2005;103:259–62.
65. Ghafari M, Baigi V, Cheraghi Z, Doosti-Irani A. The Prevalence of Asymptomatic Bacteriuria in Pregnant Iranian women:A Systematic Review and Meta-Analysis. Rosenfeld CS, ed. PLoS One. 2016;11(6):e0158031. https://doi.org/10.1371/journal.pone.0158031.
66. Danesh Shahraki A, Pishva E, Mirbaha S, Arabzadeh A. The prevalence of asymptomatic Bacteruria in pregnant women with and without gestational diabetes. J Isfahan Med Sch. 2011;28(118):1214–22.
67. Mojahedi S, Baradaran H, Kordi M. Validity of urine analysis in diagnosis of asymptomatic bacteriuria in pregnancy. J Mashhad School Nurs Midwifery. 2000;4(11):32–8.
68. Daneshyar E, Mosavibahar SH, Alikhani MY. Association Between Asymptomatic Bacteriuria And Some emographic Variables in Pregnant Womenr Refered to Health Centers Affilited to Hamadan Univ Med Sci. sjimu. 2010;18(3):53–60.
69. Keshavarz M, Babaee G. Prevalence of Asymtomatic bacteriuria and drug sensitivity pattern inPregnant women. Med Sci J Islamic Azad Univ Mashhad. 2005;3(11):137–42.
70. Sujatha R, Nawani M. Prevalence of asymptomatic bacteriuria and its antibacterial susceptibility pattern among pregnant women attending the antenatal Clinic at Kanpur, India. J Clin Diagnostic Res. 2014;8(4):DC01–3.
71. Cunningham F, Leveno K, Hauth J, et al. Williams Obstetrics. 23rd ed. New York: McGraw-Hill Professional; 2009. p. 489–91.
72. Onu FA, Ajah LO, Ezeonu PO, Umeora OUJ, Ibekwe PC, Ajah MI. Profile and microbiological isolates of asymptomatic bacteriuria among pregnant women in Abakaliki, Nigeria. Infect Drug Resistance. 2015;8:231–5.

73. Imade PE, Izekor PE, Eghafona NO, Enabulele OI, Ophori E. Asymptomatic bacteriuria among pregnant women. N Am J Med Sci. 2010;2(6):263–6 PubMed.
74. Thakur A, Baral R, Basnet P, Rai R, Agrawal A, Regmi MC, et al. Asymptomatic bacteriuria in pregnant women. JNMA. 2013;52(192):567–70.
75. Tadesse S, Kahsay T, Adhanom G, Kahsu G, Legese H, G/Wahid A, et al. Prevalence, antimicrobial susceptibility profile and predictors of asymptomatic bacteriuria among pregnant women in Adigrat General Hospital, Northern Ethiopia. BMC Res Notes. 2018;11(1):740.
76. Ronald AR, Pattullo AL. The natural history of urinary infection in adults. Med Clin North Am. 1991;75(2):299–312.
77. Ahmed F, Molla E, Eriso F. Prevalence and associated F infections among pregnant antenatal medical hospital, Borena zone. Merit Res J Med Sci. 2016;4(1):068–75.
78. Foxman B. Epidemiology of urinary tract infections:incidence, morbidity, and economic costs. Am J Med. 2002;113(1):5–13.
79. Nicolle LE. Asymptomatic Bacteriuria and bacterial interference. Microbiol Spectr. 2015;3:1–25.
80. Hooton TM, Scholes D, Stapleton AE, Roberts PL, Winter C, Gupta K, et al. A prospective study of asymptomatic bacteriuria in sexually active young women. N Engl J Med. 2000;343:992–7.
81. Kunin CM, Deutscher R, Paquin A. Urinary tract infection in school children: an epidemiologic, clinical and laboratory study. Medicine (Baltimore). 1994; 43:91–130.
82. Mabbett AN, Ulett GC, Watts RE, Tree JJ, Totsika M, Ong CLY, Wood JM, Monaghan W, Looke DF, Nimmo GR, Svanborg C, Schembri MA. Virulence properties of asymptomatic bacteriuric Escherichia coli. Int J Med Microbiol. 2009;299:53.
83. Suriano F, Gallucci M, Flammia P, Musco S, Alcini A, Imbalzanot G, Dicuonzo G. Bacteriuria in patients with an orthoptic ileal neobladder:urinary tract infection or asymptomatic bacteriuria? Brit J Urol Internat. 2007;101:1576–9.
84. Hernandez JG, Sunden F, Connolly J, Svanborg C, Wullt B. Genetic control of the variable innate immune response to asymptomatic bacteriuria. PLoS One. 2011;6:e28289.
85. Szweda H, Jóźwik M. Urinary tract infections during pregnancy - an updated overview. Dev Period Med. 2016;20(4):263–72.
86. De Wals P. Immunization strategies for the control of serogroup C meningococcal disease in developed countries. Expert Rev Vaccines. 2006;5(2):269–75.
87. Mathai E, Thomas RJ, Chandy S, Mathai M, Bergstrom S. Antimicrobials for the treatment of urinary tract infection in pregnancy: practices in southern India. Pharmacoepidemiol Drug Saf. 2004;13(9):645–52.

Permissions

All chapters in this book were first published by BioMed Central; hereby published with permission under the Creative Commons Attribution License or equivalent. Every chapter published in this book has been scrutinized by our experts. Their significance has been extensively debated. The topics covered herein carry significant findings which will fuel the growth of the discipline. They may even be implemented as practical applications or may be referred to as a beginning point for another development.

The contributors of this book come from diverse backgrounds, making this book a truly international effort. This book will bring forth new frontiers with its revolutionizing research information and detailed analysis of the nascent developments around the world.

We would like to thank all the contributing authors for lending their expertise to make the book truly unique. They have played a crucial role in the development of this book. Without their invaluable contributions this book wouldn't have been possible. They have made vital efforts to compile up to date information on the varied aspects of this subject to make this book a valuable addition to the collection of many professionals and students.

This book was conceptualized with the vision of imparting up-to-date information and advanced data in this field. To ensure the same, a matchless editorial board was set up. Every individual on the board went through rigorous rounds of assessment to prove their worth. After which they invested a large part of their time researching and compiling the most relevant data for our readers.

The editorial board has been involved in producing this book since its inception. They have spent rigorous hours researching and exploring the diverse topics which have resulted in the successful publishing of this book. They have passed on their knowledge of decades through this book. To expedite this challenging task, the publisher supported the team at every step. A small team of assistant editors was also appointed to further simplify the editing procedure and attain best results for the readers.

Apart from the editorial board, the designing team has also invested a significant amount of their time in understanding the subject and creating the most relevant covers. They scrutinized every image to scout for the most suitable representation of the subject and create an appropriate cover for the book.

The publishing team has been an ardent support to the editorial, designing and production team. Their endless efforts to recruit the best for this project, has resulted in the accomplishment of this book. They are a veteran in the field of academics and their pool of knowledge is as vast as their experience in printing. Their expertise and guidance has proved useful at every step. Their uncompromising quality standards have made this book an exceptional effort. Their encouragement from time to time has been an inspiration for everyone.

The publisher and the editorial board hope that this book will prove to be a valuable piece of knowledge for researchers, students, practitioners and scholars across the globe.

List of Contributors

Jiawei Chen, Guihao Zhang, Yang Chen, Jialei Zhong, Weina Huang, Jiarong Zeng and Peng Wu
Department of Urology, Nanfang Hospital, Southern Medical University, Guangzhou 510515, China

Jie Zhao
School of Pharmaceutical Sciences, Southern Medical University, Guangzhou, China

Ying Cao
Department of Endocrinology and Metabolism, Nanfang Hospital, Southern Medical University, Guangzhou 510515, China

Joongwon Choi and Deok Hyun Han
Department of Urology, Samsung Medical Center, Sungkyunkwan University School of Medicine, 81 Irwon-ro, Gangnam-gu, Seoul 06351, South Korea

Kyung Jin Chung
Department of Urology, Gachon University Gil Medical Center, Gachon University School of Medicine, 21, Namdong-daero 774beon-gil, Namdong-gu, Incheon 21565, South Korea

Seol Ho Choo
Department of Urology, Ajou University Medical Center, Ajou University School of Medicine, 164, World cup-ro, Yeongtong-gu, Suwon 16499, South Korea

Jun Miyazaki and Mizuki Onozawa
Department of Urology, International University of Health and Welfare, 6-1-14 Kounodai, Ichikawa City, Chiba 272-0827, Japan

Satoshi Takahashi
Department of Infection Control and Laboratory Medicine, Sapporo Medical University School of Medicine, S1 W16, Chuo-ku, Sapporo 060-8543, Japan

Yuka Maekawa and Mitsuru Yasuda
Department of Urology, Gifu University Graduate School of Medicine, 1-1 Yanagido, Gifu City 501-1194, Japan

Koichiro Wada
Department of Urology, Okayama University Graduate School of Medicine, Dentistry and Pharmaceutical Sciences, 2-5-1 Shikata-cho, Kita-ku, Okayama 700-8558, Japan

Yuji Maeda
Department of Urology, Public Central Hospital of Matto Ishikawa, 3-8 Kuramitsu, Hakusan-shi, Ishikawa 924-0865, Japan

Takuro Masaki and Akito Yamaguchi
Department of Urology, Harasanshin Hospital, 1-8 Taihaku-machi, Hakata-ku, Fukuoka City, Fukuoka 812-0033, Japan

Masahiko Suzuki
Department of Urology, Kasumigaura Medical Center, 2-7-14 Shimotakatsu, Tsuchiura City, Ibaraki 300-0812, Japan

Yasuyuki Sakai
Department of Urology, National Cancer Center East, 6-5-1 Kashiwanoha, Kashiwa-shi, Chiba 277-8577, Japan

Tomokazu Kimura
Department of Urology, Faculty of Medicine, University of Tsukuba, Tennodai 1-1-1, Tsukuba City, Ibaraki 305-8575, Japan

Manabu Takai
Department of Urology, Kizawa Memorial Hospital, 590 Shimokobi, Kobicho, Minokamo, Gifu 505-8503, Japan

Kensaku Seike
Department of Urology, Chuno Kosei Hospital, 5-1 Wakakusadori, Seki-city, Gifu 501-3802, Japan

Yun-lin Ye, Hai-tao Liang, Kang-hua Xiao, Xia Zheng and Zi-ke Qin
Department of Urology, Sun Yat-sen University Cancer Center, State Key Laboratory of Oncology in South China, Collaborative Innovation Center for Cancer Medicine, Guangzhou 510060, Guangdong, China

Lei Tan
Department of Urology, Sun Yat-sen University Cancer Center, State Key Laboratory of Oncology in South China, Collaborative Innovation Center for Cancer Medicine, Guangzhou 510060, Guangdong, China
Department ofUrology, the First Affiliated Hospital of Sun Yat-sen University, Guangzhou 510080, Guangdong, China

Dan Xiong
Department of Urology, Sun Yat-sen University Cancer Center, State Key Laboratory of Oncology in South China, Collaborative Innovation Center for Cancer Medicine, Guangzhou 510060, Guangdong, China
Medical Laboratory of The Third affiliated Hospital of Shenzhen University, Shenzhen 518000, Guangdong, China

Samara Carollyne Mafra Soares and Fabia Cheyenne Gomes de Morais Fernandes
Student in the Graduate Program in Collective Health, Health Science Faculty of Trairi, Federal University of Rio Grande do Norte (UFRN), Natal, Brazil

Katarina Márcia Rodrigues dos Santos
Undergraduate student in Nursing, Health Science Faculty of Trairi, Federal University of Rio Grande do Norte (UFRN), Natal, Brazil

Isabelle Ribeiro Barbosa and Dyego Leandro Bezerra de Souza
Graduate Program in Collective Health, Universidade Federal do Rio Grande do Norte/ Federal University of Rio Grande do Norte. Programa de Pós-Graduação em Saúde Coletiva, Avenida Senador Salgado Filho 1787, CEP: 59010-000 Lagoa Nova, Natal, RN, Brazil

Longlong Fu, Jianfeng Xu, Fang Zhou, Xiaowei Wang and Ying Guo
National Health Commission Key Laboratory of Male Reproductive Health, National Research Institute for Family Planning, Beijing 100081, China
Department of Male Clinical Research/Human sperm bank, National Research Institute for Family Planning & WHO Collaborating Center for Research in Human Reproduction, Beijing 100081, China

Qi An, Yue Tong and Yiqun Gu
National Health Commission Key Laboratory of Male Reproductive Health, National Research Institute for Family Planning, Beijing 100081, China
Department of Male Clinical Research/Human sperm bank, National Research Institute for Family Planning & WHO Collaborating Center for Research in Human Reproduction, Beijing 100081, China
Graduate School of Peking Union Medical College, Beijing 100730, China

Wenhong Lu
National Health Commission Key Laboratory of Male Reproductive Health, National Research Institute for Family Planning, Beijing 100081, China
Graduate School of Peking Union Medical College, Beijing 100730, China

Xiaowei Liang
Department of Male Clinical Research/Human sperm bank, National Research Institute for Family Planning & WHO Collaborating Center for Research in Human Reproduction, Beijing 100081, China

Kaishu Zhang
Department of Reproductive Medicine, The Afliated Hospital of Qingdao University, Qingdao, Shandong 266000, People's Republic of China

Ying Liu
Institute of Pediatric Research, Children's Hospital of Soochow University, Suzhou, Jiangsu Province 215025, China

Judith Wiltink, Arto E. Boeken Kruger and Daan J. Reesink
Department of Urology, Tergooi Hospital Hilversum, Rijksstraatweg 1, 1261 AN Blaricum, The Netherlands

Peter M. Huisman
Department of Radiology, Tergooi Hospital, Rijksstraatweg 1, 1261 AN Blaricum, The Netherlands

Tycho M. T. W. Lock
Department of Urology, University Medical Center Utrecht, Heidelberglaan 100, 3584 CX Utrecht, The Netherlands

Akihiro Kanematsu, Takahiko Hashimoto, Michio Nojima and Shingo Yamamoto
Department of Urology, Hyogo College of Medicine, Mukogawacho 1-1, Nishinomiya, Hyogo 663-8501, Japan

Shiro Tanaka
Department of Clinical Biostatistics, Graduate School of Medicine Kyoto University, Yoshida Konoecho, Sakyo, Kyoto 606-8501, Japan

Wang Zhenxing
Basic Medical College, Guizhou Medical University, Guiyang 550004, China
Department of Urology, Guizhou Provincial People's Hospital affiliated to Guizhou Medical University, Guiyang 550002, Guizhou, China

Sun Zhaolin, Yang Xiushu, Luo Guangheng and Tian Ye
Department of Urology, Guizhou Provincial People's Hospital, No. 83 East Zhongshan Road, Guiyang 550002, Guizhou, China

Shen Lei
Department of Surgical Operation Laboratory, Zunyi Medical University, No. 6 West Xuefu Road, Zunyi, Xinpu New District, China

Su Zhiyong
Department of Urology, Guizhou Medical University, No. 9 Beijing Road, Guiyang, Guizhou, China

Liu Hongming
Department of Urology, Zunyi Medical University, No. 6 Xuefu West Road, Xinpu New District, Zunyi, Guizhou, China

Kang Sup Kim
Department of Urology, Incheon St. Mary's Hospital, College of Medicine, The Catholic University of Korea, 59, Dongsu-ro, Bupyeong-gu, Incheon 21431, Republic of Korea

Woong Jin Bae and Sae Woong Kim
Department of Urology, Seoul St. Mary's Hospital, College of Medicine, The Catholic University of Korea, 222, Banpo-daero, Seocho-gu, Seoul 06591, Republic of Korea
Catholic Integrative Medicine Research Institute, College of Medicine, The Catholic University of Korea, 222, Banpo-daero, Seocho-gu, Seoul 06591, Republic of Korea

Moo Yeon Lee
Adams Urology Clinic, 513, Teheran-ro, Gangnam-gu, Seoul 06169, Republic of Korea

Robin Schaffar, Samaksha Pant, Christine Bouchardy, Hyma Schubert and Elisabetta Rapiti
Geneva Cancer Registry, Global Health Institute, University of Geneva, Geneva, Switzerland

Omar Alhunaidi, Bader Akroof, Abdullatif Al-Terki and Ali Alamiri
Urology Department, Al-Amiri hospital, Kuwait City, Kuwait

Abdulrahman A. Ahmad
Urology Department, Adan hospital, Hadiya, Kuwait

Ahmed R. EL-Nahas
Urology Department, Al-Amiri hospital, Kuwait City, Kuwait
Urology and Nephrology Center, Mansoura University, Mansoura, Egypt

Feras Al-Ajrawi
Urology Department, Al-Farwaniya hospital, Sabah Al Nasser, Kuwait

Mohamed El-Shazly
Urology Department, Menoufia University, Al Minufya, Egypt

Emanuele Rubilotta, Matteo Balzarro, Antonio D'Amico, Maria Angela Cerruto, Silvia Bassi and Walter Artibani
Department of Urology, Azienda Ospedaliera Universitaria Integrata (AOUI), Piazzale Aristide Stefani, 1, 37126 Verona, Italy

Chiara Bovo
Healthcare Department Administrator, Azienda Ospedaliera Universitaria Integrata (AOUI), Verona, Italy

Valerio Iacovelli, Daniele Bianchi and Enrico Finazzi Agrò
Department of Experimental Medicine and Surgery, Urology Unit, Tor Vergata University, Rome, Italy

Huitao Wang, Jianhe Liu, Kewei Fang, Changxing Ke, Yongming Jiang, Guang Wang, Tongxin Yang, Tao Chen and Xin Shi
Department of Urology, The Second Affiliated Hospital of Kunming Medical University, No.374, Dianmian Avenue, Yunnan 650101, People's Republic of China

Petra Anheuser
Klinik für Urologie, Albertinen-Krankenhaus, Hamburg, Germany
Urologische Klinik AK Wandsbek, Hamburg, Germany

J. Kranz
Klinik für Urologie und Kinderurologie, St.-Antonius Hospital, Eschweiler, Germany

E. Stolle
Institut für diagnostische und interventionelle Radiologie, Albertinen-Krankenhaus, Hamburg, Germany

D. Höflmayer and F. Büscheck
Institut für Pathologie, Universitätsklinikum Eppendorf, Universität Hamburg, Hamburg, Germany

S. Mühlstädt
Universitätsklink und Poliklinik für Urologie, Martin-Luther-Universität, Halle-Wittenberg, Halle (Saale), Germany

G. Lock
Klinik für Innere Medizin II, Albertinen-Krankenhaus, Hamburg, Germany

K. P. Dieckmann
Klinik für Urologie, Albertinen-Krankenhaus, Hamburg, Germany
Hodenzentrum Hamburg, Asklepios Klink Altona, Hamburg, Germany

Tsung-Hsin Chang and Chih-Chiao Lee
Department of Urology, Mackay Memorial hospital, No.92, Sec. 2, Zhongshan N. Rd., Zhongshan Dist, 10449 Taipei City, Taiwan (Republic of China)
Mackay Medical College, No.46, Sec. 3, Zhongzheng Rd., Sanzhi Dist, 252 New Taipei City, Taiwan (Republic of China)

Lei Wang, Xiao-fei Wang, Guo-feng Sun and Jia Chen
Department of urology, Peking University Shougang Hospital, Peking University Health Science Center, Beijing 100144, China
Peking University Wu Jieping Urology Center, Peking University Health Science Center, Beijing 100144, China

Ying-chao Qin
Department of General Surgery, Shuangqiao Hospital in Chaoyang District, Beijing 100024, China

Cun-hai Shang
Department of Medical Imaging, Peking University Shougang Hospital, Peking University Health Science Center, Beijing 100144, China

Ning-chen Li
Department of urology, Peking University Shougang Hospital, Peking University Health Science Center, Beijing 100144, China
Peking University Wu Jieping Urology Center, Peking University Health Science Center, Beijing 100144, China
Peking University Wu Jieping Urology Center, Peking University Shougang Hospital, 9# Jinyuanzhuang Road, Shijingshan District, Beijing 100144, China

Karim Courtemanche, Peter Chan and Wassim Kassouf
Division of Urology, McGill University Health Center, 1001 Blvd Decarie, room E02.4366, Montreal, Quebec H4A 3J1, Canada

Bernhard Haid
Department of Pediatric Urology, Hospital of the Sisters of Charity, Ordensklinikum Linz, Seilerstätte 4, 4020 Linz, Austria
Department of Urology, Ludwig Maximilians University, Marchioninistraße 15, 81367 Munich, Germany

Josef Oswald
Department of Pediatric Urology, Hospital of the Sisters of Charity, Ordensklinikum Linz, Seilerstätte 4, 4020 Linz, Austria

Daniela Reider and Nikolaus Romani
Department for Dermatology and Venereology, Medical University Innsbruck, Anichstraße 35, 6020 Innsbruck, Austria

Helga Fritsch and Felix Nägele
Section for clinical and functional Anatomy, Medical University Innsbruck, Müllerstraße 59, 6020 Innsbruck, Austria

Anne-Françoise Spinoit
Department of Urology, University Clinic Gent, Corneel Heymanslaan 10, 9000 Gent, Belgium

Elisabeth Pechriggl
Department of Plastic, Reconstructive and Aesthetic Surgery, Medical University Innsbruck, Innerkoflerstraße 1, Innsbruck, Austria

C. S. North
The Altshuler Center for Education & Research at Metrocare Services, The University of Texas Southwestern Medical Center, 1250 Mockingbird Lane, Suite 330, Dallas, TX 75247-4914, USA
Department of Psychiatry, The University of Texas Southwestern Medical Center, 5323 Harry Hines Blvd., Suite NE5.102, Dallas, TX 75390-9070, USA

B. A. Hong
Department of Psychiatry, School of Medicine, Washington University School of Medicine, St. Louis, MO, USA

H. H. Lai
Departments of Surgery and Anesthesiology, Division of Urologic Surgery, Washington University School of Medicine, St. Louis, MO 63110, USA

D. H. Alpers
Department of Internal Medicine, Division of Gastroenterology, Washington University School of Medicine, St. Louis, MO 63110, USA

Dong Zhang, Yue Cheng, Kerong Wu, Qi Ma, Junhui Jiang and Zejun Yan
Department of Urology & Nephrology, Ningbo First Hospital, The affiliated hospital of ZheJiang University, 59, Liuting Street, Ningbo, Zhejiang, China

Fang Yong, Wei Jinhuan, Yao Haohua, Chen Wei, Mo Jiacong, Luo Junhang and Wang Wenwei
Department of Urology, First Affiliated Hospital of Sun Yat-sen university, Guangzhou 510080, China

Lin Juan
Department of Pediatrics, Third Affiliated Hospital of Sun Yat-sen university, Guangzhou 510630, China

Chi-Fang Chen and Li-Chen Chen
Department of Urology, MacKay Memorial Hospital, No.92, Sec. 2, Zhongshan N. Rd., Zhongshan Dist, Taipei City 10449, Taiwan

Marcelo Chen
Department of Urology, MacKay Memorial Hospital, No.92, Sec. 2, Zhongshan N. Rd., Zhongshan Dist, Taipei City 10449, Taiwan
School of Medicine, MacKay Medical College, No.46, Sec. 3, Zhongzheng Rd., Sanzhi Dist, New Taipei City 252, Taiwan

Tzu-Ying Tang
Department of Pathology, Tamsui branch, MacKay Memorial Hospital, No.45, Minsheng Rd., Tamsui Dist, New Taipei City 25160, Taiwan
School of Medicine, MacKay Medical College, No.46, Sec. 3, Zhongzheng Rd., Sanzhi Dist, New Taipei City 252, Taiwan

Chih-Wei Chen, Chin-Ho Lee and Yi-Ming Wang
Department of Radiology, Kaohsiung Medical University Hospital, Kaohsiung Medical University, No. 100, Ziyou 1st Rd., Sanmin District, Kaohsiung City 80756, Taiwan, Republic of China

Tsung-Yi Huang
Department of Urology, Kaohsiung Medical University Hospital, Kaohsiung Medical University, Kaohsiung City, Taiwan

Defu Lin, Pei Liu, Guannan Wang, Weiping Zhang and Ning Sun
National Center for Children's Health, Beijing, China
Department of Urology, Beijing Children's Hospital affiliated to Capital Medical University, No.56 Nanlishilu Rd, West District, Beijing, China

Su Jin Kim
Department of Urology, Seoul St. Mary's Hospital, The Catholic University of Korea College of Medicine, Seoul, Republic of Korea
Current address: Department of Urology, Yonsei University Wonju College of Medicine, Wonju, Republic of Korea

Jayoung Kim
Departments of Surgery and Biomedical Sciences, Cedars-Sinai Medical Center, Los Angeles, CA 90048, USA
Department of Medicine, University of California Los Angeles, Los Angeles, CA 90095, USA

Hana Yoon
Department of Urology, Medical Research Center, Ewha Womans University School of Medicine, Seoul, Republic of Korea

Marilena Gubbiotti
Department of Surgical and Biomedical Sciences, Uro-Oncology Section, University of Perugia, S. Maria della Misericordia Hospital, 06132 Perugia, Italy
Istituto Serafico di Assisi, Centro di Ricerca "InVita", 06081 Assisi, Perugia, Italy

Antonella Giannantoni
Department of Medical and Surgical Sciences and Neuroscience, Urology Section, University of Siena, Siena 53100, Italy

Simona Cantaluppi, Anna Chiara Coluccia, Fabio Ghezzi and Maurizio Serati
Department of Obstetrics and Gynecology, University of Insubria, Varese 21100, Italy

Frank Christoph and Martin Schostak
University of Urology, Otto-von-Guericke-Universität, Magdeburg, Leipziger Str. 44, 39120 Magdeburg, Germany

Franziska Herrmann, Peter Werthemann, Thomas Janik, Christian Klopf and Steffen Weikert
Department of Urology, Vivantes Humboldt Klinikum Berlin, Am Nordgraben 2, 13509 Berlin, Germany

Umberto Maestroni and Francesco Ziglioli
Department. of General and Specialty Surgery, Urology Unit, University Hospital of Parma, Parma, Italy

Marco Baciarello, Valentina Bellini, Giada Maspero and Elena Bignami
Department of Medicine and Surgery, Anesthesia, Critical Care and Pain Medicine, University of Parma, Parma, Italy

Raffaele Dalla Valle
Department of Medicine and Surgery, Hepatobiliary Surgery Unit, University of Parma, Parma, Italy

Simona Cataldo
Department of Medicine, Endocrinology and Metabolic Diseases Unit, University Hospital of Parma, Parma, Italy

Maokun Sun, Shuai Guo, Wenyi Ma and Ruili Sun
Department of Urology, Liaocheng People's Hospital, Liaocheng, Shandong, China

Wanting Xu
Liaocheng Food and Drug Administration, Liaocheng, Shandong, China

Haiyue Xu
Division of Molecular Pharmaceutics and Drug Delivery, The University of Texas at Austin, College of Pharmacy, Austin, TX, USA

Ikenna I. Nnabugwu
Department of Surgery, College of Medicine, University of Nigeria Ituku-Ozalla, KM 20 Enugu-PortHarcourt Highway, Enugu PMB 01129, Nigeria
Department of Health Administration and Management, University of Nigeria Enugu Campus, Enugu, Nigeria

Fredrick O. Ugwumba and Emeka I. Udeh
Department of Surgery, College of Medicine, University of Nigeria Ituku-Ozalla, KM 20 Enugu-PortHarcourt Highway, Enugu PMB 01129, Nigeria

Solomon K. Anyimba and Louis T. Okolie
Department of Surgery, University of Nigeria Teaching Hospital Ituku-Ozalla, Enugu, Nigeria

Milad Azami
Faculty of Medicine, Ilam University of Medical Sciences, Ilam, Iran
Department of Obstetrics & Gynecology, Women's Reproductive Health Research Center, School of Medicine, Tabriz University of Medical Sciences, Tabriz, Iran

Shamsi Abbasalizadeh
Department of Obstetrics & Gynecology, Women's Reproductive Health Research Center, School of Medicine, Tabriz University of Medical Sciences, Tabriz, Iran

Zahra Jaafari
HIV/STI Surveillance Research Center, and WHO Collaborating Center for HIV Surveillance, Institute for Futures Studies in Health, Kerman University of Medical Sciences, Kerman, Iran

Mansour Masoumi
Department of Urology, Faculty of Medicine, Ilam University of Medical Sciences, Ilam, Iran

Masoumeh Shohani
Department of Nursing, Faculty of Nursing and Midwifery, Ilam University of Medical Sciences, Ilam, Iran

Gholamreza Badfar
Department of Pediatrics, Behbahan Faculty of Medical Sciences, Behbahan, Iran

Leily Mahmudi
Faculty of Medicine, Dezful University of Medical Sciences, Dezful, Iran

Index

www.ingramcontent.com/pod-product-compliance
Lightning Source LLC
LaVergne TN
LVHW082144200926
848484LV00008B/2105